PEDIATRIC ORTHOPAEDIC

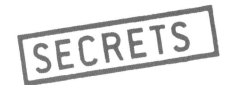

PEDIATRIC ORTHOPAEDIC

SECRETS

Third Edition

Lynn T. Staheli, MD
Professor of Orthopedics
Department of Orthopedics
University of Washington
Consulting Orthopedist
Children's Hospital and Regional Medical Center
Seattle, Washington

Kit M. Song, MD
Assistant Director of Orthopedic Surgery
Associate Professor of Orthopedic Surgery
University of Washington
Children's Hospital and Regional Medical Center
Seattle, Washington

MOSBY

ELSEVIER

MOSBY
ELSEVIER

1600 John F. Kennedy Boulevard, Suite 1800
Philadelphia, PA 19103-2899

Pediatric Orthopaedic Secrets
Third Edition

ISBN-13: 978-1-4160-2957-1
ISBN-10: 1-4160-2957-5

NOTICE

Knowledge and best practice in this field are constantly changing. As new research and experience broaden our knowledge, changes in practice, treatment and drug therapy may become necessary or appropriate. Readers are advised to check the most current information provided (i) on procedures featured or (ii) by the manufacturer of each product to be administered, to verify the recommended dose or formula, the method and duration of administration, and contraindications. It is the responsibility of the practitioner, relying on his or her own experience and knowledge of the patient, to make diagnoses, to determine dosages and the best treatment for each individual patient, and to take all appropriate safety precautions. To the fullest extent of the law, neither the Publisher nor the Editor assumes any liability for any injury and/or damage to persons or property arising out or related to any use of the material contained in this book.

Library of Congress Cataloging-in-Publication Data

Pediatric orthopaedic secrets / [edited by] Lynn T. Staheli, Kit M. Song.– 3rd ed.
    p.; cm.
    ISBN 1-4160-2957-5
    1. Pediatric orthopedics–Examinations, questions, etc.   I. Staheli, Lynn T.
    II. Song, Kit M.
    [DNLM: 1. Orthopedic Procedures–Examination Questions.   2. Adolescent.
    3. Child.   4. Infant.   WS 18.2 P3701 2007]
    RD732.3.C48P43 2007
    618.92'70076–dc22

23801573

2006033345

Senior Acquisitions Editor: James Merritt
Developmental Editor: Stan Ward
Project Manager: Mary Stermel
Marketing Manager: Alyson Sherby

Working together to grow
libraries in developing countries

www.elsevier.com | www.bookaid.org | www.sabre.org

ELSEVIER   BOOK AID International   Sabre Foundation

Printed in China.

Last digit is the print number: 9 8 7 6 5 4 3 2 1

CONTENTS

IV. ACUTE PROBLEMS

V. SPORTS-RELATED INJURIES

VI. LOWER-LIMB PROBLEMS

VII. FOOT AND ANKLE PROBLEMS

VIII. KNEE AND TIBIA PROBLEMS

IX. HIP PROBLEMS

X. SPINE AND NECK PROBLEMS

XI. SHOULDER PROBLEMS

XII. UPPER LIMB PROBLEMS

XIII. ARTHRITIS

XIV. TUMORS

XV. INFECTIONS

CONTRIBUTORS

Benjamin Alman, MD
Canadian Research Chair; A.J. Latner Professor and Chair of Orthopaedic Surgery; Vice Chair of Research, Department of Surgery, University of Toronto; Head, Division of Orthopaedic Surgery and Senior Scientist, Program in Developmental Biology, The Hospital for Sick Children, Toronto, Ontario, Canada

Elizabeth A. Aronson, APN, MNSc
Orthopaedic Specialty Nurse and Registered Nurse Practitioner, Department of Pediatric Orthopaedics, Arkansas Children's Hospital, Little Rock, Arkansas

James Aronson, MD
Professor, Departments of Orthopaedics and Pediatrics, University of Arkansas for Medical Sciences; Chief of Orthopaedic Surgery, Arkansas Children's Hospital; Director, Laboratory for Limb Regeneration Research, Arkansas Children's Hospital Research Institute, Little Rock, Arkansas

David D. Aronsson, MD
Professor, Department of Orthopaedics and Rehabilitation, University of Vermont College of Medicine; Chief, Pediatric Orthopaedics, Fletcher Allen Health Care; Medical Director, Orthopaedic Program, Division for Children with Special Health Needs, Department of Health, State of Vermont, Burlington, Vermont

Amir M. Atif, MD
New York University, New York, New York

Donald S. Bae, MD
Instructor in Orthopaedic Surgery, Harvard Medical School; Department of Orthopaedic Surgery, Children's Hospital of Boston, Boston, Massachusetts

Severino R. Bautista, Jr., MD
Divison of Orthopaedic Surgery, Children's Hospital of Philadelphia, Philadelphia, Pennsylvania

James H. Beaty, MD
Professor, University of Tennessee–Campbell Clinic, Department of Orthopaedic Surgery; Chief of Staff, Campbell Clinic, Memphis, Tennessee

Nadire Berker, MD
Professor of Physical and Rehabilitation Medicine, VKV American Hospital, Istanbul, Turkey

Robert M. Bernstein, MD
Department of Orthopaedics, University of California at Los Angeles School of Medicine; Director of Pediatric Orthopedic Surgery, Cedars-Sinai Medical Center, Los Angeles, California

Wesley Bevan, MBChB, FRACS
Department of Orthopedics, Medical University of South Carolina, Charleston, South Carolina

Terri Bidwell, MD, FRACS

Richard E. Bowen, MD
Shriners Hospitals for Children—Los Angeles Unit, Los Angeles, California

Michael T. Busch, MD
Vice-Chairman of Orthopaedic Surgry, Surgical Director of Sports Medicine, Children's Healthcare of Atlanta, Atlanta, Georgia

Noelle Cassidy, MB
Shriners Hospital for Children of Los Angeles, Los Angeles, California

Henry G. Chambers, MD
Clinical Associate Professor, Department of Orthopedic Surgery, University of California at San Diego; Senior Orthopedic Surgeon, Rady Children's Hospital of San Diego, San Diego, California

Paul D. Choi, MD
Children's Orthopaedic Center, Children's Hospital Los Angeles, Assistant Professor of Clinical Orthopaedics, University of Southern California School of Medicine, Los Angeles, California

Mary Williams Clark, MD
Clinical Professor, Orthopaedics and Pediatrics, Michigan State University; Chief, Pediatric Orthopedics, Sparrow Regional Children's Center; Sparrow Hospital, Lansing, Michigan

N. M. P. Clarke, ChM, FRCS
Professor, Consultant Orthopaedic Surgeon and Reader, Southampton General Hospital, Southampton, United Kingdom

Paul Connolly, MD
Department of Orthopaedic Surgery, University of Iowa Hospital, Iowa City, Iowa

Ernest U. Conrad III, MD
Professor, Department of Orthopedics and Sports Medicine, University of Washington School of Medicine; Director, Department of Orthopedics, Children's Hospital and Regional Medical Center, Seattle, Washington

Alvin H. Crawford, MD, FACS
Professor of Orthopaedics and Pediatrics, University of Cincinnati College of Medicine; Director, Spine Center, Children's Hospital Medical Center, Cincinnati, Ohio

R. Jay Cummings, MD
Associate Professor of Orthopedics, Mayo Medical School; Vice President, Physician Practices, Nemours Children's Clinics of Florida, Jacksonville, Florida

Jon R. Davids, MD
Chief of Staff and Medical Director, Motion Analysis Laborator, Shriners Hospital for Children, Greenville, South Carolina

Jose Fernando De la Garza, MD
Head, Pediatric Orthopedic Division, Trauma and Orthopedic Service, Universidad Autonoma de Nuevo Leon; Ortho Centro de Traumatologia, Ortopedia, y Microcirugia Articular SC, Monterrey, Mexico

S. K. DeMuth, DPT
Assistant Professor, Department of Biokinesiology and Physical Therapy, University of Southern California, Los Angeles, California

Mohammad Diab, MD
Chief, Paediatric Orthopaedic Surgery; Associate Professor of Orthopaedic Surgery and
Paediatrics, University of California at San Francisco, San Francisco, California

Frederick R. Dietz, MD
Professor, Department of Orthopaedic Surgery and Rehabilitation, University of Iowa,
Iowa City, Iowa

Matthew B. Dobbs, MD
Department of Pediatric Orthopaedic Surgery, Washington University School of Medicine,
St. Louis, Missouri

John P. Dormans, MD
Department of Orthopedic Surgery, Children's Hospital of Philadelphia, Philadelphia,
Pennsylvania

Robert E. Eilert, MD
Professor of Orthopaedic Surgery, University of Colorado School of Medicine; Chair, Department
of Orthopaedics, Children's Hospital, Denver, Colorado

Nathan K. Endres, MD
Sports/Shoulder Fellow, Harvard Shoulder Service; Brigham and Women's Hospital;
Massachussetts General Hospital, Boston, Massachusetts

Marybeth Ezaki, MD
Professor of Orthopaedic Surgery, University of Texas Southwestern Medical School; Director of
Hand Surgery, Charles Seay Hand Center, Texas Scottish Rite Hospital for Children, Dallas, Texas

John R. Fisk, MD
Professor, Department of Orthopaedic Surgery, Southern Illinois University School of Medicine,
Springfield, Illinois

John M. Flynn, MD
Children's Hospital of Philadelphia, Philadelphia, Pennsylvania

Edilson Forlin, MD, MSc, PhD
Pediatric Orthopaedic Surgeon, Hospital Pequeno Principe and Hospital das Clinicas UFPR,
Curitiba–PR; President of Brazilian Pediatric Orthopaedic Society, Curitiba, Brazil

James G. Gamble, MD, PhD
Professor, Department of Orthopaedic Surgery, Stanford University Medical Center; Packard
Children's Hospital at Stanford, Stanford, California

Mark C. Gebhardt, MD
Carl J. Shapiro Department of Orthopaedics, Beth Israel Deaconess Medical Center, Boston,
Massachusetts

Michael J. Goldberg, MD
Department of Orthopedics, Children's Hospital and Regional Medical Center, Seattle,
Washington

Ryan C. Goodwin, MD
Department of Orthopaedic Surgery, Cleveland Clinic Foundation, Cleveland, Ohio

J. Eric Gordon, MD
Department of Orthopaedic Surgery, Washington University School of Medicine, St. Louis
Children's Hospital; St. Louis Shriner's Hospital for Crippled Children; Barnes-Jewish Hospital;
Missouri Baptist Medical Center, St. Louis, Missouri

H. Kerr Graham, MD, FRCS (Ed), FRACS
Professor of Orthopaedic Surgery, Royal Children's Hospital, University of Melbourne; Murdoch Children's Research Institute; Clinical Centre of Research Excellence in Gait and Rehabilitation, Melbourne, Australia

Alfred D. Grant, MD
Clinical Professor, New York University School of Medicine, New York University Medical Center, New York University-Hospital for Joint Diseases, and Bellevue Hospital and Medical Center, New York, New York

Neil E. Green, MD
Professor of Orthopaedics, Vanderbilt Medical Center; Division of Pediatric Orthopedics, Vanderbilt Children's Hospital, Nashville, Tennessee

Walter B. Greene, MD
Professor of Orthopaedic Surgery, Department of Orthopaedic Surgery, University of Missouri at Columbia School of Medicine, Columbia, Missouri

J. A. Herring, MD
Chief of Staff, Texas Scottish Rite Hospital for Children; Professor of Orthopedic Surgery, University of Texas Southwestern Medical School, Dallas, Texas

John E. Herzenberg, MD, FRCSC
Head of Pediatric Orthopaedics, Co-Director, International Center for Limb Lengthening, Sinai Hospital, Baltimore, Maryland

Sevan Hopyan, MD, FRCSC
Assistant Professor, Division of Orthopaedic Surgery and Program in Developmental and Stem Cell Biology, The Hospital for Sick Children, Toronto, Ontario, Canada

John Charles Hyndman, MD
Professor of Surgery, Dalhousie University Faculty of Medicine; Head, Department of Orthopaedics, IWK Grace Health Centre, Halifax, Nova Scotia, Canada

Lori A. Karol, MD
Professor, Department of Orthopaedic Surgery, University of Texas Southwestern Medical School; Staff Orthopaedic Surgeon, Texas Scottish Rite Hospital for Children, Dallas, Texas

Joseph G. Khoury, MD
Staff Orthopedic Surgeon, Shriners Hospitals for Children, Erie, Pennsylvania

Christopher K. Kim, MD
Director, Residency Program in Orthopaedics, Medical College of Georgia; Uniformed Services University of the Health Sciences, Augusta, Georgia

Shyam Kishan, MD
Staff Orthopedic Surgeon, Shriners Hospitals for Children, Erie, Pennsylvania

Ken N. Kuo, MD
National Health Research Institutes, National Taiwan University Hospital, Taipei, Taiwan; Rush University Medical Center, Chicago, Illinois

Randall T. Loder, MD
Garceau Professor of Orthopaedic Surgery, Indiana University School of Medicine; Director of Orthopaedic Surgery, Riley Children's Hospital, Indianapolis, Indiana

Scott J. Luhmann, MD
Assistant Professor, Pediatric Orthopaedic Spine and Sports Surgery, Department of Orthopaedic Surgery, Washington University School of Medicine, St. Louis, Missouri

William G. Mackenzie, MD
Co-Director, Muscular Dystrophy Association Clinic at the Alfred I. duPont Hospital for Children, Wilmington, Delaware

Richard E. McCarthy, MD
Clinical Professor, Department of Orthopaedics, University of Arkansas for Medical Sciences; Arkansas Children's Hospital, Little Rock, Arkansas

Peter L. Meehan, MD
Clinical Associate Professor of Orthopaedic Surgery, Emory University School of Medicine, Atlanta, Georgia

Vincent S. Mosca, MD
Pediatric Orthopedic Surgeon, Former Director Department of Orthopedics, Children's Hospital and Regional Medical Center; Associate Professor of Orthopaedics and former Chief of Pediatric Orthopaedics, Department of Orthopaedics and Sports Medicine, University of Washington School of Medicine, Seattle, Washington

Colin F. Moseley, MD, CM
Clinical Professor of Orthopaedics, University of California at Los Angeles; Chief of Staff, Shriners Hospitals for Children, Los Angeles, California

Kevin M. Neal, MD
Department of Pediatric Orthopaedics, Nemours Children's Clinic, Jacksonville, Florida

Blaise A. Nemeth, MD, MS
Assistant Professor (CHS), Department of Pediatrics and Department of Orthopedics and Rehabilitation, University of Wisconsin School of Medicine and Public Health, Madison, Wisconsin

Kurt Nilsson, MD
Intermountain Orthopaedics, Boise, Idaho

Kenneth Noonan, MD
Department of Orthopedics and Rehabilitation, University of Wisconsin School of Medicine and Public Health, Madison, Wisconsin

William L. Oppenheim, MD
Professor of Orthopedics, Department of Orthopedic Surgery, UCLA/Orthopedic Hospital, Geffen UCLA School of Medicine, UCLA Medical Center, Los Angeles, California

Dror Paley, MD, FRCSC
Director, Rubin Institute for Advanced Orthopedics, Co-Director, International Center for Limb Lengthening, Sinai Hospital, Baltimore, Maryland

Klaus Parsch, MD
Professor Emeritus of Orthopaedic Surgery, University of Heidelberg, Heidelberg, Germany; Chief Surgeon Emeritus, Department of Orthopaedics, Pediatric Center Olgahospital, Stuttgart, Germany

Hamlet A. Peterson, MD
Emeritus Professor of Orthopedic Surgery, Mayo Clinic College of Medicine; Emeritus Head, Division of Pediatric Orthopedics, Mayo Clinic, Rochester, Minnesota

Peter Pizzutillo, MD
Director, Orthopaedic Surgery, St. Christopher's Hospital for Children; Professor of Orthopaedic Surgery and Pediatrics, Drexel University College of Medicine, Philadelphia, Pennsylvania

Maya E. Pring, MD
Children's Hospital of San Diego, San Diego, California

William Puffinbarger, MD
Assistant Professor, Department of Orthopedic Surgery and Rehabilitation, University of Oklahoma Health Sciences Center, Oklahoma City, Oklahoma

Ryan M. Putnam, MD
Clinical Instructor, Department of Orthopedic Surgery, University of Vermont College of Medicine; Fletcher Allen Health Care, Burlington, Vermont

Chris Reilly, MD
Assistant Professor, Department of Orthopedics, University of British Columbia; British Columbia Children's Hospital, Vancouver, British Columbia, Canada

B. Stephens Richards, MD
Assistant Chief of Staff, Texas Scottish Rite Hospital for Children; Professor of Orthopaedic Surgery, University of Texas Southwestern Medical Center, Dallas, Texas

James O. Sanders, MD
Chief of Staff, Shriners Hospitals for Children, Erie, Pennsylvania

Perry L. Schoenecker, MD
Professor, Orthopedic Surgery, Washington University School of Medicine; Chief of Staff, Shriners Hospital for Children; Chairman, Pediatric Orthopaedics, St. Louis Children's Hospital; Barnes-Jewish Hospital; Missouri Baptist Medical Center, St. Louis, Missouri

Elizabeth K. Schorry, MD
Associate Professor, Cincinnati Children's Hospital Medical Center, Division of Human Genetics, Cincinnati, Ohio

Dalia Sepúlveda, MD
Coordinator, Orthopedic and Trauma Department, University of Chile; Chief, Reconstruction Surgery Unit, Roberto del Río Hospital, Santiago, Chile

Kevin Shea, MD
Intermountain Orthopedics; St. Luke's Children's Hospital; Center for Orthopedics and Biomechanics Research, Boise State University, Boise, Idaho; Adjunct Associate Professor, Department of Orthopedics, University of Utah, Salt Lake City, Utah

David D. Sherry, MD
Director, Clinical Rheumatology; Attending Physician, Pain Management, The Children's Hospital of Philadelphia, University of Pennsylvania, Philadelphia, Pennsylvania

Jeffrey S. Shilt, MD
Associate Professor, Residency Program Director, Department of Orthopaedic Surgery, Wake Forest University Health Sciences Center, Winston-Salem, North Carolina

David L. Skaggs, MD
Children's Hospital of Los Angeles, Los Angeles, California

Kit M. Song, MD
Assistant Director of Orthopedic Surgery, Associate Professor of Orthopedic Surgery, University of Washington; Children's Hospital and Regional Medical Center, Seattle, Washington

David A. Spiegel, MD
Division of Orthopaedic Surgery, Children's Hospital of Philadelphia, Philadelphia, Pennsylvania

Paul D. Sponseller, MD
Riley Professor and Head, Department of Pediatric Orthopaedics, Johns Hopkins Medical Institutions, Baltimore, Maryland

Lynn T. Staheli, MD
Professor of Orthopedics, Department of Orthopedics, University of Washington; Consulting Orthopedist, Children's Hospital and Regional Medical Center, Seattle, Washington

Carl L. Stanitski, MD
Professor Emeritus of Orthopedic Surgery, Medical University of South Carolina, Charleston, South Carolina

Deborah Stanitski, MD
Professor Emeritus of Orthopedic Surgery, Medical University of South Carolina, Charleston, South Carolina

Peter M. Stevens, MD
Professor, Department of Orthopedics, University of Utah School of Medicine, Salt Lake City, Utah

J. Andy Sullivan, MD
Don H. O'Donoghue Professor and Endowed Chair, Department of Orthopedics, University of Oklahoma College of Medicine; Oklahoma University Medical Center, Oklahoma City, Oklahoma

Terry J. Supan, CPO
Orthotic and Prosthetic Associates, Springfield, Illinois

Michael Sussman, MD
Staff Surgeon, Former Chief of Staff, Shriners Hospital for Children; Clinical Professor of Orthopaedic Surgery, Oregon Health and Science University, Portland, Oregon

George H. Thompson, MD
Professor of Orthopaedic Surgery and Pediatrics, Case Western Reserve University School of Medicine; Director of Pediatric Orthopaedics, Rainbow Babies and Children's Hospital, Case Medical Center, Cleveland, Ohio

Stephen J. Tredwell, MD
Professor and Head, Division of Pediatric Orthopedics, Department of Orthopedics, University of British Columbia; British Columbia Children's Hospital, Vancouver, British Columbia, Canada

Inge Falk van Rooyen, MBChB, FRCA
Assistant Professor, University of Washington School of Medicine; Attending Physician, Department of Anesthesiology, Children's Hospital and Regional Medical Center, Seattle, Washington

Charles Douglas Wallace, MD
Medical Director of Orthopedic Trauma, Children's Hospital and Health Center; University of California Hillcrest Medical Center, San Diego, California; University of California Thornton Hospital, La Jolla, California

Peter M. Waters, MD
Professor of Orthopaedic Surgery, Harvard Medical School; Associate Chief of Orthopedic Surery, Children's Hospital, Boston, Massachusetts

Hugh G. Watts, MD
Clinical Professor of Orthopaedics, University of California at Los Angeles; Adjunct Associate Professor, Department of Biokinesiology and Physical Therapy, University of Southern California; Orthopedic Staff, Shriners' Hospitals for Children, Los Angeles Unit, Los Angeles, California

Stuart L. Weinstein, MD
Ignacio V. Ponseti Chair and Professor of Orthopaedic Surgery, Department of Orthopaedic Surgery, University of Iowa Hospital, Iowa City, Iowa

Dennis R. Wenger, MD
Director, Pediatric Orthopedic Training Program, Children's Hospital of San Diego; Clinical Professor of Orthopedic Surgery, University of California at San Diego, San Diego, California

David E. Westberry, MD
Pediatric Orthopaedic Surgery, Shriners Hospital for Children: Greenville, Greenville, South Carolina

Kaye E. Wilkins, DVM, MD
Professor, Departments of Orthopaedics and Pediatrics, University of Texas Health Science Center at San Antonio, San Antonio, Texas

James G. Wright, MD, MPH, FRCSC
Professor, Departments of Surgery, Public Health Sciences, and Health Policy, Management and Evaluation, University of Toronto; Surgeon-in-Chief, Robert B. Salter Chair of Surgical Research and Senior Scientist, Population Health Sciences, Research Institute, The Hospital for Sick Children, Toronto, Ontario, Canada

Selim Yalçin, MD
Professor of Orthopaedic Surgery, Marmara University School of Medicine and VKV American Hospital, Istanbul, Turkey

PREFACE

Pediatric orthopaedics is an important subspecialty. Musculoskeletal problems in children are common and may account for up to 20% of the office visits for primary care providers of children. Poorly planned evaluation and management are not only costly to the health care system but can also lead to harm to the child. As training for this area is limited, resources such as *Pediatric Orthopaedic Secrets* may help to close the gap.

This latest edition of *Pediatric Orthopaedic Secrets* continues the excellent tradition of the *Secrets Series* and expands upon prior editions by highlighting key points and principles that are important in the assessment and management of children with orthopaedic problems.

The contributors to this book are recognized as experts and leaders in their field and were selected not only for their knowledge but also in recognition of their ability as educators. We appreciate the eager participation of so many learned authors and are especially grateful to them for their enthusiasm in continuing this vital work of education. The authors have given us scientifically based, child-oriented, and practical tips to use in our practices.

Lynn T. Staheli, MD
Kit M. Song, MD

Acknowledgment

We would like to express our appreciation to Tracy Anderson, whose tireless efforts kept the collaborative efforts of over 90 authors moving ahead during the preparation of this book.

TOP 100 SECRETS

These secrets are 100 of the top board alerts. They summarize the basic concepts, principles, and most salient details of pediatric orthopaedics.

1. Congenital anomalies derive from genetic, teratogenic, or mechanical problems during development.

2. Deformations are more readily treatable by simple methods than dysplasias, which often require complex surgical or medical treatment.

3. Acute osteomyelitis presents as fever and progressive pain in a limb, typically near a joint. Septic arthritis should be suspected in a patient experiencing exquisite pain with any passive motion of the presumably infected joint.

4. Clues in the history of amplified musculoskeletal pain include a minor injury that subsequently becomes increasingly painful. The pain is either minimally responsive or not responsive to conservative management with pain or anti-inflammatory medications.

5. Because x-rays are two-dimensional, at least two x-rays at 90 degrees to each other must be taken to understand the three dimensions of an injury or deformity.

6. Gait analysis cannot tell a surgeon whether to operate on a child with cerebral palsy but may assist the surgeon in clarifying which muscles or bones require surgical treatment and which do not.

7. An accurate diagnosis provides a clear prognosis. Discuss all treatment options, be honest about your uncertainty, and find the best treatment based on the best evidence.

8. You need to develop appropriate relationships with all members of the family, particularly the child.

9. Without some help from medical professionals, many children with disabilities will not achieve their maximum potential for participation in society. Do not define people by their impairments.

10. For an upper respiratory infection, wait 1–2 weeks after cessation of symptoms before performing surgery. For a lower respiratory infection, wait at least 4–6 weeks after cessation of symptoms.

11. Intravenous conscious sedation for fractures generally combines narcotics and benzodiazepines. Narcotics provide good analgesia, and the benzodiazepines provide relaxation and some degree of amnesia.

12. The four Ps are signs that a cast is too tight: pain, pallor, paresthesias and possible numbness, and paralysis or paresis. Tight casts can be prevented by sufficient padding, bivalving, splitting the padding to the skin, and elevating the limb to prevent dependent edema and inflammatory swelling.

13. Splints and orthotics should be prescribed for a specific purpose and length of time, with periodic reassessment of their effect over time. Ongoing use of splints and orthotics needs to be monitored for possible adverse effects upon function or the creation of skin irritation or breakdown.

14. The family, as well as the child, can benefit from physical and occupational therapy.

15. The best shoe is one that simulates barefootedness. The major problems now are pointed toes and high heels for girls and cowboy boots for boys.

16. A carefully executed and timely joint aspiration can give precious information for diagnosis and treatment of the joint or other systemic diseases.

17. Trauma is the most common cause of injury and death in children worldwide. Traumatic accidents are most often due to poorly designed equipment, mismatch of equipment to child size, and inexperience of the child in avoiding dangerous situations.

18. Orthopaedic injuries account for a significant proportion of injuries in the pediatric polytrauma setting—up to 34% in one series. These are rarely life-threatening but can place the patient at risk for long-term morbidity.

19. Because children's bones have less density and more cartilage, they are more flexible, and injury to underlying soft structures can occur without visible damage to the bones.

20. By far, the most common and serious complication of damage to the growth plate is premature complete or partial growth plate closure. There is no way to reestablish growth following complete growth plate closure.

21. The most important early sign of compartment syndrome is severe pain.

22. Accurate recognition and referral for suspected child abuse may prevent subsequent abuse in up to 50% and death in up to 15% of cases.

23. The physis and its state of maturity are the keys to understanding the pattern of fractures in the foot and ankle in children and adolescents. The physis, when open, is the weak link in the bone-ligament interface and, when stressed, fails before the ligament. In adolescents, the physis is closed and the injury resembles that seen in adults.

24. Long-term results of meniscectomy in children are poor, and repair should be attempted when possible.

25. Proximal tibial fractures in younger children will often temporarily grow into valgus. The capacity for remodeling malunion or overgrowth of shortening due to tibial shaft fractures is age-dependent.

26. The treatment of femur fractures should be individualized. Options for treatment are varied and depend on the patient, the fracture type, and the surgeon's experience. Although remodeling does occur, aim for an anatomic reduction. Be prepared to revise the position early if the results are not satisfactory.

27. Displaced hip and acetabular fractures should be reduced and fixed with age- and size-appropriate devices. Most isolated pelvic fractures in younger children can be treated nonoperatively.

28. Children tend to get more upper cervical spine injury due to increased head size and more-horizontally oriented facet joints. Almost all cervical spine injuries in children tend to displace on a standard spine board because of the relatively larger size of a child's head.

29. Because the medial end of the clavicle closes very late (i.e., 22 years of age or later), you must have a high index of suspicion for medial physeal separation in patients with an apparent sternoclavicular dislocation.

30. Extension supracondylar fractures have a higher incidence of complications, including nerve injuries, vascular injuries, and compartment syndrome. The most common problem associated with inadequate treatment of extension supracondylar fractures is a cubitus varus deformity.

31. If a child is suspected of having a wrist or forearm fracture, a careful physical examination should be performed and radiographs that include the area of tenderness should be obtained.

32. In general, replantation should be considered in digital amputations in children.

33. The medical history is the most cost-effective component of the preparticipation screening evaluation.

34. Stress fractures result from a disruption of the normal continual process of bone remodeling, in which the resorption component becomes more prevalent than bone deposition. This disruption is triggered by an abrupt increase in biomechanical stress.

35. An overuse injury results from a repetitive action, such as throwing or swimming, that exerts too much stress on the bones, growth plates, muscles, and muscle origins and insertions. It is often associated with poor mechanics and can be prevented by avoiding overuse of the upper extremity and learning proper mechanics.

36. The most common physeal fracture pattern from an inversion injury of the ankle is a Salter-Harris type I injury. These injuries are often nondisplaced and result in a normal-looking bone (with soft tissue swelling). The diagnosis of fracture is based primarily on the physical examination findings. When in doubt, assume and treat for a nondisplaced physeal fracture.

37. In a growing child, always plan correction based on the predicted leg-length discrepancy at maturity, not the present discrepancy. Failure to observe this rule is the most common source of error.

38. History and physical exam are key to understanding the extent of the problem with leg aches. Occasionally, leg aches are early signs of significant importance.

39. The most common causes of limp are trauma, infection, inflammation, and tumor. The differential diagnosis is age-specific.

40. Performing a rotational profile provides the information necessary to establish an accurate diagnosis in children with intoeing or out-toeing. This diagnosis is essential in management to provide a prognosis, to deal with the concerns of the family, and to provide the child with any necessary treatment.

41. When evaluating children and adolescents with bowed legs or knock knees, the clinician should be aware of the benign natural history of normal variants (i.e., physiologic varus or valgus).

42. Pathologic conditions that persist and progress may cause gait disturbance and joint damage; surgical intervention is warranted. The first line of defense is to consider guided growth, reserving osteotomy for recalcitrant conditions.

43. It is important to differentiate between flexible and rigid flat feet. Tarsal coalition is an important cause of a rigid flatfoot in children and adolescents.

44. The most important consideration when choosing which bunion operation to perform is whether the metatarsophalangeal (MTP) joint is subluxated. Surgical treatment for a juvenile hallux valgus deformity with a subluxated MTP joint must include a distal soft tissue realignment.

45. Toe deformities may be congenital, developmental, or resulting from neuromuscular imbalance. The treatment depends upon the symptoms (e.g., pain, skin breakdown, or alteration in shoe wear), the presence of functional problems, and, to a lesser extent, on cosmesis.

46. The majority of uncomplicated puncture wounds of the foot may be managed in the emergency department with local wound care. Routine prophylactic antibiotics are controversial. These injuries may be complicated by a retained foreign body, and a small subset of cases will become infected (causing cellulitis or osteomyelitis) and will require surgical debridement and antibiotics.

47. The only error that can be made in treating metatarsus adductus is manipulation without stabilizing the hindfoot. Even no treatment will result in a functionally normal, painless foot, regardless of severity.

48. Proper correction of clubfoot by manipulation is not difficult, time-consuming, or lengthy. The manipulation itself requires less than a minute and is not painful. Over 95% of clubfeet can be corrected this way within 2 months. Even after complete correction, clubfoot has a strong tendency to recur if proper bracing is not maintained.

49. Flexible flatfoot is a normal foot shape that is present in most children and a high percentage of adults. The longitudinal arch elevates in most children through normal growth and development. Surgery for flatfoot is rarely indicated.

50. The cavus foot deformity is a manifestation of a neuromuscular disorder with muscle imbalance until proven otherwise. Diagnosis and treatment (if possible) of the underlying neuromuscular disorder must precede treatment of the cavus foot deformity.

51. Toe-walking is normal in toddlers up to about 3 years of age. A simple and fast treatment in a 2-year-old child with idiopathic toe walking consists of percutaneous lengthening of the Achilles tendon, followed by a below-knee cast for 4 weeks.

52. Knee pain equals hip pain until proven otherwise. Clinical examination of the hip must be included in a knee examination.

53. The most common physical finding in adolescents with anterior knee pain is hamstring contracture. Perthes' disease, slipped capital femoral epiphysis, and osteoid osteoma are among the proximal lesions that commonly cause referred pain to the knee.

54. Many cases of congenital hyperextension of the knee resolve spontaneously or with minimal treatment. For congenital dislocation or subluxation of the knee, active treatment and surgical reduction are often necessary.

55. Indications for surgical correction of Blount disease are age older than 3 years at the initial visit, noncompliance with the brace, and marked obesity, especially for bilateral involvement. Valgus osteotomy should be performed before stage IV because, at this stage, a bone bridge may produce recurrence.

56. In children with congenital pseudoarthrosis of the tibia, unilateral anterolateral bowing is noticed in the first year of life. In most patients, a nontraumatic fracture occurs by 2–3 years of age. The principles of most surgical techniques are resection of the dysplastic segment, correction of the deformity, and provision of adequate apposition of the bone at the defect.

57. Hip pain is often referred to the anterolateral thigh. If a child presents with knee pain, be sure to evaluate the hip.

58. The very important distinction between transient synovitis and septic arthritis is, in the first instance, clinical. The patient with transient synovitis is not sick, and, if there is a fever, it is usually low-grade. Investigations such as the white blood cell count tend not to be elevated as much as they would be in the case of acute infection.

59. Developmental dysplasia of the hip (DDH) is a continuum of disorders, from radiographic dysplasia to frank dislocation. Ortolani-positive hips in the newborn do not require imaging prior to initiation of treatment in the Pavlik harness. Teratologic and late-presenting hip dislocations are usually fixed dislocations, requiring surgical reduction.

60. In the short run, the natural history of Legg-Calvé-Perthes is very favorable. Most patients go through adolescence and most of adulthood with either no symptoms or mild transient aches and pains. By the fifth decade, half the patients will have developed degenerative arthritis and will be in need of hip replacement.

61. Always obtain both anteroposterior (AP) and lateral radiographs of both hips when evaluating children with known or suspected slipped capital femoral epiphysis (SCFE).

62. The treatment of SCFE is considered urgent, and the child should be immediately referred to an orthopaedic surgeon so that fixation can be performed rapidly.

63. The most common cause of back pain in adolescents is muscle strain. Scoliosis is rarely responsible.

64. Bracing is the only nonsurgical intervention for which evidence exists that it may arrest the progression of scoliosis. Surgery should be considered only for curves greater than 50 degrees.

65. Kyphotic deformity presenting at a young age may progress rapidly and lead to neurologic abnormalities. Early referral to an orthopaedic specialist with an interest in pediatric conditions is advisable.

66. Whereas infants with congenital muscular torticollis with a palpable nodule have an 8–10% risk of requiring surgical intervention, infants without a nodule have only a 3% risk of surgical intervention.

67. Newborn brachial plexus palsy is an increasingly common condition related to the general trend for obesity in modern populations.

68. With the diagnosis of congenital cervical fusion comes a mandatory obligation to exclude genitourinary anomalies (usually by abdominal ultrasonography) and cardiovascular anomalies by competent medical examination. Hearing should be tested in preschool children.

69. The most effective approach to the patient with complex regional pain syndrome is to prepare and apply the full resources of a comprehensive pain service and then to withdraw the components that are unnecessary. Delayed aggressive management will have a deleterious effect on the final outcome.

70. The use of full-thickness skin grafts should be considered in the release or reconstruction of syndactyly.

71. Reconstructions of thumb abnormalities are generally attempted since functional gains can be significant.

72. For a patient with acquired hand problems, do not waste time and money by ordering magnetic resonance imaging (MRI) before consulting the person to whom you will be referring the patient. MRI may not be needed, or the critical information may not be obtainable by that study.

73. Do not aspirate hand masses in children.

74. Despite the enhanced vascularity of the hand, some form of decompression of purulent fluid is necessary to allow adequate antibiotic penetration into the confined space of septic joints. The gold standard is surgical arthrotomy with irrigation and drainage.

75. The aim of treatment in juvenile rheumatoid arthritis (JRA) is to control the synovitis. In children with a limited number of joints involved, intra-articular corticosteroid injection is most useful.

76. Children with JRA with more-widespread joint involvement require early treatment with methotrexate. Anti–tumor-necrosis-factor (TNF) agents are next used and may be able to halt erosions.

77. Children with systemic JRA may require oral or parenteral corticosteroids and aggressive anti-inflammatory and immunosuppressive therapy under the care of a pediatric rheumatologist.

78. MRI is the best image study for bone infection. Biopsy and culture should always be performed during surgical exploration for bone infections. The results determine treatment in cases of atypical pathogens.

79. It is important to understand the natural history of specific bone tumors so that overtreatment and undertreatment can be avoided. After the staging work-up is completed and a differential diagnosis is formulated, a biopsy is often indicated.

80. Soft tissue lesions that are small and superficial are more likely to be benign, whereas large lesions deep to the fascia are more likely to be malignant, but there are exceptions to both rules.

81. Osteomyelitis is different in children than that adults, primarily because the physis serves as a structural barrier to metaphyseal circulation in long bones.

82. The typical child with septic arthritis is irritable and may go limp with weight-bearing or may refuse to use the involved extremity. Fever is an inconsistent finding, but in subcutaneous joints, one should be able to detect an effusion, increased warmth, soft tissue swelling, and possibly erythema.

83. To a variable degree, all septic joints will have a painful, limited range of motion and will be tender to palpation. The joints will be held in the position of maximal comfort.

84. Needle aspiration of the subperiosteal space and metaphyseal bone at the site of maximum tenderness in an attempt to isolate the causative organism is highly recommended to determine an adequate antibiotic treatment for atypical infections.

85. Parents and therapists often rate walking as their primary goal for the pediatric patient, but communication, which impacts socialization and education, is much more important than walking. Independence in activities of daily living is the second key issue.

86. In children with spina bifida, the orthopaedic surgeon needs (1) to obtain extension posture for standing and walking, (2) to provide lower extremity alignment for bracing, and (3) to correct deformities that lead to skin breakdown.

87. Daily administration of corticosteroids will significantly and dramatically alter the natural history of Duchenne's muscular dystrophy.

88. Arthrogryposis multiplex congenita (AMC) or amyoplasia is a diagnosis of exclusion as there are more than 150 different syndromes that have multiple congenital contractures.

89. Only the distal form (e.g., in the hands, feet, or face) of arthrogryposis multiplex congenita has hereditary factors. It is an autosomal dominant disorder. All other forms are sporadic.

90. A physical examination of *all* of the parts of the body, including a manual muscle test of the parts, is a necessary minimum for evaluating a child with poliomyelitis.

91. As in most areas of limb lengthening, the best treatment for fibular hemimelia is somewhat controversial. Conversion to Syme's amputation almost uniformly results in a very functional child. However, newer methods of limb lengthening make limb salvage a viable option for most degrees of fibular hemimelia.

92. Syndromes are characteristic groups of birth defects caused by dysregulation of pathways that lead to limb and organ development. They may be due to genetic aberrations or fetal environmental factors. A careful examination and history with an open mind by the observer can lead to an accurate diagnosis in many cases.

93. Establishing the etiology of the short stature is critical to understanding what interventions may or may not be effective in trying to gain more height.

94. Spinal deformities pose the greatest surgical challenge in the osteochondrodysplasias. The management of other deformities in these disorders must be influenced by patient demands, which may support a less-aggressive approach.

95. Neurofibromatosis type I (NF-1) is a progressive, multisystem disease that will lead to significant disability if not treated. A team approach is most effective in managing the multidimensional problems of this condition.

96. Osteogenesis imperfecta (OI) is usually a clinical diagnosis made by a combination of physical and radiographic findings. In most cases, OI is not readily confused with other entities. In questionable cases, diagnosis may be confirmed by DNA testing.

97. The major factors affecting bone mineral homeostasis can be thought of as the *three 3s*, intra- and extracellular levels of three ions (calcium, phosphorus, and magnesium), which are regulated by three hormones (parathyroid hormone, calcitonin, and 1,25-dihydroxyvitamin D) and act upon three tissues (bone, intestine, and kidney).

98. The most common orthopaedic treatment in hemophiliacs is open or arthroscopic synovectomy for recurrent hemarthrosis. Soft tissue lengthening or osteotomy is used for deformities. Nihilistic treatment of lower-extremity fractures is essential when appropriate.

99. The most common presenting symptom in patients with leukemia (up to 18%) is musculoskeletal pain (i.e., aching in bones, joints, and the spine).

100. Persistent extremity pain beyond 4–6 weeks and night pain in teenagers are concerning symptoms that should raise suspicion about an occult malignancy.

GROWTH AND DEVELOPMENT

Sevan Hopyan, MD, FRCSC, and Benjamin Alman, MD

1. **What is mesoderm? What is it good for?**

   Mesoderm is one of the three germ layers established by the embryonic process of gastrulation. Mesoderm is the tissue that gives rise to the musculoskeletal tissues. Undifferentiated mesoderm cells are called mesenchyme.

2. **What is neurulation? What happens when it is incomplete?**

   Neurulation is the process of dorsal closure of the neural tube. This proceeds from the center to both ends. A failure of this closure at the caudal end results in spinal dysraphism, ranging from spina bifida occulta to myelomeningocele.

3. **What is the significance of the notochord?**

   The notochord is a midline longitudinal tissue that is deep to the neural tube. It is crucial for organizing the longitudinal axis of the embryo. Persistence of the notochord beyond development may lead to chordoma in later life.

4. **When does spinal and limb patterning occur?**

   Organogenesis, including pattern formation of the spine and limbs, takes place during the second month of gestation.

5. **What are somites? What happens when they do not segment properly?**

   Somites are midline paired segmented condensations of mesenchyme that form in a head-to-tail order. Improper somite formation or segmentation leads to spinal anomalies such as congenital scoliosis or Klippel-Feil syndrome in the cervical spine.

6. **How does the spinal canal develop? What can go wrong?**

   The spine forms from three anlagen for each vertebra: an anterior centrum that forms most of the vertebral body, and two posterior anlagen that unite to form the pedicles, facets, laminae, and spinous processes. If the so-called neurosynchondroses between these anlagen fuse prematurely, spinal stenosis results. This can lead to neurogenic claudication symptoms in spinal dysplasias and achondroplasia.

7. **What is the filum terminale? Why does it normally separate?**

   The filum terminale is the attachment of the lower end of the spinal cord to the region of the lumbosacral junction. During the last trimester and beyond, the spinal cord and the spinal column grow differentially. Failure of the filum to separate normally from the spinal canal can lead to the tethered cord syndrome.

8. **Where do dermatomes get their pattern?**

   Dermatomes, myotomes, and sclerotomes are derived from somites. These structures generate dermal, muscular, and skeletal tissues, respectively, which retain their head-to-tail pattern during development.

9. **How do the limb buds develop?**

   Limb buds arise from flank mesoderm surrounded by ectoderm. They have two special organizing centers: an apical ectodermal ridge (AER) and a mesenchymal progress zone (PZ), both of which are essential for outgrowth and pattern. The most important effector molecules expressed by the AER and by the PZ are fibroblast growth factors and sonic hedgehog, respectively.

10. **From where do the tissues of the limb bud come?**
Cells that will form the skeleton and tendons are derived from the limb bud mesenchyme, whereas muscle cells migrate into the limb secondarily from the somite.

11. **How does the limb skeleton form? What can go wrong?**
Mesenchyme condenses and then forms a cartilaginous template, or anlage, in a proximal-to-distal sequence. A failure of formation of skeletal parts can occur in a transverse or longitudinal pattern due to genetic alterations or teratogens. Intrauterine constriction bands can subsequently destroy a well-formed limb segment.

12. **What are aplasias, amelia, and dysplasias?**
Aplasia and amelia refer to the failure of formation of a given structure and occur during embryogenesis. Dysplasia refers to the improper subsequent development of a given structure and occurs during the fetal or postnatal periods.

13. **What is common about the processes by which joints form and digits separate?**
Programmed cell death, or apoptosis, initiates formation of a cavity between adjacent skeletal anlagen. Fetal motion subsequently elaborates formation of the joint. Interdigital apoptosis is also necessary for the separation of digits. Failure of appropriate apoptosis can lead to synostosis (e.g., congenital proximal radioulnar fusion or tarsal coalition) or syndactyly.

14. **Do the limbs reorient themselves after they are initially formed?**
The upper limbs rotate externally and the scapulae descend caudally to their final position. The lower limbs rotate internally, which results in spiraled dermatomes and the twisted hip capsule, which has greater capacity in external rotation.

15. **What are the two types of bone formation?**
- **Endochondral:** Condensed mesenchyme differentiates to a cartilage template, or anlage, which is subsequently followed by replacement of the template by bone. This process occurs in tubular bones.
- **Membranous:** Mesenchyme transforms directly into bone. This process occurs in most flat bones.

16. **How are the cells of the cartilaginous template organized?**
Chondrocytes differentiate longitudinally from the two metaphyses of a long bone toward the center of the diaphysis. They differentiate from a resting state to a proliferating state to a postmitotic, hypertrophic state, after which they undergo programmed cell death. The matrix they leave behind becomes calcified and subsequently is replaced by bone laid down by invading osteoblasts.

17. **From where does a growth plate come? What can go wrong?**
The growth plate is the residual cartilaginous template that has been diminished by the expansion of the primary ossification center. Abnormal growth plate function can lead to a diverse group of metaphyseal dysplasias. These may be secondary to genetic, nutritional, or mechanical etiologies.

18. **What are the two kinds of growth plates?**
- **Physis:** Primarily responsive to compression forces
- **Apophysis:** Primarily responsive to traction forces

19. **What are the segments of a long bone?**
    - **Diaphysis:** The shaft
    - **Metaphyses:** The flared ends between the physis and the diaphysis
    - **Physis:** The growth plate
    - **Epiphysis:** The area between the physis and the articular surface

20. **What is an ossification center?**
    This is the site at which a cartilaginous or mesenchymal template is initially replaced by bone. In a long bone, the primary ossification center occurs in the center of the diaphysis and expands toward both metaphyses. Secondary ossification centers form within epiphyseal cartilage, mostly postnatally.

KEY POINTS: GROWTH AND DEVELOPMENT

1. The complex three-dimensional human is derived from a single cell by a fascinating process regulated by the genome.

2. Congenital anomalies derive from genetic, teratogenic, or mechanical problems during development.

21. **What is an osteon? How does it change with time?**
    An osteon is a longitudinally oriented tunnel surrounded by osteocytes within diaphyseal bone. Primary osteons mostly form postnatally and are gradually replaced by stronger secondary and tertiary osteons as the bone is remodeled in response to physiologic stresses.

22. **What are the two basic types of bone growth?**
    - **Longitudinal:** Elongation through the growth plate
    - **Latitudinal:** Circumferential, appositional growth by the periosteum (surrounding the diaphysis and metaphysis), the zone of Ranvier (surrounding the physis), and the perichondrium (surrounding the cartilaginous epiphysis)

23. **What are special features of a child's bone that are relevant to injury?**
    - Relatively elastic, so comminution is uncommon.
    - Thick periosteum is often intact on the concavity of a fracture (i.e., greenstick fracture).
    - Metaphyseal cortex is relatively porous and can buckle under compression.
    - Growth plates are weak points with subsequent risk of growth arrest.
    - Bone is weaker than tendon, so avulsion fractures are more common than tendon rupture.
    - Great healing capacity, so nonunion is uncommon following closed fractures.

24. **What does epiphysiodesis mean?**
    Epiphysiodesis is closure of the growth plate by a bony bridge connecting the metaphyseal bone with epiphyseal bone. This process normally occurs at skeletal maturity but may occur prematurely following injury, infection, or surgery. The consequences may be shortening or angular deformity, secondary to partial physeal growth.

25. **Where does a growth plate fail when it is fractured?**
    Mostly through the hypertrophic zone, leaving the resting and proliferating zones intact.

26. **Why does the Salter-Harris type of growth plate fracture correlate with the likelihood of subsequent growth arrest?**
Because the resting and proliferating zones of the growth plate are increasingly injured with the higher grades of fracture.

27. **How does a malunited bone remodel?**
Bone is laid down in the concavity and is resorbed from the convexity, causing the bone to straighten in time.

BIBLIOGRAPHY

1. Buckwalter JA, Ehrlich MG, Sandell LJ, Trippel SB: Skeletal Growth and Development: Clinical Issues and Basic Science Advances. Chicago, American Academy of Orthopaedic Surgeons, 1998.
2. Kaplan KM, Spivak JM, Bendo JA: Embryology of the spine and associated congenital abnormalities. Spine J 5:564–576, 2005.
3. Lord MJ, Ganey TM, Ogden JA: Postnatal development of the thoracic spine. Spine 20:1692–1698, 1995.
4. Tickle C: Patterning systems—From one end of the limb to the other. Dev Cell 4:449–458, 2003.
5. Wolpert L, Beddington R, Jessell TM, et al: Principles of Development. New York, Oxford University Press, 2002.

CHAPTER 2

ETIOLOGY OF ORTHOPAEDIC DISORDERS

James G. Gamble, MD, PhD

1. **What is the meaning of the word *etiology*?**

   Etiology refers to the ultimate cause of something. The Oxford English Dictionary defines *etiology* as the branch of medical science that investigates the causes and origin of diseases: it is the scientific exposition of the origin of any disease. Without an understanding of the etiology of a disease, we are stuck with an empirical approach to treatment. Consider the following common pediatric orthopaedic conditions: adolescent idiopathic scoliosis, Legg-Calvé-Perthes disease, osteochondritis dissecans, and talipes equinovarus. In 2006, we know no more about the etiology of these conditions than was known in 1906, but the outcomes of our contemporary treatments are more favorable due to the empirical research of our predecessors.

2. **What are seven major disease categories, or etiologies, of pediatric orthopaedic disorders?**

   When considering the differential diagnosis of a pediatric orthopaedic condition, seven major disease categories can help to organize your thinking. Ask yourself if the condition falls into one of the following categories:
   - Congenital
   - Developmental
   - Genetic
   - Traumatic
   - Neoplastic
   - Infectious/Inflammatory
   - Metabolic

3. **Are the seven disease categories mutually exclusive?**

   No. An orthopaedic disorder may be classified as neoplastic (such as osteosarcoma) but have a genetic etiology (due to mutations in a tumor suppressor gene). As more information becomes available about the human genome, it is certain that more diseases will be shown to have a genetic basis.

4. **What is the difference between a congenital and a developmental disorder?**

   The word *congenital* refers to a condition existing at or before birth, implying that the condition was acquired during the embryonic or fetal part of intrauterine gestation. Spina bifida is a congenital disorder. The word *developmental* refers to a disorder that appears after the neonatal period. For instance, Scheuermann's kyphosis is a developmental disorder of the spine.

5. **Why is it important to use the term *developmental* and not *congenital* when referring to hip dysplasia?**

   Hip dysplasia may be present at birth, but it also may develop after the neonatal period. Take the case of a 6-month-old girl with hip dysplasia. It is impossible to tell whether the dislocation was present at birth or appeared at 1 week or 1 month. That is why we call it *developmental dysplasia of the hip* (DDH). If the condition is erroneously called *congenital hip dislocation*, as was done in the past, then by definition the condition would have been present at birth, and the clear implication is that the doctor missed the condition. A more accurate term is *developmental dysplasia of the hip*, reflecting our understanding that the dislocation may occur in the prenatal, the natal, or the postnatal period.

6. **Why do we not use the term** *birth defect*, **as was used in the past, when referring to congenital disorders?**
   The term *birth defect* is an old medical term occasionally encountered in the literature of the 19th and early 20th centuries. Today, we find the term to be offensive, prejudicial, and socially unacceptable because of the negative connotations associated with the word *defect*. If something is defective, it is assumed by many to be inferior. People with congenital disorders are not inferior; they are only different. It is preferable to use the term *congenital disorder* when referring to a condition present at birth.

7. **What is the frequency of children born with a congenital disorder?**
   The frequency has remained stable over the past decade and stands at the surprisingly high rate of approximately 4.5%.

8. **What is the difference between a congenital disorder and a genetic disorder?**
   A *congenital disorder* is one that is present at birth. A *genetic disorder* is one that results from an alteration of the DNA sequence of the individual's genome. In theory, all genetic disorders are congenital. However, in certain conditions, such as Duchenne's muscular dystrophy, the children are phenotypically normal until the age of 3–4 years, so it would be confusing to call the condition *congenital*. If the phenotype is apparent at birth, for example by a rigid talipes equinovarus, we classify the condition as congenital.

9. **What is the human genome?**
   The human genome is the specific sequence of nucleotide molecules (i.e., adenine, guanine, cytosine, and thymine) making up the huge polymer of deoxyribonucleic acid in the nucleus of our cells. Our DNA is separated into two sets of 23 chromosomes. Thus, the human genome is the DNA blueprint for the making and maintaining of every human life.

10. **Approximately how big is the human genome?**
    The human genome contains roughly 3.2 billion nucleotides, and each human cell—except the red blood cell—contains them. A billion is a huge number! In the United States, a billion is a thousand million, but in Great Britain a billion is a million million, what we in the United States would call a trillion. The human genome is 3200 million nucleotides. If the sequence of the human genome were written in book form, the book would be a novel of a million pages, with 32,000 letters on each page. Each human cell contains approximately 30,000 genes, but only a small fraction of those genes are expressed in any one cell type.

11. **What is proteomics? What does it have to do with the etiology of disease?**
    Proteomics is the study of all the interactions of proteins in a cell. Proteomics tells us what metabolic pathways are active and when they are active during the life cycle of a cell. The etiology of many human diseases stems from a dysfunction of cellular proteomics.

12. **What genes are responsible for the basic design of the human body?**
    Homeotic genes are responsible for basic body design, such as the division into a head, chest, abdomen, and extremities. These genes establish a molecular coordinate system throughout the primitive embryonic cells that defines the basic body plan.

13. **Name three orthopaedic disorders that are caused by genetic abnormalities.**
    Examples of disorders caused by genetic mutations include achondroplasia, Marfan syndrome, and osteogenesis imperfecta.

14. **What is the etiology of achondroplasia?**
    A mutation in the gene for fibroblast growth factor receptor 3 (FGFR3) causes achondroplasia. This mutation is a simple change in which arginine substitutes for glycine at codon 380 (G380R). This small genotypic change results in a large phenotypic difference.

15. **What is the etiology of Marfan syndrome?**
    The etiology of Marfan syndrome, an autosomal dominant disorder of connective tissue, is a mutation in the fibrillin 1 gene, located on chromosome $15q^{21.1}$.

16. **What is the embryonic period, and why is it so important to the etiology of pediatric orthopaedic conditions?**
    The embryonic period is the first 8 weeks of gestation. This is the time of basic pattern formation in the embryo and is the time when all the major organ systems form. Any extrinsic perturbation during this time, such as a chemical or physical insult, can result in severe structural disorders to the child.

17. **What is the difference between growth and development?**
    Growth is an increase in the physical size of an organ, system, or organism. Development is an increase in the complexity. Development can include both growth and differentiation. We recognize growth and development as the sequential changes that occur as an infant matures into an adult.

18. **What is differentiation?**
    Differentiation is a change from a pluripotential cell to a highly specialized cell. Embryonic stem cells offer so much medical promise because they can differentiate into any type of cell. Cells such as neurons, osteocytes, or chondrocytes no longer have this ability.

19. **What are the four major classes of disorders of growth and development?**
    - Malformation
    - Disruptions
    - Deformations
    - Dysplasias

20. **What are malformations?**
    Malformations are structural disorders that result from an interruption of normal organogenesis during the second month of gestation. Examples include myelomeningocele, syndactyly, and polydactyly.

21. **What are disruptions of growth and development?**
    Disruptions are structural disorders that result from extrinsic interference with normal growth and development. An example would be a congenital constriction band.

22. **What is the difference between deformations and dysplasias?**
    - **Deformations** are structural disorders resulting from either mechanical pressure or muscular activity. Examples would be supple metatarsus adductus, physiologic bowing of the tibia, and medial femoral torsion.
    - **Dysplasias** are structural disorders caused by genetic or cellular abnormalities. Examples include osteogenesis imperfecta, achondroplasia, and spondyloepiphyseal dysplasia.

23. **Why is it important to differentiate deformations from dysplasias?**
    Deformations are relatively easy to treat by removing the deforming mechanical force or by providing an effective counterforce such as corrective casting or bracing. Dysplasias are not

corrected by simple mechanical measures and may require complex medical and surgical management.

24. **What are metameres?**
Metameres are segmental collections of sclerotome cells in the area where the embryonic spine forms. The meters are separated into distinct cranial and caudal portions.

25. **What is a metameric shift?**
In a metameric shift, a resegmentation of cells occurs, such that the cranial portion of the inferior sclerotome combines with the caudal portion of the directly superior sclerotome to form the vertebral bodies of the spine.

26. **Why are renal anomalies commonly associated with congenital scoliosis and other spinal anomalies such as Klippel-Feil syndrome?**
In the embryo, there is a close spatial and temporal relationship of vertebral body formation and nephrogenesis. Any insult to the embryo can affect both systems.

27. **Why does the cervical spine have eight nerves but only seven vertebral bodies?**
During the metameric shift, the cranial portion of the first cervical sclerotome combines with the fourth occipital sclerotome to form the base of the skull. The caudal portion of the first sclerotome combines with the cranial portion of the second sclerotome to form the atlas. This resegmentation essentially removes one sclerotome from the cervical spine.

28. **What are the two major types of malformations that involve the vertebral bodies?**
Disorders of formation cause wedged vertebrae, hemivertebrae, and butterfly vertebrae. Disorders of segmentation cause unsegmented bars, laminar synostosis, and block vertebra.

29. **Why do rib anomalies commonly accompany vertebral anomalies?**
The same sclerotomal cells that give rise to the vertebral body also give rise to the ribs. Any disturbance that affects the vertebral body will also affect the ribs at that level.

KEY POINTS: ETIOLOGY OF ORTHOPAEDIC DISORDERS

1. Understanding the etiology of disorders helps organize one's thinking about natural history and treatment.

2. Congenital disorders may arise from disorders of apoptosis (i.e., programmed cell death), dysfunction of cellular proteomics, metameric shift, and other alterations of genetic expression.

3. Deformations are more readily treatable by simple methods than dysplasias, which often require complex surgical or medical treatment.

30. **What is apoptosis? What is the etiology?**
Apoptosis is the process of programmed cell death. A gene called *reaper* is responsible for initiation of apoptosis. The gene product is a small peptide that causes release of lysosomal enzymes into the cell, resulting in cellular suicide.

31. **Name two common orthopaedic conditions that result from a disorder of apoptosis.**
Failure of apoptosis in the embryonic hand or foot causes syndactyly, and failure of apoptosis in the embryonic knee results in incomplete cavitation, causing synovial folds called plicae.

32. **What is the physis?**
The physis is the growth plate sandwiched between the epiphysis and the metaphysis. The physis is the histologic site of longitudinal bone growth. The physis can be divided into four distinct histologic zones of unique cellular structure: the reserve zone, the proliferative zone, the hypertrophic zone, and the metaphyseal zone.

33. **What causes bone growth?**
Under the influence of pituitary growth hormone, bones grow in length at the physis by the process of endochondral bone formation. Bones grow in girth by the process of intramembranous bone formation. Growth hormone is released at night, so we assume bones grow at night. This makes sense since many children have leg pains in the night, which we call "growing pains."

34. **What is the difference between endochondral and intramembranous bone formation?**
Endochondral bone formation results when osteoblasts collect on a cartilaginous precursor and replace the matrix with bone. Intramembranous bone forms when osteoblasts differentiate into osteocytes and begin to form bone without a cartilaginous precursor.

35. **What takes place at the cellular level when bones grow in length?**
Chondrocyte hyperplasia, hypertrophy, and maturation result in bone growth. The length achieved by chondrocyte hyperplasia and hypertrophy is maintained by deposition of calcium salts within the cartilaginous matrix, followed by remodeling, resorption, and ossification.

36. **What does the Hueter-Volkmann law have to do with the etiology of progressive adolescent genu varum?**
The Hueter-Volkmann law states that compressive forces inhibit bone growth, and tensile forces stimulate bone growth, at the physis. An adolescent with a varus alignment has increased compressive forces on the medial side and increased tensile forces on the lateral side, contributing to inhibited medial growth relative to the lateral part of the physis.

THE SICK CHILD

Ryan C. Goodwin, MD

1. **What are the local exam physical findings in an ill child with acute hematogenous osteomyelitis or septic arthritis?**

   Pain, swelling, mild erythema, and warmth over the affected bone or extremity. Asymmetry of joint motion may be indicative of a joint effusion or synovitis, which, if extremely painful, may be indicative of septic arthritis. Global swelling of the affected extremity may reflect an extensive infection. Local bony tenderness occurs early in the disease process. The most frequent site of infection is the metaphysis of lower-extremity long bones (the tibia and femur account for two-thirds of cases), although it can occur in any bone.

KEY POINTS: COMMON CONDITIONS THAT PRODUCE MUSCULOSKELETAL SYMPTOMS IN A SICK CHILD

1. Septic arthritis

2. Acute osteomyelitis

3. Leukemia

4. Sickle cell crisis

5. Ewing's sarcoma

6. Juvenile rheumatoid arthritis

7. Child abuse

---

2. **What diagnostic tests are useful in acute osteomyelitis and septic arthritis?**

   The white blood cell count, erythrocyte sedimentation rate (ESR), and C-reactive protein (CRP) levels are usually elevated. Bone findings on plain x-rays are typically normal early in the disease process. Periosteal reaction may be seen later into the disease process—at least 7–10 days after symptoms begin. Soft tissue swelling that obliterates the muscle planes can on occasion be seen before bone changes. (It is helpful to have a comparison radiograph of the opposite extremity.) Large-bore needle aspiration of the subperiosteal space and metaphyseal bone within a centimeter of the physis performed under general anesthesia yields pus, which confirms the diagnosis and may identify an organism. Joint aspiration should be performed emergently if septic arthritis is suspected. This can be done by ultrasound guidance or in the operating room with x-ray or arthrogram. The pus and any other fluid should be sent immediately to the laboratory for Gram stain and culture. Blood cultures will yield an organism in 50% of cases. Magnetic resonance imaging (MRI) may be useful in the early diagnosis of osteomyelitis. Signal changes in the marrow suggestive of edema are an early clue to the diagnosis. Fluid collections, joint effusions, and abscesses can be seen on MRI, which has become an excellent adjunct study when the symptoms are localized. Bone scan is also helpful when the sick child limps but a specific location for the presumed infection is not yet identified.

3. **Describe the treatment of acute osteomyelitis.**
Treatment consists of empirical or organism-directed intravenous antibiotics, with the affected extremity at rest. Early conversion to oral therapy is possible if a good early clinical response is noted. Infections that progress to abscess require surgical drainage and debridement with longer courses of intravenous therapy. Acute-phase reactants such as ESR and CRP typically normalize with appropriate therapy.

4. **What is the treatment of septic arthritis?**
Septic arthritis requires urgent drainage and lavage of the affected joint. Drilling of the adjacent metaphyses for drainage is occasionally performed. Organism-directed antibiotic therapy of longer duration (6 weeks or greater) is the rule. Acute-phase reactants typically normalize with appropriate therapy.

5. **Describe the presenting symptoms of an ill child with systemic-onset juvenile rheumatoid arthritis (JRA).**
Intermittent fever and joint pain suggest the diagnosis of systemic JRA. Systemic-onset JRA can occur at any time from infancy to adulthood. There is no age or sex predilection for systemic-onset JRA, unlike the other forms of childhood JRA. High, spiking fever is the key finding, which by definition must exceed 39.38°C. Initially, the fever may be erratic, but usually there is a daily or twice-daily pattern. The peak fever is characteristically present in the late afternoon to evening; by morning, the child feels better and has a normal temperature. Severe arthralgias and myalgias accompany the fever spikes. Cervical spine stiffness is common.
   A characteristic rash frequently occurs with the fevers. The rash is classically nonpruritic, pink to salmon-colored, macular or maculopapular, and evanescent. The rash is seen most frequently on the trunk, on the proximal extremities, and in the axillae when the child is febrile. It tends to be migratory, with individual lesions disappearing within hours and leaving no residua.
   The joint pain in JRA typically improves with use of the affected joint. Morning stiffness is commonly reported and improves as the day progresses. These children are often quite ill while febrile and feel surprisingly well during the rest of the day. The child may have lymphadenopathy, hepatosplenomegaly, and pleural or pericardial effusions, as well as frank arthritis. The diagnosis of systemic-onset JRA requires the presence of arthritis for a minimum of 6 weeks; however, high fevers associated with a rash and arthritis in a sick child result in earlier diagnosis.

KEY POINTS: INITIAL WORK-UP OF THE CHILD WITH MUSCULOSKELETAL SYMPTOMS

1. Careful history and physical exam

2. Plain x-rays

3. Complete blood cell count with differential

4. Erythrocyte sedimentation rate and C-reactive protein

5. Additional studies (e.g., computed tomography [CT], magnetic resonance imaging [MRI], bone scan, skeletal survey, etc.), ordered based on the specific clinical scenario

6. **What are the local findings in systemic-onset JRA?**
Any number of joints may be involved in systemic-onset JRA. The arthritic joints often look worse than they feel. The finding may only be swelling, although most involved joints have some

combination of warmth, pain, and tenderness. As a rule, children walk on these joints despite the presence of fusiform swelling, warmth, discomfort, and limitation of motion. There is generally greater active and passive motion and less pain than is found in joint swelling caused by infection or trauma. Tenderness is diffuse and nonfocal. Atrophy and weakness of the adjacent muscles (suggesting chronicity) may be present at the time of diagnosis.

7. **Which laboratory tests should be ordered for the diagnosis of systemic-onset JRA?**

As with any sick child, the complete blood cell count (CBC), ESR, and CRP are the cornerstone of the laboratory tests with suspected JRA. Unfortunately, laboratory tests are of little value since no single laboratory test can be used to make a definitive diagnosis of systemic JRA. The ESR is usually elevated. The CBC is important in screening for neoplasia. The white blood cell count (WBC) should be normal or elevated (it can be very high in systemic-onset JRA, at 40,000 WBC/mm^3 or greater). Low platelet count or WBC may indicate leukemia or systemic lupus erythematosus. The hematocrit is usually normal or slightly low in chronic arthritis. Antinuclear antibody (ANA) and rheumatoid factor (RF) are only rarely positive in systemic-onset JRA. The ANA is more likely to be positive in more-focal JRA. A positive ANA is a marker for those children at high risk for developing asymptomatic uveitis.

8. **What are the radiographic findings of joints with JRA?**

Early radiographs in JRA are not diagnostic. They usually show only soft tissue swelling, effusion, and osteopenia of the adjacent bone. They are, however, very helpful in ruling out other diagnoses (e.g., trauma, neoplasia, and osteomyelitis).

9. **What are the presenting musculoskeletal symptoms in an ill child with leukemia?**

Leukemia is the most common cancer of childhood and usually affects young children. Most children appear systemically ill at presentation. All organ systems are eventually involved, although the initial symptoms of leukemia often involve only the musculoskeletal system. Diffuse, nonspecific musculoskeletal (i.e., bone) pain is present in 20–30% of children with acute leukemia. It usually results from distention of the medullary cavities due to the rapid proliferation of hematopoietic tissue. Frequent sites of pain are the long bones and the spine. Sympathetic joint effusions can sometimes be present and can mimic the appearance of an infectious process. Although the diffuse symptoms make the initial diagnosis difficult, one should be suspicious of leukemia in sick children with obscure bone pain.

10. **What radiographic findings appear in a child with leukemia?**

X-rays are usually normal. When they are abnormal, generalized osteopenia is seen most typically. In actively growing bones (usually the distal end of the femur and the proximal end of the tibia), metaphyseal bands (i.e., the leukemic lines) appear as radiolucent transverse bands next to the growth plate. These radiolucent bands are due not to the infiltration of leukemia cells, but rather to a disturbance in formation of bone in the growth plate. With progression of the disease, lytic areas develop, which may be demarcated or moth-eaten in appearance. The lytic lesions may involve the metaphyses of long bones, the skull, the pelvis, and the tubular bones of the hands and feet. There may be associated subperiosteal new bone formation, suggesting acute osteomyelitis.

11. **What are the laboratory findings in a child with acute leukemia?**

The WBC may be elevated, depressed, or, in some instances, normal. Severe anemia is common. When the hemoglobin is 9 grams per 100 milliliters or less, leukemia must be ruled out. Blast forms are often seen in the peripheral blood smear, but their absence does not exclude leukemia. The ESR is often elevated. Lactate dehydrogenase and uric acid, which are markers of rapid turnover of lymphocytes, may be elevated and are helpful in making the diagnosis. Relative thrombocytopenia is often seen. Platelet counts should ordinarily be elevated in acute infections. A low normal or low platelet count is suggestive of leukemia.

12. **What is acute rheumatic fever? How does it present in a sick child?**
Acute rheumatic fever (ARF) is an autoimmune reaction that occurs 2–4 weeks after infection with β-hemolytic group A streptococci in children 5–15 years of age. Musculoskeletal sequelae include arthritis, which is characteristically acute and painful and involves the peripheral joints in a migratory, asymmetric pattern. The joints are exquisitely tender, red, and hot, and the arthritis typically migrates from joint to joint over a period of days. The rapid decrease in joint symptoms with aspirin or nonsteroidal anti-inflammatory drug therapy is almost diagnostic. A similar clinical picture of inflammatory arthritis may be associated with carditis, chorea, erythema marginatum, subcutaneous nodules, and fever. These associated features and a history of previous streptococcal infection are key in making the diagnosis.

13. **What is Ewing's sarcoma? How does it present?**
Ewing's sarcoma is a malignant bone tumor that occurs between the ages of 5 and 25 years. It is rare in African Americans and Asians and is usually located in the diaphysis of a long bone. Pain and swelling are common at the site of tumor, and the pain is often present at least 1 month prior to the diagnosis. The presentation often mimics that of an infection, and systemic symptoms such as fever, malaise, and weight loss, combined with physical findings of local warmth, inflammation, and swelling, are common. An elevated ESR and WBC and a mottled appearance of the involved bone on radiographs also confuse this diagnosis with infection. The femur is most commonly involved, followed by the tibia, the fibula, and the humerus. A translocation involving chromosomes 11 and 22 or 21 and 22 is frequently present and is essentially diagnostic of the condition.

14. **Describe the plain radiographic appearance of Ewing's sarcoma.**
Ewing's sarcoma is seen radiographically as an aggressive bone-destroying lesion. Diffuse and permeative or moth-eaten destruction of the diaphyseal bone, extension of the tumor through the cortex into the surrounding soft tissue, and periosteal reaction are all apparent. Periosteal reaction is commonly seen and has been described classically as "onionskin" in appearance. It may also produce a Codman's triangle or sunburst appearance. A large, noncalcified, soft tissue mass is frequently present. The bone destruction may be minimal in comparison to the soft tissue mass, although the cortex may appear to be destroyed. All of these findings suggest an aggressive bone tumor that has rapidly penetrated the cortex and elevated the periosteum, but they are not pathognomonic for Ewing's sarcoma.

15. **What clinical scenarios are suggestive of child abuse?**
   - Changing history or history inconsistent with the injury
   - Delay in seeking treatment
   - Long bone fractures in children <1 year of age (non-walking)
   - Multiple fractures in various stages of healing
   - Pathognomonic fractures (rib, skull, corner fracture)

16. **What clinical tools and skills are helpful in making the diagnosis of abuse and in instituting treatment?**
Efficient diagnosis and management of the abused child requires a multidisciplinary approach. Pediatric hospitalists and social work professionals are invaluable in caring for these children. The assessment of a potentially abused child should include an interview with the child whenever possible. It should be conducted in a safe, quiet, and nonthreatening environment. Approaching the family in a nonthreatening manner is often helpful as well in facilitating care for the child. Mortality rates in battered children approach 3%. Reinjury rates of battered children are extremely high (at 30–50%); therefore, proper identification and treatment of these cases is essential.

BIBLIOGRAPHY

1. Cassidy JT, Ross PE: Textbook of Pediatric Rheumatology, 4th ed. Philadelphia, W.B. Saunders, 2001.

2. Fink CW, Nelson JD: Septic arthritis and osteomyelitis in children. Clin Rheum Dis 12:423–435, 1986.

3. Green NE, Edwards K: Bone and joint infections in children. Orthop Clin North Am 18:555–576, 1987.

4. Hering JA (ed): Tachdjian's Pediatric Orthopaedics, 3rd ed. Philadelphia, W.B. Saunders, 2002, pp 1841–1860.

5. Levesque J, Marx R, Bell B: A Clinical Guide to Primary Bone Tumors. Philadelphia, Williams & Wilkins, 1998.

6. Rogalsky RJ, Black GB, Reed MH: Orthopaedic manifestations of leukemia in children. J Bone Joint Surg Am 68A:494–501, 1986.

7. Schaller JC: Juvenile rheumatoid arthritis. Pediatr Rev 18:337–349, 1997.

8. Sponseller PD (ed): Orthopaedic Knowledge Update—Pediatrics 2, AAOS, 2002.

9. Stollerman GH: Rheumatic fever. Lancet 349:935–942, 1997.

10. Wenger DR, Pring ME, Rang M (eds): Rang's Children's Fractures, 3rd ed. Philadelphia, Lippincott Williams & Wilkins, 2005, pp 11–25.

CHAPTER 4

AMPLIFIED MUSCULOSKELETAL PAIN

David D. Sherry, MD

1. **What is amplified musculoskeletal pain?**

   Every child suffers musculoskeletal pain from time to time. A child with amplified musculoskeletal pain has an amplified pain response, so the pain he or she experiences is much greater than one would expect. Additionally, most of these children have disproportional dysfunction. A child with knee pain will not bend the knee, will be completely non-weight-bearing, and will not even tolerate bedcovers touching the knee. Because of the pain, the child will miss school for weeks at a time and will even need help dressing.

2. **Who gets amplified musculoskeletal pain?**

   Most (80%) are females between 9 and 18 years old, with the average being 12 years old. It is rare before the age of 6 years.

3. **What causes amplified pain?**

   These pains can be initiated by trauma or inflammation, such as tendinitis or arthritis; however, they seem to be related to psychological factors in the majority of children.

4. **If it is due to psychological factors, is the pain "just in the child's head"?**

   No. Pain is a personal experience, and these children suffer tremendously. Each person's psychological makeup influences the way in which he or she experiences and copes with pain.

5. **Are there different kinds of amplified musculoskeletal pain?**

   There are several patterns of amplified musculoskeletal pain, depending on the location of the pain, associated symptoms, and physical findings. The names used to describe the clinical variations are legion, and all are somewhat unsatisfactory. It may not be useful to label each variation, but when confronted with a child in pain, delineating the pattern in your own mind may help you make the diagnosis. The most common patterns are as follows:

   - **Psychogenic or idiopathic musculoskeletal pain:** This is the most common form. It may be constant or intermittent, well-localized or diffuse, and may involve multiple sites. The pain is disproportionate and is characterized by allodynia, marked dysfunction, an incongruent affect, and absence of signs of overt autonomic dysfunction.
   - **Reflex neurovascular dystrophy, reflex sympathetic dystrophy, or complex regional pain syndrome, type 1:** This pattern usually involves a single site. Lower extremities are more frequently involved than upper extremities, and the pain is usually constant. The characteristics of the pain are identical to those of psychogenic musculoskeletal pain, but there are signs of overt autonomic dysfunction; that is, the limb is cold and cyanotic and can be edematous. Less-common signs are perspiration changes or dystrophic skin changes (i.e., thickened, waxy, hairy skin).
   - **Fibromyalgia:** This is characterized by widespread pain (involving more than half the body) that lasts more than 6 months. On examination, 11 of 18 possible trigger points are reported to be painful to digital palpation. These children report more feelings of depression, have unrestful sleep, and have other associated pain symptoms such as headaches, chest pains, and abdominal pains.

- **Hypervigilance:** These children seem to pay too much attention to normal body sensations and interpret these sensations as painful. These pains are usually short-lived and do not significantly interfere with function but cause the child great anxiety.

6. **What are some clues in the history of amplified musculoskeletal pain?**
   Frequently, the patient has a minor injury that subsequently becomes increasingly painful. Commonly, the child presents in an emergency department days after the injury because the parents suspect a fracture. The pain is either minimally responsive or not responsive to conservative management with pain or anti-inflammatory medications. Immobilization frequently makes it worse. There may be a history of color changes (purple) and temperature changes (cold). The pain may be so intense that clothing or bedcovers are intolerable. The pain prohibits activities of daily living such as attending school, interferes with mental concentration, and is reported to be much more severe than the pain experienced by children with organic disorders such as arthritis.

   On a 10-point scale, most patients will report their pain to be near 10 or even higher. There is an absence of symptoms that would suggest infection. Interestingly, children with lower-extremity pain frequently crawl around their homes rather than walk; this is exceedingly rare, if not completely absent, in children with arthritis.

7. **Is there anything to be learned from the past history?**
   These children are described as slow healers (possibly taking 6 months or more to recover from an uncomplicated fracture) or have had similar prolonged painful experiences in the past. An occasional child will report hundreds of musculoskeletal injuries, such as spraining his or her ankle every week, or even every day.

8. **What should one inquire about in the family history?**
   Similar pain or chronic pain, such as fibromyalgia, in family members or even friends *is not uncommon.*

9. **Is there anything to be learned from the social history?**
   Most of these children are in the midst of multiple traumatic life events, such as parental divorce, a change in schools, a change in family membership, and the loss of significant people in their lives. Physical and sexual abuse is seen in about 10% of cases and needs to be discussed in the appropriate setting.

10. **What physical examination findings should one seek?**
    Important things to look for include inappropriate child / parent (usually mother/daughter) interactions, incongruent affect, belle indifférence, allodynia, signs of autonomic dysfunction, compliance, and fibromyalgic tender points. Rule out inflammation, infection, and neurologic dysfunction.

11. **What do you mean by mother/daughter interaction?**
    Most of the mothers and daughters seen in these cases are inappropriately close and overinvolved in the emotional lives of each other.

12. **What do you mean by *incongruent affect*?**
    Most, but not all, of these children report that the pain rates a 10 on a scale of 1–10 (or even a 20) and yet will be smiling and will manifest no pain behaviors.

13. **What do you mean by *belle indifférence*?**
    The child has the appearance of being unconcerned about the amount of pain and dysfunction he or she has.

14. **What do you mean by *allodynia*?**
Severe pain in response to a stimulus that normally is not interpreted as noxious. Test for this by either lightly touching the skin or gently pinching the skin between your thumb and forefinger. During either maneuver, the child will report severe pain, with or without pain behaviors such as wincing. Repeatedly check the location of the border of the area of skin that is painful. Commonly, the border will vary by as much as 6–8 cm.

15. **What are the signs of autonomic dysfunction?**
    - Cyanosis
    - Coolness
    - Edema
    - Increased perspiration
    - Dystrophic skin

    Autonomic signs need to be checked both before and after exercising the limb since they may become manifest after use. The limb will be cool and cyanotic, purple, or ruddy in color and can be quite mottled. Sometimes the pulse is decreased. Occasionally, the limb will be diffusely edematous; the joints will not be swollen. Rarely, it will be clammy or there will be dystrophic skin changes (i.e., waxy, hairy, thick skin).

16. **What are the fibromyalgia tender points?**
    - The insertion of the suboccipital muscle at the base of the occiput
    - The lateral transverse cervical processes of C6 or C7
    - The mid-upper border of the trapezius
    - Above the medial border of the scapular spine
    - The second costochondral junction
    - Two centimeters distal to the lateral epicondyle
    - The gluteal muscle fold
    - One centimeter posterior to the greater trochanter
    - One centimeter proximal to the medial knee joint mortise

    In addition to the trigger points, you should check control points such as the center of the forehead, the muscles of the midforearm, the left thumbnail, and the midshin (Fig. 4-1).

17. **How do you know if a trigger point is truly tender?**
You apply 4 kg of pressure with the flat surface of the thumb, held perpendicular to the body. The patient may or may not wince but needs to indicate verbally that the pressure caused definite pain, not just discomfort.

18. **What are other signs of fibromyalgia?**
Fibromyalgia is widespread body pain lasting longer than 3 months, involving more than half the body, in which 11 of 18 trigger points are painful to digital palpation. Children with fibromyalgia also frequently report feeling depressed and unrested in the morning, even if they sleep late.

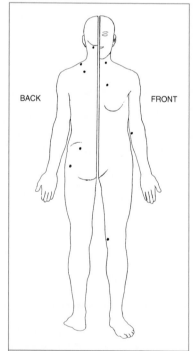

BACK · FRONT

Figure 4-1. Tender points in children with the fibromyalgia variant of disproportional musculoskeletal pain. Tenderness in 11 of 18 points is required for diagnosis.

19. **What tests are indicated?**
   If you are sure of the diagnosis, no tests are indicated. If you are unsure, make certain that acute-phase reactant levels are not elevated (i.e., the erythrocyte sedimentation rate and the C-reactive protein level) and that the complete blood cell count (CBC) and radiographs are normal. If still unsure, obtain a three-phase bone scan. This can confirm the diagnosis by showing decreased blood flow to the involved limb and decreased uptake in the delayed images. The bone scan can be normal, in which case it is reassuring that you are not missing a small, hidden osteoid osteoma or an occult fracture. Rarely, the bone scan will show increased spotty uptake, which is characteristic of reflex neurovascular dystrophy in adults.

20. **What is the treatment for amplified musculoskeletal pain?**
   The treatment is intense exercise therapy that is focused on function and desensitizing painful skin. We administer 5–6 hours of aerobic therapy (one-on-one physical therapy and occupational therapy plus pool therapy) daily, although many children will respond to a smaller dose of exercise therapy. Exercises should focus on the disability. Stair-climbing, jumping activities, biking, and walking are used for those with leg involvement; wall washing, writing, typing, throwing, and gripping are used for those with upper-extremity involvement. What hurts the most is what we emphasize. We acknowledge the pain but encourage the child to complete the exercises in much the same way a coach motivates a player. Changing the activity frequently helps keep the child interested, along with having specific goals of performance (e.g., beating the last time or number of repetitions). We reinforce the idea that the pain does not indicate tissue damage but is an abnormal amplified response and needs to be worked through.

21. **What about other modalities, medications, and surgery?**
   We do not recommend any modalities such as transcutaneous nerve stimulation, ultrasound, nerve blocks, sympathectomies, or medications. We have found that if the child is dependent on us to fix the pain, the recurrence rate is much higher.

22. **How does one desensitize painful skin?**
   Rub it with a towel or lotion, possibly with cornmeal added, for 2 minutes at a time. Repeat this two or three times during the day. Care needs to be taken to ensure that there is no skin breakdown.

23. **How long does it take for improvement to be seen?**
   Within a few days, most children will have a significant increase in function, although the pain may increase. It will gradually decrease over time. The intense exercise program is usually followed daily for the first week and, in most, can be decreased to 2–3 days a week the following week. Thereafter, the child graduates to a daily home program that takes about 40 minutes to complete. Most require 2 full weeks of daily therapy, and occasionally a child will require more than a month. For most, the daily home program can be stopped after a month, after which the child is encouraged to participate in normal activities such as sports, dance, and physical education class. This helps decrease the emphasis on illness and promotes the idea that he or she is healthy.

24. **What about the psychological aspects?**
   Stresses may be caused by family, school, or friends. Marital discord may be covert, so the parents may not report strife. School can be a major source of stress; most of these children work hard to be excellent students and to please others without getting their own needs met.

25. **Are these children depressed?**
   Few of these children are clinically depressed. About half of children with the fibromyalgia variant are depressed, however, which is one of the distinguishing features of that condition.

26. **Can these children also have a concurrent conversion reaction?**
Up to 40% of children with amplified musculoskeletal pain will have a conversion reaction. Conversion reactions, by themselves, are not associated with pain. The conversion reaction can take the form of paralysis, shaking, seizures, stiffness, or a sensory abnormality such as numbness or blindness.

27. **What is the outcome?**
The vast majority (80%) of the children are completely without symptoms within a month or two. Another 15% have only mild or intermittent pain and are fully active. About 5% continue to have disabling pain and require psychotherapy before they can become better. About half of such children, in our experience, do seek appropriate psychological care and eventually are free of pain.

28. **How can one prevent a recurrence?**
It is most important to recognize that a recurrence is happening. The pain may or may not feel like the first episode and may be at a different site. Clues are allodynia, marked dysfunction, and increasing pain over time. The second episode may not necessarily have the same manifestations as the first episode. It is imperative to exercise the limb as soon as a recurrence is thought to be starting, even if it was initiated by injury. Desensitization early on is helpful for those with allodynia. Most children will not want to repeat an intense exercise program and will work hard on the home program to avoid a full recurrence.

29. **Can amplified musculoskeletal pain involve the back or jaw?**
Yes. It is harder to diagnose, but the basic principles are the same.

30. **What signs do you find in children with amplified musculoskeletal pain of the back?**
Children can manifest the same signs described by Waddell et al regarding nonorganic back pain in adults:
- **Distracted straight-leg-raising:** Back pain when the hip is flexed to 90 degrees with knee extended when supine, but not when seated; rarely positive in children
- **Axial loading:** With patient standing, pressure on the head causes back pain
- **Passive rotation:** Back pain is reported when twisting the patient at the ankles and knees while keeping the back in one plane, causing no real back rotation
- **Nonanatomic tenderness or regional pain:** Half the back
- **Nonanatomic allodynia**: Common in children
- **Overreaction:** Exaggerated wincing, loud ouches, or collapsing

31. **How do children with intermittent amplified musculoskeletal pain present? How do you treat it?**
They look entirely well and are without pain or dysfunction. The history reveals that after activity, there is such pain that the child cannot function for hours to days. Often, there is a history of allodynia while the pain lasts, and rarely there is a history consistent with overt autonomic dysfunction.

The treatment is the same; that is, intense exercise daily. Most children do very well after exercising daily for a week and suffer no further episodes of postactivity amplified musculoskeletal pain.

32. **How do you treat children with hypervigilance?**
Recognizing the diagnosis, avoiding any further testing, and offering reassurance are all that are needed in most cases. Occasionally, a home exercise program is prescribed, which is to be carried out when the child is feeling the pain. It is important to evaluate these children a few months later to reaffirm the diagnosis.

33. **What if the child has an underlying illness or injury?**

A child with an underlying condition needs to have that condition addressed while the exercise program is started. If the underlying condition is active, such as arthritis, it should be aggressively treated. If it is inactive without organic sequelae, such as reactive arthritis, it should be ignored. If it is associated with musculoskeletal sequelae, such as cerebral palsy or destructive arthritis, the exercise program will have to be modified but should still focus on regaining baseline function and desensitization. Pool therapy is quite helpful for children who are normally nonambulatory.

34. **How do I explain amplified musculoskeletal pain to the child and parents?**

The child should be told that the nerves going to the blood vessels are working too much, and that is causing the amplification of the pain. The exercise therapy retrains these nerves so that blood flow is restored. Function comes back first, and then the pain subsides. Occasionally, the pain will stop instantaneously.

KEY POINTS: AMPLIFIED MUSCULOSKELETAL PAIN

1. If the child hurts too much given the history and psychical examination, think about amplified musculoskeletal pain, especially in adolescent girls.

2. Do not tell the child that the pain is not real or is in his or her head, but rather say that the pain is amplified so it hurts more than one would expect.

3. Mobilize early and aggressively with functional activities and exercises, and desensitize areas painful to touch.

4. Explore the role that psychological stress may play in amplified musculoskeletal pain by inquiring about recent and past stressful life events.

BIBLIOGRAPHY

1. Sherry DD: Pain syndromes. In Isenberg DA, Miller J III (eds): Adolescent Rheumatology. London, Martin Dunitz, 1998, pp 197–227.

2. Sherry DD, Wallace CA, Kelley, C, et al: Short- and long-term outcome of children with complex regional pain syndrome type I treated with exercise therapy. Clin J Pain 15:218–223, 1999.

3. Waddell G, McCulloch JA, Kummel E, Venner RM: 1979 Volvo Award in Clinical Science. Nonorganic physical signs in low-back pain. Spine 5:117–125, 1980.

4. Wolfe F, Smythe HA, Yunus, MB, et al: The American College of Rheumatology 1990 criteria for the classification of fibromyalgia: Report of the multicenter criteria committee. Arthritis Rheum 36:160–172, 1990.

CHAPTER 5

DIAGNOSTIC IMAGING

Maya E. Pring, MD, and Dennis R. Wenger, MD

1. **What is the imaging method of choice for assessing developmental dysplasia of the hip (DDH) in an infant younger than 3 months of age?**
   Hip ultrasonography is now widely accepted as the method of choice for imaging the infant hip to rule out DDH. The use of hip sonography to diagnose hip dysplasia in infancy was developed by Graf of Austria. His method emphasizes angular measurement of acetabular landmarks in addition to assessment of hip position. Harcke, of Delaware, developed a dynamic approach that assesses the hip under motion in several positions. Modern study methods synthesize these two concepts into a single comprehensive study.

2. **Should all infants have an ultrasound of the hips?**
   In some countries, infants are routinely screened with ultrasound to rule out dysplasia. In the United States, only children who are at risk for hip dysplasia or who have an abnormal physical exam are referred for ultrasound. There is little international agreement as to whether routine ultrasound examination of all infant hips is the best way to spend a health care budget.
   - **Risk factors:** First born females, breech delivery, family history of DDH, metatarsus adductus, and torticollis
   - **Abnormal physical exam findings:** An unstable hip (i.e., Ortolani or Barlow positive), unequal thigh folds, apparent femoral length discrepancy (i.e., a positive Galeazzi test), and unequal hip abduction

3. **What are the most common uses of diagnostic ultrasonography in children's orthopaedics?**
   Ultrasonography is the method of choice for detecting early DDH before the femoral head ossifies (for ages 3–6 months). Other uses include evaluation of a possible imbedded foreign body, detection of joint effusion (especially the hip joint), and evaluation of soft tissue masses. Ultrasonography can be used to evaluate physeal fractures in young children. It can also be used for guiding interventions including hip aspiration, cyst aspiration, and foreign body removal.

4. **When is a bone scan ordered?**
   In osteomyelitis, the plain films may be negative until 7–10 days after the onset of symptoms. Early diagnosis is greatly aided by use of a three-phase bone scan. The study is also a good screening tool for the child with occult back or limb complaints and is very useful for early diagnosis of conditions such as discitis and sacroiliac joint infections. It can also be used to assess the activity of a bone tumor and to look for metastases.

5. **What is the injected substance that lights up on a bone scan? On a white blood cell labeled scan?**
   Diphosphonates labeled with radioactive technetium (i.e., Tc 99m) are injected prior to a bone scan and will accumulate in areas of increased bone turnover or calcification. Fracture, spondylolysis, osseous tumor, and osseous infection will all light up.
   White cells can be tagged with a radioactive tracer (i.e., indium or technetium) and injected. The white cells will then accumulate in areas of infection. This study can help differentiate fracture from infection in complex circumstances.

6. **What are the three phases in a three-phase bone scan?**
   - **Initial:** Perfusion phase (tracer is delivered to perfused tissues)
   - **Second:** Blood pool phase
   - **Delayed:** (2–4 hours after injection) Tracer accumulates in tissues with active turnover of phosphates (usually bone undergoing turnover or growth)

7. **How can osteomyelitis be differentiated from cellulitis with a bone scan?**
   On the three-phase bone scan, cellulitis demonstrates increased uptake in the immediate perfusion and blood pool images. Normal activity is demonstrated on delayed images. Osteomyelitis often has abnormal activity in all three phases but is most specifically positive on the delayed image.

8. **When will a bone scan have cold spots (i.e., decreased uptake)?**
   If there is decreased blood flow to a region, the bone scan will be cold in that area, indicating Perthes' disease, avascular necrosis (AVN), bony abscess, or cysts. Always remember to look for areas of decreased uptake as well as hot spots. An acute severe osteomyelitis with the pus under pressure may have a cold bone scan.

9. **When is single photon emission computed tomography (SPECT) used?**
   A SPECT scan can be used in conjunction with a bone scan. With this technique, sectional images of the body can be obtained in the sagittal, coronal, and axial planes. The SPECT scan is used effectively to detect spondylolysis and to search for small lesions such as osteoid osteoma.

10. **What are some of the advantages of computed tomography (CT) over plain x-ray?**
    CT uses x-rays to produce tomographic images or slices through the subject; the overlap of structures is eliminated. CT has much higher contrast resolution, and the images can be reconstructed to provide three-dimensional images versus the two-dimensional images of plain films.

11. **The new multislice CT scanners are faster and give much better resolution and improved three-dimensional images. What is a drawback to this imaging study?**
    The radiation exposure necessary to get the improved images is higher than the standard helical CT.

12. **When are three-dimensional CT studies useful?**
    Three-dimensional reconstruction of routine axial CT images allows enhanced imaging of complex structures. The edit function allows removal of any structure in the image for direct visualization of a single part (e.g., removing the femoral head so the entire acetabulum can be visualized). That part can also be rotated in space for three-dimensional evaluation. These capabilities aid in the evaluation and preoperative planning of many orthopaedic conditions, as follows:
    - **Hip:** Dysplasia, avascular necrosis, or proximal femoral deformity (congenital or following slipped capital femoral epiphysis [SCFE], Perthes' disease, or AVN)
    - **Spine:** Congenital spine deformities, fractures, or dislocations
    - **Intra-articular fractures:** At any joint

13. **What is the best imaging study to evaluate soft tissue tumors?**
    Magnetic resonance imaging (MRI).

14. **What tissues are bright or have high-signal intensity on T1-weighted MRI images?**
    Fat (i.e., lipoma), subacute hemorrhage (i.e., hematoma), and gadolinium enhancement.

15. **What tissues are dark or have low-signal intensity on T2-weighted images?**
    Cortical bone, matrix mineralization, fibrous tissue, air (i.e., abscess), some foreign bodies (polymethylmethacrylate [PMMA] and hardware), acute hemorrhage, pigmented villonodular synovitis (PVNS), hemosiderin, and old hemorrhage.

KEY POINTS: DIAGNOSTIC IMAGING

1. Ultrasound is a safe and versatile method of imaging that is used for evaluation of many different musculoskeletal problems.

2. Musculoskeletal infections can be surgical emergencies—it is important to know which imaging studies to order if infection is a concern.

3. CT scans allow evaluation of bony problems (fractures, tumors, deformity) in three dimensions.

4. MRI is the best study to evaluate soft tissues such as ligament, tendon, labrum, meniscus, and articular cartilage.

5. PET scans are used for evaluation of tumors and metastases.

---

16. **What is the best study to evaluate a triangular fibrocartilage complex (TFCC) tear in the wrist, a superior labrum anterior-to-posterior (SLAP) lesion in the shoulder, or a labral tear in the hip?**
    The joint can be injected with dilute gadolinium prior to MRI for an MRI arthrogram that shows the contours of intra-articular structures and tears within these structures.

17. **How are meniscal tears graded on MRI?**
    - **Grade 1:** A rounded or amorphous signal that does not disrupt an articular surface
    - **Grade 2:** A linear signal that does not disrupt an articular surface
    - **Grade 3:** A rounded or linear signal that disrupts an articular surface (a grade 3 signal is, by definition, a tear)

18. **What foot and ankle pathology is best studied with MRI?**
    Tendon pathology (Achilles, posterior tibial tendon, flexor hallucis longus [FHL], and peroneal tendons), osteochondritis dissecans lesions of the talus, AVN, tumors (i.e., synovial sarcomas), ligament injuries, and sinus tarsi syndrome.

19. **When is a positron emission tomography (PET) scan indicated?**
    PET scanning is very useful for evaluation of tumors. The 2-deoxy-2-fluoro-D-glucose (FDG) is a metabolic tracer that will be taken up by tissues with an increased glycolytic rate (usually pathologic tissue).

BIBLIOGRAPHY

1. Graf R: Fundamentals of sonographic diagnosis of infant hip dysplasia. J Pediatr Orthop 4:735–740, 1984.
2. Grissom LE, Harke HT: Developmental dysplasia of the pediatric hip with emphasis on sonographic evaluation. Semin Musculoskelet Radiol 3:359–370,1999.
3. Jaramillo D, Connolly LP: Imaging techniques and applications. In Morrisy RT, Weinstein SL (eds): Lovell and Winter's Pediatric Orthopaedics, 5th ed. Philadelphia, Lippincott Williams & Wilkins, 2006, pp 63–98.
4. Johnson TR, Steinbach LS: Essentials of Musculoskeletal Imaging. Rosemont, IL, American Academy of Orthopaedic Surgeons, 2004.
5. Potter HG: Imaging beyond conventional radiology. In Orthopaedic Knowledge Update 6. Rosemont, IL, American Academy of Orthopaedic Surgeons, 1999, pp 81–88.
6. Pring ME, Wenger DR, Rang MD (eds): Rang's Children's Fractures, 3rd ed. Philadelphia, Lippincott Williams & Wilkins, 2005.
7. Resnick D: Bone and Joint Imaging. Philadelphia, W.B. Saunders, 1989.
8. Schmidt AH, Kallas KM: Imaging considerations in orthopaedic trauma. In Beaty JH, Kasser JR (eds): Rockwood and Green's Fractures in Adults, 6th ed. Philadelphia, Lippincott Williams & Wilkins, 2006, pp 353–388.

CHAPTER 6

GAIT ANALYSIS

Lori A. Karol, MD

1. **What is a gait laboratory? Who works there?**

   A gait laboratory, more appropriately termed a *movement science laboratory*, is an area where movement can be objectively assessed. A typical gait lab includes motion picture cameras and infrared cameras linked to computerized tracking equipment. Reflective markers are taped to anatomic landmarks of the subject's body. The markers are tracked by special cameras that relay information about the location of the markers to a computer system. The data on the computer are then processed, resulting in the quantification of movement of the trunk and extremities, termed *kinematics*.

   Most movement science laboratories are staffed by engineers, kinesiologists, and physical therapists. An orthopaedic surgeon typically provides medical direction for a movement science laboratory. Some labs also employ computer programmers who develop special models for the measurement of body movement.

2. **Describe the typical gait cycle.**

   The gait cycle begins at foot contact, which in normal gait may be called *heel strike*. Stance phase accounts for 60% of the gait cycle and is divided into single-leg stance and two periods of double-leg stance, one at the beginning of stance before the opposite limb leaves the ground, and the other at the end of stance, when the opposite limb has finished the swing phase and has contacted the floor again. Swing phase is the period of time when the limb is off the floor, representing 40% of the normal gait cycle.

3. **What are cadence parameters?**

   Cadence parameters are time and distance data that can be measured in a gait analysis laboratory. Walking speed can be accurately measured and compared to data from normal age-matched individuals. Cadence is the number of steps taken per minute. Step length is the distance between the two feet during double-limb support and is measured from the heel of one foot to the heel of the contralateral foot. Stride length is the amount of distance, measured in meters, from one initial contact until the next initial contact of the same limb. Stride length is, therefore, the distance covered by a left plus a right step.

4. **What are kinematics?**

   Kinematics are the objective measurements of joint position and joint motion in three planes during gait. An example of kinematics is knee flexion and extension during walking. Kinematics are plotted on a graph versus time, with the delineation between stance and swing phase noted vertically on the graph.

5. **What are kinetics?**

   Kinetics are the study of the forces generated during gait. As a patient walks across a force plate embedded into the floor of a gait laboratory, forces are measured and combined with kinematic measurements to calculate ground reaction forces, joint moments, and powers.

   Moments are forces acting at a distance from the axis of rotation of a joint. An example of a moment is the varus/valgus moment at the knee, which can be quantified and is abnormal in patients with tibia vara. Joint powers are energy generated or absorbed during gait. An example of power generation is the burst of power at the ankle as the gastrosoleus fires concentrically and the foot pushes off the floor at the end of stance phase. An example of power absorption occurs at the hip at the transition from double-limb to single-limb stance, when the abductors fire eccentrically to limit pelvic drop and to prevent Trendelenburg gait.

6. **Can muscle function be assessed with gait analysis?**
   Dynamic electromyography (EMG) is frequently included during the assessment of the gait of a patient. Large superficial muscles can be monitored with surface electrodes taped to the skin, whereas smaller or deeper muscles such as the tibialis posterior require needle electrodes inserted into the muscle. The patient walks while wearing the electrodes, and the activity of a muscle during the gait cycle can be identified. Dynamic EMG can be collected simultaneously with kinematics so that the activity of a given muscle can be compared to the joint motion at a specific time. If a muscle is firing inappropriately during the gait cycle, transfer of the muscle may help improve the efficiency of gait.

7. **How can efficiency of gait be measured?**
   The easiest way to measure efficiency of gait is by assessing heart rate during walking. Patients with diminished walking speed and tachycardia are inefficient walkers. These patients have increased energy expenditure during gait. A precise method to assess energy expenditure is with an oxygen-consumption monitoring system. The patient is asked to wear a tightly sealed mask over his or her nose and mouth. This mask analyzes expired air. Oxygen consumption can then be calculated as the amount of oxygen required during walking per unit of time, and this can be compared to the patient's oxygen consumption during quiet sitting. Oxygen cost takes walking speed into account as it is the oxygen consumed per distance walked. Patients with abnormal gait have increased oxygen consumption and increased oxygen cost. Normal values exist for comparison of a patient's data.

8. **What is a pedobarograph?**
   A pedobarograph is a pressure-sensitive plate that is embedded into the floor of the movement science laboratory. It contains multiple sensors that measure the pressure exerted by segments of the foot during gait. A pedobarograph can identify areas of abnormally increased pressure and the line of progression of pressure through the foot during stance phase.

9. **What are the rockers?**
   Stance phase can be further subdivided into three segments. First rocker is the period of time immediately after initial contact, when the ankle plantar flexes gently and the foot comes to rest on the floor. Second rocker occurs during midstance and is characterized by progressive dorsiflexion of the ankle as the body moves forward over the plantigrade foot. Ankle plantar flexion leads to heel rise during third rocker, when the gastrosoleus fires and the ankle pushes the limb off the floor at the end of the stance phase.

10. **Can any patient be tested in a movement science laboratory?**
    Any patient of any age who can walk and is cooperative can be tested, but there are some limitations as to the type of information that can be obtained from different patient groups. Kinematic, EMG, and oxygen-consumption data can be collected from patients who use walkers and crutches, but kinetic information can only rarely be obtained because the assistive devices interfere with the force plates. Similarly, very small children cannot clear the force plate with their opposite feet.

11. **What are typical uses for gait analysis?**
    The most frequent use of gait analysis is in the preoperative assessment of children with cerebral palsy. Current surgical treatment of gait abnormalities in cerebral palsy consists of single-event multilevel surgery, known as SEMLS. This entails surgical lengthening, release, or

transfer of multiple muscles or tendons, often combined with osteotomies. Gait analysis is used in many of these patients to best identify which muscles require surgery and which gait abnormalities are compensatory and therefore can be spared, and also to assess the rotation of the limbs during gait.

KEY POINTS: GAIT ANALYSIS

1. Gait analysis is the study of joint motion, forces, muscular activity, energy expenditure, and plantar pressure during walking.

2. Kinematics describes joint position and movement in the sagittal, coronal, and transverse plane during the gait cycle.

3. Abnormal gait can result from spasticity, contractures, lower-extremity deformity, joint instability, or weakness, and it results in increased energy requirements during walking.

4. Gait analysis data are most frequently used in the preoperative assessment of children with cerebral palsy who are scheduled for single-event multilevel lower-extremity surgery.

12. **Can the decision to perform surgery be based solely on gait analysis data?**
No. Although gait data may help a surgeon confirm or fine-tune a surgical plan for the treatment of a child with cerebral palsy, it should not be used in isolation. The clinical examination of the child, the behavior and development status of the child, the rehabilitative capacity of the child, and the desired goals of the child and family are equally important in deciding what gait deviations are significant and what types of surgery may be helpful.

13. **Is gait analysis limited to neuromuscular patients?**
No. Many labs are actively testing other groups of patients, both for clinical purposes and for research. Gait analysis can be used to assess the design of orthoses and prostheses. Cadence parameters, kinematics, kinetics, and oxygen consumption can be measured as patients wear different braces so that the orthosis or prosthetic limb that allows the gait to be the fastest and most efficient, and also allows the most normal joint motion, can be used.
   Gait analysis is also used in sports labs to improve performance, in studies of geriatric patients to decrease potential for falling, and as an outcome measure for the treatment of orthopaedic conditions such as clubfoot, slipped capital femoral epiphysis, and limb deficiencies. Recently, it has been used in the assessment of upper-extremity motion for patients with upper-extremity contracture or weakness.

14. **Are gait data always reliable, or are there possible sources of error?**
No, they are not always reliable. Gait data are as objective as possible, but there are some limitations. First of all, it is assumed that patients walk with their usual gait during testing in the movement science laboratory. This is not always the case, however. Children may alter their gait either due to irritation from wearing the markers or from nervousness due to the unfamiliar testing environment and the multiple cameras. It is important to ask the parent if the child is walking in a manner similar to his or her gait at home.
   Secondly, accurate kinematic data rely on precise placement of the reflective markers over anatomic landmarks. It is difficult to place markers reproducibly on patients who are obese or who have severe contractures. Markers may fall off during testing of patients with fixed foot deformities or those with significant adduction contractures and scissoring of the lower extremities.

Finally, the most commonly used computer programs for processing kinematic and kinetic data assume normal skeletal anatomy. Routine kinematics are inaccurate for patients with significant orthopaedic abnormalities such as hip fusions, proximal femoral focal deficiency, or rotationplasties. More-advanced computer modeling has been used to assess joint motion in such patients.

BIBLIOGRAPHY

1. Davids JR, Ounpuu S, DeLuca PA, Davis RB: Optimization of walking ability of children with cerebral palsy. Instr Course Lect 53:511–522, 2004.

2. DeLuca PA, Davis RB, Ounpuu S, et al: Alterations in surgical decision making in patients with cerebral palsy based on three-dimensional gait analysis. J Pediatr Orthop 17:608–614, 1997.

3. Gage JR, De Luca PA, Renshaw TS: Gait analysis: Principles and applications with emphasis on its use in cerebral palsy. Instr Course Lect 45:491–507, 1996.

4. Wren TA, Rethlefsen S, Kay RM: Prevalence of specific gait abnormalities in children with cerebral palsy: Influence of cerebral palsy subtype, age and previous surgery. J Pediatr Orthop 25:79–83, 2005.

III. MANAGEMENT

PHILOSOPHY OF CARE

James G. Wright, MD, MPH, FRCSC

CHAPTER 7

1. **What factors go into a treatment decision?**
   - The treatment must be necessary. The condition being treated must have the potential to produce problems.
   - The treatment should be effective in altering the course of the disease.
   - The benefits of the treatment should exceed the risks and the negative psychologic effects.
   - The treatment chosen must be better than alternative treatments.

2. **What are the major responsibilities of the physician?**
   - Establish a correct diagnosis.
   - Explain your findings in understandable words to the parents and, if the child is old enough, to the patient as well.
   - Deliver care in a competent fashion.

3. **What must you know about the natural history?**
   Do not suggest active treatment if the natural history will allow spontaneous resolution.

4. **What are the main reasons that parents choose doctors?**
   - Good human relations: the doctor has explained enough, and the patient and the family have felt themselves to be the center of interest
   - Competence and good service

5. **Is there a risk of overtreatment?**
   Yes. Just because someone *could* have an operation does not mean they should, and just because someone *may* give them an operation does not mean they should.

6. **How do I avoid just "doing something"?**
   Relatives and friends can cause a parent to wonder whether a condition is normal and whether it needs treatment. It may be helpful to have photos or radiographs of similar cases, demonstrating that many conditions do well without "doing something."

7. **Give a common example of the risk-to-benefit ratio.**
   Radiographs taken of mobile flatfeet or asymptomatic spines that are clinically straight are a waste of money and bear the risk of radiation exposure.

8. **How do I instill confidence in the child's family?**
   First, accept the child as a partner. If the child is very unhappy in consultation, try to find a diversion before concentrating on your examination. A chat about a doll or a football team can break the ice.

   If you have pictures of similar cases ready (e.g., a lengthening procedure with an Ilizarov apparatus), this is helpful for the parents. If you know families who have gone through the same procedure, you might ask them to contact each other. Parent associations are also available for some conditions in some regions.

9. **What is the purpose of a diagnosis?**
   A diagnosis is intended to place a patient into a category that has prognostic significance for some future meaningful clinical outcome.

10. **What is the intent of treatment?**
    Treatment is intended to, on average, positively affect the patient's prognosis.

11. **What will treatment accomplish?**
    Treatment is intended to improve current symptoms, such as pain and disability, or to prevent future problems, such as the treatment of dislocated hips to prevent arthritis.

12. **In choosing a treatment, how do you balance wanting to achieve the best outcomes versus maximizing family and parental satisfaction?**
    The primary aim of the physician is to improve health. Once that is established and ensured, parental satisfaction should be addressed.

13. **What is patient satisfaction?**
    Patient satisfaction has two components:
    1. **Satisfaction with treatment:** Dependent primarily on the outcome of treatment
    2. **Satisfaction with care:** Dependent on the family's view of the doctor (e.g., how the doctor treats them) and the care setting and delivery (e.g., parking, food, and surroundings)

KEY POINTS: PHILOSOPHY OF CARE

1. Focus care on the family and their needs.

2. An accurate diagnosis provides a clear prognosis.

3. Discuss all treatment options, be honest about your uncertainty, and find the best treatment based on the best evidence.

4. If things do not go well, fully disclose and spend more time with the family.

14. **How do you deal with different cultures?**
    You need to be sensitive that different cultures have different rituals, different expectations, different modes of communication, and different family dynamics. Spending time talking with families is the best way to address these issues.

15. **What do you do if you make an error?**
    - Express your regret over the event.
    - Fully disclose the error to family.
    - Engage other team members to support the family.
    - Determine how to ensure that the error never occurs again.

16. **What is the most important thing you can do to prevent errors?**
    Communication among team members and with the family. Meet to talk about cases. Call your anesthetist about the case. Ensure that you are on a first-name basis with the whole team and that they feel valued and comfortable.

17. **What do you do if a complication occurs?**
    - Keep your focus on the reasons for doing the surgery.
    - Address the complication, but also try to preserve a successful surgical outcome.
    - Visit the family twice daily on the ward, and call them frequently.

18. What do you say if you are uncertain?
Tell patients that you are uncertain. Always be truthful.

BIBLIOGRAPHY

1. Rang M: Children's Fractures. Philadelphia, J.B. Lippincott, 1974, pp 67–68.
2. Staheli LT: Philosophy of care. Pediatr Clin North Am 33:1269–1275, 1986.

CHAPTER 8

THE PHYSICIAN–PARENT RELATIONSHIP

James G. Wright, MD, MPH, FRCSC

1. **What are the essential steps of a surgical consultation?**
   Although the best approach for assessing children will vary by physician, patient, and illness, the following elements must be included:
   - **Initial evaluation and presumptive diagnosis:** Includes a thorough history, physical exam, review of imaging and laboratory studies that are available, and a plan for any further consults or imaging and laboratory data needed
   - **Re-evaluation and treatment plan:** Includes a review of new data to confirm presumptive diagnosis and an outline of the treatment plan, with alternatives
   - **Presurgical evaluation:** Includes reviewing of previous discussion, answering questions, and obtaining informed consent

2. **How do you help child and parent decide about appropriate treatment?**
   The process of deciding on treatment is called *shared decision-making*. The essential elements are ensuring that families understand the risks and benefits of no treatment and the risks and benefits of all treatment options including surgery. The discussion may differ according to families' different styles of decision making; some want complete control, some want a shared decision, and others want physicians to make the decision.

3. **How should you handle a family with what seems like an endless series of questions?**
   Sit down, close the door, look relaxed. Take the time to ensure you have addressed all their concerns. Having spent that initial time, if subsequent visits are relatively brief, parents will trust that they have received sufficient attention; in the long-term, it actually saves you time.

4. **When should you see parents again after an initial evaluation for a serious disorder?**
   Arrangements should be made to have a follow-up discussion, preferably face-to-face, within 1–2 weeks of the initial evaluation for a serious problem. A telephone conversation should be used only when a direct discussion is not possible.

5. **When should you make specific recommendations for surgery?**
   In general, final decisions about surgery should not be made at the initial visit. The family and the patient should return at least one (if not two) additional time so that questions can be answered before surgery is scheduled. Often, the families feel rushed and believe that they have inadequate information to make a final decision after only one visit with the doctor. A copy of the consultation letter, including a discussion of treatment options and their risks and benefits, can be copied to the family.

6. **How do you handle parents and patients that live a long distance away when significant treatment is necessary or a problem arises?**
   It is best to see the patient back to discuss any issues directly. If this is not practical, speaking on the telephone with both parents on extensions or using a speaker phone is a possibility. Developing a relationship with the patient's primary care provider is important and may allow follow-up visits, radiographs, or minor treatments to be performed by him or her.

7. **Should you keep records of telephone calls?**

   All telephone calls concerning patient care must be documented, with a copy placed in the patient's chart. This prevents forgetting or misinterpreting what has been said.

8. **How do you speak to families with a language barrier?**

   The ideal situation is to use a formal translator who has a medical background. Err on the side of using a translation service because patients, parents, and guardians who know a little English may appear or claim to understand complex discussions even if they do not. Asking for them to repeat the important aspects of the discussion back to you will help to gauge how much they really know. Written material or drawings can be very helpful. Phone-based interpreters are also available for patient histories, informed consent, and other important discussions. Try to avoid using a child as a translator.

9. **During preoperative discussion, is patient satisfaction more reliant on discussion of technical issues or on the process of communication?**

   The way in which the surgeon communicates is more important in the decision-making process than the discussion of technical issues. Effective communication and a good relationship with parents or guardians and their child are excellent techniques to minimize the chance of legal action.

10. **Should you encourage parents or guardians to investigate their child's problem?**

    Yes, but you should encourage them to return with the information they have obtained so that you may help them to interpret it. This avoids confusion, especially with new information, such as that obtained from the Internet, that is not peer-reviewed and often is not well referenced. Other sources of information include talking to other families with the condition or who have had the surgery. Primary care physicians can also provide useful information and advice for families.

11. **What is the significance of both parents showing up?**

    Although it may take longer than usual to address the issues of both parents, hear out both parents. Some of your questions should be directed to each parent or guardian, as well as the child, to ensure no one dominates the conversation.

12. **How do you talk to a parent or guardian who arrives with the grandparents?**

    Speak to the mother and father as much as possible, even if the grandparent dominates the conversation. Much like both parents bringing the child to the clinic appointment, the attendance of the grandparents may signify a higher degree of familial concern.

13. **How do you talk with a grandparent who brings the child without the parent or guardian?**

    This can be a potentially hazardous situation. This is an excellent time to do a little extra listening and a little less talking so as not to interfere with the relationship you have with the parents. Dictating a letter to the parents to review the discussion that you had with the grandparent may also help decrease potential confusion.

14. **What situations can arise with divorced or separated parents?**

    Sometimes one parent thinks that the other parent is not taking good care of the child or has not received good medical advice. You need to get more than the usual amount of history in this situation. If possible, try to hear the other side by involving the other parent. The information in this situation may be very biased. Listen a great deal and be careful about specific recommendations. Try not to take sides or make judgments. It is very important that legal custody of the child is verified prior to initiation of any treatment.

15. **How do you handle a parent who is hypercritical of treatment by other physicians?**

    Obtain a careful history and the exact names of the physicians who have treated the child. Offer to call the other physician directly to see what treatment has been done or offered. Although honesty is the best policy, unless asked, avoid direct comments on care delivered by other care providers. Although flattering to think that the family wants to see you, you can very easily be added to the list of physicians who have displeased the parents.

16. **What should you do if parents or guardians seem uncertain about treatment decisions?**

    Provide time for families to deliberate. Suggest talking to their primary care doctor or to other families who have had surgery. Liberally offer the option of a second opinion. Discuss second opinions openly with them and offer to make your notes and x-rays available. If second opinions are not discussed and the second opinion is different from yours, the family will be reluctant to come back and discuss the situation with you. If you have already brought up the subject, they will feel more comfortable returning to you. Emphasize to the family that your goal is that their child receive the best treatment. Ultimately, it is their decision of which treatment and surgeon they choose.

17. **What should you do if parents or guardians are angry or agitated?**

    Close the door. Sit down. Appear relaxed. Let them address all their issues in a nonrushed fashion. If they leave agitated, call them that evening or no later than the next day. Try to determine what the issues are, and document the conversation. Showing your concern and interest is probably the best thing that you can offer them at such a time.

18. **Should you review the radiographs with the parents or guardians?**

    Yes, in all instances, the radiographs should be shown to the family and explained. Others can easily obtain radiographs for review, so it is better for you to explain the details that the family needs to see and understand. If you do not show them the x-rays, they are sometimes concerned that there is a major problem that you do not want them to see.

19. **Are children fearful of physicians who wear white coats?**

    No. Fifty-four percent of children actually prefer physicians who wear white coats. Parents were poor predictors of what their children would prefer.

20. **How do you examine a fearful child?**

    Do not look directly at the child. Sit or crouch down to look less imposing. Talk constantly to the parents without changing your focus to the child. Examine the child on the parents' lap. Start distally at the feet by laying your hands on the child, even if the area of interest is more proximal. Lean your body away from the child. For some things, such as range of motion, a parent can do that while you stand across the room. Often, a better exam of a young child can be obtained while the child is being held by the parents.

KEY POINTS: THE PHYSICIAN-PARENT RELATIONSHIP

1. A family needs time to develop a complete understanding of their child's condition and the plans and outcomes of treatment.

2. You need to develop appropriate relationships with all members of the family, particularly the child.

3. Extra time spent with the family early on improves the relationship with the family and saves your time in the long run.

21. **If an older child (such as a teenager) signs the consent, does the parent or guardian also need to sign?**

The consent laws vary by jurisdiction. Some areas have no age of consent and rely only on documenting competency. In any case, an explanation should be provided for children old enough to understand. In jurisdictions where there is an age of consent, the child may sign the consent form (referred to as an assent), but the parent or guardian must also sign.

22. **Are parents solely responsible for the decision to treat their impaired infants?**
No. The "Baby Doe rules" passed during the Reagan administration mandated treating impaired newborns unless they are permanently comatose, treatment would prolong death, or treatment would not be effective.

23. **Are physicians required to report suspected child abuse or neglect?**
Yes. This is true in all 50 states and Canada. If abuse or neglect is suspected, contact the child abuse team and admit the child to hospital until the issue is resolved.

24. **How common is child abuse?**
Child abuse is common and may be fatal.

25. **Is the father the most common perpetrator of child abuse?**
No. Both the mother and father account for the abuse in 21% (each) of the cases. Other common perpetrators include the boyfriend of the mother (9%), the babysitter (8%), and the stepfather (5%).

26. **What is Munchausen syndrome by proxy?**
A deceptive action is taken toward a child (such as intentional poisoning) to simulate a medical disorder. Mortality is 10%.

27. **What do you do when children become adults?**
At some age, children become adults and should be referred to an adult facility and an adult surgeon. Families need to be told well in advance, and appropriate transfer of care and relevant health information needs to occur.

28. **How do you respond to email requests for information?**
If emails request comments or recommendations on care from patients unknown to you, politely decline to comment and provide information on how they can obtain appropriate treatment. For information requests from your own patients, be careful not to compromise your clinical care when you really need to talk to and examine patients in person. In addition, you must inform families that emails are not confidential and they accept that risk in emailing you.

29. **What happens if patients miss reappointments?**
You must make reasonable attempts to contact them to ensure they have appropriate care (because sometimes families forget or do not understand the need to return).

BIBLIOGRAPHY

1. Barrett TG, Booth IW: Sartorial eloquence: Does it exist in the pediatrician-patient relationship? Br Med J 309:1710–1712, 1994.

2. Bradbury E: Psychological issues for children and their parents. In Buck-Gramcko D (ed): Congenital Malformations of the Hand and Forearm. London, Churchill Livingstone, 1998, pp 49–56.

3. Deber RB, Kraetschmer N, Irvine J: What role do patients wish to play in treatment decision making? Arch Intern Med 156:1414–1420, 1996.

4. Dobyns JH: Helping parents to decide what is best for their child. Hand Clin 6:551–554, 1990.

5. Fell JME, Rylance GW: Parental permission, information and consent. Arch Dis Child 66:980–981, 1991.

6. Hickson GB, Federspiel CF, Pichert JW, et al: Patient complaints and malpractice risk. JAMA 287:2951–2957, 2002.

7. Johnson CF: Abuse and neglect of children. In Behrman RE, Kliegman R, Jenson HB (eds): Nelson Textbook of Pediatrics, 16th ed. Philadelphia, W.B. Saunders, 2000, p 111.

8. McCarthy JJ, McCarthy MC, Eilert RE: Children's and parents visual perception of physicians. Clin Pediatr 38:145–152, 1999.

9. Morrow J: Making moral decisions at the beginning of life: The case of impaired and imperiled infants. JAMA 284:1146–1147, 2000.

10. Stanford TC: Medical Malpractice. A Primer for Orthopaedic Residents and Fellows. Rosemont, IL, American Academy of Orthopaedic Surgeons, 1993, pp 25–30.

11. Weinstein JN: The missing piece: Embracing shared decision making to reform health care. Spine 25:1–4, 2000.

INTEGRATING THE CHILD WITH A DISABILITY INTO SOCIETY

Mary Williams Clark, MD

CHAPTER 9

1. Why is this chapter necessary?

Without some help from medical professionals, many children with disabilities will not achieve their maximum potential for participation in society.

2. What are the everyday issues facing the young person with a significant physical difference?

Communication, mobility, and independence in self-care (i.e., activities of daily living [ADLs], such as getting in and out of bed, dressing, hygiene, and eating), as well as a lack of role models; the lack of self-esteem; and the lack of access to buildings, public and private transportation, educational and vocational opportunities, and recreation. It is important to ask patients and their families about the above activities and to note any problems or concerns.

3. Who can help with communication?

Evaluation and recommendation of appropriate communication devices are usually arranged through speech and language specialists, with the help of occupational therapists and, sometimes, rehabilitation engineers. They may be part of the rehabilitation team in the school or in the medical or rehabilitation center; most of these centers have outpatient programs to which you can refer your patient. If your patients are having problems getting help, start with the closest department of speech pathology.

4. Who can help with mobility aids?

Crutches and walkers are most easily obtained from durable medical equipment (DME) vendors. All equipment is ordered by prescription—usually by an orthopaedist or physiatrist, but they may need to receive an approval (or referral to "evaluate and treat") from the patient's primary care physician. Therapists fit and train in use of the equipment.

Braces (i.e., orthoses) are necessary for many young people with disabilities. They almost always need to be custom-made by orthotists or therapists and rechecked for fit and any skin reactions. Therapists should teach function with the braces, including proper donning and doffing, using steps and ramps, and getting up and down from chairs and the floor, where appropriate.

Wheelchairs and cushions need to be ordered with the particular patient's size, ability to push, type of transfers, necessary height, and so on in mind. Therapists and DME vendors can help you and the patient select appropriate options.

For complex needs, adaptive seating specialists are available, usually at medical or rehabilitation centers. These specialists also offer evaluation for power chairs, scooters, and custom supportive seating. Power chairs are now lighter, quieter, and easier to maneuver than before, and the controls are programmable.

5. Who can help with ADLs?

Occupational and physical therapists, speech and language pathologists, and rehabilitation nurses. Children need tune-ups as they reach different ages and stages. Some children with significant disabilities will need ongoing therapy for ADL function and mobility as outpatients;

this therapy is usually available in the community. Therapists are also available through school systems for monitoring education-related functions (e.g., mobility, communication, and bathroom use), but it is unusual to accomplish actual training in the school setting as most school districts have a limited number of therapists.

6. **Who can help with education?**
Special education teachers and psychologists can evaluate children with intelligence quotient (IQ) testing (appropriately modified if necessary) to diagnose learning disabilities and to determine other aspects of appropriate school placement. Early intervention is available in all states, usually up to age 3 and usually with in-home services; the name for these services varies from state to state. Early intervention units and developmental clinics can be found through pediatricians.

Physical accessibility is legally mandated for all publicly funded schools but may not have actually been instituted (see below). Parents have the right to be present and to have input into individual education programs (IEPs) if their child is eligible for special education.

U.S. Public Law 94–142 was enacted in 1975 and became effective in late 1977. It was the first U.S. federal law to mandate appropriate education in "the least restrictive environment" for all children with disabilities. In 1986, P.L. 99–457 mandated early intervention services for infants and children under 3 years of age. P.L. 101–476 further updated and specified the provisions of P.L. 94–142 and is titled the "Individuals with Disabilities Education Act" (IDEA). (*See* Question 12 and the websites at end of this chapter regarding P.L. 101–336, the Americans with Disabilities Act.)

These laws are still necessary and important: many obstacles exist, and openness to students with differences varies among school districts, often relating directly to the principal's attitude.

7. **Are there any specific school-related problems?**
   - **Inappropriate placement:** A child may be placed in a setting that is too restrictive for her or his intellectual or physical capabilities or mainstreamed into a situation beyond his or her capabilities.
   - **Inappropriate "solutions":** These may include football players carrying a student up and down the stairs instead of using an elevator, or reorganization of room and floor class assignments.
   - **Inappropriate fears:** These may include not allowing children to go out for recess with their classmates, to climb gyms or swings, or to try out for a sport.
   - **Inappropriate rewards:** A's "because she works so hard" or "it's hard for him" do not help prepare the child for the real world.

8. **How do families access special services through the schools?**
Through primary or specialist physician referral. Or families themselves can contact special education services and request evaluation of their child for special services. The exact mechanisms vary from state to state and among school districts.

9. **What about role models and self-esteem? They don't teach that in medical school!**
You can help self-esteem every day that you see children in your office by saying hello to them by name and by talking directly to them, as well as to their parents or caregivers. Ask them about their situations, even if they can just give you a yes or no, verbally or otherwise. For role models, see the response to Question 10—observing or (even better) being involved in sports and other community programs can provide role models.

10. **Who can help with social and recreational opportunities?**

Social opportunities arise for children and teenagers with physical differences in the usual ways—for example, neighborhoods, schools, and places of worship—but are also facilitated by *access* (*see* Question 12) as well as attitude. As Clark has observed, if physicians and their colleagues encourage the parents of these children, early in their lives, "to see her as capable, emphasize all the things he can do...to consider them normal children who happen to have their differences, that is the picture of themselves they will grow up with...and they will develop the self-esteem and self-confidence they need."

Service or assistance animals are available and trained to assist in many ways that significantly improve independence for people, including children, with many different impairments. Although they are working animals and not pets, they also provide chances for social interaction and normalization for those for whom they work.

Therapeutic recreation specialists, or recreation therapists, and adapted physical educators know community resources. These may range from camping to wheelchair basketball to adaptive winter sports. Both informal recreational and competitive sports opportunities are available in most areas of the country (*see* website suggestions at the end of this chapter).

Camp experiences also offer activities, fun, and many opportunities for interaction with others. They can also provide opportunities for camp counselor jobs. There are increasing numbers of camps with experiences for those with differences, including international opportunities (*see* the list of websites at end of this chapter).

Clark MW: Things To Remember: For Families of Children with Congenital or Early-Acquired Amputations. Available at *http://amp-info.net/i-canart.htm#clark*; originally published in *In Motion*, the official magazine of the Amputee Coalition of America. Quoted material used with permission.

11. **Who can help with vocational rehabilitation?**

All U.S. states have an Office or Division of Vocational Rehabilitation (OVR or DVR). Counselors are available to evaluate and help patients aged 16 and older. There are also many independent living units and organizations, and they may have more help available than some OVRs, which may be overworked and understaffed.

12. **What is the Americans with Disabilities Act (ADA)?**

The ADA (U.S. P.L. 101–336) is a complex law that was enacted in 1990. It has five titles, or sections, as follows. Title I covers employment, prohibiting discrimination in terms or conditions of employment for qualified disabled individuals. Title II covers public service and requires that services offered by public entities (including public transportation) be available and accessible to everyone. Title III covers public accommodation or "goods, services, privileges, benefits, and accommodations offered to the general public." Any new construction open to the public occupied after January 26, 1993 must be accessible. Titles IV and V address telecommunication and miscellaneous provisions, respectively.

The 2006 ADA Internet home page (*see* the list of websites at the end of chapter) now offers a free CD-ROM related to technical assistance.

As of August 11, 2005, the U.S. Department of Justice completed agreements (for situations not compliant with the ADA standards) in 128 localities, in all 50 states, the District of Columbia, and Puerto Rico. The online map of the United States showing these localities demonstrates how few areas have specifically corrected problems and how much more room there is to continue improvements. Two strategies that will help include:

- **Quoting the ADA** to individual business owners, local government officials, school boards, and so forth
- **Advocating for and with** those who need better access wherever you see a need

KEY POINTS: INTEGRATING THE CHILD WITH DISABILITY INTO SOCIETY

1. Without some help from medical professionals, many children with disabilities will not achieve their maximum potential for participation in society.

2. It is important to ask patients and their families about communication, mobility, and independence in self-care, as well as issues of lack of role models, lack of self-esteem, and lack of access to buildings, public and private transportation, educational and vocational opportunities, and recreation.

3. Do not define people by their impairments.

4. Special education teachers and psychologists can evaluate children with intelligence quotient (IQ) testing (appropriately modified if necessary) to diagnose learning disabilities and to determine other aspects of appropriate school placement.

13. **Define impairment, disability, and handicapped.**
In 1980, the World Health Organization (WHO) published the International Classification of Impairments, Disabilities, and Handicaps, in which they defined these terms. *Impairment* is "any loss or abnormality of psychological, physiologic, or anatomic structure or function." *Disability* is "any restriction or lack of ability [resulting from an impairment] to perform an activity in the manner or within the range considered normal for a human being." Under federal law in the United States, an individual is *handicapped* if he or she "has an impairment that substantially limits one or more of life's activities," and the 1993 American Medical Association (AMA) Guide to the Evaluation of Permanent Impairment states that "an impaired individual who is able to accomplish a specific task with or without accommodation is *neither* handicapped nor disabled with regard to that task" [emphasis added].

14. **How can I avoid saying things that will offend people who have differences?**
People who have physical differences vary in opinion about the use of the words *handicapped*, *disabled*, and *impaired*. Some of them think that some or even all of these words are insulting or demeaning and would prefer more neutral terms such as *a difference*. The WHO and AMA guidelines are very useful for written communication, but they are not much help for spoken language.
The first rule is to think of and mention the person *as a person first*, and then, *if* necessary and relevant, her or his condition: they are people who happen to have a certain condition, for example, "a young woman with cerebral palsy" or "a young man who uses a wheelchair." (Never say "wheelchair-bound." In reality, people who use wheelchairs move, or are moved, in and out of them; they use them like one uses a car.) *Do not define people by their impairment.*
The United Cerebral Palsy Association points out that "People with cerebral palsy and other disabilities have the same rights as everyone else in this world—the right to fall in love, to marry, to hold down a competitive job, to acquire an adequate and appropriate education. Above all, they have a right to self-esteem. Please insure these rights by referring to people with disabilities in terms that acknowledge ability, merit, dignity."

WEBSITES

1. **www.ada.gov:** Americans with Disabilities Act (P.L. 101–336); ADA information line: toll-free phone, 800-514-0301; TDD, 800-514-0383.

2. **www.usdoj.gov/crt/ada/publications.htm:** ADA publications, available free from the U.S. Department of Justice; also available from the ADA information line listed above.

3. **www.ada.gov/aprjun05.htm#Anchor-49575:** ADA site including information about mediation services and reports of actual cases resolved by mediation without filing a lawsuit.

4. **www.ncd.gov/resources.htm:** National Council on Disability and Resources, with links to state agencies.

5. **www.evolt.org/article/Accessibility_Laws_In_Canada/4090/28074/index.html:** All Canadian provinces have a human rights commission, with links from this site to the provincial details.

   For children and young adults and their caregivers: Information and support, including groups, and listservs:

6. **www.amp-info.net:** Connects to I-CAN, a listserv for families of children with limb loss or absence; also provides online mentors and access to other families to respond to questions and concerns from new families.

7. **www.amputee-coalition.org:** Amputee Coalition of America. See also *In Motion,* their monthly magazine; *First Step,* published for new amputees, in its 4th edition in 2005; *Expectations,* in its 1st edition in 2004, designed specifically for amputee children (congenital or acquired) and their families; and their sponsored online magazine, *Youth Amputee E-Zine.*

8. **www.arthritis.org:** Arthritis Foundation; includes information about diagnosis, treatment, and activities for children with arthritis.

9. **www.avenuesforamc.com:** *Avenues,* a newsletter about arthrogryposis multiplex congenita.

10. **www.biausa.org/children.htm:** Brain injury.

11. **www.dsusa.org:** Disabled Sports USA; includes information about the Paralympics and regional sport organizations.

12. **www.easterseals.com/site/PageServer:** For children with any disabilities; includes information about activities and camps.

13. **www.eparent.com:** *Exceptional Parent* magazine; for all children's disabilities and special healthcare needs.

14. **www.makoa.org/travel.htm#camps:** Information for travel with children with differences; includes many countries.

15. **www.mdausa.org:** Muscular Dystrophy Association; information and clinics for children and young adults with the many forms of muscular dystrophies.

16. **www.mysummercamps.com/camps/Special_Needs_Camps:** Lists 24 subcategories of special needs; links to global camp options (nb: the capitalized letters in the URL are necessary).

17. **www.nichcy.org:** National Dissemination Center for Children with Disabilities; information about many children's diseases and disabilities, including discussions about assistive technology for education.

18. **www.nscd.org:** National Sports Center for the Disabled.

19. **www.oif.org:** Osteogenesis Imperfecta Foundation.

20. **www.sbaa.org:** Spina Bifida Association of America.

21. **sdog.danawheels.net:** Assistance and service dogs.

22. **www.spinalcordinjury.org/kids.htm:** For children with spinal cord injury (last modified in 2001).

23. **www.tbi.org:** For traumatic brain injury survivors.

24. **www.ucpa.org:** United Cerebral Palsy Association; has up-to-date information about state support for Medicaid and other opportunities.

25. **www.umabroad.umn.edu/access/specific sites/index.shtml:** Accessibility for students at overseas sites, published by the University of Minnesota.

ANESTHESIA

Inge Falk van Rooyen, MBChB, FRCA

CHAPTER 10

1. **How long should the nothing-by-mouth (NPO) period last?**
   - **Formula:** 6 hours prior to surgery
   - **Breast milk:** 4 hours prior to surgery
   - **Clear fluids or juice (no pulp):** 2 hours prior to surgery

   Chewing gum, sucking candy, or one bite of a cookie are all frequently treated as a full meal. Surgery will be postponed to accommodate a 6-hour NPO period to allow full gastric emptying. Gastric physiologic reflexes stimulate secretion of gastric acid during mastication of any substance in the mouth.

2. **Why is surgery canceled or delayed if the NPO period is not adhered to?**
   Aspiration of gastric contents is possible. This creates the risk for aspiration pneumonia, which may be fatal, depending on the volume aspirated or the hydrogen ion concentration (pH) of the gastric content. Normal gastric emptying occurs, for a combination of protein, carbohydrate, and fat, within a period of 6 hours. During periods of physiologic stress (i.e., pain), gastric emptying is usually delayed. Special anesthesia techniques have to be employed for emergency surgery to minimize this risk as much as possible.

3. **What is informed consent?**
   This is the information discussed with the parents, patient, or both, in terms that the family understands. It details the preoperative medications, anesthesia risks, plan, and postoperative pain management. Consent has to be given by the legal guardian. Legal advice should be sought during special guardianship issues. These should be documented and available to the staff who will treat the patient prior to anesthesia and surgery.

4. **What is the physical status classification of the American Society of Anesthesiologists (ASA)?**
   - **Class 1:** Healthy patient; no medical problems
   - **Class 2:** Mild systemic disease
   - **Class 3:** Severe systemic disease, but not incapacitated
   - **Class 4:** Severe systemic disease that is a constant threat to life
   - **Class 5:** Moribund; not expected to live 24 hours, irrespective of operation
   - **Class 6:** Organ donor

   An "E" is added to the status number to indicate that the procedure is done as an emergency case, rather than an elective operation.

5. **What are the main anesthesia risks for a patient undergoing surgery?**
   - Aspiration of gastric content
   - Allergic reaction to inhalation agent or any pharmacologic agents used intraoperatively (Malignant hyperthermia is a rare inherited disorder of muscle metabolism and has to be ruled out prior to giving an inhalation anesthetic.)
   - A physiologically detrimental interaction of a disease that the patient suffers from with concomitant cardiac, respiratory, and central nervous system (CNS) depression, related to

the anesthesia (Renal function, glucose metabolism, and temperature regulation are additional important factors that need vigilant attention as this may lead to cardiac arrest.)
- Recent changes to the patient's health that make him or her vulnerable to laryngospasm and bronchospasm (This generally refers to recent upper-airway respiratory tract infections.)
- Nausea and vomiting
- In cases in which a patient may be difficult to intubate, chipped teeth, and minor lip lacerations
- Temporary neuropraxia related to difficulty in patient positioning, prolonged surgery, or the inability to fully protect areas, leaving superficial nerves vulnerable to prolonged pressure
- Blindness, a rare complication associated with prolonged spinal surgeries in the prone position

The overall objective or the preoperative evaluation by the anesthesiologist is to reduce perioperative morbidity and mortality of the above factors.

6. **Why are anesthesiologists concerned about colds in children before surgery?**
Upper respiratory infections (URIs) are the most common illnesses affecting children younger than 5 years of age. (Reported incidence of URI is 24% in this age group.) Children younger than 1 year of age have an average of 6.1 respiratory illnesses per year. Children between 1 and 5 years old have an average of 4.7–5.7 respiratory illnesses per year. In children with a URI, there is an increased incidence of the following problems during and after surgery:
- **Laryngospasm** during induction of and emergence from anesthesia
- **Bronchospasm,** because viral URI will initiate wheezing more commonly in children than in adults, whether or not they have a history of asthma (Children younger than 5 years old with preexisting asthma or with respiratory syncytial virus are more prone to developing bronchospasm.)
- **Coughing** due to increased airway secretion and hyperreactivity (Coughing can infrequently cause silent regurgitation and aspiration.)
- **Reduction in oxygen saturation** intra- and postoperatively owing to the above mentioned factors, and also owing to lung atelectasis and reduction of functional residual capacity (FRC)

7. **Should routine surgery be canceled in all cases of runny nose?**
No. When possible, communication directly with an anesthesiologist will help to confirm cancellation of the surgery. The risks and benefits of each surgical procedure will be considered carefully in each case. Also, not every runny nose is due to a URI; it can be due to allergic rhinitis. Inquire if the child has allergies or if there is a family history of allergy.

8. **How can I diagnose a URI?**
In general, two of the following criteria must exist:
- Sore or scratchy throat
- Sneezing
- Rhinitis
- Fever (mild)
- Congestion
- Malaise
- Nonproductive cough
- Laryngitis

Sneezing and runny nose do not necessarily indicate a URI, however. If in doubt, ask the mother if she feels that the patient has a URI.

9. **Bottom line: In which groups of children with a URI should routine surgery definitely be canceled?**
- Patients younger than 1 year of age
- Patients with lower respiratory infection
- Those with signs of overt viremia or bacteremia

- Patients awaiting operations of long duration that necessitate insertion of an endotracheal tube (ET) (because of increased incidence of intraoperative bronchospasm and postextubation croup)
- Operations that involve surgery to the trachea in which prolonged coughing will rupture the sutures

10. **How long must I wait before performing surgery on patients with a suspected respiratory tract infection?**
- **Upper respiratory infection:** 1–2 weeks after cessation of symptoms
- **Lower respiratory infection:** At least 4–6 weeks after cessation of symptoms

11. **How is perioperative fluid managed in children?**
There are two types of fluids the body requires: maintenance and replacement. A balanced salt solution (BSS) such as lactated Ringer's or Plasma-Lyte is commonly used for fluid maintenance. The amount of fluid can be estimated using simple formulas.

12. **How is fluid requirement calculated?**
- 4 mL/kg/hr for the first 10 kg of body weight
- 2 mL/kg/hr for the next 10 kg
- 1 mL/kg/hr for any weight of more than 20 kg (i.e., a 30-kg child will receive 70 mL/hr)
This allows a good estimation of maintenance fluids. The same formulas are used to determine the volume of fluid required to cover the NPO period (i.e., replacement fluids). Blood lost is best replaced by blood products in children under 2 years of age undergoing *major* surgery.

13. **What is the estimated blood volume (EBV) in children?**
See Table 10-1.

TABLE 10-1. ESTIMATED BLOOD VOLUME (EBV) BY AGE	
Age	EBV (mL/kg)
Neonate (preterm)	100
Neonate (term)	90
Infant up to 1 year of age	80
Child 1 year or older	70

14. **What criteria are used to assess the need for blood transfusion in children?**
Healthy children can compensate for acute volume loss of 25–30% before any changes in blood pressure are observed. This fact may result in inadequate and untimely blood transfusion. The most reliable early signs of hypovolemic shock in children are persistent tachycardia, poor capillary refill time (i.e., 2 seconds), and diminished pulse pressure.

Intraoperatively, one may allow the hematocrit to drop to between 21% and 25% before starting blood transfusion. However, blood has to be immediately available. If the patient is hemodynamically unstable despite what seems to be adequate hydration, blood transfusion should be started at the beginning of the procedure, or earlier.

Patients with high thoracic spinal pathology, such as meningomyelocele, may require blood transfusion much earlier than other patient populations. In this group of patients, all efforts must be made to not challenge the cardiovascular system. Poor control of the autonomic nervous system in this group of patients increases the risk of life-threatening hemodynamic instability.

Postoperatively, if the patient does not exhibit clinical signs of anemia (such as postural hypotension and dizziness), the hematocrit level can be allowed to drop to 18–20%.

15. How does one identify a patient at risk for bleeding?
One has to take an accurate medical history. This identifies current medications taken (e.g., anticoagulants, nonsteroidal anti-inflammatory agents, and aspirin), excessive unexplained previous intraoperative blood loss, and medical conditions associated with bleeding disorders.

16. How helpful are clotting function screening tests?
Asymptomatic patients are missed. Moreover, abnormal clotting function tests and prolonged bleeding times are not always associated with clinical hemorrhage. Common tests include the following:

1. Measurement of the intrinsic and common clotting pathways
   - **Partial thromboplastin time (PTT):** Normal range is 40–100 seconds.
   - **Activated PTT (APTT):** Produces more consistent results than PTT; normal range is 25–35 seconds.
   - **Activated clotting time (ACT):** Normal range is 90–120 seconds; frequently used intraoperatively to measure heparin therapy.
2. Measurement of the extrinsic and common pathways
   - **Prothrombin time (PT):** Normal range is 10–12 seconds.
   - **International normalized ration (INR):** Used to improve the consistency of oral anticoagulant therapy; standard dose is 2.0–3.0; high dose is 2.5–3.5.

Patients undergoing major surgery that requires massive blood transfusion need ongoing monitoring of their coagulation status. Patient-specific blood products are required (e.g., whole blood, fresh frozen plasma, cryoprecipitate, or specific factors) to treat coagulopathies that prevent surgical hemostasis.

17. What are the different types of myopathies?
Myopathies (i.e., primary diseases of muscle fibers) are divided into three groups, according to muscle biopsy examination:

- Segmental necrosis of muscle fibers (e.g., muscular dystrophies such as Duchenne's muscular dystrophy [DMD] or Becker's muscular dystrophy)
- Structural defects of muscle fibers (e.g., myotonic dystrophy or congenital myopathies)
- Disorders of conduction function within muscle fibers or at the neuromuscular junction (e.g., myasthenia gravis)

18. What are the coexisting organ system dysfunctions in these groups of patients?
Cardiac abnormalities
- Electrocardiogram (ECG) abnormalities are seen in 90% of patients, as demonstrated by a progressive decrease in R-wave amplitude.
- Mitral valve prolapse and regurgitation have been documented in 20% of affected individuals and are due to papillary muscle dysfunction.

Cardiomyopathy
- Usually confined to the wall of the left ventricle, cardiomyopathy is responsible for the high incidence of cardiac arrhythmias.
- Ultimately, profound right ventricular dysfunction is also possible, leading to congestive cardiac failure.
- Cardiomyopathy is more common in Duchenne's muscular dystrophy.

Cardiac conductive system abnormality
- More often seen in myotonic dystrophy, this results in dysrhythmias and atrioventricular block.

- The severity of cardiac lesions may not correlate with duration or severity of skeletal muscle disease. Also, restricted activity may mask compromised unstressed cardiac function.

Restrictive respiratory disease

- This is seen due to degeneration of inspiratory, expiratory, and diaphragmatic muscle fibers.
- Patients are more prone to aspiration of secretions owing to ineffective and weak cough and, hence, are more prone to pneumonia.

19. **What preoperative investigations are necessary in patients with myopathy?**
    - **ECG**
    - **Echocardiography and radionuclide studies:** Indispensable in elucidating anatomic abnormalities (e.g., left ventricular wall thickness or mitral valve prolapse)
    - **Chest x-ray:** To detect cardiomegaly, diaphragmatic elevation, and pulmonary disease (e.g., infiltrates and mediastinal shifts secondary to scoliosis)
    - **Pulmonary function testing:** Greatest reduction occurs in vital capacity (The reduction of vital capacity to 30–40% of the predicted normal usually indicates the need for postoperative ventilatory support.)

20. **What are the anesthetic risks associated with these groups of patients?**
    - **Malignant hyperthermia (MH) syndrome:** This is an inherited myopathy characterized by a hypermetabolic state upon exposure to triggering agents. If untreated, it leads to death. Patients with myopathy (especially DMD) are susceptible to MH; this could be due to shared skeletal muscle disease or gene aberration. (Triggering agents include all potent inhalational agents and succinylcholine.)
    - **Cardiac rhythm disturbance**
    - **Postoperative ventilatory failure**

21. **Why are anesthesiologists concerned about cervical spine disease and trauma?**
    - Cervical spine abnormality may result in permanent neurologic damage during positioning of the patient's head during endotracheal intubation.
    - Airway management or intubation may be made more difficult when the cervical spine is fused due to disease or previous surgery.

22. **What do anesthesiologists seek during preoperative evaluation of the cervical spine?**
    Cervical spine stability. If the cervical spine is unstable, movement (e.g., mask ventilation or intubation) may result in loss of normal alignment of the vertebrae, compression of the cord, and possibly permanent neurologic injury. The most common patients at risk are:
    - Trauma victims
    - Patients with Down syndrome

23. **What radiologic examinations are important?**
    This depends in part on the disease process:
    - Patients with congenital diseases and those with chronically acquired disease (e.g., rheumatoid arthritis) require lateral spine films in neutral position with flexion and extension views.
    - The acute trauma patient should have lateral, anteroposterior, and odontoid views in neutral position. If findings are equivocal, then a computed tomography (CT) scan or magnetic resonance imaging (MRI) may be necessary.
    - In preschool children, plain radiographs of the spine are difficult to interpret because of incomplete ossification of the spine. Hence, a CT scan is the first-line investigation in this age group.

24. **What is the best way to manage the airway in patients with cervical spine instability?**
There is not one good method. There are many different approaches for intubation of the trachea. All have significant advantages and disadvantages. Whatever technique of intubation is used, the goal should be to eliminate neck and head movement during intubation and subsequent positioning. Flexion and extension have to be avoided.

25. **What methods are used to immobilize the neck during intubation?**
   - Manual in-line stabilization, preferably by a neurosurgeon or an orthopaedic surgeon
   - Halo traction or vest
   - Cervical collars, which are least effective (they do not prevent neck movement during intubation) and must not be relied on during intubation

26. **What conditions are associated with cervical spine abnormality?**
Congenital
   - **Down syndrome:** 20% incidence of atlanto-occipital instability
   - **Goldenhar's syndrome:** Craniovertebral abnormalities; may limit head extension
   - **Klippel-Feil syndrome:** Fused cervical vertebrae and spinal cord compression
   - **Achondroplasia:** Decreased head extension caused by abnormalities at the atlanto-occipital joint and the upper cervical spine such as scoliosis, neurofibromatosis, and spondyloepiphyseal dysplasia
   - **Mucopolysaccharidoses:** Morquio's, Hurler's, Hunter's, Scheie's, and Sanfilippo's syndromes

Acquired
   - Rheumatoid arthritis
   - Ankylosing spondylitis
   - Still's disease
   - Psoriatic arthritis
   - Reiter syndrome
   - Trauma

27. **What is acute pain?**
Acute pain refers to pain of short duration (usually 3–7 days) and is usually associated with surgery, trauma, or an acute illness.

28. **Why should we as physicians strive for good management of acute pain?**
Effective pain management has been shown to improve mortality and morbidity rates and immune function. Pain is a form of stress and causes release of stress hormones, which cause catabolism and impaired tissue healing. The value of preemptive analgesia in certain conditions is well known. For example, patients who undergo amputation under a regional block have a decreased incidence of phantom pain.

29. **Why has acute pain in children been undertreated?**
   - Lack of ability to assess pain in nonverbal children
   - Our fear of respiratory depression and use of narcotic analgesia
   - The wrong assumption that the pain pathways are not developed in babies, and, therefore, babies do not feel pain

30. **How is acute pain assessed in children?**
Age-appropriate pain assessment is essential. Both subjective and objective assessment tools may be utilized, depending on patient age and clinical status. Ideally, pain assessment tools must be introduced before surgery or before the occurrence of pain. In our institution (the Texas Scottish Rite Hospital for Children), we use the Visual Analog Scale (VAS; Fig. 10-1)

for patients older than 7 years and the Objective Pain Scale (Table 10-2) for younger children and older noncommunicative children (e.g., children with cerebral palsy).

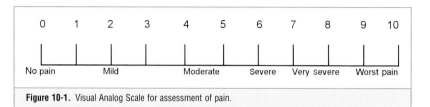

0	1	2	3	4	5	6	7	8	9	10
No pain		Mild		Moderate		Severe	Very severe		Worst pain	

Figure 10-1. Visual Analog Scale for assessment of pain.

TABLE 10-2. OBJECTIVE PAIN SCALE

Observation	Criteria	Points
Blood pressure	±10% preoperatively	0
	>20% preoperatively	1
	>30% preoperatively	2
Crying	Not crying	0
	Crying; responds to TLC	1
	Crying; doesn't respond to TLC	2
Movement	None	0
	Restless	1
	Trashing	2
Agitation	Asleep or calm	0
	Mild	1
	Hysterical	2
Verbal evaluation	Asleep or no pain	0
	Mild pain (cannot localize)	1
	Moderate pain (can be localized)	2

TLC = tender loving care.

31. **What methods are used in the management of pediatric acute pain?**
    1. **Patient-controlled analgesia (PCA):** In hospitalized patients 5–6 years or older with postoperative acute pain, PCA is the most commonly used technique. Loading doses are necessary before initiation of PCA. I usually use morphine in a loading dose of 0.1–0.2 mg/kg. The PCA is then programmed as follows:
       - **Dose:** 0.02–0.03 mg/kg
       - **Lock-out:** 5–10 minutes (usually 8 minutes)
       - **Maximum hourly dose:** 0.75–0.1 mg/kg
    2. **Continuous intravenous (IV) infusion:** This is used when PCA or regional anesthesia is not indicated. Preloading before continuous infusion is necessary. I usually use morphine in a loading dose of 0.1–0.2 mg/kg and then use a continuous IV infusion of morphine at

0.01–0.03 mg/kg/hr. The infusion rate is slowly titrated to provide adequate pain relief. The infusion rate is then reduced by 10% every 12–24 hours if the patient is comfortable.

3. **Sliding scale methadone:** Methadone is an effective medication in the treatment of pain. Because it has a plasma half-life of 15–30 hours, methadone provides analgesia for a much longer period. Methadone doses are the same as those of morphine. It is an alternative drug when a true allergy to morphine exists. The loading dose for methadone is 0.1–0.2 mg/kg IV, and then the patient is assessed every 2 hours. The following regimen is followed:
   - 0.08 mg/kg methadone IV every 2–4 hr for severe pain
   - 0.05 mg/kg methadone IV every 2–4 hr for moderate pain
   - 0.025 mg/kg methadone IV every 2–4 hr for minor pain

   Remember that the half-life is very long; therefore, reduce the dose or increase the time interval between doses, or both, if methadone is to be used for more than 24 hours.

4. **Oral route:** The oral route is used when the patient has not received an NPO order (Tables 10-3 and 10-4).

5. **Epidural analgesia:** An extremely effective method of pain control in most postoperative patients. It provides good pain relief with smaller doses of narcotic and local anesthetic

TABLE 10-3. COMMONLY USED ORAL OPIATES

Medication	Ingredients	Usual Dosage
Codeine elixir + acetaminophen (i.e., codeine elixir with Tylenol)	Codeine (12 mg/5 mL) + acetaminophen (12 mg)	0.5–1.0 mg/kg PO every 4 hr prn
Codeine tablets + acetaminophen (i.e., Tylenol No. 3)	Codeine (15 mg/tablet) + acetaminophen (300 mg)	1–2 tablets PO every 4–6 hr prn
Morphine sulfate oral solution	Morphine sulfate (2 mg/mL)	0.3 mg/kg PO every 4 hr prn
Oxycodone + acetaminophen (i.e., Percocet)	Oxycodone (5 mg) + acetaminophen (325 mg)	1–2 tablets PO every 4 hr prn
Hydrocodone + acetaminophen (i.e., Vicodin)	Hydrocodone (5 mg) + acetaminophen (500 mg/tablet)	1–2 tablets PO every 4 hr prn
Hydrocodone + acetaminophen (i.e., Norco)	Hydrocodone (5, 7.5, or 10 mg) + acetaminophen (325 mg)	1–2 tablets PO every 4 hr prn
Propoxyphene N + acetaminophen (i.e., Darvocet)	Propoxyphene N100 or N50 + acetaminophen (650 mg)	1–2 tablets PO every 4 hr prn

PO = postoperative, prn = when necessary.

TABLE 10-4. COMMONLY USED NONSTEROIDAL ANTI-INFLAMMATORY DRUGS

Ketorolac (used as an adjuvant for acute pain management)	Bolus 0.5 mg/kg (max 30 mg) IV; then 0.5 mg/kg (max 30 mg) IV every 6 hr for 24–48 hr
Ibuprofen (i.e.,Motrin)	8 mg/kg PO every 6 hr for 24–48 hr

IV = intravenously, PO = by mouth.

and less sedation than those of IV narcotics. The most common insertion sites for epidural analgesia are caudal (for newborns to children 6 years old), lumbar (for patients older than 6 years), and thoracic (for patients with specific indications such as anterior spinal fusion). In our institution, we use continuous-infusion epidural analgesia for all age groups. The three most commonly used epidural infusions are the following:

- **Hydromorphone (i.e., Dilaudid):** 20 mg/mL 1 0.1% bupivacaine for postoperative pain management after posterior or anterior spine fusion
- **Fentanyl:** 2 mg/mL 1 0.1% bupivacaine after all lower periphery surgery in patients older than 6 months
- **Fentanyl:** 1 mg/mL 1 0.05% bupivacaine in infants younger than 6 months old

32. **Does regional anesthesia mask compartment syndrome?**
One of the complications of proximal tibial osteotomy is compartment syndrome, which is characterized by pain, neurologic dysfunction, decreased sensation, decreased motor function, and swelling. When local anesthetics or narcotics are used in regional anesthesia, they interrupt the pain pathways. Local anesthetic alone also interrupts motor and sensory pathways. Therefore, the first two signs of compartment syndrome can be masked by regional technique. Marked increases in analgesic requirements may suggest the presence of compartment syndrome.

33. **Are there any benefits to the use of nonpharmacologic methods of acute pain management?**
Nonpharmacologic methods, such as relaxation, biofeedback, recreational therapy (i.e., methods such as distraction), hypnosis, and acupuncture, can improve the quality of pain control and should be utilized when appropriate.

34. **What is the key to the success of an acute pain service?**
- Must be a multidisciplinary team, which can include an anesthesiologist, a pediatrician, a pediatric pain nurse, a psychologist, a physical therapist, and a recreational therapist
- Must implement appropriate assessment techniques
- Must closely monitor the vital signs and pain scores every 2–4 hours
- Must be able to recognize and treat the side effects of each modality, such as nausea and vomiting, itching, urinary retention, and, most importantly, respiratory depression

35. **What is latex allergy?**
Latex allergy was first described by Nutter in 1979 as "contact dermatitis" following the use of rubber gloves. Since then, many manifestations of latex allergy have been reported, such as urticaria, rhinitis, conjunctivitis, asthma, angioedema, anaphylaxis, and intraoperative cardiovascular collapse.

36. **What is the pathophysiology of latex allergy?**
Latex allergy is due to a type 1 reaction (i.e., hypersensitivity or an anaphylactic reaction). Initial exposure to the antigen (i.e., latex) develops sensitization. Reexposure to the antigen causes it to bind the immunoglobulin E (IgE) antibodies on the surfaces of mast cells and basophils. This causes the release of mediators such as histamine, prostaglandins, eosinophilic chemotactic factor of anaphylaxis (ECFA), leukotrienes, kinins, and platelet-activating factor (PAF). The clinically observable signs of allergy are urticaria, bronchospasm, laryngeal edema, hypotension, and cardiovascular collapse.

37. **Who are high-risk patients for latex allergy?**
- Patients with spina bifida (18–40%) and congenital urologic abnormality who have been in contact with latex through repeated urinary catheterizations, use latex gloves during bowel evacuation, and have had repeated surgeries

- Physicians, nurses, and dental personnel, all of whom are chronically exposed to latex products
- Individuals who have a history of atopy (35–85% of those with latex allergy have a history of atopy)
- Patients with a history of allergy to balloons, rubber gloves, and bananas

KEY POINTS: ANESTHESIA

1. Surgery should be postponed to accommodate 6 hours of NPO to allow full gastric emptying.

2. For an upper respiratory infection, wait 1–2 weeks after cessation of symptoms before performing surgery.

3. For lower respiratory infection, wait at least 4–6 weeks after cessation of symptoms before performing surgery.

4. ECG, echocardiography, radionuclide studies, chest x-ray, and pulmonary function testing should be performed in patients with myopathy before performing surgery.

5. If the cervical spine is unstable, movement in the surgical patient (e.g., mask ventilation or intubation) may result in loss of normal alignment of the vertebrae, compression of the cord, and possibly permanent neurologic injury.

6. Effective pain management has been shown to improve mortality and morbidity rates and immune function.

---

38. **Are there any tests available to identify latex allergy?**
    - Skin-prick testing
    - Radioallergosorbent test (RAST), performed on the patient's serum (this test detects and quantifies IgE antibodies)

39. **How do you manage the patient at high risk for latex allergy?**
    Preoperatively
    - Have an increased index of suspicion.
    - Obtain a detailed medical history (e.g., the family history of allergies, allergies to foods or drugs, and previous problems).
    - Do an allergy evaluation for high-risk patients (e.g., those with spina bifida).
    Intraoperatively
    - Avoid using latex surgical gloves and any latex-containing materials that may come into contact with the patient.
    - Most latex hypersensitivity reactions occur about 30 minutes after the induction of anesthesia (range is 10–290 minutes). Anaphylactic reactions vary in severity from mild bronchospasm and desaturation, which may be self-limiting, to severe life-threatening episodes of bronchospasm and cardiovascular collapse.

40. **How is an anaphylactic reaction managed?**
    1. Discontinue infusion of anesthetic agents, blood, or antibiotics.
    2. Administer 100% O_2 with positive-pressure ventilation.
    3. Administer IV fluid (normal saline) to maintain blood pressure.

4. Administer epinephrine (3–5 mg/kg bolus, followed by 1–4 mg/kg/min of epinephrine infusion as required).
5. Administer an antihistamine (i.e., diphenhydramine, 0.5–1.0 mg/kg IV).
6. Utilize β-agonist inhalers when necessary.
7. Administer steroids (i.e., hydrocortisone, 1 gm, or dexamethasone, 4–20 mg, IV).
8. Administer bicarbonate for severe persistent acidosis.
9. Do not extubate the patient since there can be severe laryngeal edema. Allow time for edema to subside.
10. Obtain blood for RAST.

41. **When do anesthesiologists employ the technique of total intravenous anesthesia (TIVA)? What is a concern regarding its use?**
Propofol is an induction agent that may be used as an alternative to a volatile anesthetic agent, to provide maintenance of anesthesia during surgery. This is a useful alternative technique specifically for patients that have a sensitivity to volatile anesthesia or have a severe illnesses like malignant hyperpyrexia (where volatile anesthesia agents have to be avoided entirely).

A limited number of deaths have been related to high-dose propofol infusions in the intensive care unit (ICU) in critically ill patients. This has been related to infusion doses of more than 5 mg/kg/hr for more than 48 hours in the pediatric population. Features of the syndrome include cardiac failure, rhabdomyolysis, severe metabolic acidosis, and renal failure. Patients susceptible to the propofol infusion syndrome usually suffer from either acute neurological disease or inflammatory illnesses. As a measure to prevent this syndrome, patients should be monitored and limited in their exposure to the above dose of propofol. The syndrome may be triggered when propofol is used in conjunction with steroids and in the presence of catecholamines.

Alternative sedative agents should be considered where appropriate and are possible since the introduction of dexmedetomidine.

BIBLIOGRAPHY

1. Berry FA (ed): Anesthetic Management of Difficult and Routine Pediatric Patients, 2nd ed. New York, Churchill Livingstone, 1990.
2. Breucking E, Mortier W: Anesthesia in neuromuscular diseases [review]. Acta Anaesthesiol Belg 41(2):127–132, 1990.
3. Nguyen DH, Burus MW, Shapiro GG, et al: Intraoperative cardiovascular collapse secondary to latex allergy. J Urol 146:571–574, 1991.
4. Nutter AF: Contact urticaria to rubber. Br J Dermatol 101:597–600, 1979.
5. Porter SS (ed): Anesthesia for Surgery of the Spine. New York, McGraw-Hill, 1995.
6. Ready L, Ashburn M, Caplain R, et al: Practice guidelines for acute pain management in the peri-operative setting. A report by the American Society of Anesthesiologists Task Force on Pain Management, Acute Pain Section. Anesthesiology 82:1071–1081, 1995.
7. Schreiner MS, O'Hara I, Markakis DA, Politis GDb: Do children who experience laryngospasm have an increased risk of upper respiratory tract infection? Anesthesiology 85:475–480, 1996.
8. Suderman VA, Crosby ET: Elective intubation in the unstable cervical spine patient. Can J Anaesth 37:S122, 1990.
9. Sullivan M, Thompson WK, Hill GD: Succinylcholine-induced cardiac arrest in children with undiagnosed myopathy. Can J Anaesth 41:497–501, 1994.

CHAPTER 11

POSTOPERATIVE MANAGEMENT

David D. Aronsson, MD, Nathan K. Endres, MD, and Ryan M. Putnam, MD

1. **A 9-year-old boy with a displaced fracture of the distal radius and ulna was successfully treated by closed reduction under anesthesia in the operating room. What type of cast do you recommend to maintain the reduction?**
   Fractures of the distal third of the forearm are the most common fractures in children; yet, the method of immobilization after closed reduction remains controversial. Some investigators have recommended an above-the-elbow cast, whereas others have proposed a below-the-elbow cast. In a recent blinded, randomized, controlled trial involving 102 children with a mean age of 8.6 years, there was no difference between an above-the-elbow cast and a below-the-elbow cast with respect to the initial fracture angulation, postreduction angulation, reangulation during cast immobilization, and angulation of the fracture at the time of cast removal. The authors concluded that below-the-elbow casts perform as well as above-the-elbow casts in maintaining reduction of fractures in the distal third of the forearm in children, and the complication rates are similar.

2. **A 3-month-old boy with a congenital clubfoot deformity that was treated by serial casting according to the technique described by Ponseti recently had a percutaneous Achilles tenotomy. What do you recommend for postoperative management?**
   The postoperative management of a congenital clubfoot that was treated by the Ponseti technique of serial casting and Achilles tenotomy includes a long-leg cast, with the foot positioned in 15 degrees of dorsiflexion and 70 degrees of abduction for 3 weeks to allow the Achilles tendon to heal in this position. The cast is removed at the end of 3 weeks, and the patient is fitted with a foot abduction orthosis (FAO), also called a Denis Browne bar. The orthosis consists of a metal bar with two custom-fitted straight-last shoes attached to its ends (as sold by MJ Markell Shoe Co, Yonkers, NY), separated by a distance adjusted to 1 inch more than the width of the shoulders. The affected foot (i.e., the clubfoot) is turned out 70 degrees, and the unaffected foot is turned out 45 degrees. The family is instructed to have the boy wear the FAO full time (approximately 23 hours a day) for the first 2–4 months after casting and then part time (i.e., nighttime and naptime) for 2–4 years. Several investigators have reported an increased recurrence rate in patients who failed to wear the FAO according to the recommended guidelines.
   In a recent study including 30 patients with 44 clubfeet, 30 clubfeet were cared for by families who were compliant with the postoperative recommendations and did not require any further treatment, whereas 8 of the 14 clubfeet (57%) cared for by families who were noncompliant needed further treatment.

3. **A 13-year-old boy with an unstable (acute) slipped capital femoral epiphysis (SCFE) had a hip joint hematoma aspiration and closed reduction with single-screw fixation. What do you recommend for postoperative management?**
   The frequency of postoperative complications, particularly osteonecrosis and progression of the slip, is higher in patients with an unstable SCFE. The lateral epiphyseal vessels provide most of the blood supply to the epiphysis. The lateral epiphyseal vessels enter the epiphysis posterosuperiorly and anastomose with the vessels from the round ligament at the junction of

the medial and central thirds. If multiple pins or screws are placed in the posterosuperior quadrant, the lateral epiphyseal vessels may be damaged. The other problem with multiple pins or screws is that, although they may look well positioned on the images, one pin or screw may have penetrated the femoral head into the joint. This unrecognized pin or screw penetration causes chondrolysis. Single screw fixation decreases the risk of damage to the lateral epiphyseal vessels and of unrecognized screw penetration. In a patient with an unstable SCFE, one screw may not provide rigid fixation, and two screws may increase the risk of osteonecrosis and chondrolysis. In either case, having the affected limb be non-weight-bearing through the use of crutches for 6–8 weeks is recommended to prevent progression.

4. **A 6-year-old boy had a closed reduction and percutaneous pinning for a displaced (Gartland type III) supracondylar humerus fracture. When do you recommend a follow-up evaluation with radiographs?**
Follow-up evaluation with radiographs should take place when the pins are removed.

Up to 75% of pediatric fractures occur in the upper extremity, with supracondylar humerus fractures accounting for the majority of fractures around the elbow. Despite the recent trend from nonoperative management to surgical stabilization for displaced supracondylar humerus fractures, complications, including pin tract infections, iatrogenic neurovascular injury, pin migration that necessitates a return to the operating room for removal, and loss of reduction, continue to plague clinicians caring for patients with displaced supracondylar humerus fractures.

A recent study, involving 104 patients with displaced supracondylar humerus fractures, compared the frequency of complications between two groups of 52 patients each. The first group had the initial postoperative evaluation with radiographs within 10 days of closed reduction and percutaneous pinning; the second had the initial postoperative evaluation with radiographs after 10 days of pin placement. The overall complication rate for the series was 7.7%, or 8 out of 104, with 6 complications in the early follow-up group and 2 complications in the late follow-up group.

The authors concluded that clinical and radiographic evaluation of routine displaced supracondylar humerus fractures requiring closed reduction and percutaneous pinning may be safely delayed until pin removal.

5. **A 7-year-old boy with a displaced fracture of the distal radius and ulna is treated by closed reduction and application of a well-molded splint using intravenous conscious sedation. What type of monitoring do you recommend during recovery, and when do you recommend that the patient be discharged?**
Intravenous conscious sedation for fractures generally combines narcotics and benzodiazepines. Narcotics provide good analgesia, and the benzodiazepines provide relaxation and some degree of amnesia. Narcotics provide analgesia by reversibly binding to opioid receptors; in higher doses, they may have sedative properties. Benzodiazepines are primarily sedatives that provide hypnosis, anxiolysis (i.e., anxiety relief), muscle relaxation, and some retrograde amnesia, but they have no analgesic properties. Narcotics and benzodiazepines act synergistically to induce a deep level of sedation and analgesia. The preferred route of administration is intravenous, to allow easier titration. Monitoring is mandatory during intravenous sedation and recovery, and the administering physician should ideally be trained in pediatric life support. The drug dosage, time, and route of administration must be documented, and there must be an assistant who can continuously monitor the patient. Vital signs and pulse oximetry should be monitored continuously during the procedure and then at routine intervals, usually every 5 minutes, until the following discharge criteria are met:
1. Cardiovascular functioning is normal, with a patent, stable airway.
2. The patient is arousable, and protective reflexes are intact.
3. The patient can talk (if age-appropriate).
4. The patient can sit up (if age-appropriate).

5. Very young or disabled children should be returned to their presedation level.

6. Hydration is adequate.

Discharge usually occurs about 80 minutes after administration of intravenous conscious sedation. Contraindications include a history of apnea or airway disease, altered mental status, hemodynamic instability, or age less than 2 months.

6. **A 9-year-old boy with type IV osteogenesis imperfecta (OI) has been treated with bisphosphonates to decrease pain and the frequency of fractures. He had an olecranon fracture that was treated by open reduction and internal fixation. Would postoperative management include stopping the bisphosphonates?**

No.

Bisphosphonates, both oral and intravenous, inhibit bone resorption. Bisphosphonates are currently indicated for the symptomatic treatment of children with OI. They provide considerable improvement in the quality of life of the patients, increasing bone mineral density and physical activity while the fracture rate decreases and chronic pain improves dramatically.

A recent study followed seven patients with OI for 2 years prior to starting treatment with either pamidronate (1.5–3.0 mg/kg per treatment cycle) or alendronate (a single daily dose of 5 mg for subjects 30 kg and under or 10 mg for subjects above 30 kg). The seven patients sustained 24 fractures during the 2 years prior to treatment and 20 fractures during the 2.5 years after the start of treatment. Only 1 fracture showed signs of nonunion after 6 months, and that occurred in a patient who was receiving bisphosphonate treatment.

Some reports suggest that there is no influence of bisphosphonate treatment on fracture healing, whereas others show a delay of fracture healing in animal models.

The authors concluded that treatment with bisphosphonates at the doses currently recommended did not appear to interfere with fracture healing in their small group of children.

7. **An 11-year-old boy had a resection of a calcaneonavicular tarsal coalition with interposition of the extensor digitorum brevis muscle. The anesthesiologist believes that postoperative popliteal fossa blockade (PFB) would be beneficial for postoperative pain control. What do you recommend?**

Regional anesthetic techniques have gained popularity in recent years for postoperative pain management of pediatric orthopaedic patients. Caudal epidural blockade has been the modality of choice for many centers, secondary to technical ease and familiarity. Although the technique is generally safe and effective, adverse effects have been reported. The more serious problems result from inadvertent intravascular or intraosseous injection with cardiovascular and central nervous system toxicity, whereas less-serious sequelae include urinary retention and unnecessary sensory blockade of the contralateral extremity.

Effective analgesia for foot and ankle surgery requires blockade of the sciatic nerve or its branches and the common peroneal and tibial nerves. The saphenous nerve may need to be addressed for procedures on the medial side of the foot. Popliteal fossa nerve blocks have been used for intraoperative anesthesia and postoperative analgesia for lower-extremity orthopaedic procedures in adults.

In a recent study, 20 children, ranging in age from 6 months to 12 years, who were having foot and ankle surgery, received a PFB of 0.7–0.75 mL/kg of 0.2% ropivacaine, administered under anesthesia. Five patients had surgical procedures that involved the medial aspect of the foot. In these patients, the PFB was supplemented with a saphenous nerve block at the ankle. Nineteen patients experienced significant pain relief, with none requiring supplemental intravenous analgesic agents during the first 8 postoperative hours. The duration of analgesia ranged from 8–12 hours, without any complications.

PFB is a reasonable alternative that is safe and effective in providing postoperative pain control in children after foot and ankle surgery.

KEY POINTS: POSTOPERATIVE MANAGEMENT

1. Below-the-elbow casts perform as well as above-the-elbow casts in maintaining reduction of fractures in the distal third of the forearm in children, and the complication rates are similar.

2. The postoperative management of a congenital clubfoot treated by the Ponseti technique includes a long-leg cast, with the foot positioned in 15 degrees of dorsiflexion and 70 degrees of abduction for 3 weeks. After the cast is removed, the patient is fitted with a foot abduction orthosis (FAO).

3. The frequency of postoperative complications, particularly osteonecrosis and progression of the slip, is higher in patients with an unstable slipped capital femoral epiphysis (SCFE).

4. Intravenous conscious sedation for fractures generally combines narcotics and benzodiazepines.

5. Several studies have suggested that waterproof cast liners can improve hygiene and allow water activities in patients with stable fractures or sprains.

8. **A 5-year-old boy with a distal radius and ulna fracture was treated by closed reduction and splint application under conscious sedation. At the 2-week follow-up appointment, the radiographs show satisfactory alignment with early callus formation. The parents ask if their son can have a waterproof cast. What do you recommend?**

The patient should be given a waterproof cast.

Fractures during childhood are common. Boys have a 40% risk and girls a 25% risk of sustaining a fracture by age 16 years. The treatment of many of these fractures includes immobilization in a cast. Standard casts usually include cast padding over a cotton tubular stockinette. Moisture is absorbed and retained, which may cause skin irritation. Parents report that standard casts often cause itching, have a foul smell, and are very difficult to keep dry. Several studies have suggested that waterproof cast liners can improve hygiene and allow water activities in patients with stable fractures and sprains.

A recent study involving 127 children treated with waterproof casts reported that a survey of the children and parents revealed that 79% were very satisfied, 21% were satisfied, and none were dissatisfied with the waterproof casts. When the casts were removed, there was no difference in skin irritation between casts exposed to salt water and those exposed to fresh water.

The advantages of waterproof casts include improved patient satisfaction, improved hygiene, decreased skin irritation, and the ability to swim and to receive hydrotherapy. The only disadvantage appears to be a slight increase in the cost of the materials. In waterproof casts, a waterproof cast liner replaces the stockinette and cast padding. The waterproof cast liner is designed to repel liquid while permitting evaporation.

9. **A 10-year-old boy has a temperature of 38.6°C on the second postoperative day after an elastic nailing of a femur fracture. How should this be evaluated?**

For pediatric orthopaedic patients, the authors have concluded that the incidence of postoperative fever is high and fever does not reliably predict complications. A routine septic work-up should not be undertaken on the basis of fever, and fever should not delay discharge from the hospital.

The presence of fever during the postoperative period often causes considerable worry and consternation by nursing staff, physicians, and parents. Several investigators have reported that a postoperative febrile response is a poor predictor of complications in patients having nonorthopaedic procedures.

In a study involving 174 pediatric orthopaedic surgical patients, 127 (73%) had a postoperative fever of 38°C or higher. A postoperative fever was associated with longer procedures; the average surgical duration of the febrile surgical patient was 3.1 hours, compared to 1.7 hours in the afebrile group. Patients who had surgery without a formal incision such as percutaneous pinning were found to have a 42% incidence of fever, compared to a 78% incidence for patients who had open procedures. As a result of fever, 10 septic work-ups were initiated, and only one patient was found to have pneumonia to explain the postoperative fever.

The normal human body core temperature varies up to 1°C each day, and vigorous activities such as running a marathon may increase the core temperature up to 4°C without untoward sequelae. Fever is most commonly thought to be associated with infection, but other causes include trauma, anesthesia, surgery, allergic reaction, thrombosis, gout, transfusion, constipation, atelectasis, and drug reactions.

10. **A 10-year-old boy with cerebral palsy and spastic quadriplegia had bilateral varus rotational osteotomies for subluxating hips, with a satisfactory postoperative course. Two weeks after the operation, he presented to the emergency room with decreased appetite, emesis, decreased bowel sounds, abdominal distention, tachypnea, and tachycardia. What do you recommend?**
The boy should be watched carefully for signs of gastric rupture.

Children with cerebral palsy and spastic quadriplegia often have dysphagia, gastroesophageal reflux, and reduced bowel motility. Several investigators have reported a high complication rate after hip osteotomies in nonambulatory patients with cerebral palsy, particularly if the patient had a gastrostomy or tracheostomy. Gastric rupture without preceding trauma is uncommon in children.

A recent study reported three cases of postoperative gastric rupture following orthopaedic surgical procedures. All children had cerebral palsy with spastic quadriplegia and were nonambulatory, and all three cases were fatal. The gastric rupture occurred an average of 30 days after the operation. All patients presented with acute abdominal distention, with the patients subsequently becoming acutely unstable. The histologic evidence suggests that the acute gastric rupture developed rapidly during the postoperative period, rather than representing a slow, insidious process of long-standing duration.

Careful postoperative monitoring can improve survival by identifying signs of impending gastric rupture, including gastric distention, decreased tolerance of feeding, and early signs of sepsis, including tachycardia. Awareness of this rare but highly lethal complication is essential for the orthopaedist caring for postoperative patients with cerebral palsy.

11. **A 13-year-old girl presents to the emergency room 4 weeks after scoliosis surgery complaining of increasing back pain. A C-reactive protein (CRP) is drawn and measures 4.0 mg/dL. How should this be interpreted?**
A recent study examined the response of CRP following pediatric orthopaedic surgery. The authors found that in all patients, the CRP returned to normal by 3 weeks. This patient has a CRP that is still elevated 4 weeks after the operation, so a work-up for possible infection should be seriously considered.

12. **A 6-year-old boy had a closed reduction and percutaneous pinning for a supracondylar humerus fracture. At a follow-up appointment 4 weeks after the operation, the pins are removed and the family asks if he would benefit from physical therapy. What do you recommend?**
Physical therapy is not necessary.

Parents often ask if physical therapy is necessary for rehabilitation of the arm following a closed reduction and percutaneous pinning of a supracondylar humerus fracture. Most parents want their child to return to full activities as soon as possible, but they are reluctant to put their child through a treatment program that may cause discomfort unless it is beneficial. The indications for physical therapy following a closed reduction and percutaneous pinning for a supracondylar humerus fracture are not clear in the literature.

A recent prospective randomized study was performed to assess the effectiveness of physiotherapy in improving the elbow range of motion after such fractures. The authors studied two groups of 21 (without physical therapy) and 22 (with physical therapy) children with supracondylar humeral fractures treated by open reduction and internal fixation with Kirschner wires. Postoperative follow-up at 12 and 18 weeks showed a significantly better elbow range of motion in the group treated with weekly physiotherapy, but there was no difference in elbow motion after 1 year. The authors concluded that postoperative physiotherapy is unnecessary in children with supracondylar humeral fractures without associated neurovascular injuries.

13. **A 13-year-old girl had a posterior spinal arthrodesis with segmental spinal fixation with autograft and allograft bone for adolescent idiopathic scoliosis. On the first postoperative day, she is hypotensive, with diminished urinary output. Do you recommend a bolus of intravenous fluids?**
Not necessarily.

The syndrome of inappropriate secretion of antidiuretic hormone (SIADH) is a well-known clinical entity associated with spinal and cardiovascular surgery and is characterized by a striking reduction in postoperative urinary output, despite no evidence of hypovolemia. It consists of (1) hyponatremia with associated serum hypo-osmolality, (2) persistent renal loss of sodium, (3) absence of clinical evidence of hypovolemia, (4) inappropriately concentrated urine, (5) normal renal function, and (6) normal adrenal function.

A recent study involving 10 children and adolescents who had a spinal arthrodesis for scoliosis or spondylolisthesis compared preoperative and postoperative levels of serum sodium, serum osmolality, urine sodium, urine osmolality, and serum antidiuretic hormone (ADH). All patients had SIADH, with peak levels of ADH developing within a few hours of surgery, resulting in reduction of urinary output on the day of surgery, with a gradual resolution over the next 3 days.

SIADH must be considered in the differential diagnosis of oliguric patients who have had spinal surgery. Urine and serum osmolalities can be measured to document SIADH. The treatment of choice is fluid restriction as liberal administration of hypotonic crystalloid can perpetuate respiratory distress.

14. **A 12-year-old boy had a plantar release with a plantar-based opening wedge osteotomy of the medial cuneiform to correct a pes cavus deformity. The anesthesiologist believes that epidural analgesia may help for postoperative pain control. What do you recommend?**
Postoperative pain control in children is a difficult problem, with physiologic and psychologic ramifications that can disrupt the family and prolong the hospital stay. It has finally been documented, as patients already knew, that the traditional method of on-demand narcotics for postoperative pain control is inferior to a continuous administration.

A recent study reported a dramatic improvement in postoperative pain control in patients treated by continuous epidural analgesia. Patient-controlled morphine analgesia in children resulted in a higher narcotic requirement for adequate pain control than continuous epidural analgesia.

The use of fentanyl has been shown to reduce the requirement for supplemental analgesia. Several investigators have reported that epidural narcotics provide longer-lasting pain relief than bupivacaine and have recommended a continuous infusion of bupivacaine (up to a maximal dose of 0.5 mg/kg/hr) combined with fentanyl (up to a maximal dose of 1 mg/kg/hr).

The complications of continuous epidural analgesia include catheter dislodgement, pruritus, nausea, vomiting, respiratory depression, and urinary retention. If a Foley catheter is placed during the operation, it is recommended to continue the catheter until the epidural medication is discontinued. It is important to be aware that continuous epidural analgesia may mask the early physical findings in a patient who is developing a compartment syndrome. If the patient is at risk for developing a compartment syndrome, continuous epidural analgesia for postoperative pain control is not recommended.

BIBLIOGRAPHY

1. Angel JD, Blasier RD, Allison R: Postoperative fever in pediatric orthopaedic patients. J Pediatr Orthop 14:799–801, 1994.
2. Blasier RD: Anesthetic considerations for fracture management in the outpatient setting. J Pediatr Orthop 24:742–746, 2004.
3. Bohm ER, Bubbar V, Hing KY, Dzus A: Above- and below-the-elbow plaster casts for distal forearm fractures in children. J Bone Joint Surg Am 88:1–8, 2006.
4. Jones MD, Aronsson DD, Harkins JM, et al: Epidural analgesia for postoperative pain control in children. J Pediatr Orthop 18:492–496, 1998.
5. Keppler P, Salem K, Schwarting B, Kinzi L: The effectiveness of physiotherapy after operative treatment of supracondylar humeral fractures in children. J Pediatr Orthop 25:314–316, 2005.
6. Loder RT, Aronsson DD, Dobbs MB, Weinstein SL: Slipped capital femoral epiphysis. J Bone Joint Surg Am 82:1170–1188, 2000.
7. Ponce BA, Hedequist DJ, Zurakowski D, et al: Complications and timing of follow-up after closed reduction and percutaneous pinning of supracondylar humerus fractures: Follow-up after percutaneous pinning of supracondylar humerus fractures. J Pediatr Orthop 24:610–614, 2004.
8. Register BC, Hansel DE, Hutchins GM, et al: Postoperative gastric rupture in children with cerebral palsy. J Pediatr Orthop 25:280–282, 2005.
9. Shannon EG, DiFazio R, Kasser J, et al: Waterproof casts for immobilization of children's fractures and sprains. J Pediatr Orthop 25:56–59, 2005.
10. Thacker MM, Scher DM, Sala DA, et al: Use of the foot abduction orthosis following Ponseti casts: Is it essential? J Pediatr Orthop 25:225–228, 2005.
11. Tobias JD, Mencio GA: Popliteal fossa block for postoperative analgesia after foot surgery in infants and children. J Pediatr Orthop 19:511–514, 1999.

CHAPTER 12

CASTS

Alfred D. Grant, MD, and Amir M. Atif, MD

1. What are casts used for?

Casts are most often used for immobilization when treating fractures, severe joint sprains, or muscle strains. Temporary immobilization of an injured part can prevent further soft tissue damage. Cast immobilization is used frequently after surgery to permit healing without unwanted motion.

Use for positioning is most often prescribed for patients in paralytic states to position a part to enhance function. Similarly, casts can be used to rest a joint while allowing function, such as for patients in inflammatory states.

One of the most common uses in children is for corrective casting, such as for clubfoot. In this situation, the casts are not the corrective device but are used to hold the position obtained during manipulation. Such casts can be applied serially, repeatedly reapplying the cast after manipulation until correction of the deformity is achieved. The technique of Ponseti, a successful conservative program for the serial casting of clubfeet, has been used with increasing frequency. It has reduced the extent and frequency of need for surgical correction.

Another use of casts in children is for tone reduction in cases of cerebral palsy. These short-leg casts that position the toes in dorsiflexion are controversial and lack hard scientific evidence of benefit; yet, they are popular in some therapeutic circles.

2. How are casts applied?

Casts are applied either in a circular manner encompassing a part or as splints.

Circular casts are more rigid, more easily contoured, less apt to change shape, more protective, and are thought to be more permanent. Splints are applied as layers of casting material placed on one or more sides of a limb. They tend to be less secure and less permanent. Splints are most often used either to allow for expansion such as swelling, as can be seen in the acutely injured or operated limb, or in cases in which removable immobilization is desired, such as night splinting for positioning.

Casts and splints are rarely applied directly to the skin. Various types of padding are placed on the skin. They come in rolls that are applied either directly on the skin or over a layer of stocking-like material named *stockinet*. The most common of these materials are sheet cotton and a nonwoven batting named *Webril*. These both disintegrate when they are wet, making them undesirable when used with waterproof casting materials such as fiberglass. In such instances, synthetic material, which is stable when wet and dries easily, is advised. One manufacturer has recently produced a padding that does not absorb moisture but still permits the skin to breathe, allowing for the evaporation of moisture. This material, Gortex, is more difficult to apply but has an advantage when treating children who may get casts wet with water or urine. This material has allowed children to swim and has improved hygiene in infant hip spicas.

3. What is the composition of casting material?

The most commonly used material is plaster of Paris. It is composed of calcium sulfate hemihydrate imbedded in gauze rolls of different widths. Fiberglass casting material has become popular. Urethane material is embedded in knitted fiberglass rolls. Each of these materials is activated to harden by immersion in water.

4. **What are the differences among various casting materials?**

Plaster of Paris is easiest to work with and can be readily molded but is much weaker than fiberglass. Plaster of Paris is the most forgiving of casting materials. It spreads apart easily in its hardened state when split longitudinally. Once it is spread, it tends to stay in the enlarged state since it does not have a memory. Plaster is the most easily wedged of all materials. It is inexpensive and is the most readily available material. One of the materials most commonly used in children is Gypsona plaster, a very quick-setting, fine-textured material. Other plasters, however, can serve the same purpose.

Fiberglass casts are lighter, harder, more radiolucent, and water-resistant, allowing swimming and showering. However, fiberglass casting material is difficult to apply due to stickiness, requiring gloves and a lubricant such as Vaseline to facilitate application. The most common types are Delta-Lite and Scotchcast. Some of the stickiness can be reduced by adding silicone to the fiberglass-knitted material. Examples are Delta-Lite S and Scotchcast Plus. If a circular fiberglass cast is split longitudinally and spread, it tends to return to its original state, having a memory. Thus, to expand a fiberglass cast, it must be split on two sides and then spread on both sides; alternatively, if split only along one line, small wedges, usually plastic, are used to keep the split open.

Hybrid casts are combinations of several layers of plaster, which allows the cast to be well molded, and several layers of fiberglass, which significantly increases strength.

There are **other materials**, such as Hexalite, that are thermoplastic. They are more difficult to use, are weaker, and have little benefit when compared to the previous materials. Theoretically, thermoplastic casts or splints can be heated and remolded to different positions. However, this is rarely done. Therapists frequently use thermoplastic materials as temporary splints acting as temporary braces, such as foot dorsiflexion and knee extension splints for night use.

5. **What occurs when casts harden?**

Plaster changes its chemical composition:

$$CaSO_4 \bullet H_2O + H_2O = CaSO_4 \bullet 2H_2O$$

The reaction gives off heat. Thus, casts are hot when applied. The temperature can vary depending on the temperature of the water and the room and on the cast thickness. The cast should not be covered until it is dry. Setting time depends on the material. Plaster casts set in 2–8 minutes, depending on type. Complete drying can take 24 hours. Thick casts can take up to 72 hours to completely dry.

Fiberglass comes as a prepolymer urethane resin, which reacts with water to become cured polyurethane. Fiberglass casts set within 4–5 minutes, and weight bearing can begin after 20 minutes.

6. **How are casts removed?**

With special cast cutters. They look like rotating saws but are not; they vibrate. If the motion used to cut the cast is simply in and out, not pulling, it will cut the hard cast but not the underlying padding or skin (when pushed against the soft material). Strips of plastic or a tongue blade can be slipped under the cast to further protect the skin.

7. **When casts are used to treat fractures, are there special guidelines?**

- Casts are used to immobilize a fracture or fractured part.
- To immobilize a limb segment or part, the cast should extend across the joints above and below the fracture.
- The cast is not used to reduce a fracture but to hold the position, either of an undisplaced fracture or that obtained by manipulation.
- Failure to immobilize the joints above and below can result in displacement of the fracture.

- Unstable fractures may displace in a cast under the following conditions: (1) as a result of muscle forces, (2) because the fracture has no intrinsic stability (i.e., comminution), and (3) because room within a cast will permit displacement as swelling decreases.
- Contouring and molding the cast enhances stability of the fracture.
- Initial circular casting of fresh fractures is dangerous (see below). Therefore, these casts must be split or the initial immobilization should be done with splints.
- Radiographs should be obtained before and after cast application to ensure and document proper treatment position.
- The neurologic and vascular condition of the limb must be examined and documented before and after cast application.
- Fractures that cannot be satisfactorily managed in a cast or splint are usually unstable. Stability can be achieved in such instances by introducing pins into the boney structures adjacent to the fractures and incorporating these pins into the cast. In other instances, surgical intervention may be necessary.

8. **Can casts be applied over damaged skin, wounds, and surgical incisions?**
   Yes, if access to the involved skin is provided. This can be done with removable splits or by providing a window in the circular cast over the area needing inspection. If a window is used, it should be replaced after observation or treatment of the skin to prevent swelling or window edema.

9. **What major problem can occur in using a cast?**
   A cast that is too tight can cause serious neurovascular compromise. The four Ps are signs that a cast is too tight: pain, pallor, paresthesias and possible numbness, and paralysis or paresis.

10. **How do you prevent a tight cast?**
    - Use sufficient padding.
    - Split the cast on both sides, and spread the cast to allow for swelling (i.e., bivalving).
    - Split the padding to the skin.
    - Elevate the limb to prevent dependent edema and inflammatory swelling.

11. **Are there other problems in using a cast?**
    A cast that is too loose can result in displacement of a fracture. This occurs after initial swelling subsides in treating acute injuries. Casts must be replaced or adjusted to prevent this occurrence.

    Pressure by the cast over boney prominences can lead to irritation and decubitus ulceration. This is prevented by extra padding over these areas, such as the head of the fibula, the anterosuperior iliac spine, and the malleoli.

    A cast that is too tight across the abdomen (e.g., in a hip spica) can cause superior mesenteric artery compression at the level of the third part of the duodenum. This can result in an acute abdominal crisis, gangrene of the bowel. Any suggestion of acute abdominal symptoms must be taken seriously!

    Displacement of bones can occur from inadequate immobilization when both adjacent joints are not immobilized. Immobilizing both joints may not always be practical. However, in such instances, frequent checking of the fracture position is necessary. Examples are when a hip joint or a shoulder joint is not immobilized in treating an injury to the thigh or arm. Obviously, if the hip or shoulder were immobilized, it would require that the casting material go across part of the trunk. If you decide not to do that, careful observation of the fracture is critical.

12. **What should you remember at all times about a cast?**
    Pay attention to the patient's complaints! A properly casted limb is comfortable and warm, has moving joints distally (e.g., digits) and proximally, and has normal color. Splints used to protect a joint or to position a part should also be comfortable.

13. **Are there new ways to care for a cast?**
Showering has been made easier (although with cost). A plastic bag with a tight tape at the top will work. There is now a latex cover, called XeroSox, that works with a vacuum system to seal the cast against water. See the website www.waterproofcast.com for source information.
Casts can be kept clean with cloth covers, made for both adults and children, from the companies Zula and Cast Soxs. Interestingly, knitted toe covers can be made at home. The website www.fiberspray.com/pmkn/toecover gives detailed knitting instructions.

KEY POINTS: CASTS

1. Casts used to immobilize (e.g., for fractures or after surgery) should go across the joints above and below the part.

2. Casts can be too tight, which can cause permanent damage. Know the signs of a tight cast (i.e., the four Ps: pain, pallor, paresthesias, and paralysis or paresis).

3. Casts used for acute injuries should be split or bivalved (i.e., cut along both sides), including the padding.

4. Padding over boney prominences (e.g., malleoli or the fibula head) prevents pressure sores.

5. Instruct the patient not to stick pencils, knitting needles, or other implements inside casts to scratch the skin. The skin may be penetrated and can become infected.

14. **Is there any way to control the itching?**
Antihistamines, such as Benadryl, may work. Sometimes hitting the outside of the cast over the spot can help. A product called Cast Blast, a spray can of talc with a long thin nozzle, can spray the talc down the cast. Objects such as pencils and knitting needles must not be inserted down the cast. They may severely damage the skin and cause infection.

15. **What do you do if a coin, pencil eraser, or other foreign object falls into the cast?**
It is tempting to leave the object alone, but there is a danger. Such objects have slowly eroded through the different layers of skin. The result can vary from a tattoo of the coin to a severe ulcer. A window should be made in the cast to remove the object. If the object is radiopaque, a film will help localization. If not, hopefully the patient can guide you.

16. **Are there websites that are regularly updated that give information on cast care?**
The site www.castroom.com gives updated information about all kinds of casts, types, and materials. *Cool Cast Facts* is an excellent place for children to learn about casts, why they are used, their problems and uses, and so on. It is especially kid friendly. This website, www.kidshealth.org/kid/feel_better/things/casts.html, is sponsored by the Nemours Foundation. The website www.arthroscopy.com has an excellent section on casts, cast care, and warning signs after cast and splint application. The American Academy of Orthopaedic Surgery has information at www.aaos.org/wordhtml/pteduc/castcare.htm.

17. **Does traveling with a cast require special care?**
Traveling in a car can be a problem of dependency (i.e., keeping the limb down), particularly during the acute and postacute periods (e.g., injury, fracture, or surgery), when swelling is a problem. The lower limb should be elevated across the seating surface (use the backseat);

a forearm or hand should be elevated across the seat back. Children in a hip spica should have a car seat with the sides notched or absent (e.g., the Cosco Buster Seat).

Air travel can be a problem because of swelling associated with the pressure changes from varying altitudes. In instances in which swelling has been a problem when keeping the cast dependent or during the acute and or postacute period, circular casts should be bivalved or splints should be used, with increased padding to accommodate the swelling.

18. **When is weight bearing permitted? What walking devices are used?**
Weight bearing is usually permitted when a fracture is stable (such as with lateral ankle fractures), a soft tissue injury is in advanced healing (i.e., after 2–3 weeks), and after unstable fractures have healed to the point of stability, as seen from healing on radiographs.

Devices for walking vary; older methods include a stirrup, a rubber cast heel, and a section of bicycle tire. Each of these is satisfactory, but they have been replaced by the cast shoe. These shoes consist of some type of rubber or foam in a rocker shape, held to the cast by a Velcro closing cloth or vinyl cover over the foot portion of the cast. Their greatest conveniences are ease of removal for bedtime as well as for replacement.

BIBLIOGRAPHY

1. Chapman DR, Bennett JB, Byran WJ, Tullos HS: Complications of distal radial fractures: Pins and plaster treatment. J Hand Surg Am 7:509–512, 1982.
2. Cusick BD: Splints and casts: Managing foot deformity in children with neuromotor disorders. Phys Ther 68:1903–1912, 1988.
3. Gill JM, Bowker P: A comparative study of the properties of bandage-form splinting materials. Engin Med 11:125–134, 1982.
4. Hutchinson DT, Bassett GS: Superior mesenteric artery syndrome in pediatric orthopedic patients. Clin Orthop 250:250–257, 1990.
5. Keenan WNW, Clegg J: Intraoperative wedging of casts: Correction of residual angulation after manipulation. J Pediatr Orthop 15:826–829, 1995.
6. Kowelski KL, Picher JD Jr, Bickley B: Evaluation of fiberglass versus plaster of Paris for immobilization of fractures of the arm and leg. Mil Med 167:657–661, 2002.
7. Martin PJ, Weimann DH, Orr JF, Bahrani AS: A comparative evaluation of modern fracture casting materials. Engin Med 17:63–70, 1988.
8. Walker JL, Rang M: Forearm fractures in children: Cast treatment with the elbow extended. J Bone Joint Surg Br 73:299–301, 1991.
9. Wolff CR, James P: The prevention of skin excoriation under children's hip spice casts using the Goretex Pantaloon. J Pediatr Orthop 15:386–388, 1995.

CHAPTER 13

ORTHOSES (BRACES AND SPLINTS)

John R. Fisk, MD, and Terry J. Supan, CPO

1. **What is an orthosis?**

   Frequently referred to as a brace, *orthosis* is the preferred term applied to a vast array of devices that are applied externally to different regions of the body for support, control, or correction. An orthosis (or plural, orthoses) is the device. An *orthotist* produces the device. The term *orthotic* is the adjective applied to these devices. An orthosis is an external force system that can support, correct, or improve the function of a body segment.

2. **Who is an orthotist?**

   An orthotist is a health care professional schooled in the field of brace manufacturing and certified by his or her professional society; an orthotist also may be licensed by the state. Orthotists are much more than skilled technicians; they are consultants and members of the rehabilitation team responsible for the care of an individual with a musculoskeletal disability.

3. **What is the history of splinting and bracing?**

   Splinting, the temporary external support of an extremity, probably had its beginning with the early treatment of fractures. Hippocrates described in detail the closed reduction and splinting of fractures. Galen, in the second century, proposed the use of braces for scoliosis and kyphosis. Early braces were manufactured by armorers. Polio required a vast expansion of brace treatment. Early devices were made of leather and iron. Modern materials, including plastics and carbon fiber, are lighter and more cosmetic.

4. **Is there a difference among the terms *splint, brace,* and *orthosis*?**

   Splints generally are temporary devices used for the support of a body segment. They may be used for stabilizing a fracture or for providing comfort to an injured part. Splints can be made from any available material. They may be premade of plastic or aluminum, or they may be a folded magazine or pillow used to stabilize a broken arm on the way to the emergency department. Lower-temperature plastic splints are usually for short-term use. *Brace* is a popular term of antiquated use. The preferred term, as indicated earlier, is *orthosis*. An orthosis is more long-lasting and purposeful than a splint, providing support, correction, or improved function of a body part.

5. **How are different orthoses described or named?**

   Orthoses are named after regions of the body, including the desired function; they can also be named after a city, an individual, or the manufacturer. Examples include ankle-foot orthosis (AFO), the hip-knee-ankle-foot orthosis (HKAFO), and the thoracolumbosacral orthosis (TLSO). The Milwaukee brace is perhaps the most famous brace named after a city. The Blount brace is named for a person. The Rhino cruiser is named for the manufacturer.

6. **What are the uses for orthoses?**

   Orthoses are designed to support, correct, or improve function of the body part for which they are constructed. A lower limb orthosis provided to a person with postpolio paralysis can support a joint lacking muscle control. It can also improve the function of the individual by allowing him or her to bear weight on the limb and walk. A spinal orthosis can correct a spinal deformity. The functional walking of a child with cerebral palsy can be improved by the control that an AFO may provide.

7. **What principles govern orthotic use?**
Orthoses function by contact with the body part that they are designed to influence. They exert control by pressure, using sound biomechanical principles and three-point contact. The broader the surface area of contact, the more comfortable they are; therefore, they follow the principle of total contact. Lower-limb orthoses should be designed to meet Gage's principles of efficient gait: stability in stance, clearance in swing, prepositioning of the foot in terminal swing, adequate step length, and energy conservation.

8. **How are orthoses prescribed?**
The orthotic prescription is a document that clearly communicates a patient's needs from the prescriber to the certified orthotist. The prescription writer, generally a physician, must understand the specific disability, the overall condition of the patient, the abnormal biomechanical or physiologic conditions, and the area where the orthosis is to function and assist. The prescription communicates this information to the orthotist so he or she may design an appropriate device as a treatment or remedy for a specific patient's pathologic condition. It includes the name, age, and gender of the patient; the diagnosis and purpose; and the extent of the orthosis. The orthotist will then evaluate the patient, applying his or her professional expertise to the production of an appropriate device.

9. **How are orthoses made?**
Custom-made orthoses are usually fabricated over a model created by making a cast of the patient, taking detailed measurements of the patient, or scanning the patient for a CAD/CAM (computer-aided design, computer-aided manufacturing) model. Premade, custom-fitted orthoses usually come in kits (composed of individual parts) that are assembled by the orthotist. Mass-produced devices like fracture braces and fabric splints are sized by gross measurements and are adjustable with straps. Custom-made splints for a variety of purposes (usually provided by occupational therapists) may be directly formed on the patient with low-temperature plastics.

10. **What problems can arise from orthotic use?**
The two main problems with any orthosis can be improper fit and the patient's reluctance to wear the device. Fitting problems usually come from excessive pressure over bony areas; change in body shape due to growth, edema, or weight change; or excessive (uncontrolled) muscle contraction. These must be evaluated and corrected by the orthotist. Expectations for correcting a deformity may exceed the ability of an orthosis, causing discomfort or skin irritation. If the functional goals of the orthosis do not match the patient's perceived needs, the patient will reject the orthosis for a number of reasons, such as appearance, bulk, or weight. Good communication among the physician, the orthotist, and the patient can improve compliance.

KEY POINTS: ORTHOSES

1. Orthotists are certified professionals who not only can manufacture orthoses but also can advise and guide physicians in appropriate orthotic functions and uses.

2. Orthoses and splints should be prescribed for a specific purpose and length of time, with periodic reassessment of their effect over time.

3. Ongoing use of orthoses or splints needs to be monitored for possible adverse effects on function or the creation of skin irritation or breakdown.

11. **For how long should orthoses be worn each day?**

An orthosis designed to improve muscle function or to provide joint stability is necessary only when the individual will be ambulating, usually during the daytime. Containment or corrective orthoses, such as fracture orthoses and scoliosis orthoses, are usually prescribed for full-time use. Sports orthoses, such as knee or ankle braces, are usually used only during athletic activity.

12. **What is the evidence for effective orthotic management?**

Most evidence of effective orthotic management is subjective but quite self-evident. A patient who has a drop-foot condition using a dorsiflexion assist AFO walks with a more natural heel-to-toe gait. The total contact orthosis provides compressive forces to immobilize the fracture site while allowing removal for improved hygiene. The effectiveness in scoliosis has been well documented for select deformities in a number of studies. Finally, the International Society of Orthotics and Prosthetics and the American Academy of Orthotists and Prosthetists have been conducting consensus conferences and state of the science conferences to examine the objective evidence in support of existing orthotic management for different types of physical disabilities. The reports from these conferences will be the basis for future research.

BIBLIOGRAPHY

1. American Academy of Orthopaedic Surgery: Atlas of Orthoses and Assistive Devices. St. Louis, Mosby, 1997.
2. Bowker P: Biomechanical Basis of Orthotic Management. Boston, Buttterworth-Heinemann, 1993.
3. Gage JR: Gait Analysis in Cerebral Palsy. London, Mac Keith Press, 1991, pp 61–95.
4. International Society for Prosthetics and Orthotics: Consensus Conference Report: Cerebral Palsy, Copenhagen, 1995.
5. International Society for Prosthetics and Orthotics: Consensus Conference Report: Poliomyelitis, Copenhagen, 2003.
6. International Society for Prosthetics and Orthotics: Consensus Conference Report: Stroke, Copenhagen, 2003.

CHAPTER 14

PHYSICAL AND OCCUPATIONAL THERAPY

S. K. DeMuth, DPT, and Hugh G. Watts, MD

1. **What is physical therapy?**

   Physical therapy developed from the need for rehabilitation of persons injured in World War I and grew rapidly during and after World War II. Involvement with children came from needs identified during the polio epidemics after World War II. According to the American Physical Therapy Association (APTA) *Guide to Physical Therapist Practice*, physical therapists perform the following:
   - Diagnose and manage movement dysfunction and enhance physical and functional abilities
   - Restore, maintain, and promote not only optimal physical function but also optimal wellness and fitness and optimal quality of life as it relates to movement and health
   - Prevent the onset, symptoms, and progression of impairments, functional limitations, and disabilities that may result from diseases, disorders, conditions, or injuries

2. **What is occupational therapy?**

   Occupational therapy also developed out of the need to rehabilitate those injured by war. Occupational therapy, as defined by the American Occupational Therapy Association, is the therapeutic use of self-care, work, and play activities to increase independent function, to enhance development, and to prevent disability. It may include the adaptation of tasks or the environment to achieve maximum independence and to enhance quality of life. Occupational therapy provides people with the "skills for the job of living."

3. **Is there a subspecialty of children's physical or occupational therapy?**

   How often have we been told that children are not small adults? This truth is no less valid for physical or occupational therapy. Although therapists used to dealing with adults are not incompetent with children, those dealing with children and their families all the time are better able to understand what a child should be able to do at a given stage of development and what that child's and family's needs are in the home or school. A physical therapist may choose to complete a specialist certification in pediatrics (becoming a pediatric certified specialist [PCS]), sponsored by the APTA.

4. **What is the difference between occupational therapy and physical therapy?**

   Sometimes the margins between the two fields are blurred. This blurring is more common when working with children than with adults. Over the decades, occupational therapy has focused on assisting people with their ability to succeed at school or work, their adaptive behavior, the rehabilitation of upper-extremity injuries, and the management of upper-limb prosthetics. Physical therapy has tended to focus on walking and mobility with or without adaptive equipment such as braces and wheelchairs, the rehabilitation of trunk and lower-extremity injuries, and lower-limb prosthetics. Since many children have both upper- and lower-extremity problems, sometimes the occupational therapist will look after both, and sometimes the physical therapist will.

5. **What does physical therapy have to do with children's orthopaedics?**

   Physical therapists are knowledgeable in assessing children's problems with motor function. This involves not only the assessment of muscle strength by manual testing and range of motion assessment but also the assessment of a child's ability to manage age-appropriate activities of daily living (ADLs). Physical therapists are very involved in the care of children with movement disorders such as cerebral palsy and have an interest in the child's integration in the community. As such, they are concerned with the child's role in the family, the home, the school, and the community. The treatment recommendations of the physical therapist and the pediatric orthopaedist should be complementary and should support the family's wishes as much as possible.

6. **What do occupational therapists have to do with children's orthopaedics?**
Occupational therapists have a strong background in assessing children's developmental difficulties. They usually make such assessments using standardized tests. In addition, occupational therapists have a strong interest in ensuring that the child with developmental disabilities is able to manage age-appropriate ADLs. Obviously, children with upper-extremity injuries and deformities are appropriate for occupational therapy assessment. Occupational therapists, too, can be very helpful in assessing the child's function in the home, school, and community. The treatment recommendations of the occupational therapist and the pediatric orthopaedist should be complementary and should also support the family's wishes. Children and their families benefit from a team approach.

7. **Is there only one category of occupational therapist or physical therapist?**
No. There are registered occupational therapists and certified occupational therapy assistants (COTAs). These assistants provide occupational therapy services under the supervision of a registered occupational therapist. The same is true for physical therapy. There are licensed physical therapists and physical therapy assistants (PTAs). Assistants provide care under the supervision of a licensed physical therapist. Occupational therapists, COTAs, physical therapists, and PTAs have all received their education at accredited colleges or universities. Occupational and physical therapy aides are trained on the job and have not received any formal education in therapy.
   Physical therapists must have either 2 years of postgraduate education, earning a master's degree (MPT), or 3 years of postgraduate education, earning a doctorate (DPT). By 2020, the APTA expects all educational programs to offer the doctoral degree. Occupational therapists may have a BS in occupational therapy, a master's (i.e., Master of Science [MS], Master of Occupational Therapy [MOT], or Master of Arts [MA]), or a doctorate of occupational therapy (OTD). Both professions also have numerous members with PhD degrees working in research and teaching.

8. **For which children should you order physical therapy?**
Children who have had an injury or recent operation would be greatly assisted by the physical therapist in learning how to use crutches or a walker, for example. They would be taught not only to be able to go from one point to another but also how to go up and down stairs and how to transfer from a chair to a bed, toilet, and car. Children with cerebral palsy and other developmental disabilities frequently benefit from their contact with physical therapists.

9. **Children are very agile. Do they really need to learn how to use crutches?**
Children can learn to use crutches easily if they have normal coordination and are provided with properly fitted ones. Both of these factors are not always present. It is important that the child knows how to safely ascend and descend stairs. If the child is going to use the crutches for a long time, adjustment for growth and safety issues such as prevention of nerve damage due to crutch palsy should be raised with the child and family.

10. **You have a child who could use a wheelchair. Who should be asked for advice?**
For a small child whose parents want a convenient way to get the child around while shopping, a stroller may be all that is needed. At other times a **properly fitted** wheelchair may be the

answer. For some children, a powered chair may be needed, but not if the home does not have the space to make it useful. The physical therapist is the one who usually helps with the decision and the fitting.

11.   **For which children should you order occupational therapy?**
Children who have had an injury or recent operation would be greatly assisted by the occupational therapist in learning how to feed or dress, for example. They would be taught how to chew or swallow as well as how to use adapted utensils and how to use specific strategies to dress themselves without assistance from an adult. Children with cerebral palsy and other developmental disabilities, especially those associated with sensory or behavioral abnormalities such as autism, frequently benefit from their treatment by occupational therapists.

12.   **What role do the therapists play in splinting and bracing?**
Occupational therapists have expertise in making splints to improve function or to prevent deformity, especially for the upper extremities. Physical therapists are knowledgeable about the use of braces to enhance function, especially of the lower extremities. There are also certified hand therapists, and these therapists can be either physical or occupational therapists who have chosen to specialize in caring for children with hand injuries or abnormalities.

13.   **You have a child with a new limb prosthesis. Who would help the child with training in its use?**
That depends. As a general rule, occupational therapists work with children with upper-extremity prostheses, whereas physical therapists work with the lower-extremity prostheses. But limb deficiencies in most children are of congenital origin, and 30% of them have a loss of multiple limbs. Therefore, there may need to be some overlap.

14.   **Is the child the only one to benefit from physical or occupational therapy?**
Obviously, the tone of the question implies otherwise. The family can receive tremendous help from the therapist. They can learn what to expect from the child and how to rearrange home furnishings to facilitate the care of the child, and they can receive advice on appropriate equipment and management of learning and behavior.

15.   **What kinds of range of motion exercises are there for children?**
Passive range of motion is an exercise in which the therapist or parent does the moving of the joint without the active involvement of the child. Active exercises are those in which children are doing the motion themselves, albeit usually with additional encouragement by the therapist or parents. Active assisted exercises are those in which the child moves the joint through a range of motion, but the therapist or parent is assisting and supporting the child's limb. Both the child and the therapist or parent have some control over the amount of motion. Active resisted exercises are those in which the child does the motion, with the parent or therapist resisting the activity.
    Because children are small and their muscles can be easily overpowered, caution has to be used so that a child does not get injured. With this in mind, there is very little place for passive exercises in children except where there is no motor ability whatsoever.

16.   **What other kinds of exercises are there for children?**
There are many therapeutic approaches to teaching children how to move or perform various tasks. Most are based on current motor control and motor learning theory. The important point is that there is no one approach that solves all the problems, and therapy approaches continue to evolve and change as new knowledge is provided by research. Occupational therapists and physical therapists often use standardized tests of development or motor ability such as the

Alberta Infant Motor Scale, the Gross Motor Function Measure, the Pediatric Evaluation of Disability Inventory, the School Function Assessment, and the Sensory Integration and Praxis Tests to document change and to make treatment recommendations.

17. **Getting children to do exercises can be like having them clean up their rooms. How would you suggest avoiding such turmoil?**

With children, exercises should be modified into game playing. Using ball kicking, for example, as a means of strengthening the quadriceps muscle in the leg is preferable to going through the often-frustrating activity of encouraging a child to straighten and bend the knee.

But these game-like exercises must be appropriate for the stage of development that a child has reached. At what age does a normal child learn to hop on one leg? This is where the expertise of a children's therapist comes in. In addition, the therapist needs to know what activities are likely to sustain attention in a child at a given age. A normal child usually learns to hop on one leg at around 3–3½ years of age.

18. **Do these exercises need to be done only in the presence of the therapist?**

Certainly not. There are not enough therapists or days in the week to have the exercises limited to direct hands-on treatment. A major role of the therapist is to teach the parents how to help the child to do the appropriate exercises. This is usually done by demonstration and is reinforced by illustrations to take home as a reminder. The therapist may see a child fairly frequently to reinforce the teaching, but not necessarily to help the child with the exercises directly.

19. **The role of therapy may be more obvious in children with purely mechanical problems such as osteogenesis imperfecta. But what can physical or occupational therapy do for a child with cerebral palsy?**

A child with cerebral palsy may benefit by maintaining the range of motion of the extremities and also with muscle strengthening where appropriate and particularly with learning coping skills to manage ADLs.

20. **What aspects of cerebral palsy are unlikely to benefit from physical or occupational therapy?**

Fixed contractures of joints are not amenable to correction by exercises. In some places, physical therapists are mandated to apply plaster casts. In such situations, serial casting may be used to overcome fixed contractures. Although there has been a great deal of interest, there is no scientific evidence that physical therapy is able to reduce spasticity. Both physical therapists and occupational therapists assist these children and their caregivers with the use of adaptive equipment or environmental modifications in order to maximize their participation in activities required for play or school.

21. **Why do they have occupational and physical therapists working in the school systems?**

It is often in the school setting that evidence of a central nervous system disorder is first seen, when demands are made for specific activities that take place at school. Therapists are then asked by teachers to assess such children. This may provide the child's introduction into the medical system. A therapist can help the teachers to help the children in their daily activities, making sure that the activities are indeed possible and that equipment needed to help the child is available.

22. **What are the indicators for occupational therapy referral of a school student?**

The guidelines published by the California Department of Education are a good place to start. They suggest that children with the following characteristics be referred to occupational therapy:

- Difficulty in learning new motor tasks
- Poor organization and sequencing of tasks

- Poor hand use (including writing and tool use)
- Difficulty in accomplishing tasks without the use of adaptive equipment, environmental modifications, or assistive technology
- Unusual or limited play patterns
- Deficits in adaptive self-help or feeding skills in the educational setting
- Poor attention to tasks
- Notable over- or under-reaction to textures, touch, or movement

23. **What are the indicators for a referral for physical therapy in the schools?**
The same guidelines suggest that children with the following characteristics should be referred to physical therapy:
- Delayed gross motor skills
- Difficulty in learning new motor tasks
- Unusual walking or movement patterns
- Difficulty in moving or moving safely in the school environment
- Difficulty in maintaining an appropriate sitting posture
- Poor balance or falling frequently
- Difficulty in accomplishing tasks without the use of adaptive equipment, environmental modifications, or assistive technology
- Postural or orthopaedic abnormalities
- Reduced endurance or excessive fatigue

24. **What exactly is the Individuals with Disabilities Education Act (IDEA)?**
This act guarantees that no child can be excluded from a free and appropriate public education. Legislation was originally passed in 1975 and has been amended several times since. The name *IDEA* was part of the 1990 amendment, and services have continued to be expanded, with the most recent amendments in 1997. Children with disabilities from birth to 21 years of age can receive special education services and related services (i.e., occupational therapy and physical therapy) at school. Children from birth to 3 years of age can receive early intervention services including educational and therapeutic services in their homes or wherever their families would prefer to receive intervention. The federal government defines 13 categories of disabilities as eligible for special education and related services: autism, combination deafness and blindness, deafness, hearing impairment, mental retardation, multiple disabilities, orthopaedic impairments, other health impairments, serious emotional disturbance, specific learning disability, speech or language impairment, traumatic brain injury, and visual impairments including blindness.

25. **What does all that have to do with children's orthopaedics?**
Children with orthopaedic problems often have associated diagnoses and may need the services of therapists outside of the setting of the hospital or clinic.

26. **What is an Individualized Education Program (IEP)?**
This is a working document required under IDEA for special education students from 3 through 21 years of age that documents their eligibility for services; their level of present functioning; appropriate goals, objectives, services, and service providers; and other specifics. When the written IEP is accepted and signed by the parent or legal guardian, it becomes the legal document ensuring compliance with provision of service. The IEP team refers to all the members, including the parents, who provide services to special education students.

27. **What are some other terms you are likely to see on a therapist's report that you may not understand?**
When you get reports, therapists naturally will use their own jargon. It not always clear to a physician what these jargon terms mean. We have mentioned ADLs (activities of daily living).

These are tasks that individuals engage in on a regular basis so that they can function and be sustained in the environments in which they operate.

Some other jargon terms not too familiar to a physician might be worth reviewing. *Fine motor skills* are the types of skills that require precise controlled movement of the hands to perform an activity. They are contrasted with *gross motor skills,* an example of which is walking. *Motor planning* is the ability of the brain to conceive, organize, and carry out a sequence of unfamiliar actions. *Visual perception and integration* is the ability to use visual information to recognize, recall, and discriminate the meaning of what you see.

KEY POINTS: PHYSICAL AND OCCUPATIONAL THERAPY

1. Not just the child, but the family, too, can benefit from physical therapy and occupational therapy.

2. A child's work is to play. Therapy needs to incorporate play.

3. There are pediatric occupational therapy and physical therapy specialists, just as in orthopaedic surgery.

4. Exercises do not always have to be done by direct service (i.e., with the therapist in attendance).

5. Cooperation among the team (i.e., the pediatric orthopaedist, the physical therapist, and the occupational therapist) sharing complimentary goals enhances the likelihood of success.

28. What is meant by *modalities*?
Therapists use the term *modalities* to mean externally applied physical agents such as hot packs, or ultrasound and cold using ice packs or ice massage. Whirlpool units are often used in the hospital setting to provide heat and exercise as well as wound care.

29. What is the role of these modalities in children?
You have to be a little cautious in using some of these agents in children. For example, there is experimental evidence that open epiphyses can be damaged by ultrasound. Therefore, ultrasound is generally not used in children. Young children and those with developmental delays may not be able to communicate readily. It is possible that excessive heat could be applied using some of the other modalities. These same cautions are needed with manual therapy techniques (including mobilization and manipulation), which are generally not used with children.

30. What is meant by architectural barriers?
A good exercise is to spend a part of a day moving around and living your life in a wheelchair. You will find that even thick rugs on the floor can be an impediment, let alone steps, the absence of ramps, or the absence of elevators. Although there are laws mandating the elimination of architectural barriers in public buildings, private homes and apartments can present enormous difficulties. For example, the doors into most bathrooms are too narrow for a wheelchair to be pushed through. Keep that in mind the next time you are in a hurry to relieve an overstretched bladder.

31. What is the role of biofeedback in children?
Biofeedback is just a matter of using some physical end result of effort to signal back to a child the outcome of the child's work. One simple example is when electromyographic (EMG) leads are placed over the muscles on the upper-extremity amputation stump of a child. These leads

are attached to the transmitter of a radio-controlled toy automobile. The child then learns to drive the car around by using muscle contractions. This training can be used prior to fitting a child with an upper-extremity myoelectric prosthesis. Other biofeedback systems are used for less obvious outcomes such as relaxation.

32. **Does physical therapy have a role in teaching body mechanics in children's orthopaedics?**

Yes. The most important role may be teaching parents how to lift their children properly so that the parents do not injure their own backs as their children grow heavier.

33. **What about the role of physical therapists in motion analysis laboratories?**

The role of motion analysis laboratories (or gait labs) has grown as a means of documenting the pre- and postoperative status of children. This is particularly so with children with musculoskeletal problems secondary to cerebral palsy. These labs are also used in assessing children with other musculoskeletal problems, such as those with myelodysplasia (spina bifida) or amputations. Such studies may include energy consumption assessments. Many such gait laboratories are managed by physical therapists who have been specially trained in the field. As with all such laboratory tests, the findings need to be carefully integrated with the child's physical examination.

34. **What is the role of physical therapists in aerobic conditioning exercises in children?**

In the past, such activity has been confined to the treatment of adults. As our focus on the problems of obesity of adulthood sharpens, we recognize that patterns established by children, especially in their teenage years, continue into adulthood. The problems of osteoporosis may begin with bad childhood habits. As a consequence, there is a greater interest in involving children in fitness programs such as Fit Kids, established by the APTA. Occupational therapists have also become more involved in assisting children with behavioral approaches to deal with obesity.

WEBSITES

1. **www.aota.org:** American Occupational Therapy Association (AOTA).

2. **www.apta.org:** American Physical Therapy Association (APTA).

3. **www.pediatricapta.org:** APTA Section on Pediatrics.

CHAPTER 15

SHOES FOR CHILDREN

Lynn T. Staheli, MD

1. **Is going without shoes okay for infants and children?**
   Barefoot is a natural and healthy state for the foot at any age. Barefoot people have stronger feet with fewer deformities than those who wear shoes. Shoes may also cause skin problems such as plantar hidradenitis or allergic reactions.

2. **What are the benefits of wearing shoes?**
   Shoes, like other clothing, are worn for appearance and protection. Shoes protect the foot from cold, sharp objects, and the eyes of those who do not like the appearance of the bare foot.

3. **What are the harmful effects of wearing shoes?**
   This depends on the shoe. Stiff shoes make the foot weaker and increase the frequency of flat feet. Tight shoes can cause deformities of the toes.

4. **Does the growing foot need support?**
   No. A supportive shoe limits movement, makes the foot weaker, and lowers the long arch. The foot should be allowed to move freely and to develop mobility and strength. We would think it ridiculous to place the hand in a rigid glove.

5. **Are shoes corrective?**
   Shoes are not corrective and have never been shown to correct any deformity.

6. **When should an infant be first fitted for shoes?**
   Usually parents fit shoes sometime during the first year. This is a clothing issue. The infant will do well in stockings around the house. Soft shoes can be fitted for appearance or to protect the foot when outside.

7. **What shoes are best for the toddler?**
   Soft, flexible shoes are best. Because the infant foot is chubby, sometimes a high-top shoe is helpful just to keep the shoe on the foot.

8. **What shoes are best for the teenager?**
   Shock-absorbing shoes reduce overuse injuries. Thick-cushioned soles make walking more comfortable.

9. **How do we know if new shoes fit properly?**
   They should be comfortable and should provide about a fingerbreadth of room for growth. It is preferable that the shoes be too large rather than too small. Sometimes shoes are sold without sufficient room for growth, shortening the useful life of the shoe.

10. **What are the features of a good shoe?**
    The five *F*s (Fig. 15-1) summarize the features of a good shoe:
    - **Flexible:** The shoe should allow as much free motion as possible. As a test, make certain that the shoe can be easily in the patient's hand.

- **Flat:** Avoid high heels that force the foot forward, cramping the toes.
- **Foot-shaped:** Avoid pointed toes or other shapes that are different from that of the normal foot.
- **Fitted generously:** Better to be too large than too short.
- **Friction, like skin:** The sole should have about the same friction as skin. Soles that are slippery or adherent can cause the child to fall. Slide the shoe across a flat surface and compare that with running your hand on the same surface. The resistance to sliding should be about the same.

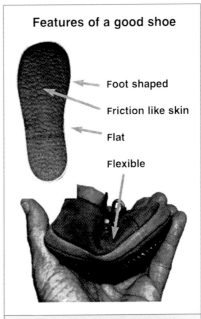

Features of a good shoe

- Foot shaped
- Friction like skin
- Flat
- Flexible

Figure 15-1. The five Fs: Features of a good shoe.

11. **How often should shoes be replaced?**

    In the growing child, shoes are nearly always outgrown before being worn out. Foot growth occurs earlier than growth of the rest of the body and is completed before adolescence.

12. **Can outgrown shoes be safely worn by younger siblings?**

    Hand-me-downs are okay. Minor alterations in the shape of the shoe will not damage the younger sibling's foot.

    However, note that fungal skin infections can be passed in the shoe.

13. **Are expensive shoes best for the child's foot?**

    Provided that the shoe meets the criteria of a good shoe, the price is not important. It is often useful to emphasize this point to parents as some equate the quality of parenting to the quality of the shoes.

14. **Does asymmetric shoe wear indicate a foot problem?**

    Not necessarily. If wear is asymmetric, examine the child's feet. Children with normal feet often will show asymmetric shoe wear.

15. **Do stiff shoes, orthotics, or inserts prevent or correct flat feet?**

    No. The belief that the foot needs support and that the arch would fall unless supported by inserts was once common. We now know that this concept is wrong. A stiff shoe actually increases the incidence of flat feet. As one would expect, the stiff shoe, by limiting mobility, makes the foot weaker. This weakness results in a loss of the dynamic component of arch maintenance in a flatter foot.

16. **Do shoe wedges or inserts help with intoeing or out-toeing?**

    No. In the past, countless children wore various wedges on their shoes to correct a rotational problem. When we studied this by applying various wedges to children's shoes and measuring the effect on the foot progression angle, we found that the wedges made no difference in how much the child toed in or out.

17. **Are shoe wedges helpful in managing bow legs or knock knees?**
    No. In the past, sole wedges were commonly prescribed for these conditions. Now we know that the improvement in these conditions was due simply to natural history.

18. **Are orthotics useful in managing bunions in children?**
    No. This has been studied and found not to be useful.

19. **Is there any harm in prescribing shoe modifications for children?**
    Yes. Shoe modifications are often uncomfortable, limit play, and are embarrassing. In addition, they can impart in the child a sense that he or she is defective. We found that adults who wore shoe modifications as children had significantly lower self-esteem than control subjects. They remembered the experience of wearing the devices as unpleasant.

KEY POINTS: SHOES FOR CHILDREN

1. Shoes are not corrective.

2. Shoes function like other clothing to protect the foot and to enhance appearance.

3. Shoes should allow the foot free mobility.

4. Shoes can help by being shock-absorbing.

5. Shoe modifications may be helpful in providing shock-absorbing qualities and with inserts to distribute load more evenly.

20. **Are inserts useful in reducing abnormal shoe wear?**
    Sometimes. Inserts such as heel cups may reduce the frequency of the shoe's breaking down. The cost, discomfort, and inconvenience for the child and the possible effect on the child's self-image make this approach to excessive shoe wear questionable. It is usually best for the parents to buy a sturdier shoe.

21. **When are shoe inserts useful?**
    Shoe inserts and orthotics are useful to redistribute the load bearing on the sole of the foot. Children with stiff, deformed feet may benefit from orthotics that are recessed under prominences. This is most useful in children with clubfeet, who often have excessive loading under the base of the fifth metatarsal.

22. **Are arch supports or orthotics useful in managing growing pains?**
    Controversial. Growing pains are common and resolve without treatment with time. The value of orthotics in changing the natural history has never been studied. I do not treat growing pains with shoe inserts because of possible long-term harmful effects on the child, the cost for the family, and doubts regarding effectiveness.

23. **What should I do if families insist on some treatment?**
    Prescribe a healthy lifestyle for the child (e.g., physical activity, limited television time, and healthy foods). Avoid mechanical interventions as these can be unpleasant for the child and can cause possible long-term adverse psychological effects.

BIBLIOGRAPHY

1. Driano AN, Staheli LR, Staheli LT: Psychosocial development and "corrective" shoewear use in childhood. J Pediatr Orthop 18:346–349, 1998.

2. Rao UB, Joseph B: The influence of footwear on the prevalence of flat foot: A survey of 2300 children. J Bone Joint Surg Am 74:525–527, 1992.

3. Sim-Fook L, Hodgson A: A comparison of foot forms among the non-shoe and shoe-wearing Chinese population. J Bone Joint Surg Am 40:1058–1062, 1958.

4. Wenger DR, Mauldin D, Speck G, et al: Corrective shoes as treatment for flexible flatfoot in infants and children. J Bone Joint Surg Am 71:800–810, 1989.

CHAPTER 16

JOINT ASPIRATION AND INJECTION

Ken N. Kuo, MD

1. **What is joint aspiration or injection?**
   Joint aspiration or injection is a procedure that introduces a syringe needle into a joint (i.e., arthrocentesis) and withdraws its content for diagnostic purposes or injection for therapeutic purposes.

2. **What equipment is required for joint aspiration or injection?**
   - Syringes, with size dependent on the size of the joint to be aspirated and the amount of material to be injected
   - A 18- to 22-gauge 1.5-inch straight needle with a short bevel. In the hip of a larger person, a 3.5-inch spinal needle may be required. (The gauge of the needle used partly depends on the viscosity of the fluid aspirated.)
   - Sponges, sized 4 × 4
   - Topical antiseptics including tincture of iodine or Betadine stick and 70% alcohol wipes
   - Sterile barrier and sterile gloves
   - Local anesthetic (such as 1% plain lidocaine) and a 3-mL syringe with a 22-gauge needle
   - Plain or anticoagulated sterile fluid collection vials or test tubes
   - Culture tubes, as needed
   - A fluoroscopic x-ray machine or ultrasonographic machine

3. **What are the indications for joint aspiration or injection?**
   - **Diagnostic purposes:** Diagnosing different diseases such as septic arthritis, inflammatory disorders and arthritis, traumatic arthropathy, and certain metabolic maladies
   - **Decompression:** Decompression of acute traumatic hemarthrosis, septic arthritis, or a large effusion secondary to inflammatory disease
   - **Therapeutic purposes:** Includes intra-articular injection of therapeutic agents

4. **What are contraindications to joint aspiration or injection?**
   - Soft tissue cellulitis or soft tissue abscess in the path of needle entrance since needle insertion may introduce the pathogen into the joint
   - Pathologically uncontrolled bleeding tendency such as aspiration of hemarthrosis in a patient with hemophilia or in one receiving active anticoagulative therapy
   - The path of the needle goes through tumorous tissue

5. **What are the precautions during joint aspiration or injection?**
   - Avoid passing the needle through a vascular area.
   - Avoid obvious nerve trunk structures.
   - Do not wiggle the needle tip in the joint because it may damage intra-articular structures such as articular cartilage. It may also cause unnecessary bleeding.
   - Make sure the needle tip is completely in the joint before injection takes place to avoid injection into soft tissue space.
   - Observe strict sterile techniques.

6. **What is the best site of needle entrance?**
So long as one observes the above-mentioned indications, contraindications, and precautions, it is generally acceptable to perform the aspiration where the fluid can be most easily seen and felt (Fig. 16-1). The location for entrance to each joint is different, depending on its specific anatomic structure. Fluoroscopic or ultrasonographic imaging may be used for guidance in a difficult joint.

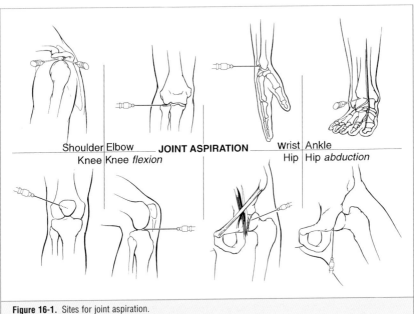

Figure 16-1. Sites for joint aspiration.

7. **What is the approach for shoulder joint aspiration?**
The shoulder joint can be approached through either the anterior or the lateral aspect, just below the acromial process. The needle should enter the joint directly. Avoid sticking the needle directly into the convex contour of the humeral head.

8. **What is the approach for elbow joint aspiration?**
The elbow joint can be easily entered from the posterolateral aspect to avoid the medial neurovascular structure. The needle should enter the space between the lateral humeral condyle and the radial head. The structure can be palpated with the forearm in supinated position. At the time of aspiration, the elbow can be placed in flexion and the forearm in pronation.

9. **What is the approach for wrist joint aspiration?**
The easiest one is the dorsal radial approach. The needle can be inserted distal to Lister's tubercle at the joint line. The wrist should be kept in pronated position and slight ulnar deviation. Care should be taken not to puncture the extensor tendons. Other approaches are radial entrance at the tip of the radial styloid and ulnar entrance at the tip of the ulnar styloid.

10. **What is the approach for finger joint aspiration?**
With the finger or thumb slightly flexed and distracted (by pulling the finger or thumb distally), the needle can enter from either the dorsal ulnar or the dorsal radial angle.

11. **What is the approach for hip joint aspiration?**

The hip joint is the most difficult joint to approach. The patient should be placed under general anesthesia or heavy sedation with local anesthesia. Unless the patient is very thin and in the hands of a very experienced physician, fluoroscopic or ultrasonographic guidance is often required. The approach can be medial, anterior, or lateral.

- **Medial approach:** The needle enters just below the adductor longus in the groin and advances in the cephalad direction. The needle tip enters the joint through the anteroinferior joint capsule. The hip can be placed in abduction, external rotation, and slight flexion to facilitate the procedure.
- **Anterior approach:** The needle enters anteriorly about one finger width lateral to the femoral artery pulse and distal to the inguinal ligament. The needle advances posteriorly, with cephalad and medial direction. It enters the joint through the anterior joint capsule.
- **Lateral approach:** The needle enters the area proximal to the tip of the greater trochanter. The needle advances medially and in a slightly cephalad direction. It enters the joint through the lateral joint capsule. This approach travels the longest distance and is not practical in larger patients.

12. **How can I be sure the needle is in the hip joint?**

- Rotate the hip joint gently. You should feel the needle scratching on the femoral head. If it is fixed, the needle may have penetrated the articular cartilage of the acetabulum or the femoral head.
- Use fluoroscopic or ultrasonographic observation to ensure that the tip of the needle is between the femoral head and the acetabulum.
- Use an obturator during needle insertion to avoid soft tissue plugging the needle lumen.
- If there is no fluid aspirated, inject 0.5–1 mL of normal saline, and then disconnect the syringe. The saline will backflow quickly when the needle tip is in the joint.
- Confirm negative hip aspiration by injecting arthrographic dye.

13. **What is the approach for knee joint aspiration?**

Commonly, the joint can be approached in two ways, superolateral or anteromedial:

- **Superolateral approach:** One can insert the needle just under the superolateral corner of the patella, with the knee in full extension. The needle is advanced medially into the suprapatellar pouch or slightly distally into the patellofemoral junction.
- **Anteromedial approach:** With the knee in 90 degrees of flexion, one can insert the needle into the triangle formed by the patellar tendon, the medial femoral condyle, and the medial tibial plateau. The needle will go straight into the medial knee joint.

KEY POINTS: JOINT ASPIRATION AND INJECTION

1. Joint aspiration is an important orthopaedic management tool for joint problems in children.

2. A carefully executed and timely joint aspiration can give precious information for diagnosis and treatment of the joint or other systemic diseases.

3. With the assistance of modern fluoroscopic and ultrasonographic images, one can add accuracy of the needle placement in the joint.

4. Intra-articular injection can offer direct treatment of intra-articular disease when properly utilized.

14. **What is the approach for ankle joint aspiration?**
    The ankle joint can be easily and safely entered anterolateral to the dorsalis pedis pulse. The needle enters proximal to the talus in a straight posterior direction into the ankle joint. In a smaller child, precautions should be taken not to enter the distal tibial epiphyseal plate, which is only a short distance from the joint line.

15. **What is the approach for toe joint aspiration?**
    With the toe in slight flexion and distracted by being pulled distally, the small needle can enter dorsomedially or dorsolaterally.

16. **What should I observe and test once the joint fluid has been aspirated?**
    You should describe the general characteristics of the gross appearance. The aspirated fluid is inspected for viscosity by the string test, looking for clarity, color, and the presence of blood or fat droplets. The aspirated fluid is then placed in different containers and sent for laboratory tests, depending on the differential diagnosis. In general, testing often includes a cell count with differential, an immunologic test for arthritis, and analysis of glucose and protein. A smear for Gram stain and a bacterial culture are ordered when infection is suspected.

BIBLIOGRAPHY

1. Park AL, Dlabach JA: Infectious arthritis. In Canale ST (ed): Campbell's Operative Orthopaedics, 10th ed. St. Louis, Mosby, 2003, pp 685–711.
2. Pfenninger JL: Infection of joints and soft tissue: Part I and Part II: general guidelines and guidelines for specific joints. Am Fam Physician 44:1196–1202, 1991.
3. Pfenninger JL: Infection of joints and soft tissue: Part II: Guidelines for specific joints. Am Fam Physician 44:1690–1701, 1991.
4. Staheli LT: Fundamentals of Pediatric Orthopedics, 3rd ed. Philadelphia, Lippincott, Williams & Wilkins, 2003, pp 153–164.
5. Tachdjian MO: Clinical Pediatric Orthopedics: Art of Diagnosis and Principles of Management. East Norwalk, CT, Appleton & Lange, 1997, pp 200–204.

CHAPTER 17

PREVENTION OF INJURY

Severino R. Bautista, Jr., MD, and John M. Flynn, MD

1. **What is the most common cause of death in children worldwide?**
   Trauma is the major cause of death in children over 1 year of age and the major cause of morbidity among children of all ages. It is estimated that approximately 20% of worldwide fatalities in children under the age of 15 (i.e., 650,000 child deaths) are traced to unintentional injuries due to road traffic injuries, drowning, falls, burns, and poisonings. Those who suffered injuries that did not result in death often had permanent disabilities. Environment plays a crucial role in both the occurrence and the severity of an injury. Most injuries take place in or near a child's home, where unsafe play areas and play apparatuses may be found.

2. **Why are children more vulnerable to injuries than adults?**
   The relative small size of children makes it difficult for motorists to see them, increasing their risk of being run over. Behaviorally, children explore things by touching and putting them in their mouths; impulsive behavior may lead to unintentional injuries. Older children often seek new adventures with immature and poor judgment and can be exposed to situations that may lead to serious injury.

3. **How common are farm injuries?**
   Farm injuries are an important cause of mortality and morbidity worldwide. Farm children are exposed to work-related injury even if they are not directly involved in work activities. Every year, it is estimated that more than 100,000 children younger than 20 years of age are seen in various emergency departments due to farm injuries. More than 50% of victims die before reaching a hospital. Boys outnumber girls 3:1, and head injuries occurred in 64% of fatalities. The most common causes of agricultural injury are due to tractor and farm machinery, followed by injuries from animals, falls, and burns. Extremity fractures are the most common injuries, with the upper extremity being more frequently involved than the lower. Amputations are the most common cause of long-term morbidity, the result of 40% of farm injuries.

4. **How can farm injuries be prevented and minimized?**
   By encouraging the compilation of data concerning farm trauma in children and thus increasing awareness of the problem. Guidelines, such as those provided by the North American Guidelines for Children's Agricultural Tasks (NAGCAT), have provided educational intervention to assist farm parents and workers in appropriate and safe work for their children. Encourage the use of safety devices on augers and power take-offs, and support public awareness campaigns to discourage children from sitting on the fenders of tractors and riding dangerous equipment. Other strategies include parental education with regard to the physical and emotional capabilities of children, environment and mechanical protection, technical education, and adult supervision.

5. **What is the epidemiology of bicycle trauma in North America?**
   The greatest number of injuries to children occur when they are actually riding the bikes. Broken arms and wrists are common. The accident rate in the United States for bicycle injuries is 200 minor injuries per 100,000 bicyclists each year, 85 severe injuries per 100,000 bicyclists each year, and 2 fatal bicycle accidents per 100,000 bicyclists each year.

6. **What age group is most vulnerable to death and injury from bicycle riding?**
    Children ages 10–14 years and those under age 5 years are five times more likely to be injured in a bicycle-related crash than older riders. Children in these age groups represent 36% of all bicycle riders but have a death rate of more than two times the death rate of all bicycle riders. Male riders aged 10–14 years have the highest death rate from bicycle-related head injury at all ages. Ninety percent of all deaths involving bicycles are secondary to collision with a motor vehicle. Head injuries are the most common cause of death and the most common reason for hospitalization. Bicyclists actually have a higher incidence of severe head injuries than motorcyclists.

7. **What is the most common risk factor responsible for bicycle injuries in children under 10 years of age?**
    Children under 10 years are most frequently injured in midblock rideouts. This occurs when the child rides out of the end of a driveway in the middle of a block into oncoming traffic.

8. **In the age group of 11- to 19-year-olds, what is the most common cause of bicycle accidents?**
    Falling off the bike and colliding with a fixed object such as a wall or with another bicycle.

9. **What is the most common musculoskeletal injury resulting from a bicycle accident? How can it be prevented?**
    Eighty-five percent of all bicycle injuries involve the shoulder or upper extremity. "Bicycle shoulder" may occur when the bicycle is suddenly stopped and the rider is thrown over the handle bars. Bicyclists can try to prevent this problem by keeping a tight grip on the handle bars and being taught to roll with the bike, allowing it to absorb some force of the fall. Emphasis should be given to using protective safety equipment such as helmets and elbow pads to minimize injuries.

10. **What can be done to decrease the incidence of bicycle injuries?**
    Since most injuries result from rider error, rider-skill courses may be of value. Riding on the right side of the road with traffic, as well as learning the rules of the road and obeying all traffic laws, can decrease chances of being hit by a motor vehicle. Wearing a properly fitted helmet at all times and using reflective material and a visible light when riding at night can decrease the rate of injury. Use of designated bicycle trails also decreases injury rates.

11. **Does the use of helmets by motorcyclists and bicyclists decrease the mortality rate in accidents?**
    The death rate for motorcycle accidents was 15 per 10,000 in the 1960s and has now fallen to 1–16 per 10,000 in areas enforcing universal helmet laws. Bicycle helmets can effectively reduce serious head injuries by up to 85%.

12. **Have automobile restraint systems prevented morbidity and mortality in children?**
    Infant car seats properly restrained and placed in the rear seat, facing the rear, will protect an infant. From 1975–2004, it is estimated that safety belts saved 195,382 lives, of which 7472 were children. In 2004 alone, seat belts were estimated to have saved 15,434 lives, of which 451 were children under the age of 5 years. In 2004, 7810 vehicle passengers aged 14 years and younger were involved in fatal crashes. Fifty percent of fatal injuries were unrestrained.

13. **When, where, and how are restraint systems used?**
    All states require that all children wear seat belts whenever traveling in a vehicle. In 2005, there was 82% compliance with seat belt usage among Americans, compared to 71% in 2000. This increase in seat belt use has prevented an estimated 540 fatalities and 8000 serious injuries

and has saved $1.8 billion in economic costs. Approved safety profiles based on weight and height are as follows:

- **<20 lb:** Rear-facing infant seat
- **20–40 lb:** Forward-facing toddler seat
- **40–60 lb:** Booster seat with lap belt
- **>60 lb:** Regular lap belt
- **>48 in:** Shoulder strap with belt

14. **Are air bags effective in preventing injury in children?**

The air bag has been very effective in reducing trauma in adults and teenagers. In young children, however, the force of the explosion of the bag has the potential to cause sudden hyperextension of the cervical spine, and in younger children the bag may obstruct breathing. Children under the age of 12 years are safest when properly placed and buckled in the back seat of a motor vehicle. This will prevent any possible trauma from the sudden explosion of the bag.

15. **How common are playground injuries?**

Fractures were the most commonly reported injury on public and home playground equipment. Most fractures involve the elbow, forearm, and wrist and occur on public equipment such as climbing equipment, swings, and slides. A study conducted for the U.S. Consumer Safety Commission revealed that more than 200,000 children under the age of 14 years were seen in emergency rooms for playground-related injuries from 1998 to 1999. It is estimated that about 17 children each year under the age of 15 years die from injuries sustained at playgrounds (according to the 1990–2000 census). The majority of deaths are caused by strangulation, and the rest result from falls to the playground surface.

16. **What preventive measures can be taken to minimize falls for children?**

It is difficult to modify children's behavior; hence, the environment needs to be adapted. Playground modification, including guidelines for playground equipment, has contributed to a decrease in falls at playgrounds. The use of rubber or shredded rubber provides the best material to absorb the impact of falls. The use of wood chips or sand around playground equipment provides minimal protection and has been shown to be ineffective in cushioning falls enough to decrease injury rates. In high-rise apartment buildings, the incidence of falls out of windows can be minimized by window guards and window modifications. Falls down stairs have been reduced by discouraging the use of infant walkers.

17. **Why are playground guidelines focused on height and construction?**

The height of playground equipment is the most important contributing factor to most severe nonfatal injuries. There is no consensus on safe playground height, but it is recommended that equipment heights should range from 1.5 to 4.0 m. Replacing unsafe playground equipment with safe equipment, according to established standards, has been shown to decrease injuries almost by half.

18. **What areas of prevention must take top priority in preventing spinal cord injuries in children?**

Prevention programs should focus on the most common causes of spinal cord injury in children: motor vehicle accidents, gunshot injuries, and contact sports such as hockey and football. Improvements in motor vehicle child restraints have been helpful. A high degree of suspicion for cervical spinal cord injury is warranted in children with sporting injuries or signs of abuse. Modification of athletic rules, such as abolishing checking from behind in hockey and spearing in football, can decrease the incidence of spinal cord trauma in sports.

19. **What anatomic and biomechanical differences account for the different patterns of spinal injuries seen in children, compared to adults?**

The ligaments, discs, and surrounding tissue structures are less elastic and the musculature is more developed in adults, as compared to children. These important features make the pediatric spine more resilient to injury. Spinal injuries in the very young child are not common as compared with older children and adults. The relatively large head size of children and the horizontally oriented facets in the upper cervical spine with increased laxity make spinal cord injury without radiographic abnormality more common in children than in adults.

20. **Is it possible to prevent atlantoaxial spinal cord injury in children with marked ligamentous laxity?**

Atlantoaxial instability occurs in a number of syndromes characterized by marked ligamentous laxity. For instance, children with Down syndrome are at higher risk in sports where there may be hyperflexion of the cervical spine. The American Academy of Pediatrics has suggested these guidelines for minimizing trauma to the atlantoaxial region:

- All children with Down syndrome who desire to train or compete in at-risk sports should first obtain flexion-extension radiographs of the lateral cervical spine to determine the atlantodens interval (ADI).
- If the ADI is greater than 4.5 mm or if odontoid dysplasia is present, at-risk sports should be avoided and regular follow up should begin.
- If the ADI is greater than 4.5 mm and abnormal neurologic signs are present, it is recommended that the child be evaluated for C1–C2 fusion.

21. **How is it possible to prevent further cervical trauma during the transport of infants with cervical spine injuries?**

In the emergency care of children with spinal cord injury, the spine must be stabilized to prevent further damage to the spinal cord. Upper-cervical spine injuries are more common in infants due to the larger size of their heads and the horizontal orientation of the facet joints. These factors exert forces on the upper aspect of the cervical spine. When transporting these infants, the transport board should have a cutout in order to accommodate the occiput so that flexion of the head is minimized.

22. **What is the major problem that prevents spinal-cord–injured children from regaining their full potential?**

The greatest barriers to regaining a full and productive life are impairments and disabilities secondary to the spinal cord injury, such as severe scoliosis, chronic renal infection, or pressure sores. These can be prevented through a good orthopaedic rehabilitation program, proper hygiene, and an improved understanding of stable seating.

23. **How common are spinal cord injuries?**

It is estimated that there are 32 spinal cord injuries per million population, or 11,0000 injuries in the United States, per year. Of these, 82% are male and 18% are female, with 52% resulting in paraplegia and 47% in quadriplegia. The most rapidly increasing cause of injuries is penetrating injury and violence (i.e., gunshot injury), with vehicular accident injuries decreasing in number.

24. **Why are all-terrain vehicles such a major hazard to inexperienced childhood riders?**

The three-wheeled all-terrain vehicle is very unstable and easily tipped over by the inexperienced driver. As a result of their involvement in thousands of deaths and severe injuries, this vehicle was banned in 1988 in North America. There have been recommendations to ban the four-wheel all-terrain vehicle due to its propensity to flip backward, causing severe closed head injuries and paraplegia. Injuries that most commonly require medical care are orthopaedic, head, and facial injures. Injury prevention can be increased by not having children less than 16 years of age use the vehicle, using protective gear for the head and eyes, and avoiding nighttime driving, driving under the influence of alcohol, or having a passenger on the vehicle.

25. **In most major trauma centers in North America, what is the most common cause of amputation in young children? How can it be prevented?**
The most recent studies of amputations have revealed that the power lawn mower now accounts for the majority of amputations in children less than 10 years of age. Young children should not be allowed to ride on lawn mowers, either alone or accompanied by an adult. Injury can be due to loss of mower stability, blade contact, and layout and function of mower controls, as well as running over or backing over children. Each year, approximately 9400 children younger than 18 years are brought to emergency departments for lawn-mower–related injuries. Changing the design of lawn mowers to improve safety, issuing appropriate age and maturity guidelines for mower operators, and distributing proper education to avoid and prevent accidents related to lawn mowers can help prevent these injuries.

26. **What is the major cause of skiing accidents in children and adolescents?**
Most catastrophic pediatric skiing injuries result from collisions with stationary objects. The two high-risk groups are beginners and experienced male skiers. The main reasons for such injuries are excessive speed and loss of control. Lower-extremity injuries have decreased over the past decade with improved equipment, but upper-extremity injuries have not. Most injuries result from impact with the snow surface or a bending or twisting motion of the lower extremities during falls. The injury rate is highest in beginners, with 20–40% of total injuries occurring in children under 16 years of age.

27. **What activities predispose to stress fracture of the pars interarticularis in adolescent athletes?**
Over the past decade, there has been an increased interest by North American adolescent athletes in highly competitive sports such as gymnastics, weightlifting, and figure skating, as well as traditional team sports such as hockey and football. This has resulted in increased training and competition time. Participation to an extreme (i.e., hours of practice daily with frequent stressful competition) may be required of the adolescent athlete to excel at a national level. All of these training exercises, as well as the actual sport, involve frequent flexion and extension of the lumbar spine. The L5 pars interarticularis experiences considerable stress over a small area. The cross-sectional area of the pars at L5 measures 0.75 cm^2, for a total cross-sectional area of 1.5 cm^2 for each neural arch. It has been demonstrated by Hutton and coworkers that *in vitro* cyclical stress loading will produce fractures of the pars after as few as 1536 cycles at a force of 570 ± 190 newtons in a vertebral column taken from a 14-year-old child. The tensile and sheer forces across the pars interarticularis in normal flexion and extension have been calculated to be on the order of 400–630 N. Thus, it is quite conceivable that with numerous flexion-extension movements, such as in the training of a gymnast, this area of the vertebrae is indeed exposed to the dangers of fatigue fracturing.

28. **How can this injury be prevented in high-level adolescent athletes?**
Parents and coaches must take responsibility for preventing injuries in child athletes by understanding each individual's health needs, recognizing dangerous field conditions, and ensuring the use of protective athletic equipment. Since abnormal stress such as vigorous training involving multiple flexion-extensions of the lumbar spine does increase the incidence of microfractures, coaches should be taught to avoid extensive exercising involving these training methods. Persistent back pain in athletes involved in high-level competitive sports, such as gymnastics, should never be dismissed since identification of the fatigue fracture at an early stage may facilitate healing using a lumbosacral orthosis. It should be emphasized that

oblique radiographs may not show the lesion, and a bone scan is often necessary to demonstrate the increased uptake in the region of the stress fracture in the pars interarticularis. Stretching and age-appropriate training are also essential in preventing injuries.

KEY POINTS: PREVENTION OF INJURY

1. Trauma is the most common cause of injury and death in children worldwide.

2. Traumatic accidents are most often due to poorly designed equipment, mismatch of equipment to child size, and inexperience of the child in avoiding dangerous situations. Education of parents and children and a better design of equipment can decrease the incidence of injuries.

3. Children with suspected cervical spine injuries should be immobilized on size-appropriate equipment and followed closely.

4. Small children should be kept away from all power equipment such as lawnmowers and farm equipment. These are the most common causes of amputations in children.

29. **What risk factors can predispose female athletes to anterior cruciate ligament (ACL) injury?**
With increased participation of the female athlete in organized sports has come an increasing number of sports injuries. Risk factors such as lower-limb alignment, intercondylar notch shape and width, ligament size, joint laxity, hormonal effects, and muscle strength predispose girls to ACL injury. It has been suggested that strength training programs target the hips, trunk, and knees, as well as increase knee flexion and decrease knee valgus flexion. Specific jump-training programs combined with weight training, plyometrics, and stretching can help decrease the incidence of injury. Lastly, prescreening of female athletes may help identify those at risk for injury and start them on quadriceps and hamstring strengthening and knee-stabilizing exercises.

30. **How is it possible to reduce and prevent the incidence of recurrent fractures of the lower extremities in children with severe osteogenesis imperfecta or in children with osteoporosis secondary to paraplegia?**
Severe osteogenesis imperfecta and disuse osteoporosis may result in frequent fracturing of lower-extremity bones when the child assumes upright weight bearing. To prevent such breaking and to provide simple comfortable standing, specialized orthosis, such as vacuum pants, can be used. This can be augmented by standing devices such as the standing frame and the parapodium for young children to allow the child to safely bear weight. Bone densitometry studies of the tibia have revealed an increase in both mineral content and bone density above that expected for growth alone in patients with osteogenesis imperfecta, who can safely bear weight with these devices. In older children, this can be facilitated by intramedullary rodding of the femur and tibia in order to provide more intrinsic support and, again, to facilitate weight-bearing and the stimulation of new bone formation through Wolff's law.

31. **How can the increasing epidemic of gunshot trauma in children be minimized and prevented?**
The majority of such injuries are due to children obtaining handguns in the home. Preventing this requires input not only from the pediatric care teams but also from public health officials, social workers, and child-protection teams. All children with these injuries should be admitted to

a hospital for appropriate social service and child-protection-team intervention. Education of the whole family is required, including children, whenever there is a gun in the home. Areas of the country characterized by high rates of firearm ownership have the highest rate of unintentional firearm injury to children. Some types of firearm control may minimize gunshot injuries in children. Many states have passed laws regulating firearms, but no law was associated with a statistically significant decrease in firearm homicide rates.

Glatt K: Child-to-child unintentional injury and death from firearms in the United States: What can be done? J Pediatr Nurs 20:448–452, 2005.

Rosengart M, Cummings P, et al: An evaluation of state firearm regulations and homicide and suicide death rates. Inj Prev 11(2):77–83, 2005.

32. How are ice cream trucks implicated in injuries to children?

Ice cream trucks have tremendous appeal to children. Children become unaware of their surroundings and are drawn to the music and bells of the ice cream trucks, making them a dangerous attraction. These trucks are large and box-like. When they park on the side of the street, they block the vision of both the child customer and the driver of the passing motor vehicle. Obstructed vision is an important etiologic environment problem in the majority of pedestrian versus motor vehicle accidents involving children.

33. What can be done to minimize injuries sustained with sledding?

The combination of high speed, an uncontrollable sled, and an unsafe environment can lead to severe internal injuries, head trauma, and extremity fractures in children. The collision of sledders with stationary objects or moving cars is the most frequent cause of severe morbidity. Injuries can be kept to a minimum by selecting a safe sledding location, by proper positioning of the sledder, and with the use of safety-standard equipment such as flexible metal runners, protective guards, and an intact steering mechanism; the use of inner tubes, saucers, or disks should be avoided.

34. How can injuries to children participating in in-line skating be minimized?

A recent review of in-line skating has revealed that upper-extremity injuries are common in children and beginners, especially in the pediatric age group. Injuries can be minimized by wearing protective gloves, wrist guards, knee pads, and helmets; by riding on smooth surfaces without traffic; and by providing supervision and training.

35. How can pediatric firework injuries be prevented?

In the year 2000, it was reported that 9000 people were treated for firework-related injuries. This was a decrease from the 12,000 injuries reported in 1990. Children less than 14 years of age have a high rate of injury, which is believed to be due to their innate curiosity and limited understanding of the dangers involved in handling such devices. It is believed that the decline in injury rates from 1990–2000 was due to increased restriction on the sale and use of fireworks by minors. Enforcement of existing laws and introduction of new restrictions on distribution and the power of fireworks have been recommended to further reduce the number of injuries from these devices.

36. How can injuries from horseback riding be minimized?

The most serious injuries from horseback riding are to the spine and head, with common injuries ranging from bruises, strains, and sprains to fractures of the upper extremities. Most injuries can be prevented or minimized by having riders wear riding helmets. Novice riders should take lessons and should be supervised on all occasions. The horse should be matched to the rider's age, skill, experience, and size. Children should consider using safety stirrups that break away from the horse as well as wearing proper riding attire. Novice riders are advised to ride on open terrain and to avoid stunts and jumps.

BIBLIOGRAPHY

1. Baker SP, O'Neill B, Ginsburg MJ, Li G: The Injury Fact Book, 2nd ed. New York, Oxford University Press, 1992.

2. Bernardo L, Gardner M, Rogers K: Pediatric sledding injuries in Pennsylvania. J Trauma Nursing 5:34–39, 1998.

3. Bull MJ, Sheese J: Update for the pediatrician on child passenger safety: Five principles for safer travel. Pediatrics 106:1113–1116, 2000.

4. Committee On Injury and Poison Prevention: Lawn mower related injuries to children. Pediatrics 107:1480–1481, 2001.

5. Cushman R: Injury prevention: The time has come. CMAJ 152(1):21–23, 1995.

6. Drkulec JA, Letts M: Snowboarding injuries in children. Can J Surg 44:435–439, 2001.

7. Flynn JM, Lou JE, Ganley : Prevention of sports injuries in children. Curr Opin Pediatr 14:719–722, 2002.

8. Flynn JM, Lou JE, Ganley F: Exercise and children's health. Curr Sports Med Rep 1:349–353, 2002.

9. Friede AM, Azzara CV, Gallager SS, Guyer B: The epidemiology of injuries to bicycle riders. Pediatr Clin North Am 32:141–151, 1985.

10. Keenan H, Bratton S: All-terrain vehicle legislation for children: A comparison of a state with a sate without a helmet law. Pediatrics 4:330–334, 2004.

11. Letts M, Kaylor D, Gouw G: A biomechanical analysis of halo fixation in children. J Bone Joint Surg 708:277–279, 1988.

12. Letts M, Monson R, Weber K: The prevention of recurrent fractures of the lower extremities in several osteogenesis imperfecta using vacuum pants. J Pediatr Orthop 8:454–458, 1988.

13. Letts M, Smallman T, Afanasiev R, Gouw G: Fractures of the pars interarticularis in adolescent athletes: A clinical-biomechanical analysis. J Pediatr Orthop 6:40–46, 1986.

14. Letts M, Stevens L, Coleman J, Kettner R: Puppetry and doll play—An adjunct of pediatric orthopaedics. J Pediatr Orthop 3:605–609, 1983.

15. Letts RM, Gammon W: Auger injuries in children. Can Med Assoc J 118:519–522, 1978.

16. Loder R, Brown K, Zaleske D, Jones E: Extremity lawn-mower injuries in children: Report by the Research Committee of the Pediatric Orthopaedic Society of North America. J Pediatr Orthop 17:360–369, 1997.

17. Mack M, Sacks J, Thompson D: Testing the impact attenuation of loose playground surfaces. Inj Prevent 6:141–144, 2000.

18. Nguyen D, Letts M: In-line skating injuries in children: A 10 year review. J Pediatr Orthop 21:613–618, 2001.

19. Rowe BH, Rowe AM, Bota GW: Bicyclists and environmental factors associated with bicycle-related trauma in Ontario. Can Med Assoc J 45–51:152, 1995.

20. Spence LJ, Dykes EH, Bohn DJ, Wesson DE: Fatal bicycle accidents in children: A plea for prevention. J Pediatr Surg 28:214–216, 1993.

21. Stover E, Keller AS, Cobey J, Sopheap S: The medical and social consequences of landmines in Cambodia. JAMA 272:331–336, 1994.

22. Stucky W, Loder RT: Extremity gunshot wounds in children. J Pediatr Orthop 11:64–71, 1991.

23. Trautwein LC, Smith DG, Rivara FP: Pediatric amputation injuries: Etiology, cost, and outcome. J Trauma 41:831–838, 1996.

24. University of Alabama National Spinal Cord Injury Statistical Center, March 2002.

EVALUATION OF THE INJURED CHILD

Severino R. Bautista, Jr., MD, and John M. Flynn, MD

1. **What are the skeletal features of the growing child that must be considered in evaluation?**

   Features unique to the growing child include the presence of perosseous cartilage in the epiphysis of long bones and growth plates or physes. The periosteum in children is much thicker, more active, and less readily torn than in adults and can be easily stripped from the bone. It has an enormous osteogenic potential that declines in the teenage years as growth ceases. Bone remodeling can occur after injury through continued physeal growth and bone remodeling. The biomechanical properties of the cartilaginous physis make injury through the growth plate highly likely as compared to ligamentous injury.

2. **How does the age of the child influence injury patterns due to falls?**

   The head is disproportionately large at birth, with a ratio of head height to total height of 1:4. Falls from a height in younger children tend to be head-first patterns, with a higher rate of head and neck injuries as well as a higher rate of upper-extremity injuries when they try to shield their fall. Older children tend to have a higher rate of lower-extremity, pelvic, and thoracolumbar spine injuries.

3. **What are some mechanical influences on growth?**

   The application of forces to the growing skeleton can improve or worsen deformities in children. Wolff's law states that bone alters its shape in response to the stresses placed on it. Hueter-Volkmann's law says that excessive compression inhibits physeal growth, but tension or distraction across the physis accelerates growth.

4. **What are important features in the history of the mechanism of injury that should be obtained from the parents or emergency rescue personnel?**

   The size of the child and the orientation of the force are important elements. Depending on the size and position of the child, different injuries may be produced. The treating physician should note whether the child was on a motor vehicle or bicycle, whether he or she was walking or running, and whether the child was wearing a helmet at the time he or she was struck. Other important features would be an estimation of the height of the fall and the type of surface that the child struck.

5. **What key elements of the history must be noted to avoid missing a case of child abuse?**

   A history of previous trauma is important. The mechanism of injury should make sense when considered in relation to the child's age and injury. Incompatibility of history with mechanism of injury greatly leads to a suspicion of child abuse. Up to 50% of long-bone fractures in children younger than 1 year and 90% in children younger than 6 months are the result of nonaccidental injury. A careful social history should be obtained, focusing on the presence of new individuals in the house, a history of substance abuse among the caretakers, and other household socioeconomic stresses. The child's skin should be thoroughly examined because cutaneous injuries (i.e., burns, contusions, lacerations, and abrasions) are the most common manifestations of child abuse. Careful, timely documentation is vital for later use of the information (e.g., in a court setting).

6. **What are common red flags seen during physical examination for children suspected of child abuse?**

An abused child may have soft tissue injuries, rib fractures, or other long-bone fractures in various stages of healing. Other red flags include femur fractures in children who are less than walking age, metaphyseal corner fractures, and a delay in seeking medical attention.

7. **How common is serious, life-threatening trauma in children?**

The World Health Organization (WHO) estimates that, worldwide, 685,000 children under the age of 15 are killed annually by unintentional injuries (approximately 20% of all childhood fatalities). Most are from road traffic injuries, drowning, burns, falls, and poisoning. Motor vehicle collisions are the leading cause of mortality for children aged 3–14 years. In all age groups, occupant injuries are the most deadly. Every day in the United States, an average of 6 children aged 14 years and younger are killed and 673 children are injured in motor vehicle crashes. Since 1994, 1479 children have died from school-transportation-related crashes (an average of 134 fatalities per year); since 1994, 182 school-age pedestrians have died in school-transportation-related crashes.

8. **What risk factors predisposes children to trauma?**

Risk factors associated with a higher likelihood of childhood injury include a lower socioeconomic status, living in an area with increased population density, maternal smoking, single-parent families, and attention deficit disorder, with the peak ages for fracture being within 6–9 years old, and with males at greater risk than females. Environmental risk factors include areas with a high volume of traffic and crime or with poorly built playgrounds, activities with motorized equipment, and an improper pediatric seating configuration in a vehicle.

9. **What are common mechanisms of serious injury in children?**

The most common mechanism of serious injury in a child is being struck by a car while walking or on a bicycle. This mechanism accounts for approximately 80% of significant injuries in children. The next-most-common mechanism is being an unrestrained passenger in a motor vehicle accident. Finally, falls, collisions with trains or other heavy equipment, injuries from lawnmowers, and injuries sustained as passengers on motorcycles make up the remaining most common mechanisms.

10. **How is force transmitted to the pedestrian struck by a vehicle?**

Force transmission has three phases: (1) vehicular bumper impact, (2) vehicular hood and windshield impact, and (3) ground impact. The initial bumper impact usually results in lower-extremity injuries such as a tibia or femur fracture. Head and torso injuries occur as the pedestrian strikes the hood and windshield. Further injuries to the head and torso can occur as the victim falls from the vehicle to the ground or is accelerated into another object.

11. **What is a lap-belt injury?**

The lap belt, when worn without the shoulder harness, predisposes the thoraco-lumbar spine to a hyperflexion injury, which in children may not only cause a typical transverse fracture through the vertebral body and spinous process (i.e., a Chance fracture) but also may result in an atypical fracture line running through the disk or the vertebral apophysis. There are often associated injuries to the abdominal viscera. Occasionally, the shoulder lap belt, when not applied properly, may produce similar forces leading to injury at the cervicothoracic junction.

12. **What are the priorities of the emergency department evaluation?**

The physical examination should be directed by the history obtained from the caregiver or emergency personnel. If the injury is of high energy, the basic ABCDE evaluation (airway, breathing, circulation, disability, exposure) should be conducted. Once the child is determined to have an adequate airway, a functional breathing exchange, a palpable pulse, a normal temperature, and adequate blood pressure, the overall neurologic status should be evaluated and all clothing should be removed to allow for full examination.

13. **What is a secondary survey?**
It is a detailed reexamination of all systems to detect non-life-threatening injury done after primary assessment. It includes careful palpation of all body regions, use of appropriate diagnostic tests, and request for pertinent radiographs, as well as abdominal computerized tomography for blunt trauma. These are then followed by repeat physical examination as soon as the patient recovers to rule out missed skeletal injury.

14. **What is the normal blood pressure value in an injured child?**
See Table 18-1.

TABLE 18-1. NORMAL VALUES FOR BLOOD PRESSURE BY AGE

Age	Blood Pressure (mmHg)	
	Systolic	Diastolic
Full-term infant	60 (45)*	35
3–10 days	70–75 (50)	40
6 months	95 (55)	45
4 years	98	57
6 years	110	60
8 years	112	60
12 years	115	65
16 years	120	65

*The numbers in parentheses refer to mean arterial blood pressure.
Data from Steward DJ: Manual of Pediatric Anesthesia. New York, Churchill-Livingstone, 1990, p 24; and Rasch DK, Webster DE: Clinical Manual of Pediatric Anesthesia. New York, McGraw-Hill, 1994, p 17.

15. **What are the normal values for heart rate in a noninjured child?**
Normal values for heart rate by age are provided in Table 18-2. In an agitated child, heart rate may increase 20–30 points more than the normal range.

16. **How does the physiologic response to trauma differ in children versus adults?**
Children have a number of physiologic differences when compared with adults that must be considered in a trauma situation. Young children have a dramatically higher metabolic rate and oxygen demand than do adults. Due to a relatively greater skin surface area, hypothermia, with its impact upon cardiac output and clotting, is a greater problem in children than in adults. Children have a smaller blood volume and will have a greater impact on their circulating blood volume for any given blood loss. Hemorrhagic shock is compensated for by tachycardia, masking significant blood loss as the blood pressure is sustained. Decompensation can occur rapidly, with profound hypotension and arrest in a child who moments ago seemed fine.

TABLE 18-2. NORMAL VALUES FOR HEART RATE BY AGE	
Age	Range (beats/min)
Newborn	110–150
1–11 months	80–150
2 years	85–125
4 years	75–115
6 years	65–110
8 years	60–110

Data from Rasch DK, Webster DE: Clinical Manual of Pediatric Anesthesia. New York, McGraw-Hill, 1994, p 16.

17. **After the initial survey is performed, how does the evaluation proceed?**
One should include a careful abdominal examination to detect injuries to the liver, spleen, pancreas, or kidney. In children, the rib cage is more pliable, abdominal muscles are not well developed, and solid organs are proportionately larger. Surface bruising from externally directed trauma or a seatbelt should be looked for. Sites of potential external bleeding are assessed. Extremity swelling, deformity, open wounds, discoloration, or crepitus is noted. Palpation of the compartments should be performed in both the upper and lower extremities. Passive range of motion can also help identify compartment syndrome. Active motor function and sensory function are important indicators of neurologic status and must be assessed at an age-appropriate level. These basic observations should be followed by an evaluation for pelvic instability.

18. **What are the key components of the spinal exam?**
The child who has a history of significant trauma and presents on a backboard should be carefully log-rolled at the end of the secondary survey. The back should be evaluated for a palpable increase in the interspinous space, flank contusions, the existence of a kyphotic or an excessively lordotic deformity, and the presence of open wounds. A careful extremity neurologic examination for sensory changes in nerve root distributions, motor strength, and reflexes at the knee, ankle, triceps, and brachioradialis then follows. Newborns and very young children are more challenging. These children may complain of occipital headache with upper-cervical injury and may cradle their head with their hands. Attention should be focused especially on the upper cervical spine in children younger than 8 years. Noncontiguous spinal injury maybe present.

19. **Are there any other essential radiographic examinations needed for children with cervical spinal injury aside from plain radiographs?**
Unique anatomic characteristics make children susceptible to cervical spine injury. The pediatric patient has open physes and apophyses, which are relatively weaker and more prone to injury than the surrounding bone. The risk of nonosseous cervical spine injury is greater in children due to this reason. Plain radiography, including anteroposterior, lateral, and open-mouth views, is commonly used to clear patients involved in trauma. However, in many cases, this is not enough to rule out cervical spine injury due to the fact that plain radiography in children younger than 8 years of age is unsatisfactory. Most views may not be definitive due to the overlap of osseous structures in the cervical spine. Computed tomography (CT) scanning is a possible tool, but its ability to detect ligaments and soft tissue injury is limited. Magnetic resonance imaging (MRI) is a better modality for detecting cervical soft tissue injury in children and for

eliminating the uncertainty commonly encountered with CT scans and plain radiographs. The criteria for using MRI were for an obtunded or nonverbal child suspected of having cervical spine injury, equivocal palin films, neurologic symptoms without radiographic findings, and an inability to clear the cervical spine within 3 days, based on testing.

20. **How should fractures initially be managed?**
Immediately after completion of the initial ABCDE evaluation and secondary survey, limbs with deformity and crepitus should be aligned and appropriately splinted. Most emergency rooms have simple cardboard or air splints available for immobilization until appropriate radiographic examination can be completed and early treatment undertaken. If the patient is to be transferred to another facility, it is advisable that either splinting with well-padded plaster splints be applied or that traction be used.

21. **Should the parents be present for the evaluation in a trauma situation?**
This depends on the parent and the situation. Parents are extremely helpful in explaining the history, particularly of the injury and past medical events, current medications, allergies, and past surgical procedures. A cooperative, calm parent can often be helpful in managing the injured awake child. For the most seriously injured children, parents are generally best served by being escorted from the room, particularly when invasive procedures are necessary.

22. **What are the scoring systems used in evaluating a child with multiple injuries?**
The new injury severity score (NISS), the injury severity score (ISS), the Glasgow Coma Scale (GCS), the pediatric trauma score (PTS), the revised trauma score, and the pediatric risk of mortality (PRISM) are all useful for individual patient management and for trauma systems research. These are reliable tools for predicting prognosis of severely traumatized children.

23. **Is there an advantage to pediatric trauma centers?**
The improved outcome for children injured by trauma who are treated at pediatric trauma centers is well documented in the literature. The American College of Surgeons (ACS) has set standards for the level of trauma care that an institution should provide to be categorized as a pediatric trauma center. Currently, there are about 59 officially verified level 1 or level 2 pediatric trauma centers. Children with severe traumatic brain injury are more likely to survive if treated in a pediatric trauma center or an adult trauma center.

24. **When should a pediatric patient be transferred to a trauma center?**
The ACS has published guidelines for referral to a pediatric trauma center (Table 18-3). Another method of determining the necessity for transfer is a PTS score of 8 or a revised trauma score of less than 11.

25. **What are the prerequisites for sedation prior to conclusion of the evaluation?**
One of the prerequisites before sedation of the injured child to manage fracture or dislocation reduction and splinting is a completed medical evaluation, including the primary survey (airway, breathing, and circulation [ABCs]), the secondary survey, and the directed evaluation of extremity injuries.

26. **Should ketamine be used in the emergency room?**
Although ketamine has been used extensively for sedation in emergency patients, careful monitoring is required. Ketamine is generally best avoided in emergency patients without a protected airway. The patients may become deeply sedated and therefore must be carefully monitored. Emergence hallucinations are more common in children older than 10 years of age. Low-dose midazolam (0.05 mg/kg) can be used with ketamine in older children to reduce the risk of emergence reactions.

TABLE 18-3. GUIDELINES FOR REFERRAL TO A PEDIATRIC TRAUMA CENTER, FROM THE AMERICAN COLLEGE OF SURGEONS COMMITTEE ON TRAUMA

- More than one body system injury
- Injuries that require pediatric intensive care unit (ICU) care
- Shock that requires more than one blood transfusion
- Fractures with neurovascular injuries
- Fractures of the axial skeleton
- Two or more major long bone fractures
- Potential replantation of an amputated extremity
- Suspected or actual spinal cord injury
- Head injuries with any of the following:
  Orbital or facial bone fractures
  Altered state of consciousness
  Cerebrospinal fluid leaks
  Changing neurologic status
  Open head injuries
  Depressed skull fractures
  Requirements of intracranial pressure monitoring
  Ventilatory support required

KEY POINTS: EVALUATION OF THE INJURED CHILD

1. Growth plates can be the cause of unique injuries in children. They can aid recovery by remodeling the deformity after injury, or they can worsen the deformity due to injury to the growth plate.

2. Child abuse needs to be a consideration in long bone fractures in nonambulatory children or in children with repeat injuries that have an incompatible history with the injury at presentation.

3. Children have smaller blood volumes than adults and better compensatory mechanisms than adults. As a result, children may seem to be initially well following major trauma but have rapid and severe decompensation.

27. **What can be done to provide sedation and pain relief for outpatient fracture management?**
    The numerous techniques available in the emergency department are grouped into blocks, sedation, and dissociative anesthesia. The American Academy of Pediatrics has come out with guidelines for monitoring patients when sedation or dissociative anesthesia is used. Blocks consists of local and regional blocks such as hematoma blocks, nerve blocks, and intravenous regional anesthesia (i.e., the Bier block). Narcotics and benzodiazepines are widely used worldwide. Narcotics provide analgesia, whereas benzodiazepines act as primary sedatives.

These drugs act synergistically to induce controlled sedation and analgesia. In using these medicines, respiratory rate and blood pressure should be monitored periodically. Naloxone is used to reverse the narcotic effect, and flumazenil is used to reverse benzodiazepine. Ketamine is a widely used form of dissociative anesthesia.

28. **What are the risks of the use of the pediatric cocktail (Demerol, Phenergan, and Thorazine [DPT])?**
The mixture of meperidine (i.e., Demerol), promethazine (i.e., Phenergan), and chlorpromazine (i.e., Thorazine) still remains widely popular for the sedation of children worldwide. The sedation can be prolonged and profound, however. Additionally, hypotension is possible, along with severe respiratory depression. Most authors feel that there are better sedation drugs available.

29. **Are local anesthetics safe to be used in children?**
Local anesthetics should be used with caution in children. Toxic levels are easily achieved in children, and, especially in young children, few are able to tolerate local anesthesia only (Table 18-4).

TABLE 18-4. MAXIMUM RECOMMENDED DOSES OF LOCAL ANESTHETICS COMMONLY USED IN CHILDREN		
	Injection Dose (mg/kg)	
Agent	Plain	With Epinephrine*
Lidocaine[†] (Xylocaine)	5	7
Bupivacaine[‡]	2.5	3
Mepivacaine (Carbocaine)	4	7
Prilocaine[§]	5.5	8.5

*The addition of epinephrine (a vasoconstrictor) reduces the rate of local anesthetic absorption into the bloodstream, permitting the use of a higher dose.
[†]For intravenous (IV) regional anesthesia (i.e., Bier blocks), the maximum lidocaine dose is 3 mg/kg. Preservative-free lidocaine without epinephrine should be used for either Bier blocks or hematoma blocks.
[‡]Due to its cardiotoxicity, bupivacaine should never be used for IV regional anesthesia or for hematoma blocks.
[§]Of the amide local anesthetics, prilocaine is the least likely to produce central nervous system and cardiovascular toxicity. However, a by-product of prilocaine metabolism may lead to severe methemoglobinemia in young children. Prilocaine is, therefore, contraindicated in children younger than 6 months old.

30. **What is the best environment for the assessment of an injured child?**
For all but the most seriously injured unconscious children, the evaluation should take place in the most comfortable environment. The child should be supine on a comfortable stretcher or bed. The area should be as quiet as possible. The parents may be present, at least for the initial part of the evaluation. Appropriate wall coverings for children are often comforting, as are stuffed animals, a warm and caring nursing staff, and a comfortable room temperature.

31. **What are some secrets to decreasing anxiety in traumatized children?**
The most important part of evaluating children is speaking directly to them and giving them age-appropriate information about what you are going to do next. If a procedure will incur some pain, you should give the child a truthful and calm explanation of when, how, and why this will

occur. The details of the screening examination of the extremities should be explained while it is being conducted. Gentleness and calmness are the critical aspects of this section of the evaluation. Once the parent and patient have had the opportunity to describe the pain in their own terms, then the physician is best prepared to manage the problem.

BIBLIOGRAPHY

1. Brownstein DR, Rivara FP: Emergency medical services for children. In Behrman RE, Kliegman RM, Jenson HB (eds): Nelson Textbook of Pediatrics, 16th ed. Philadelphia, W.B. Saunders, 2000, pp 238–244.

2. Flynn JM, Closkey RF, Mahboubi S, Dormans JP: Role of magnetic imaging in the assessment of pediatric cervical spinal injuries. J Pediatric Orthop 22:573–577.

3. Flynn J, Wildmann R: The limping child: Evaluation and diagnosis. J Am Acad Orthop Surg 9(2):89–98, 2001.

4. Jones J, Feldman K, Bruckner J: Child abuse in infants with proximal physeal injuries of the femur. Pediatr Emerg Care 20:157–161,

5. Mann DC, Rajmaira S: Distribution of physeal and nonphyseal fractures in 2,650 long-bone fractures in children aged 0–16 years. J Pediatr Orthop 10:713–716, 1990.

6. Meier R, Krattek C, Grimme K, et al: The multiply injured child. Clin Ortho Rel Research 432:127–131, 2005.

7. Mizuta T, Benson WM, Foster BK, et al: Statistical analysis of the incidence of physeal injuries. J Pediatr Orthop 7:518–523, 1987.

8. National Center for Statistics and Analysis: Traffic Safety Facts 2004.

9. National Highway Traffic Safety Administration. Traffic Safety Facts 2004: Pedestrians. U.S. Department of Transportation, 2004.

10. Ogden JA: Injury to the growth mechanisms of the immature skeleton. Skeletal Radiol 6:237–253, 1981.

11. Peng R, Bongard F: Pedestrian versus motor vehicle accidents: An analysis of 5,000 patients. J Am Coll Surg 189:343–348, 1999.

12. Peterson CA, Peterson HA: Analysis of the incidence of injuries to the epiphyseal growth plate. J Trauma 12:275–281, 1972.

13. Rivara FP, Grossman D: Injury control. In Behrman RE, Kliegman RM, Jenson HB (eds): Nelson Textbook of Pediatrics, 16th ed. Philadelphia, W.B. Saunders, 2000, pp 232–238.

14. Rodriguez-Merchan E: Pediatric skeletal trauma. Clin Orthop Rel Res 432:8–13.

CHAPTER 19

CHILD VERSUS ADULT TRAUMA: MANAGEMENT PRINCIPLES

R. Jay Cummings, MD, and Kevin M. Neal, MD

1. **What challenges exist during the evaluation of pediatric trauma patients, compared to adult patients?**

   The child may not be old enough to give an accurate history of the mechanism. The child may regress emotionally in response to the trauma, which may cause him or her to be unwilling to give details of the mechanism or to comply with the exam, making detection and localization difficult. The physician caring for the child must develop a rapport not only with the child but with the parents as well.

2. **Does trauma lead to death and disability more commonly in children than in adults?**

   Yes. Trauma is the leading cause of death in children younger than 14 years of age. It accounts for 50% of all deaths in children, compared to 10% of all deaths in the population of the United States as a whole. Up to 100,000 children sustain permanent disability each year due to accidents.

3. **Is blunt trauma or penetrating trauma more common in children?**

   Blunt. Although blunt is more common in adults as well, a greater percentage of children sustain blunt versus penetrating trauma compared to adults. Blunt trauma in toddlers and infants is often due to child abuse. In older children, vehicular accidents and falls account for the majority of multiple injuries. In teenagers, the causes of these injuries closely mirror causes of adult injury, and, unfortunately, alcohol is now considered a major factor in over one-third of vehicle-related multiple trauma cases in this age group. Motor vehicle accidents, including auto-pedestrian accidents, are the most common mechanism of injury leading to death in children and adolescents, followed in decreasing order by drowning, house fires, and homicide.

4. **What is the most common cause of death in pediatric trauma victims?**

   Head trauma. Between 30% and 70% of trauma deaths in children are due to head injury.

5. **Why are children more susceptible to head and neck trauma than adults?**

   The head represents a larger proportion of the body in children, and their neck muscles are weaker, their joint capsules are more flexible, their skulls are thinner, and their scalps are more vascular than adults. The subarachnoid space is relatively smaller than in adults, decreasing buoyancy and offering less protection. On a positive note, children recover from head and neck trauma more often and more completely than adults.

6. **What is cervical spine pseudosubluxation?**

   Pseudosubluxation is apparent anterior translation of one vertebra on another in children. This occurs most commonly at C2–C3. This is evident in 40% of children under age 7 years and in 20% of children under age 16 years. It is important to differentiate this normal variant from trauma. It is more easily seen if the x-ray was taken with the neck flexed. About 3 mm of movement of one vertebra on another is normal in children. Clinical signs such as pain, step-off, crepitance, or neurologic deficits should raise the possibility of a real injury. Soft tissue swelling will usually be present on the lateral C-spine radiograph if trauma is present. A good rule of thumb is that 7 mm of soft tissue shadow is normal at C2, and 22 mm at C7. If there is any doubt about C-spine injury, immobilization precautions should be used until further evaluation can be obtained.

7. **What is the second most common cause of death in pediatric trauma victims?**
Intra-abdominal hemorrhage. Children's livers and spleens are proportionately larger than adults, and their ribs are more flexible and do not cover as great an area of the abdominal cavity as in adults.

8. **Are there any differences in fracture patterns between victims of child abuse and victims of trauma from other causes?**
Yes. Metaphyseal corner fractures are considered characteristic of a shaken infant. (They are not seen in adults.) Rib fractures occur in only 5% of children with multiple injuries from other causes, but they are more common in abuse. Rib fractures from compressive trauma to the thorax are usually lateral. Rib fractures from child abuse are more commonly posterolateral and adjacent to the transverse processes. Incidentally, the most common fracture in child abuse is a single transverse fracture of the femur or humerus.

9. **Are pulmonary problems more or less common in pediatric trauma victims, compared to adults?**
Less common. Fat embolism, deep vein thrombosis, and pulmonary embolism are all uncommon complications in children.

10. **What type of vertebral fracture is commonly seen in children who use adult lap belts in cars instead of car seats? What injuries are associated with it?**
Chance fractures are commonly seen with improper seatbelt use. In children, the lap belt may rest across the abdomen instead of the bony pelvis, as in adults. This creates a fulcrum as the child's body is thrown forward in an accident. Chance fractures are *flexion-distraction* injuries. The spinal elements are split horizontally. There is a high association with intra-abdominal injury, especially ruptured bowel and traumatic pancreatitis. Ecchymoses in a lap belt distribution should alert the physician to this possibility.

11. **What is Waddell's triad?**
This is a classic pattern of injury in pediatric auto-pedestrian accidents. The child is hit by a car, sustaining a femur fracture at bumper-level. The body is then thrown on the hood, causing an ipsilateral chest contusion, and then the body is thrown away from the car, causing a contralateral head injury.

12. **Are clinical signs of hypovolemia as reliable in children as in adults?**
No. Children compensate much more effectively for hypovolemia. Children may lose up to 25% of their total blood volume before minimal signs of hypovolemia are present. They may lose up to 45% before they become hypotensive. Decreased blood pressure indicates a state of uncompensated shock and is indicative of severe blood loss. Tachycardia and decreased skin perfusion are earlier signs of significant blood loss in children.

13. **Other than intravenous lines, central lines, and cutdown procedures, what type of vascular access can be obtained in children under age 6 years?**
Intraosseous fluid infusion. A special needle is inserted directly into the soft bone of the child's *uninjured* metaphysis, usually in the tibia. Large amounts of crystalloid can be given in this manner.

14. **Do children maintain their body temperature as effectively as adults?**
No. Children are more prone to hypothermia. They have a higher ratio of body-surface-to–mass, their skin is thinner, and they have smaller fat stores. These factors increase heat exchange with

the environment. Hypothermia can prolong acidosis, increase coagulation time, and affect nervous system function.

15. **Should children be immobilized on adult trauma boards?**
No. Since children have a larger head size relative to the body as compared with adults, they do not fit on adult trauma boards. Children of less than age 6 years require a board with a special cutout for the posterior skull. Otherwise, their C-spine is flexed forward abnormally. If they have a C-spine injury, this flexion could lead to neurologic compromise.

16. **Are children's bones more or less dense than adults?**
They are less dense and have greater porosity, partially due to a greater number of vascular channels and partially because the bone is less mineralized than in adults.

17. **Does the density of children's bones affect the way they fail compared to those of adults?**
Yes. Because they are less dense, they may fail without actually fracturing. This is called plastic deformation (Fig. 19-1). They may also fracture incompletely. When this occurs in compression, a buckle (or torus) fracture is produced. When this occurs in tension, a greenstick fracture is produced. Comminuted fractures are less common in children. When complete fractures occur in children, they are more often associated with a high-energy mechanism.

18. **What differences exist in the periosteum of children, compared to adults?**
The periosteum in children is thicker, more vascular, and more biologically active than that of adults. Because of this, children have a greater potential to reconstitute segmental bone defects that would persist in adults.

19. **Do displaced or angulated fractures remodel better in children or in adults?**
In children. Because of their thicker, more-active periosteum and their remaining growth potential, children's bones can remodel much more than those of adults. This allows children to correct significant displacement and angulation as they grow, especially if the angulation is in the plane of motion of the adjacent joint.

20. **Do children's fractures heal faster than fractures in adults?**
In general, yes. In fact, the younger the child, the faster the bones heal. A good rule of thumb is that it takes 6 weeks for children age 5 years and older to heal a bone. For younger children, it takes the child's age in years + 1 weeks for a bone to heal.

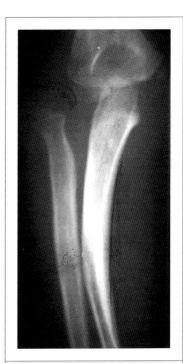

Figure 19-1. Anteroposterior x-ray of an elbow. Note the plastic deformation of the ulna, leading to dislocation of the radial head.

21. **Are delayed unions and nonunions more or less common in children than in adults?**
Less common. Again, because of children's better healing potential, delayed unions and nonunions are uncommon.

22. **Are there differences in injury patterns between children and adults that are directly related to open physes?**
Yes. Physes are made of cartilage, which is weaker than bone. The ligaments that attach near physes are often stronger than the cartilage of the physis. Therefore, injuries that would cause ligament sprains in adults often cause physeal injuries in children. A classic example is sustaining a Salter-Harris type I fracture of the lateral malleolus instead of an ankle sprain.

23. **Can children have fractures that cannot be seen on x-ray?**
Yes. Because physes are made of cartilage, they cannot be seen on x-ray. Some fractures pass through the physis without exiting the epiphysis or the metaphysis. These are classified as *Salter-Harris type I fractures*. Fractures can also pass through the portion of the epiphysis that remains unossified and may not be detectable on radiographs. Therefore, when children have pain localized to their growth centers, you must assume that a fracture exists until it is proven otherwise.

24. **Can the way children's physes ossify affect your ability to diagnose an injury?**
Yes. Epiphyses often have multiple ossification centers that begin to ossify at different times. They may also have peripheral accessory growth centers. These multiple sites of ossification are often mistaken for fractures. A radiographic atlas of normal development is helpful to rule out injury.

KEY POINTS: MANAGEMENT OF CHILDHOOD TRAUMA

1. Trauma is a major cause of pediatric death and disability in the United States.

2. Children have physiologic differences that make them more susceptible than adults to trauma.

3. Children respond differently—mentally and physiologically—to trauma.

4. Children's bones have different properties than adult bones. These include less density, the presence of growth plates, a thicker periosteum, and quicker healing times.

25. **Can children have injuries to soft structures without visible injury to the overlying bones?**
Yes. Again, because of the increased pliability of children's bones, they may give and allow damage to underlying structures without fractures occurring. Rib fractures from trauma are rare in children, but pulmonary contusions are common. Children can have cervical spinal cord injuries without radiographic abnormality (SCIWORA).

26. **Do fractures that involve the physes have any effect on growth?**
Maybe. If all goes well, the physes heal and have no effect on growth. If a fracture results in significant damage to the physis, it may lead to bone forming where the normal physeal cartilage should be. This is called a *growth arrest* or *physeal arrest*. If the damaged area is small and peripheral, the remaining normal physis may continue to grow, and this could lead to an angular deformity. If the damaged area is large, growth may cease altogether, leading to shortening of the bone.

27. **Do fractures in children that do not affect the physes have any effect on growth?**
Maybe. Most do not; however, some nonphyseal fractures are well known to affect growth. Fractures involving the femur can lead to an overgrowth phenomenon. This refers to a temporary increased rate of growth during fracture healing. Because of this growth, femur fractures in young children that are reduced end-to-end may result in the fractured leg being longer than the other leg. To avoid this, when placing a young child in a spica cast for a femur fracture, the bone should be allowed to overlap 1–1.5 cm.

28. **How long should young children be casted or splinted?**
The answer probably varies depending on the age of the patient and the nature of the fracture. However, one important point is that young children may become pain-free before their fractures are sufficiently healed. They cannot be relied upon to restrict their activity, to maintain immobilization devices, or to use assistive ambulatory devices during recovery.

29. **Do children usually require physical therapy after fracture healing?**
No. Children tend to recover their range of motion and strength more readily and rapidly than adults. Physical therapy is usually not necessary.

BIBLIOGRAPHY

1. American College of Surgeons Committee on Trauma: Pediatric trauma. In Advanced Trauma Life Support for Doctors. Chicago, American College of Surgeons, 1997, pp 353–376.
2. Tolo VT: Management of the multiply injured child. In Beaty JH, Kasser JR (eds): Fractures in Children, 5th ed. Philadelphia, Lippincott Williams & Wilkins, 2001, pp 75–89.
3. Wilber JH, Thompson GH: The multiply injured child. In Green NE, Swiontkowski MF (eds): Skeletal Trauma in Children, 3rd ed. Philadelphia, W.B. Saunders, 2003, pp 73–103.

CHAPTER 20

PHYSEAL INJURIES

Hamlet A. Peterson, MD

1. **Describe the epiphysis.**
   The epiphysis is the secondary center of ossification, located at the end of the long bone in a child. The cartilage between the epiphysis and the metaphysis is termed the *epiphyseal growth plate,* or the *physis.* Cell division and growth in the columnar and hypertrophic zones of the physis produce longitudinal growth of the bone. Damage to the physis is referred to as an *epiphyseal growth-plate injury* or, more commonly, a *physeal injury.*

2. **What are the most common causes of physeal injury?**
   The vast majority of injuries to the physis are due to fracture. Other causes of damage to the physis include infection, radiation, tumors, disuse, heat (i.e., burns), cold (i.e., frostbite), electrical and laser burns, arterial damage, and iatrogenic causes (e.g., placement of pins, screws, or staples across the physis).

3. **What is the incidence of physeal fracture?**
   Injury to the growth plate occurs in 15–20% of all fractures in children.

4. **What is the rate of physeal fracture?**
   The overall rate of physeal fracture is 365.8 fractures per 100,000 person-years for males and 181.4 fracture per 100,000 person-years for females. In a community with an average child-to-adult ratio, this is approximately 100 fractures in 100,000 total population per year.

5. **Is the incidence of physeal fracture equal in boys and girls?**
   The boy-to-girl ratio of physeal fracture is 2:1, primarily because the physes of boys remain open longer.

6. **At what ages are physeal fractures most common?**
   Girls have the highest rate of physeal fractures at ages 11–12 years; boys, at age 14 years. Since girls stop growing sooner than boys, it is uncommon for a growth-plate fracture to occur after age 15 in girls and after age 17 in boys.

7. **Which bones are most often involved in a physeal fracture?**
   The phalanges of the fingers have by far the greatest incidence of physeal fracture, followed by the distal radius. This is not surprising as each upper extremity has 14 phalanges and only 1 distal radius.

8. **What are the different types of physeal fractures?**
   The anatomic pattern of fracture of a growth plate can vary, with implications to the mechanism of injury, the treatment, and the outcome. Several classifications of physeal fractures have been developed, and there is great overlap of fracture type among the various classifications. The most recent and only statistically verified classification contains six types (Fig. 20-1).

9. **What is the anatomic basis of this classification?**
   There is a progressive increase in the amount of physeal cartilage damage from type I to type VI fracture.

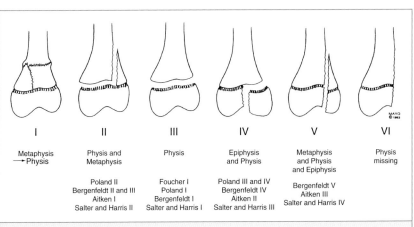

Figure 20-1. Types of physeal fractures.

10. **What is the epidemiologic significance of this classification?**
So far, type II has been found to be the most common physeal fracture, followed in order by types I, III, IV, V, and VI. Type I fracture was only recently described and often can be found only on oblique or three-quarter radiographs. In the future, it may prove to be the most common physeal fracture.

11. **What is the value of this classification with reference to treatment?**
The rates of both initial surgery to treat the fracture and late surgery to treat complications gradually progress from type I fractures (for which surgery is rarely necessary) to type VI fractures (for which surgery is always necessary).

12. **What is the prognostic value of this classification?**
The percentage of cases with a complication increases progressively from type I to type VI fractures.

13. **What is the etiology of physeal fractures?**
Statistically, falls from all sorts of activities account for 20% of physeal fractures in children. This is followed by football and bicycle accidents. Physeal fractures occur in many childhood sports, both organized and unorganized. Automobile, motorcycle, and all-terrain vehicles account for only 5% of physeal fractures.

14. **How are physeal fractures evaluated?**
History and physical examination determine the appropriate body site from which to obtain radiographs. Good-quality radiographs in at least two planes, usually anteroposterior and lateral, are required. If questions arise, radiographs in additional planes, usually three-quarter views, will help delineate the fracture. When questions persist, comparison views of the opposite uninjured extremity, as well as stress views, tomograms, arthrograms, ultrasonograms, computed tomography scans, and magnetic resonance images, can be helpful in defining the fracture.

15. **How are these fractures treated?**
In general, physeal fractures are treated by anatomic reduction and maintenance of reduction until they heal. Usually, this can be accomplished by closed reduction and immobilization.

16. **What percentage of patients require surgery?**
All physeal injuries involving an open wound require surgical debridement and irrigation. Adding these few to those injuries that require surgery to obtain adequate reduction and stabilization brings the total to 7% of all physeal fractures. The decision of whether to operate depends on the ability to obtain and maintain anatomical alignment of the growth plate to enhance the possibility of continuing normal growth.

17. **Do fractures of the physis heal in the same manner as fractures elsewhere?**
Because the fracture is through growing cartilage, physeal fractures heal much more rapidly than fractures involving only bone. Most of these fractures are stable in 3–4 weeks; stability occurs earlier in younger patients and later in older patients.

18. **How long should patients be followed after physeal fracture?**
There is no standard answer, but basically the follow-up is longer for more severe injuries, younger children (who have more growth remaining), and physes that provide more longitudinal length (i.e., the distal femur and proximal and distal tibia). These are the same factors that determine prognosis.

19. **What factors determine the prognosis?**
The prognosis depends on these factors, in descending order of importance:
- The severity of the injury, including displacement, comminution, and open versus closed injury
- The age of the patient
- The specific physis injured
- The type of fracture
- The treatment is dependent on these factors and, in itself, also has an important bearing on the prognosis.

KEY POINTS: PHYSEAL INJURY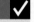

1. By far, the most common and serious complication of damage to the growth plate is premature complete or partial growth-plate closure.

2. Complete growth-plate closure ensures that the injured bone will not grow as long as the contralateral uninjured bone.

3. Partial growth-plate closure tethers growth in the damaged area, while allowing the remaining uninjured portion of the physis to grow, thus producing an angular deformity.

4. There is no way to reestablish growth following complete growth-plate closure.

5. Growth can sometimes be reestablished in partial arrest by surgically excising the bony bar and preventing bar reformation by insertion of an interposition material.

20. **What are the major complications of physeal growth-plate fractures?**
By far, the most common and serious complication of damage to the growth plate is premature complete or partial growth-plate closure. Complete growth-plate closure ensures that the injured bone will not grow as long as the contralateral uninjured bone. Partial growth-plate closure tethers growth in the damaged area while allowing the remaining uninjured portion of the physis to grow, thus producing an angular deformity. Other complications include delayed union, nonunion, infection, and avascular necrosis, all of which are infrequent.

21. **How early can growth-plate closure be detected after injury?**
It is difficult to document a premature growth-plate closure prior to 3 months after injury, even in cases in which there is a high suspicion that it will occur. Often the growth-plate closure becomes manifest several months or even years after the traumatic incident.

22. **How are growth-plate closures treated?**
There is no way to reestablish growth following complete growth-plate closure. Its treatment requires arresting the physis of the contiguous bone (as in the case of the radius and ulna and the tibia and fibula), as well as surgical arrest of the contralateral physis, surgical lengthening of the injured shorter bone, or surgical shortening of the normal longer, uninjured bone. In the case of partial arrest (i.e., bone bar), these same modalities can be used, along with osteotomy to correct angular deformity. However, growth can sometimes be reestablished in partial arrest by surgically excising the bony bar and preventing bar reformation by insertion of an interposition material.

23. **Which physeal bars respond most successfully to excision?**
Bar excision in an attempt to reestablish growth is most successful when the bar accounts for less than 50% of the total area of the physis in children who have significant growth remaining (i.e., girls aged 12 years and younger and boys aged 14 years and younger).

BIBLIOGRAPHY

1. Peterson HA: Epiphyseal Growth Plate Fractures. Springer, Heidelberg, 2007.
2. Peterson HA: Partial growth plate arrest and its treatment. J Pediatr Orthop 4:246–258, 1984.
3. Peterson HA: Physeal fractures. Part 2: Two previously unclassified types. J Pediatr Orthop 14:431–438, 1994.
4. Peterson HA: Physeal fractures: Part 3. Classification. J Pediatr Orthop 14:439–448, 1994.
5. Peterson HA: Physeal injuries and growth arrest. In Beatty JN, Kasser JR (eds): Rockwood and Wilkins' Fractures in Children, 5th ed. Philadelphia, Lippincott, Williams & Wilkins, 2001, pp 91–128.
6. Peterson HA, Madhok R, Benson JT, et al: Physeal fractures. Part I: Epidemiology in Olmsted County, Minnesota, 1979–1988. J Pediatr Orthop 14:423–430, 1994.

CHAPTER 21

PITFALLS IN TRAUMA

Randall T. Loder, MD

1. **In spite of appropriate analgesic doses, a child with a fracture of the supracondylar humerus is still experiencing severe pain. Why?**
   A compartment syndrome with impending Volkmann's ischemic contracture is highly likely. It can be associated with a traumatic lesion in the brachial artery at the level of the fracture site. Immediate orthopaedic consultation is needed to (1) reduce and stabilize the fracture, (2) assess the function of and measure the compartment pressures in the volar compartment, and (3) assess the vascular supply and viability of the hand. Following these actions, further intervention, such as release of the affected compartments or brachial arterial exploration and repair, may be urgently needed.

2. **How should a minimally displaced midshaft ulnar fracture be managed?**
   The pitfall here is the elbow joint. Innocuous-looking ulnar fractures can be associated with radial head dislocations at the elbow (i.e., Monteggia's lesion). These dislocations require, at a minimum, closed reduction and application of a long-arm cast in a position dictated by the type of radial head dislocation. Older children and adolescents often require open reduction and internal fixation. For this reason, all ulnar fractures necessitate adequate radiographs of both the elbow and the wrist.

3. **A child who sustains a nondisplaced lateral condylar fracture of the humerus is placed in a long-arm cast. What follow-up care is required?**
   Fractures of the lateral condyle must be watched closely. They may displace in the first 2 weeks after injury, and repeat radiographs are needed approximately every 5 days. These radiographs should be obtained with the patient out of the cast because a subtle displacement or shift is easily obscured by overlying shadows from the cast material. Another pitfall with lateral condylar fractures is the risk of nonunion, even when nondisplaced. Patients with these fractures must be followed for several months to ensure union and then for a few years at infrequent intervals to ensure that angular or growth deformities do not occur.

4. **What are the physical findings in a compartment syndrome?**
   Classically, the five Ps have been described: pain, paresthesias, pallor, pulselessness, and paralysis. The most important finding is severe pain or restlessness. Once pallor, pulselessness, and paralysis are present, permanent damage may have already resulted. All efforts should be made to not reach this point. A low threshold should be maintained at all times as children often will not communicate the early sign of paresthesias. If the physician has any concern, appropriate compartment pressure measurements should be taken, even if a general anesthesia is necessary. A frightened child with a fresh fracture often cannot cooperate sufficiently during the physical examination to ensure that the examiner obtains an accurate clinical assessment of the compartment's condition.

5. **A 7-month-old child presents to the emergency room with a history of falling off a couch, and radiographs are interpreted as indicating a dislocation of the elbow. What treatment is required?**
   The pitfall here is the diagnosis. Elbow dislocations in young children are essentially nonexistent. Instead, this child has sustained a displaced distal humeral physeal fracture. The distal humeral

epiphysis is still cartilaginous and not yet ossified; therefore, it cannot be seen radiographically. Thus, its displacement mimics the appearance of an elbow dislocation. To help differentiate the two, the physician should remember that a fracture of the distal humeral epiphysis is usually displaced posteromedially, whereas an elbow dislocation is usually displaced posterolaterally. My preferred method of treatment is closed reduction and percutaneous pinning in the operating room. Caution: This fracture has a high association with child abuse, and the circumstances of the accident should be explored.

6. **A 3-year-old child is injured in a motor vehicle crash. Lateral radiographs of the cervical spine obtained in the emergency room are interpreted as demonstrating a ligamentous injury at the C2–C3 level. Is this an expected finding?**
No. True ligamentous instability at the C2–C3 level in young children is extremely rare, whereas pseudosubluxation is quite common. Pseudosubluxation can be differentiated from pathologic (i.e., true) instability by using the posterior line of Swischuk (Fig. 21-1).

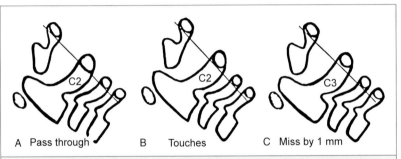

A   Pass through   B   Touches   C   Miss by 1 mm

Figure 21-1. The posterior cervical line of Swischuk is drawn from the anterior cortex of the posterior arch of C1 to the anterior cortex of the posterior arch of C3. In pseudosubluxation (or physiologic displacement) of C2 on C3, the posterior cervical line may pass through the cortex of the posterior arch of C2, touch the anterior aspect of the cortex of the posterior arch of C2, or come within 1 mm of the anterior cortex of the posterior arch of C2. In pathologic subluxation of C2 on C3, the posterior cervical line misses the posterior arch of C2 by 2 mm or more.

7. **An 8-year-old boy sustains a "minimally displaced" fracture of the medial malleolus. What type of treatment should he receive?**
The pitfalls here are both the amount of displacement and the possibility of nonunion. Fractures of the medial malleolus are rare in children; yet, they must be aggressively treated. As perfect a reduction as possible should be achieved, and the threshold for performing an open reduction and internal fixation should be very low. The risk of physeal growth arrest is much higher if an anatomic reduction is not obtained. If the fracture is truly nondisplaced, it needs to be monitored carefully to ensure that it does not displace in the first few weeks after injury and also that it proceeds to union.

8. **A 12-year-old girl presents with a displaced midshaft fracture of both bones of the forearm. After closed reduction and application of a short-arm cast, when should the child be rechecked?**
Short-arm casts have no role in the immobilization of midshaft forearm fractures of both bones. Rather, a long-arm cast is mandatory. Because this girl, at age 12 years, is nearing skeletal maturity, only minimal angulation and displacement can be permitted. Frequent checks are needed after the reduction to ensure that the fracture position remains acceptable. I typically recheck these fractures on a weekly basis for the first 3 weeks after reduction. If any shifting has

occurred, I perform either a repeat closed reduction with intramedullary stabilization or an open reduction and internal fixation.

9. **A 6-year-old boy, restrained and seat-belted, is involved in a motor vehicle crash. He is admitted to the hospital for abdominal pain and also complains of some mild discomfort of the lumbar spine, even though the abdominal computed tomography (CT) scan shows only a small hepatic hematoma. What is the cause of his back pain?**

The classic injury in a restrained lap-belted passenger is the Chance fracture, which results from forward flexion over the seatbelt, distracting the posterior vertebral elements. In adults, this type of trauma usually results in a bony fracture. In children, however, it usually results in a ligamentous injury, disrupting the interspinous ligaments, the facet capsules, the posterior longitudinal ligaments, and the intervertebral disk. Ecchymosis in the lap-belt distribution is frequently seen on physical examination, and the presence of lumbar ligamentous disruption is strongly associated with abdominal visceral injury. CT scans are usually not diagnostic since the axial CT cuts are in the same plane as the horizontal fracture or dislocation. Lateral radiographs of the spine are needed to make the diagnosis. For this reason, every child who has sustained abdominal trauma from a lap-belt injury should have radiographs taken of the thoracolumbar spine.

10. **A 14-year-old boy injures his left knee in a football game. Swelling rapidly ensues. Physical examination reveals tenderness of the medial femoral condyle and instability to valgus stress; yet, the radiographs are negative. Why?**

In children with open epiphyseal plates, athletic injuries to the knee frequently result in physeal fracture rather than ligamentous injury. This boy likely has sustained a Salter I fracture of the distal femoral physis that is nondisplaced, thus giving a "negative" radiographic appearance. Stress radiographs under controlled circumstances should be performed to determine the anatomic location of the instability and the subsequent appropriate treatment.

11. **While playing basketball, a 10-year-old boy jumps up for a rebound and his knee suddenly gives way. Physical examination reveals a markedly swollen knee. Radiographs demonstrate a chip fracture at the distal pole of the patella. What is the appropriate treatment for this fracture?**

This child has sustained a sleeve fracture of the patella. This fracture is an avulsion of a large portion of the patellar articular cartilage along with a small bony fragment. This avulsion can result in an extensor lag with considerable long-term morbidity. If the chip is truly nondisplaced, then cast immobilization is all that is required. If there is an extensor lag or if the avulsed fragment remains separated from the remainder of the patella, then surgical repair is required.

12. **A 6-year-old boy steps on a nail while wearing tennis shoes and sustains a puncture wound to the planter aspect of the foot. Ten days later, he presents to the emergency room with a complaint of increasing pain and warmth over the planter aspect of the metatarsal heads during the last 48 hours. There is slight drainage from the wound. How should this condition be managed?**

These signs and symptoms most likely indicate infection due to Pseudomonas, both a septic arthritis of the metatarsophalangeal joint and osteomyelitis of the metatarsal. The rubber soles of tennis shoes harbored Pseudomonas, which was then introduced into the foot from the puncture wound. Appropriate therapy consists of surgical debridement and intravenous antibiotics appropriate for Pseudomonas until the surgical culture results are available.

13. **An obese 14-year-old boy sustains a fall during a football game. Over the next few weeks, he complains of increasing knee pain and a limp. Knee radiographs are normal. What should the next step be in the work-up?**

    Obese adolescent children are prone to developing a slipped capital femoral epiphysis, with the initial symptoms often related to a mild episode of trauma. Hip pain is often referred to the knee, and, thus, radiographs of the hips should be obtained. Both anteroposterior (AP) and lateral pelvis radiographs are needed since early on the slip is seen only on the lateral radiograph. Up to 35% of these injuries are bilateral, with the opposite hip being asymptomatic, or silent.

14. **While playing football, a 15-year-old boy sustains a patellar dislocation with spontaneous reduction. He has a swollen knee, and radiographs demonstrate an osseous chip fracture near the patella. What does this mean?**

    During patellar dislocation, the patella rapidly impacts on the lateral femoral condyle. This may result in an osteochondral fracture of the patella. An arthroscopic examination of the knee is usually necessary to determine the extent of the injury to the patellar articular surface and the appropriate treatment (e.g., removal of the fragment, if small, or fixation of a large fragment).

KEY POINTS: PITFALLS IN TRAUMA

1. Extreme pain in children with fractures is unusual and should be seriously evaluated.

2. Do not forget to assess the radiocapitellar articulation in all children with forearm fractures.

3. Beware of innocuous-appearing physeal fractures, especially in younger children.

4. Always ensure that there is full active extension and continuity of the extensor mechanism in children with knee injuries.

5. Beware of small chips around the patella in children with knee injuries.

15. **A 10-year-old boy falls and injures his ring finger while playing soccer. Radiographs demonstrate a fracture of the distal metaphyseal portion of the middle phalanx, with slight angulation and translation. How long should the finger be splinted?**

    A simple finger splint is not adequate for this fracture! The pitfall here is the fracture location. It is far removed from the epiphyseal plate; thus, the potential for remodeling of any malunion is minimal, especially at 10 years of age. These fractures need an anatomic reduction; this may require either a closed reduction or an open reduction. Often, internal fixation after the reduction is needed to ensure that the fracture does not shift while healing.

16. **A 7-year-old boy undergoes retrograde titanium elastic nail fixation for a transverse midshaft fracture. Approximately 3 weeks later, as rehabilitation is begun, the boy complains of significant knee pain with active range-of-motion exercises. Radiographs do not document any shift in the fracture, and early healing has begun. Why does the boy experience pain?**

    Distal femoral entry points for titanium elastic nails must be carefully chosen. The entry of the nail should be 1–2 cm above the distal femoral physis, and they should be in the middle of the femur, anterior to posterior. If the nail enters too distally or too anteriorly, or both, significant interference with the patellofemoral mechanism can occur. As the child begins to actively increase knee flexion, the patella will encounter a nail that is placed too anteriorly, resulting in pain and loss of active motion. Similarly, approximately 1 cm of the nail should exit from the femur; a larger amount will become prominent and, again, will cause knee pain, reactive effusion, and interfere with patellofemoral excursion; if too little exits the femur, nail removal after fracture union will be much more difficult.

17. **A 13-year-old girl undergoes antegrade nailing of a midshaft femur fracture with a piriformis entry-point nail. One year later, she begins complaining of vague groin discomfort. Abductor muscle strength is now back to normal. Plain radiographs appear normal; the fracture has healed without complication, and there does not appear to be any radiographic abnormalities of the hip. Why does she have this pain?**

Antegrade nailing of femur fractures using a piriformis entry point in skeletally immature children (i.e., those with open physes in the proximal femur) may result in avascular necrosis approximately 1% of the time. In this instance, the occurrence of avascular necrosis must be assumed until it is proven otherwise.

BIBLIOGRAPHY

1. Beaty JH, Kasser JR (eds): Fractures in Children, 5th ed. Philadelphia, Lippincott, Williams & Wilkins, 2001.
2. Flynn JM, Hresko T, Reynolds RA, et al: Titanium elastic nails for pediatric femur fractures: A multicenter study of early results with analysis of complications. J Pediatr Orthop 21(1):4–8, 2001.
3. Letts RM (ed): Management of Pediatric Fractures. New York, Churchill Livingstone, 1994.
4. Morrissy RT, Weinstein SL (eds): Lovell and Winter's Pediatric Orthopaedics, 5th ed. Philadelphia, Lippincott, Williams & Wilkins, 2001.
5. Ogden JA (ed): Skeletal Injury in the Child, 3rd ed. New York, Springer-Verlag, 2000.

CHAPTER 22

CHILD ABUSE

William L. Oppenheim, MD, and Richard E. Bowen, MD

1. **What is child abuse?**

   Child abuse is any act or failure to act resulting in imminent risk of serious harm of a child by a parent or caretaker who is responsible for that child's welfare. This definition involves much more than the simplistic "three fractures in different stages of healing," which at one time constituted the traditional orthopaedic definition. Today, the term encompasses emotional neglect, injury resulting from supervisional neglect, starvation, and sexual abuse, as well as physical abuse. Specifically, the term *battered child syndrome* refers to cases of abuse in which a child presents with fractures and other overt physical injuries. *Shaken infant syndrome* describes brain injuries sustained by forceful shaking of the cranial contents without overt skull fracturing.

   Because fractures occur rather late in the course of physical abuse, the physician's role is to recognize nonaccidental trauma and the social milieu surrounding it and to intervene early so that further injury or neglect is prevented. The Federal Child Abuse Prevention and Treatment Act of 1974 established a National Center on Child Abuse and Neglect (NCCAN), but each state has its own definition, rules for intervention, and actions relating to child abuse.

2. **What happens to abused children eventually?**

   If unrecognized, a child returned to an abusive environment faces a 50% chance of further battering and perhaps as high as a 15% chance of death. Undetected survivors may become the next generation of child or elder abusers. When the diagnosis is recognized and appropriate intervention deployed, the vast majority of children can remain in or eventually be reunited within their families. Only in extreme cases are the children remanded to foster care.

3. **How common is child abuse?**

   Approximately 3 million "referrals" are generated across the United States each year, based on the 2004 data from the National Child Abuse and Neglect Data System (NCANDS). One half of the referrals are generated by educational or health care professionals, and the other half by family or community members. Of the reported cases, one-half were found not to involve abuse, but one-third were eventually classified as official maltreatment—approximately 872,000 children, or 11.9 per 1000 children in the population. Undoubtedly, many cases go unreported. Some health professionals are reluctant to report information gathered in an otherwise confidential manner, many do not want to become involved with the legal system, and some simply refuse to believe that otherwise normal-appearing parents would purposely injure their children.

4. **No one can be 100% sure that abuse has occurred, so why should I become involved?**

   It is usually not possible for a physician to come to a definitive conclusion regarding any one episode of trauma. However, it is not necessary to come to a definitive conclusion. Only a reasonable suspicion of abuse is necessary to trigger mandatory reporting of potential abuse or nonaccidental injury, according to most state laws.

   Since abuse most often takes place in the private confines of a home, and since small, nonvocal children are frequently involved, any legal action will of necessity involve circumstantial evidence. This requires involvement of many other professionals beyond the physician, so actual proof by the physician is neither expected nor required. In fact, physicians should not be accusatory in their approach, or their ability to elicit useful information and thus protect the child will be quickly compromised.

Failure to report your suspicions is usually punishable simply by fines, but children returned to an abusive environment frequently sustain additional injuries, and when these children are eventually sent to foster care, the new parents may sue the physician who missed or ignored the diagnosis. Settlements can be substantial and may threaten continued insurance coverage.

All states grant legal immunity to reporting physicians. Society has deemed it more important to protect innocent children than to enforce patient-physician confidentiality in this instance. This in turn may encourage over-reporting, but it effectively protects those who cannot protect themselves.

5. **Who are the common perpetrators of child abuse?**
In 80% of cases, the perpetrators are the parents.

6. **Which types of child abuse are most common?**
Although skeletal physical abuse is the realm of the orthopaedist, the majority of children being reported are victims of neglect, including severe emotional neglect and starvation. One-third of abused children will eventually be seen by an orthopaedic surgeon.

7. **What background circumstances might raise the suspicion of abuse?**
Although abuse cuts across all socioeconomic levels, there are some associations worth looking for in the history. These include the following:
- Parents who themselves were abused as children (i.e., intergenerational abuse)
- Drug and alcohol abuse on the part of parents
- Social isolation of the family
- A history of family crises
- Prior intervention
- A history of an abused sibling
- Acute severe financial pressures
- Inconsolably crying children
- Children with preexisting disabilities
- Unwitnessed injury
- History of previous injury
- Injury inconsistent with the development of the child

Most parents know exactly when their children were injured and under what circumstances. Vagueness as to how the injury took place is suspicious. The history must be consistent both with the developmental milestones and with the injury. A delay in seeking care demands an explanation. It is hard to imagine how an attentive parent could miss a fracture event, although there is a chance that a parent might not seek immediate care for a swollen limb based on financial considerations or because a minor fracture might initially be misinterpreted as a sprain. A lack of appropriate concern on the caretaker's behalf, even when the diagnosis becomes clear, should be noted in the record. Finally, small children look to their custodians for protection. A vacant, listless child who runs from a caretaker or who fails to make eye contact with him or her is quite unusual and should raise a red flag in the physician's mind.

8. **What physical findings point toward abuse?**
An old aphorism of child abuse holds that the injuries speak for the child who cannot. Most physically abused children are younger than 3 years of age. (Sexual abuse is more common after the age of 6 and most frequent in the teenage group.) Repetitive trauma, frequent bruising beyond normal play expectations, the failure to thrive syndrome, or multiple fractures with no clear cause all raise the issue of nonaccidental trauma or neglect.

Some aspects of abuse are obvious upon reflection. For example, fractures of long bones prior to the age of walking are sufficiently rare to raise concern. One-third of femur fractures in children younger than 5 years are due to nonaccidental trauma, as are two-thirds of fractures in children younger than the age of 1 year. Even after the age of walking, rib fractures, vertebral body fractures, and complex skull fractures (beyond simple linear fractures) are rarely seen in healthy children without an obvious explanation. The finding of traumatic brain injury along with other unexplained manifestations of trauma (e.g., long-bone fractures) in the absence of a significant historical traumatic event is strong evidence for abuse. Children who present with two black eyes, a torn frenulum (from a fisted uppercut), bite marks, cigarette burns, or bilateral long-bone shaft fractures reportedly sustained during normal play activities are difficult to accept as cases of accidental injury. Natural injuries tend to be irregular in character, whereas multiple injuries with linear marks are characteristic of whipping with belts, extension cords, broomsticks, and other slender objects. Similarly, circumferential marks about a limb indicate binding or restraining with ropes, chains, belts, or other cord-like objects. Examination of the genitalia can reveal evidence of sexual abuse or venereal disease.

9. **Where do burns fit into the picture of abuse?**
Soft tissue injuries are much more common than fractures, and about 20% of such injuries in abused children are caused by burns. Burns caused by cigarettes are relatively easy to spot, with their irregular concentric imprints and resultant scarring. Children who are forced to stand in a scalding hot bath for punishment demonstrate clearly delineated "stocking glove" burn patterns on their feet and legs. Flat iron or curling iron branding injuries yield similar linear-edged burns, reflecting the mirror image of the instrument, as do injuries caused when children are forced to stand on or touch a hot radiator. In contrast, when a child pulls over a hot-water kettle or bowl, the resulting injury is scattered and variable. Similarly, when young infants are dipped into scalding water, reflex flexing of the hips and knees results in popliteal sparing, a pattern quite different from that seen when children fall in and attempt to extricate themselves.

10. **How should physical findings of abuse be documented?**
Physicians should use special forms available to document suspected cases of abuse for later use in legal proceedings. Photographs can be helpful, but only if they clearly depict the actual injuries. Some states prefer that evidence technicians from the local law enforcement organization obtain such photographs, rather than the physician or hospital.

11. **What laboratory and diagnostic tests should be obtained?**
A skeletal survey remains the standard diagnostic test. The skeletal survey consists of bilateral anteroposterior (AP) films of all extremities, including the hands and feet, and AP and lateral projections of the axial skeleton and skull. Radionuclide bone scanning, though not a routine part of the work-up, may show occult fractures earlier and may highlight rib and spine fractures, which are otherwise easy to overlook. They are used when the skeletal survey is equivocal, when the child is too young to effectively localize the injuries, or when the skeletal survey is negative but clinical suspicion of abuse is high. Ultrasonographic imaging and magnetic resonance imaging (MRI) likewise may have their place in selected circumstances but are not routinely performed. Intra-abdominal injury calls for its own evaluation, including testing for hematuria, melena, and amylase and liver enzymes. A chronically low hematocrit suggests malnourishment or excessive blood loss due to fracturing. Prothrombin time (PT) and partial thromboplastin time (PTT) results will be necessary in court as the defense will raise the issue of a bleeding diathesis with easy bruisability. Levels of calcium, phosphorus, alkaline phosphatase, blood urea nitrogen (BUN), and creatinine, along with a bone density scan, may be helpful at times in ruling out metabolic or genetic diseases that may be confused with abuse. Cultures to rule out venereal disease can also be obtained, as warranted.

12. **What confirmation should be sought on radiographs?**
"Three fractures in different stages of healing" works. But the goal should be to recognize the problem before there are multiple fractures. Although certain types of fractures are suggestive of child abuse, there are no fracture types completely sensitive and specific for child abuse.

Suggestive fractures include corner metaphyseal fractures, which often result from pulling on a limb, with stretching of the periosteum and perichondrium over the growth plates. The fracture has either a "bucket handle" appearance of the physis or a "bone within a bone" appearance as the elevated periosteum lays down excessive new bone (Fig. 22-1). Unfortunately, such fractures are present in only one-quarter of child abuse cases. Other suggestive fractures are posterior or posterolateral rib fractures, which are uncommon in children (Fig. 22-2). Rib fractures are difficult to see on chest radiographs, and radionuclide bone scanning can be used to confirm their presence.

When such radiographic findings are combined with the history or lack thereof, physical findings, and a careful social services evaluation, most abuse can be recognized at this point.

13. **What should be considered in the differential diagnosis?**

Metabolic or genetic diseases such as rickets, malnourishment, and hypervitaminosis A; chronic disease processes such as renal osteodystrophy or liver disease; and complications of post-transplant steroid administration must all be considered. Osteogenesis imperfecta (OI) is a special consideration in cases of suspected abuse. Many parents of children with this syndrome, unless diagnosis is prompt, will have unfounded allegations lodged against them. This can be devastating for a family that is doing the correct thing and seeking care for a sick and frail child. OI can be recognized in 90% of cases based on the family history and findings of a helmet-shaped skull, blue sclera, prenatal fractures, thin and fragile skin, joint hypermobility, excessive sweating, discolored and breakable teeth, minimal soft tissue swelling in association with the fractures, and the gracile appearance of the bones on radiographs. Blood tests or skin biopsy with a subsequent tissue culture and collagen analysis raise the diagnostic accuracy to 95% or better.

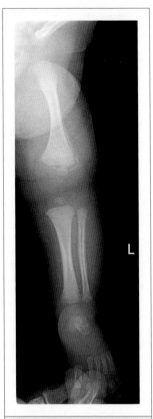

Figure 22-1. This radiograph demonstrates common metaphyseal findings after nonaccidental injury. The distal femur exhibits the "bone within a bone" appearance after a metaphyseal fracture, and the proximal medial tibia demonstrates a corner fracture. Additionally, the entire proximal tibial metaphysis has a "bucket handle" appearance.

Other conditions include physiologic periostitis, scurvy, copper deficiency, Caffey's disease, leukemia, and congenital insensitivity to pain. The spiral distal tibial fracture (or toddler's fracture) is common in children after walking age and should not be misconstrued as abuse. Although some texts suggest a high probability of abuse based on the location and character of the fracture (e.g., a spiral humeral fracture), we have not found a single isolated long-bone fracture, either transverse or spiral, to be suggestive of abuse unless accompanied by the ancillary factors mentioned in questions 7 and 8.

14. **How can you confront the parents with your suspicions and still maintain a trusting relationship with the family?**

Reporting is mandatory under the law. This should be explained to the family. At the UCLA Medical Center, only half of the children referred to the suspected child abuse and neglect

(SCAN) team are eventually confirmed as cases of abuse, in accord with the data available nationwide from the NCCAN. The fact that half of these children need to be screened to protect the other half is a price most rational parents accept. Finally, if the physician is simply not comfortable enough to handle the situation, the patient can be referred for further evaluation to a larger facility, where a SCAN team or its equivalent can be allowed to pursue the diagnosis. This removes the physician from direct confrontation with the parents but does not relieve the physician of his or her reporting obligation under the law.

Frequently, for the sake of a thorough evaluation, suspiciously injured children are admitted for their protection while investigations are carried out. If the parents do not voluntarily accept this, a legal hold can be readily obtained, but at that point the case is headed for a court hearing, rather than simple decision making by the local social services or law enforcement organization. Because of the legal and social implications for the family, only experienced and seasoned

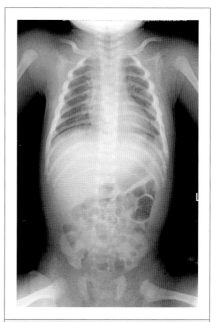

Figure 22-2. Multiple posterolateral rib fractures with associated fracture callus are seen in this chest radiograph and are suggestive of nonaccidental injury.

workers in this area should be making the final decisions for further action beyond the screening stages. The American Academy of Pediatrics supports by official policy the admission and work-up of these patients as in-patients and recommends that third-party insurance cover such care as medically necessary.

KEY POINTS: CHILD ABUSE

1. Child abuse occurs in 11.9 per 1000 children—an incidence higher than most congenital pediatric orthopaedic conditions.

2. A physician with a reasonable suspicion of abuse must report potential abuse or nonaccidental injury according to most state laws, and all states grant legal immunity to reporting physicians.

3. Accurate recognition and referral for suspected child abuse may prevent subsequent abuse in up to 50% and death in up to 15% of cases.

4. In cases of suspected child abuse, a physician should explore whether the injury is consistent with the mechanism and developmental age of the child and whether timely care was sought by the caregivers. Soft tissue injuries generally precede or accompany bony injuries and should be specifically sought and documented when examining a child with a suspicious fracture.

5. A bone survey remains the standard diagnostic test available to the orthopaedic surgeon.

15. **In the setting of multiple fractures in different stages of healing, how can child abuse be differentiated from OI in court?**

First of all, child abuse cases are rarely prosecuted, although often supervision is required of the family. When such cases are prosecuted, defending lawyers will often use this ploy, but by that time additional information is usually substantial. As noted, more than 95% of cases of OI can be diagnosed definitively through collagen analysis in combination with the clinical findings, history, and radiographic results described in question 12. Although the magnitude of precipitating trauma is small, the fractures are noted immediately. This scenario, combined with additional physical evidence and the social services reports, will usually differentiate cases of OI from child abuse. In extreme cases of abuse, removal from the home for 6 months, often by placing the child in the care of a grandparent, results in complete cessation of fractures during this period, also clarifying the diagnosis.

It has been said that carrots, gravy, and meat by themselves do not make stew, but when you put them all together, you have the requisite meal. Likewise, in child abuse, no one finding is definitive, but putting it all together usually tells the story. Some laboratories have found that collagen testing in these cases is not worthwhile. When positive, it is true that the diagnosis of OI is confirmed. Abuse, however, is not necessarily ruled out. When the test is negative, neither abuse nor the diagnosis of OI is ruled out. Remember that children with confounding and preexisting disabilities have a considerably greater chance of being abused than those without such conditions, according to the NCAAN studies.

16. **What variations on the battered-child theme are worth knowing about?**

There are many variations on the theme of child abuse. One of the more widely known is the Munchausen syndrome by proxy. A parent substitutes his or her own specimen for that of the child, so the child is subjected to medical manipulations, or the child is smothered with a pillow until he or she turns blue, and is then "rescued" by the parent just prior to the arrival of the ambulance or in-patient medical personnel. You should be wary of giving advice over the Internet in chat rooms or other venues because participants with Munchausen variants might seize the opportunity to apply valid treatment methods to otherwise normal children.

Finally, there are a series of culturally oriented folk treatments that may result in marks on the child but do not constitute abuse. The use of coins to stroke away "bad winds" (*cao gio*) in Southeast Asians may leave characteristic marks on the back of a child, and the use of suction cups to achieve similar goals leaves concentric red marks, mostly utilized by Russian immigrants. *Caida de mollera* refers to a treatment popular in the Hispanic community, in which symptoms are attributed to a fallen fontanelle and results of attempts to raise the fontanelle may be confused with the signs of shaken baby syndrome. A cultural profile should be part of the initial evaluation; severe injury is not ordinarily a feature of these folk treatments.

17. **What will you be asked in court?**

The physician will be asked to describe the fractures, to conjecture as to the force required to sustain them, to propose possible mechanisms, and perhaps to date the injuries. Soft tissue swelling resolves in 4–10 days, new periosteal bone is visible from 10–14 days, and fracture lines begin to fade by 14–21 days. Hard callous is present at 21–42 days, and remodeling of fractures occurs in the context of 6 months to several years, depending on the age of the child.

BIBLIOGRAPHY

1. American Academy of Pediatrics: Diagnostic imaging of child abuse (RE9944), American Academy of Pediatrics policy statement. Pediatrics 105:1345–1348, 2000.
2. Kocker MS, Kasser JR: Orthopaedic aspects of child abuse. J Am Acad Orthop Surg 8(1):10–20, 2000.

3. Thomas SA, Rosenfield NS, Leventhal JM, Markowitz RI: Long bone fractures in young children: Distinguishing accidental injuries from child abuse. Pediatrics 88:471–476, 1991.

4. U.S. Department of Health and Human Services Administration for Children and Families, Administration on Children, Youth and Families Children's Bureau: Child Maltreatment, 2004. Reports from the states to the National Child Abuse and Neglect Data System Available at http://www.acf.hhs.gov/programs/cb/pubs/cm04/summary.htm (as posted on November 23, 2005).

CHAPTER 23

POLYTRAUMA

Paul D. Choi, MD, and David L. Skaggs, MD

1. **How do the differences in a child's anatomy and physiology affect the overall approach to the management of a pediatric polytrauma victim?**
   One of the main differences is in the management of head injuries. Children with head injuries have greater potential for recovery than adults with similar injuries. As a result, management of orthopaedic injuries should be based on the assumption that full neurologic recovery will take place.

2. **What are the common mechanisms of injury in the pediatric polytrauma patient?**
   In contrast to the adult trauma setting, in which penetrating trauma is most frequent, blunt trauma is responsible for the majority of injuries in the pediatric polytrauma patient. Motor vehicle collisions and falls from height are most common.

3. **What anatomic differences make a child's injury unique and may alter treatment?**
   A disproportionately large head places the child at increased risk for head and cervical spine injuries. A pliable rib cage with exposed liver and spleen below its margin, as well as an unprotected large and small bowel, heighten the risk of injury to these visceral organs in the polytrauma setting. Lastly, a distended bladder becomes vulnerable to injury, especially with pelvic injuries. From an orthopaedic standpoint, the presence of open physeal growth plates in the skeletally immature child places the child at risk for growth arrest or deformity. Approximately 25% of all pediatric fractures are physeal fractures. The risk of growth arrest is reported to be 25–30% for fractures in the distal femur and distal tibia.

4. **Is there an advantage to pediatric trauma centers?**
   The literature suggests that survival rates for severely injured children are improved if the pediatric polytrauma victim is brought to a pediatric trauma center rather than a community hospital. Unfortunately, the high costs and, consequently, the sparse numbers of such centers oftentimes necessitate the use of general trauma centers for pediatric trauma care.

5. **How do you initiate the resuscitation and evaluation of the pediatric polytrauma victim?**
   The primary survey begins with the ABCs (airway, breathing, and circulation) following the advanced trauma life support (ATLS) protocol. If a child is unconscious or neck pain is present, cervical spine stabilization is also necessary. In children younger than 6 years of age, because of the relatively larger head size, special transport beds with a cutout for the occipital area are recommended to prevent flexion of the cervical spine.

6. **After an adequate airway and satisfactory oxygenation and ventilation are confirmed or established, what steps need to be taken to ensure sufficient fluid resuscitation?**
   First, intravenous access needs to be established. If the patient is hypotensive, give an initial bolus of 20 mL/kg of crystalloid solution, preferably Ringer's lactate (i.e., PlasmaLyte). If hypotension persists, consider blood transfusions. Of note, given the high physiologic reserve

of children, classic signs of hypovolemia (e.g., low blood pressure) may not be present until hypovolemia is in an advanced, critical range.

If venous access cannot be established, then intraosseous infusion is an alternative. A large-bore needle may be placed directly in the proximal tibial metaphysis in order to deliver fluids. No adverse effects on the histology of bone or the adjacent physis have been reported. Caution is necessary to avoid excessive fluid resuscitation, especially in children with head injuries, to avoid the complications associated with cerebral edema.

7. **What are the important components of a thorough secondary survey?**
    After the patient is stabilized, a complete and thorough secondary survey will include evaluations of the neurologic, abdominal, thoracic, genitourinary, and musculoskeletal systems. Important in the secondary survey is the ability to recognize that certain injuries are red flags for other types of injuries. Rib fractures can be associated with injuries to the lung parenchyma (e.g., pulmonary contusion); pelvic fractures, with genitourinary injuries; and facial injuries, with cervical spine injuries. Calcaneal fractures and femur fractures are rarely isolated injuries. Calcaneal fractures are associated with additional fractures 33% of the time, with spine fractures present in 5%. Femur fractures following motor vehicle collisions are associated with additional injuries 58% of the time, with head injuries in 14%, chest injuries in 6%, abdominal injuries in 5%, and genitourinary injuries in 4%. Cervical spine injuries are commonly multilevel (20%). Finally, the presence of a lap-belt sign (i.e., ecchymosis about the lap portion of a seatbelt) should raise one's suspicion for a lumbar spine injury.

    As the secondary survey is conducted, the child with polytrauma should be warmed appropriately. A child is particularly vulnerable to hypothermia given relatively thin skin, a lack of subcutaneous fat, and a relatively large skin-surface area.

    The secondary survey should be repeated multiple times in the polytrauma setting as it is not uncommon for some injuries to be missed initially. Additional injuries are often diagnosed weeks after injury.

8. **Given the physiologic and anatomic differences of the child, are pediatric trauma scoring systems more accurate, and therefore more helpful, in guiding trauma care?**
    Pediatric scoring systems such as the pediatric trauma score (PTS) were designed to take into account the unique physiologic and anatomic considerations in the pediatric polytrauma victim. Studies, however, have failed to demonstrate any significant advantage in these pediatric scoring systems for the purposes of triage or prognosis. In fact, trauma classification systems standard in the adult trauma setting (i.e., the injury severity score [ISS] and the trauma score [TS]) have been reported to be more accurate and superior in predicting hospital course and prognosis for the pediatric polytrauma patient. Specialized pediatric systems therefore do not appear necessary. The ISS and TS are valid, reproducible rating systems that can be widely applied in the pediatric polytrauma setting.

9. **What is the most common injury pattern in children following polytrauma?**
    Closed head injuries have been reported in 17% of children with polytrauma and are reported to be the most common cause of death and long-term impairment in children following polytrauma. A low oxygen saturation level at the time of presentation and a low Glasgow Coma Scale (GCS) score 72 hours after head injury predict poorer functional recovery. Remember, however, that, compared to an adult, a child is capable of recovering more quickly and more fully from a significant head injury. Closed head injuries can lead to spasticity, contractures, and heterotopic ossification—all of which can significantly impact the long-term orthopaedic care of children following polytrauma.

10. **How is the GCS adapted to the pediatric polytrauma victim with head injury?**

The GCS is calculated based on the best eye-opening, verbal, and motor responses. The standard scale is limited in children who are preverbal or who are in the early stages of verbal development. The GCS has been modified accordingly (Table 23-1). The GCS should be noted on arrival and should be repeated 1 hour after arrival. A GCS of less than 8 is associated with significantly lower survival rates. The 72-hour GCS motor response is predictive of later permanent disability as a sequela to head injury.

TABLE 23-1.   PEDIATRIC GLASGOW COMA SCALE

Best Eye Opening		Best Verbal Response		Best Motor Response	
				Moves spontaneously or purposefully	6
		Oriented (infant coos, babbles)	5	Localizes to touch	5
Spontaneously	4	Confused (infant irritable cries)	4	Withdraws to pain	4
To speech	3	Inappropriate words (infant cries to pain)	3	Flexion to pain	3
To pain	2	Incomprehensible sounds (infant moans to pain)	2	Extension to pain	2
None	1	None	1	None	1

11. **How do you acutely manage children with head injuries?**

The key to initial management is to maintain low intracranial pressure (ICP) (i.e., less than 30 mmHg [normal levels are <15 mmHg]). Intracranial pressure can be lowered by elevating the head of the bed to 30 degrees, lowering the partial pressure of carbon dioxide (pCO_2) by hyperventilation (especially when the patient is being mechanically ventilated), and by restricting intravenous fluid administration. Immobilizing long-bone fractures will also help as motion at the fracture site will result in elevation of intracranial pressures.

12. **What abdominal injury pattern is common in children with polytrauma?**

Abdominal injuries have been reported in 8–27% of children following polytrauma. The relative elasticity of the thoracic rib cage leaves the liver and spleen vulnerable to injury. A careful abdominal exam is vital to allow early detection of injuries to the liver, spleen, pancreas, and kidneys. Abdominal swelling, tenderness, or ecchymoses on the abdominal wall should raise suspicion. A computed tomography (CT) scan oftentimes is useful. A thorough orthopaedic evaluation of the spine, pelvis, and extremities is necessary.

13. **What types of thoracic injuries occur in the pediatric polytrauma victim?**

Thoracic injuries have been reported in 8–62% of children following polytrauma. Pulmonary contusion is the most common form of pediatric thoracic trauma. Rib fractures, pneumothorax, hemothorax, cardiac or great vessel injury (or both), and airway injury can also occur. The presence of rib fractures is often indicative of more severe chest injuries, especially injury to the underlying lung parenchyma.

14. **Are genitourinary injuries associated with a specific injury pattern in children with polytrauma?**
Genitourinary injuries have been reported in 9–24% children with pelvic fractures, especially fractures involving the anterior pelvic ring. These injuries are more common in males than in females and frequently occur at the bulbourethral level. Injuries to the bladder, prostate, kidney, vagina, and other portions of the urethra can also occur.

15. **What is fat embolism syndrome?**
Fat embolism syndrome (FES) is an uncommon but potentially fatal complication of trauma, especially after long-bone or pelvic fractures. The classic syndrome involves pulmonary, cerebral, and cutaneous manifestations and usually presents 24–48 hours after injury. Fat droplets from the fracture site may act as emboli and may become impacted in the pulmonary microvasculature and other microvascular beds such as in the brain. FES is rare in young children and uncommon in teenagers. Treatment involves supportive measures such as assistive ventilation, supplemental oxygenation, and hydration with intravenous fluids.

16. **How do the nutritional demands of a child change in the polytrauma setting?**
Injuries related to trauma increase the caloric demands on the body. Enteral or parenteral nutrition is indicated if the injured child is unable to eat for several days (e.g., in the case of a child on ventilator support). The baseline caloric needs depend on the weight and age of the child. Note that in children on mechanical ventilation, the daily energy or caloric requirements increase by 150%.

17. **What should be included in the initial radiographic evaluation for suspected polytrauma?**
Initial radiographs should include an anteroposterior (AP) view of the pelvis and a lateral of the cervical spine. In cases of suspected cervical injury, additional AP and odontoid views (in children 9 years or older) are indicated as a lateral radiograph by itself may have a false-negative rate as high as 25%. Of note, prevertebral soft tissue swelling may be a result of crying in children and may not necessarily be indicative of a cervical spine injury. Radiographs of any extremity suspicious of significant injury (i.e., one with swelling, tenderness, and ecchymosis) should also be obtained.

18. **What role does CT have in the evaluation of polytrauma?**
CT is essential in the evaluation of suspected polytrauma. In addition to its role in imaging of the head, chest, and abdomen, CT imaging of the spine and pelvis is more sensitive than plain radiographs. Only 54% of pelvic fractures identified with screening CT scans were identified on plain radiographs.

19. **What is the most appropriate radiographic evaluation for suspected cervical spine injury?**
If the initial lateral, AP, and odontoid views are normal in a child with neck pain or concern for injury, lateral flexion-extension cervical spine radiographs can be performed in order to look for instability. The child must be awake, alert, and cooperative for this study to be performed safely. Because the cervical spine of a young child is much more flexible than the cervical spine in an adult, some degree of subluxation may be considered normal. In children 12 years and younger, up to 5 mm of C1–C2 and 3 mm of C2–C3 subluxation is considered normal (compared to 3 mm of C1–C2 and 0 mm of C2–C3 subluxation in adults).

A CT scan or magnetic resonance imaging (MRI) is indicated if the dynamic lateral cervical spine radiographs cannot be obtained. Dynamic lateral cervical spine radiographs are contraindicated in children who are obtunded, intubated, or have a closed head injury. In these cases, a CT scan or MRI should be performed. MRI in particular has been reported to have superior ability in detecting most significant ligamentous and soft tissue injuries in the cervical spine. As a significant proportion of pediatric cervical spine injuries are ligamentous or soft tissue related, MRI is increasingly being advocated as the gold standard for further evaluation of the child with suspected cervical spine injury.

20. **Are there neurologic injuries unique to the child with polytrauma?**
Spinal cord injuries without radiographic abnormality (SCIWORA) can occur in children following polytrauma. These injuries can occur because of the increased elasticity of the young spine. The spinal cord is stretched or distracted, resulting in neurologic deficits in the absence of bony injury. MRI often reveals spinal cord signal change, as well as signal changes, in areas of soft tissue damage such as the interspinous ligaments.

21. **What orthopaedic injuries have the worst prognosis?**
Injuries to the spine and pelvis are associated with the most intense hospital care and the highest mortality rates (0.8% and 0.6%, respectively). Children with injuries to the spine and pelvis have an average of at least five other concomitant injuries.

22. **How should fractures of the pelvis be managed in the child with polytrauma?**
The majority of pelvis fractures are stable and can be treated nonoperatively. Unstable fractures or fractures involving the acetabulum, however, require operative stabilization. In addition, injuries with marked pubic symphysis diastasis and uncontrolled bleeding are an indication for external fixation.

KEY POINTS: POLYTRAUMA

1. Trauma is the leading cause of mortality in children over the age of 1 year in the United States and worldwide. In the United States, pediatric trauma accounts for 11 million hospitalizations, 100,000 permanent disabilities, and 15,000 childhood deaths annually. The estimated cost for the care of pediatric trauma is $1–13.8 billion annually.

2. Orthopaedic injuries account for a significant proportion of injuries in the pediatric polytrauma setting—up to 34% in one series. These are rarely life-threatening but can place the patient at risk for long-term morbidity.

3. The late diagnosis of injuries, especially orthopaedic, in children following polytrauma is not uncommon.

4. The anatomic and physiologic differences of a child necessitate a different management approach to the pediatric polytrauma victim; nevertheless, many of the principles do overlap with the management of adult polytrauma victims.

5. Outcome studies following pediatric polytrauma report high survivorship (80–95%). Quality of life, for the most part, was felt to be comparable to that of a healthy population. Nevertheless, residual impairments can be significant, with the majority of long-term impairment resulting most frequently from neurologic injury, followed closely by musculoskeletal injury.

23. **What is the significance of open fractures in the child with polytrauma?**
Ten percent of fractures in children with polytrauma have been reported to be open. The presence of an open fracture usually signifies a high-energy mechanism of injury (e.g., a motor vehicle collision) and, therefore, a higher risk of additional injuries. (Some series have noted a 25–50% risk of additional injuries to the head, chest, abdomen, or other extremities.)

24. **What is the initial management of open fractures?**
After the wound is inspected, a clean dressing should be applied to the wound. Intravenous antibiotics and tetanus prophylaxis should be initiated immediately.

25. **What is the definitive management of open fractures?**
Irrigation and debridement of tissues in the area of the open fracture is necessary. This should occur urgently if soft tissues are at risk and severe contamination is present or within 24 hours otherwise for infection prevention.
   Definitive fracture stabilization should take into consideration the need for access to the wound. Fracture stabilization should also allow weight-bearing when appropriate and preservation of the full motion of adjacent joints when possible. Fixation should not cross or span the epiphyseal plates if possible.

26. **When should the definitive treatment of orthopaedic injuries take place?**
Definitive treatment optimally should occur within 48–72 hours. Although controversial, the studies by Loder et al support the early operative stabilization of fractures. Definitive treatment within the first 2–3 days after injury resulted in shorter hospital stays, shorter stays in the intensive care unit (ICU), and shorter times on ventilator assistance. Operative complications were also reported to be lower. Early operative stabilization of fractures is also supported by literature on adults with polytrauma.

27. **With multiple fixation options available, how do you determine which fixation choice to use?**
Orthopaedic fixation options include percutaneous wires, intramedullary rods, external fixation, and internal hardware such as plates. The choice of fixation depends largely on the training, experience, and personal preference of the orthopaedic surgeon. Flexible intramedullary rods have replaced external fixation as the optimal fixation choice for fixation of long-bone fractures in the polytrauma setting. External fixation, however, continues to be useful in open fractures with significant soft tissue injury, in severely comminuted fractures with large bony defects and in fractures involving the proximal and distal regions of long bones. External fixation may also be preferred in the polytrauma patient with life-threatening injuries as it can be performed at the bedside in an intensive care setting.

BIBLIOGRAPHY

1. Galano GJ, Vitale MA, Kessler, MW, et al: The most frequent traumatic orthopaedic injuries from a national pediatric inpatient population. J Pediatr Orthop 25:39–44, 2005.

2. Kay RM, Skaggs DL: Pediatric polytrauma management. J Pediatr Orthop 26:268–277, 2006.

3. Kay RM, Tolo VT: Management of the multiply injured child. In Beaty JH, Kasser JR (eds): Fractures in Children. Philadelphia, Lippincott, Williams & Wilkins, 2006, pp 77–97.

4. Lallier M, Bouchard S, St-Vil D, et al: Falls from heights among children: A retrospective review. J Pediatr Surg 34:1060–1063, 1999.

5. Loder RT, Gullahorn LJ, Yian EH, et al: Factors predictive of immobilization complications in pediatric polytrauma. J Orthop Trauma 15:335–341, 2001.

6. Stewart DG, Kay RM, Skaggs DL: Open fractures in children: Principles of evaluation and management. J Bone Joint Surg 87A:2784–2798, 2005.

CHAPTER 24

FOOT AND ANKLE TRAUMA IN CHILDREN

William Puffinbarger, MD, and J. Andy Sullivan, MD

1. **How are fractures about the foot and ankle in children unique in comparison to their adult counterparts?**

   In children, the physes are still open, and this is the weakest part of the bone-ligament complex. When a force is applied against the foot or ankle, it can cause either a sprain or a fracture. Although serious ankle sprains can occur in children, more often the ligament remains intact and pulls off a portion of the bone. On the lateral side, this pulls off the entire fibular epiphysis with an intact physis and sometimes a very small fragment of the metaphysis. On the medial side in a very young child, usually the entire tibial epiphysis comes off with the physis and a portion of the metaphysis. Since the entire physis is usually intact in these injuries, in most instances, normal growth will resume.

2. **What classification system is used to describe children's epiphyseal fractures?**

   The Salter-Harris classification is the most useful for planning treatment and predicting outcomes in the skeletally immature patient. This system is applied to all physeal injuries and describes the relationship between the fracture and the physis. The Salter-Harris I–IV types are most frequently seen; type V is a crush injury and is rarely, if ever, demonstrated. Other systems consider the position of the foot, the force applied, and the resulting pathoanatomy (i.e., the modified Lauge-Hansen classification).

3. **Is there a fracture pattern that corresponds with age?**

   In the very young child, the injury most often occurs so that the entire epiphysis and physis are disrupted from the metaphysis. If the physis and epiphysis are intact, the articular surface is undisturbed as well. Salter-Harris III and IV medial malleolus fractures tend to occur in the latter part of the first decade of life and early part of the second. As skeletal maturity nears, the physis of the distal tibia begins to close, first medially and then laterally. A fracture may occur through the articular surface, epiphysis, and physis toward the lateral side, remaining open. This results in Salter-Harris III (i.e., juvenile Tillaux) and IV (i.e., triplane) fractures, as opposed to types I and II, which are more common in a younger child.

4. **Which factors help predict the outcome of ankle fractures in children?**

   - The Salter-Harris classification
   - How well the fracture is reduced
   - The level of skeletal maturity
   - The degree of displacement
   - Any modifier (e.g., an open fracture, a vascular injury, systemic illness, or infection)

   Salter-Harris I and II fractures are the most predictable, and the incidence of complications remains approximately the same for both, regardless of the amount of displacement. However, some type II injuries of the distal tibia that have been reduced and appear benign may develop premature growth closure; these must be followed for several years. Whenever possible, these should be reduced to near-anatomic alignment.

   Salter-Harris III and IV injuries have higher complication rates. Because they involve the articular surface and cross the physis, anatomic or near-anatomic reduction is required in addition to internal fixation to maintain the alignment. Premature closure, angular deformity, and leg-length discrepancy are more likely to result from these injuries. Particular attention must be paid to the medial malleolus, in which there is a high incidence of premature physeal closure.

5. **How are fractures about the ankle managed?**
Salter-Harris I injuries occur in the distal tibia and, more commonly, in the distal fibula. These must be differentiated from an ankle sprain. Their diagnosis is based on a history of inversion injury combined with swelling and tenderness directly over the physis, as opposed to the ligament complex. The radiograph may appear normal or show the physis slightly widened. If there is any question, the extremity should be immobilized for 3 weeks in a short-leg walking cast.

Salter-Harris II fractures of the distal tibial physis, with or without a fracture of the fibula, are not uncommon in the preadolescent and early adolescent. Most can be reduced closed and satisfactorily maintained with a long-leg walking cast, which can then be converted to a short-leg walking cast after 2–3 weeks. The fracture is typically healed in 6 weeks. Walking casts promote early healing and a rapid return to full activity and have a low complication rate.

Salter-Harris III fractures occur in the distal tibial epiphysis (i.e., Tillaux fracture). A fragment of the lateral epiphysis remains attached to the anterior tibiofibular ligament. These will often require open reduction and internal fixation of the fragment with a pin or screw. If at all possible, the fixation should not cross the physis. Fractures of the medial malleolus can be either Salter-Harris III or IV. If they are nondisplaced, they can be treated closed in a long-leg non-weight-bearing cast for 3 weeks, followed by a short-leg walking cast for 3 weeks. These are among the most unpredictable of ankle epiphyseal injuries. Near-anatomic reduction must be achieved, even if it requires open reduction or internal fixation.

Salter-Harris IV fractures include those of the medial malleolus and the so-called triplane fracture, in which the fracture lines extend into the transverse, sagittal, and coronal planes (Figs. 24-1, 24-2, and 24-3). This is best diagnosed by looking carefully at both the anteroposterior (AP) and the lateral radiographs. A computed tomographic (CT) scan will accurately diagnose and identify the pathoanatomy prior to open reduction and internal

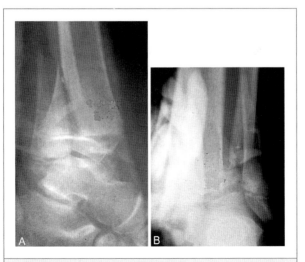

Figure 24-1. *A,* AP radiograph. *B,* Lateral radiograph of a triplane ankle fracture. The fracture lines extend through all three planes (thus the name triplane).

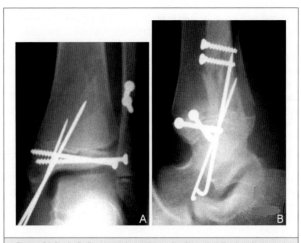

Figure 24-2. *A, B,* Postoperative radiographs. Note that fixation devices extend into the sagittal, frontal, and coronal planes.

fixation. In the past, these injuries have been associated with a high complication rate, but, if reduced well surgically, the results should be good. Because these patients are approaching skeletal maturity, physeal arrest is less likely to cause angular deformity or leg-length discrepancy. The articular surface must be reduced. These injuries should be treated for 6 weeks in a cast.

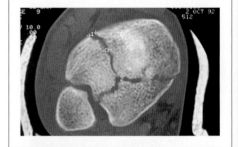

Figure 24-3. Computed tomography scan showing multiple fragments.

6. **What are the most common fractures of the foot?**

The metatarsals are the most frequently fractured, accounting for nearly 90% of fractures in one series. Most fractures of the shafts of the metatarsals can be satisfactorily treated in a short-leg walking cast for 4–6 weeks. The base of the fifth metatarsal is the point of attachment of the peroneus brevis tendon on the apophysis of the base of the fifth metatarsal. An inversion injury may avulse this apophysis. Findings include tenderness at the base of the fifth metatarsal, pain with attempted eversion against resistance, and swelling. Radiographs may show widening of the apophysis. These fractures will heal uneventfully. Immobilization with crutches and an elastic bandage until pain subsides is usually satisfactory. A period of 2–3 weeks in a short-leg walking cast can also produce favorable results.

The so-called Jones fracture is one of the proximal diaphysis of the fifth metatarsal and, although less common, can proceed to nonunion. Initially, each patient needs to be managed conservatively; immobilization in a short-leg non-weight-bearing cast should be the first form of treatment. If this results in delayed union or nonunion, operative intervention with screw fixation and bone grafting should be done. Established nonunion requires a reopening of the medullary canal.

Fractures of the toes can be treated by taping to the adjacent toe. Perhaps the only operative indication in children would be a Salter-Harris III or IV type of the proximal phalanx of the great toe. Sufficient displacement requiring operative treatment is rare.

7. What causes stress fractures? How are they managed?

"Too much, too soon." Stress fractures may result from a sudden increase or change in intensity or type of training or a change in training surface or in shoe type. These are most frequent in the metatarsals, but they can occur in the navicular and the medial sesamoid. Diagnosis requires vigilance and a high index of suspicion; initial films may be negative. Bone scan is not necessary unless you are dealing with an elite athlete who must return to competition. In most cases, immobilization in a short-leg walking cast for 2–3 weeks and repeat radiographs will show periosteal new bone, confirming the diagnosis. Again, be aware that the initial radiograph may appear normal in more than half the cases.

8. How frequent are fractures of the calcaneus? How are they treated?

They occur much less frequently than in the adult. Most occur as children approach skeletal maturity. As in the adult, these fractures are often associated with other injuries, such as fractures of the lumbar spine or pelvic injuries. Many of these involve the tuberosity of the posterior portion and will heal uneventfully with either non-weight-bearing or weight-bearing as tolerated. It is less common for them to involve the articular surface. Fractures that are intra-articular often require surgical management and reconstitution of the articular surface. Those that are minimally displaced or nondisplaced can be treated with non-weight-bearing until they heal in about 6 weeks.

9. How frequent are fractures of the talus? How are they managed in children?

Fortunately, these are rare in children and are somewhat different from the equivalent adult injury. They usually result from forced dorsiflexion and can involve the body or the neck. If they are nondisplaced, use a long-leg non-weight-bearing cast. Weight-bearing is commenced when there is some sign of healing. Displaced fractures require open reduction and internal fixation. This should be done as soon as possible as there may be embarrassment of the blood supply to the talus, which can result in avascular necrosis (AVN). Placement of a cannulated screw allows good control and compression of the fracture site. The fractures are then treated in a non-weight-bearing cast until signs of healing appear, followed by weight-bearing. These must be followed for AVN, which is the most significant complication that occurs with them. AVN can occur in either displaced or nondisplaced fractures, indicating that children may be at greater risk than adults for developing this problem. You must look for the subchondral lucency (i.e., Hawkins sign), signifying disuse osteopenia and viability of the talus.

The dome of the talus can also be injured from significant trauma. Complete AVN and destruction of the talus can occur as a result of an ankle injury with an associated high-energy Salter-Harris type III injury of the distal tibial physis. The talus is probably compressed violently against the articular surface of the tibia as a result of a high-energy injury, such as a motor vehicle accident.

Osteochondral fractures occur in children, particularly as they approach skeletal maturity. These require anatomic reduction and internal fixation.

KEY POINTS: FOOT AND ANKLE TRAUMA

1. The physis and its state of maturity are the keys to understanding the pattern of fractures in the foot and ankle in children and adolescents.

2. The physis, when open, is the weak link in the bone-ligament interface and, when stressed, fails before the ligament.

3. As the physis begins to close in adolescence, the pattern of the fractures changes, becoming that of an adult when it is fully closed.

4. The factors that determine the outcome of these injuries are as follows:
   - The Salter-Harris classification
   - How well the fracture is reduced
   - The level of skeletal maturity
   - The degree of displacement
   - Any modifier (e.g., open fracture, vascular injury, systemic illness, or infection)

---

10. Do injuries to Lisfranc's joint occur in children?

Yes. Previously unrecognized, it is now known that this tarsal-metatarsal disruption does occur and requires a precise diagnosis and anatomic reduction. A fracture at the base of the second metatarsal should raise suspicion. Some can be reduced closed but must be maintained with some type of internal fixation, such as pins or wires. The second metatarsal keys into the cuneiforms and must be reduced and stabilized. Pins may be necessary in the other metatarsals to maintain their reduction.

11. What disease processes and normal variants can be confused with fractures in children?

Children have a variety of osteochondroses that can be confused with injury. These include osteochondroses of the second metatarsal head (i.e., Freiberg's disease) and the navicular joint (Kohler's disease) and irregular ossification of the calcaneal apophysis (Sever's disease). In addition, there are a variety of accessory ossicles and sesamoids in the foot that can be mistaken for fractures. For instance, it is not unusual for the sesamoid associated with the first metatarsal to be bipartite and mistaken for a fracture of the sesamoid. The os trigonum, located immediately behind the talus, may either be an integral part of the talus or it may separate. There are also often irregularities in ossification of the epiphyses of the medial malleolus and fibular malleolus, which can be confused with fractures. All of these are distinguishable from a fracture in that they are more rounded, sclerotic, and do not have the appearance of acute fracture. When in doubt, radiographs of the opposite foot or ankle should be obtained for comparison.

12. What is the significance of a Park-Harris growth-arrest line parallel to the physis 6 months after a physeal fracture?

It signifies that a physeal arrest has not occurred. If it converges with the physis, a partial arrest has occurred.

13. What is stubbed-toe osteomyelitis?

An infected open physeal fracture of the distal phalanx of the great toe. Usually weeks to months before presentation, the child has stubbed the toe. At that time, clinically, there is elevation of the nail, disruption of the nail matrix, and bleeding from the proximal nail fold. Many do not seek formal medical care. On films, there is a physeal fracture (usually Salter-Harris I or II), which, due to the nail matrix disruption, is open, allowing bacterial contamination.

BIBLIOGRAPHY

1. Ashworth A, Hedden D: Fractures of the ankle. In Letts RM (ed): Management of Pediatric Fractures. New York, Churchill Livingstone, 1994, pp 713–734.

2. Baxter MP: Fractures and dislocations of the metatarsals and phalanges. In Letts RM (ed): The Management of Pediatric Fractures. New York, Churchill Livingstone, 1994, pp 767–788.

3. Carrol N: Fractures and dislocations of the tarsal bones. In Letts RM (ed): The Management of Pediatric Fractures. New York, Churchill Livingstone, 1994, pp 751–766.

4. Crawford AH: Fractures and dislocations of the foot and ankle. In Green NE, Swiontkowski MF (eds): Skeletal Trauma in Children, 3rd ed. Philadelphia, W.B. Saunders, 2003, pp 516–586.

5. Ertl JP, Barrack RL, Alexander AH, VanBuecken K: Triplane fractures of the distal tibial epiphysis: Long-term follow-up. J Bone Joint Surg 70A:967, 1988.

6. Jarvis JG: Tibial triplane fractures. In Letts RM (ed): The Management of Pediatric Fractures. New York, Churchill Livingstone, 1994, pp 735–750.

7. Lower extremity injuries. In Herring JA (ed): Tachdjian's Pediatric Orthopaedics from the Texas Scottish Rite Hospital for Children, 3rd ed. Philadelphia, W.B. Saunders, 2002, pp 2391–2438.

8. Price C: Management of fractures. In Morrissy RT, Weinstein SL (eds): Lovell and Winter's Pediatric Orthopaedics, 5th ed. Philadelphia, Lippincott Williams and Wilkins, 2001, pp 1401–1414.

9. Sullivan JA: Ankle and foot fractures in the pediatric athlete. In Stanitski CL, DeLee JC, Drez DD Jr (eds): The Management of Pediatric Fractures. Philadelphia, W.B. Saunders, 1994, pp 441–455.

CHAPTER 25

KNEE INJURIES

Kit M. Song, MD

1. **What are important anatomic and mechanical considerations in knee injuries in children?**

   All knee ligament origins and insertions and capsular attachments are to the epiphyses except for the medial collateral ligament and the tibial collateral insertions, which have attachments to the tibial epiphysis, the tibial metaphysis, and the fibular head. This arrangement makes the proximal tibial physis more resistant to injury than the distal femoral physis. Both are physeal growth plates and the ligaments have viscoelastic properties, and their strength is determined by the total force applied and the rate of loading. Pure ligamentous injuries are secondary to low-energy rapid-loading events, and injuries to the physis or tendon-bone junctions occur with high-energy, slow-loading events.

2. **Describe important points of the clinical evaluation of knee injuries in children.**

   - **A careful history:** This will be more vague than that for adults. Information regarding the mechanism of injury, the timing of the onset of effusion, whether a pop was felt at the time of injury, any mechanical blocking symptoms, and feelings of true instability will often be lacking.
   - **A detailed physical examination:** Always examine the uninjured knee first. If possible, examine the patient walking. Children will seldom tolerate ligamentous laxity testing or provocative maneuvers following an acute injury. In the absence of an obvious fracture, immobilization and repeat examination 1–2 weeks later are appropriate. The physical examination findings in the preadolescent will be less accurate than in adults or adolescents. A careful neurovascular examination should be performed. Always examine the hips of children presenting with knee pain. Remember that hip problems in children can cause referred pain to the knee.
   - **Selective imaging of the knee**

3. **What imaging modalities are helpful in evaluating knee injuries in children?**

   Plain radiographs remain important in evaluating knee injuries in children and can demonstrate physeal injuries and lesions that mimic meniscus injuries. Double-contrast arthrography remains useful in evaluating the pediatric knee, owing to the large amount of cartilage present prior to maturity. It has an accuracy rate of greater than 90% in experienced hands but has the great disadvantage of being invasive. Magnetic resonance imaging (MRI) has been increasingly applied to the evaluation of knee injuries. MRI is very sensitive and specific for the detection of acute injuries to the anterior cruciate ligament (ACL). The sensitivity of MRI is 95% for medial meniscus injuries and 90% for lateral meniscus injuries.

4. **What is the differential diagnosis for an acute hemarthrosis of the knee in a child?**

   For preadolescents, meniscal tears (47%), ACL injuries (47%), and osteochondral fractures (13%) account for the majority of injuries with hemarthrosis. For adolescents, ACL tears (65%), meniscus tears (45%), and osteochondral fractures (5%) account for the majority of hemarthroses.

5. **How can you differentiate a true ligament injury from a physeal injury in a child?**
Both injuries present with swelling and pain within and about the knee. Age younger than 14 years, prepubertal status, and the mechanism of injury will be the most helpful clues to suspecting a physeal injury. A nondisplaced fracture through the physis may be difficult to visualize radiographically. Oblique, comparison, and stress views may be helpful. It must be remembered that physeal fracture and ligament disruption can occur simultaneously. Evaluation of ligamentous stability after fracture management is advised.

6. **How common are knee ligament injuries in children?**
The incidence of ACL injuries is 0.3–0.38 per 1000 per year. The majority of injuries are related to the sports of football, soccer, skiing, and basketball. The incidence of avulsion of the tibial spine is estimated to be 3 in 100,000 children per year. Skeletally immature patients account for 3–4% of all ACL tears. Isolated lateral collateral ligament (LCL) injuries in children are rare and are associated with polytrauma in younger children. Isolated medial collateral ligament (MCL) injuries in children are not uncommon, but the incidence is not known. Isolated posterior cruciate ligament (PCL) injuries are rare in children.

7. **How does failure of the ACL occur in children?**
Bony avulsion of the tibial insertion of the ACLs occurs in preadolescent children. Intrasubstance tears are more common in adolescents. The mechanism of injury is generally hyperextension, sudden deceleration, or a valgus rotational force with a stationary foot.

8. **What is the natural history of the ACL-deficient knee in a skeletally immature patient?**
The natural history of ACL deficiencies in preadolescent children is not well defined, owing to the small number of such injuries. For adolescents, the natural history appears to be similar to that in young adults. Episodes of "giving way" are reported in 33–86% of subjects with ACL tears treated nonoperatively. Activity level, not age, is the primary risk factor for recurrent instability. Because adolescents are very active, conservative treatment will fail in a greater number of these patients. A relatively inactive adolescent, however, may have a very satisfactory outcome without ligament reconstruction.

9. **How are bony avulsions of the ACL insertion on the anterior tibial spine classified?**
Avulsion injuries of the ACL are classified on the basis of displacement:
- **Type I fractures:** These are minimally displaced and are best managed with cast immobilization in slight flexion.
- **Type II fractures:** These have a posterior hinge but are still attached to the tibial epiphysis. These fractures should undergo closed reduction and cast immobilization.
- **Type III fractures:** These are displaced and require open reduction and suture or screw fixation, avoiding crossing the physis.

10. **What are the management options for an isolated intrasubstance tear of the ACL in a skeletally immature child? In a skeletally mature child?**
In the absence of a torn meniscus, ACL injuries in preadolescent children are best managed with activity modification and observation. Repair of the ligament is at best controversial and will have a high rate of failure. Children with more than 1 year of growth remaining should not undergo ligament reconstruction with bone tunnels that cross the epiphyseal growth plate. For the rare situation of a prepubertal child with an intrasubstance tear and significant instability, an extra-articular reconstruction can be done (in a very young child) or a hamstring reconstruction, using a tibial tunnel and placement over the top of the femoral condyle, can be performed (in an older child).

The adolescent with an ACL disruption should be managed as an adult. It must be established that the ACL injury is an isolated one. If there is an associated meniscus tear that is repairable, an aggressive approach to reconstruction of the ACL is justified.

11. **What are the clinical findings and mechanism of injury associated with a torn PCL in a child?**
    The mechanism of injury to the PCL is a direct blow to the tibia, hyperflexion of the knee, or hyperextension of the knee. Hyperflexion injuries are associated with avulsion of the PCL origin from the femur. The posterior drawer test is usually positive, but it may be negative if Wrisberg's and Humphry's ligaments are intact.

12. **What are the treatment options for a torn PCL in a child?**
    Intrasubstance tears of the PCL in a skeletally immature child are best managed with activity modification and observation. An avulsion of the PCL origin from the femur or insertion onto the tibia is best treated with open reduction and internal fixation. Intrasubstance PCL disruptions in the skeletally mature patient should be managed as in an adult, with reconstruction if the patient is symptomatic.

13. **What is the clinical presentation of meniscal injuries in children?**
    The primary symptoms of meniscus injuries in children are pain (95%), effusion (71%), snapping (63%), giving way of the knee (63%), intermittent locking of the knee (54%), and a locked knee (7%). The symptoms may change over time. Joint-line tenderness and McMurray's test are not as reliable in children as in adults.

14. **What is the outcome of meniscectomies for a torn meniscus in children?**
    The outcome of complete meniscectomies in children is very poor, with a 60% unsatisfactory outcome at the 7-year follow-up examination. Preservation of the meniscus is important, and, whenever possible, operative repair should be done. Peripheral tears are more common in children than in adults; the repair of peripheral tears in children has a favorable outcome in 80–90% of cases. Tears of the meniscus in the avascular zone should be treated with a partial meniscectomy.

15. **What is a discoid meniscus? Where does it occur?**
    Early reports had suggested that a discoid meniscus was caused by an arrest in embryologic development with a failure of resorption of the central portion of the meniscus. Subsequent studies did not find a meniscus with a discoid morphology at any stage of fetal development. It is believed that this condition is acquired when an initially normal meniscus has abnormal peripheral attachments that lead to meniscal hypermobility and hypertrophy. The meniscus may be stable or unstable (i.e., Wrisberg's ligament), with or without meniscotibial attachments. The stable meniscus may be either complete or incomplete, depending on how much of the tibial plateau it covers. The clinical finding is a disc of meniscal cartilage covering the lateral tibial plateau. There are no reports of a medial discoid meniscus.

16. **What is the incidence of discoid meniscus?**
    There is considerable cultural variation in the incidence of discoid menisci. The reported ranges are 3–20%, with the highest incidence in the Japanese.

17. **What are the presenting symptoms and findings with a discoid meniscus?**
    Symptoms include lateral knee pain, snapping or popping within the knee, decreased extension of the knee, and episodes of giving way, with slight swelling that rapidly resolves. An asymptomatic or unstable meniscus that is popping back and forth within the knee but is not causing pain is best left untreated until it does become symptomatic. As children reach puberty, tears of the meniscus become more common. Most discoid menisci remain asymptomatic.

18. **What are the options for treatment of a symptomatic discoid meniscus?**
Excision of the torn portion of the meniscus, sculpting of the meniscus by excision of the torn central portion, or complete meniscectomy.

19. **What is the outcome of complete meniscectomy for symptomatic discoid meniscus?**
At 20-year follow-up, 75% of patients will show degenerative changes of the lateral condyle radiographically. Despite this, the majority of patients will have clinically acceptable function.

20. **What is osteochondritis dissecans?**
Osteochondritis dissecans is a lesion of bone and cartilage that results in bone necrosis and loss of continuity of the subchondral bone. This may or may not lead to loss of articular cartilage continuity. The cause of this lesion is unknown. Theories have ranged from abnormal vascular anatomy, leading to ischemic injury to bone, to existence of a normal accessory ossification center that fails to fuse with the surrounding bone.

21. **What are the most common sites for osteochondritis dissecans in the knee?**
The most common site is the lateral middle-to-posterior portion of the medial femoral condyle (57–83%). Other sites are the lateral femoral condyle (20%) and the patella (15%).

22. **What is the initial management of osteochondritis dissecans in a skeletally immature child?**
In children with open growth plates, there is a much higher potential for healing with immobilization than in adults. If the subchondral bone is intact, immobilization in a cast for 2–3 months may produce healing. This is especially true in girls younger than the age of 11 and boys younger than the age of 13. If the subchondral bone is disrupted or there is a loose fragment, immobilization is unlikely to succeed and surgical treatment should be offered.

KEY POINTS: KNEE INJURIES

1. Bony avulsion injuries can occur in prepubertal children prior to ligament failures.

2. Long-term results of meniscectomies in children are poor, and repair should be attempted when possible.

3. The diagnostic test with the greatest sensitivity and specificity for evaluation of acute hemarthrosis of the knee is a magnetic resonance imaging (MRI) scan.

23. **What are the principles of surgical treatment of osteochondritis dissecans of the knee?**
The optimal treatment is controversial. The basic concepts are as follows:
- Fragmented displaced lesions are best excised.
- Painful lesions in continuity with the surrounding bone should be drilled.
- Displaced small lesions should be excised and curetted.
- Displaced large lesions with subchondral bone attached to cartilage should be fixed, with or without bone grafting.

A wide variety of fixation devices, bone grafting techniques, and surgical approaches are available.

24. **What is Osgood-Schlatter disease?**

Osgood-Schlatter disease is an alteration in the development of the tibial tuberosity due to repeated application of tensile forces. It is generally a self-limited condition and will respond to rest. It is bilateral in 20–30% of cases. A small number of children will develop painful ossicles within the patellar tendon that will require surgical removal.

25. **How common are fractures of the tibial tubercle relative to all growth plate injuries?**

The reported incidence is 0.4–2.7% of all growth-plate injuries.

26. **What is the average age at which fractures of the tibial tubercle occur?**

The average age in most series is 14 years, and most of the patients are boys.

27. **What factors guide the management of tibial tubercle fractures?**

The degree of displacement and the size of the fragment involved. Minimally displaced small fragments can be treated nonoperatively. Displaced fragments are treated operatively with reduction and internal fixation.

BIBLIOGRAPHY

1. Beaty JH: Intra-articular and ligamentous injuries about the knee. In Rockwood CA, Wilkins KE, Beaty JH (eds): Fractures in Children, 4th ed. Vol. 3. Philadelphia, Lippincott-Raven, 1996.

2. Beaty JH, Kumar A: Fractures about the knee in children. J Bone Joint Surg 76A:1870–1880, 1994.

3. Meyers MH, McDeever FM: Fracture of the intercondylar eminence of the tibia. J Bone Joint Surg 52A:209–220, 1959.

4. Smith AD, Tao SS: Knee injuries in young athletes. Clin Sports Med 14:629–650, 1995.

5. Stanitski CL, DeLee JC, Drez D (eds): Pediatric and Adolescent Sports Medicine. Philadelphia, W.B. Saunders, 1994.

6. Stanitski CL, Harvell JC, Fu F: Observations on acute knee hemarthrosis in children and adolescents. J Pediatr Orthop 13:506–510, 1993.

7. Vahvanaen V, Aalto K: Meniscectomy in children. Acta Orthop Scand 50:791–795, 1979.

8. Vahassarja V, Kinnuen P, Serlo W: Arthroscopy of the acute traumatic knee in children. Prospective study of 138 cases. Acta Orthop Scand 64:580–582, 1993.

9. Wojtys EM (ed): The ACL Deficient Knee. American Academy of Orthopedic Surgeons, Rosemont, IL, 1994.

CHAPTER 26

TIBIAL INJURIES

Kit M. Song, MD

1. **Describe the anatomic and development features of the tibia and the fibula in the growing child.**

   The tibia develops from three ossification centers, one in the diaphysis and two in the epiphyses. The proximal epiphysis appears shortly after birth and closes at approximately 16 years of age. A secondary ossification center forms for the tibial tuberosity and appears at age 7–9 years, fusing with the remaining epiphysis in adolescence. The distal epiphysis appears in the second year of life and closes at approximately 16–18 years. There may be a secondary ossification center in the medial malleolus that appears at age 7–9 years and fuses with the remaining distal tibia by age 14–15 years. Accessory malleolar ossification centers can also be present in the medial malleolus, which can be confused with fractures. Closure of the distal tibial epiphysis is in a posteromedial-to-anterolateral direction over 1½ years. This pattern of closure creates characteristic fracture patterns.

   The distal and proximal fibular epiphyses begin to ossify at age 2 and 4 years, respectively. Distal epiphyseal closure occurs at age 16, and proximal closure is 1–2 years later. The distal fibular epiphyseal growth plate is at the same level as the tibial growth plate at birth and descends to the ankle joint by the age of 7 years.

2. **How often do fractures and injuries of the tibia and fibula occur in children?**

   The tibia and fibula are the third most commonly injured long bones in children, after the radius and ulna. Tibial fractures are the most common lower-limb fractures in children, accounting for approximately 15% of pediatric long-bone fractures.

3. **In what location and by what mechanism do most fractures and injuries of the tibia and fibula occur in children?**

   Fifty percent of fractures occur in the distal tibia. These are most common in the older child and are usually due to indirect trauma. Thirty-five percent of fractures are in the middle third. Fifteen percent involve the proximal tibia and are most common in children 3–6 years of age. Thirty percent of tibial fractures will also involve the fibula. The most common mechanism of injury is direct force from pedestrian motor vehicle injury (50%), followed by indirect twisting injuries (22%), falls from a height (17%), and motor vehicle injuries (11%). The tibia is fractured in 26% of children who are victims of child abuse.

   Fracture of the proximal fibula is uncommon and can be displaced owing to the pull of the biceps. Open reduction and internal fixation are often needed. Subluxation or dislocation of the proximal tibiofibular joint is also uncommon, but early recognition within the first week can lead to a successful closed reduction. Isolated fibular diaphyseal fractures are rare and are generally due to direct blows.

4. **What is a common deformity after treatment of proximal tibial fractures in children? What are its causes?**

   Valgus deformity after union of proximal tibial fractures is common and occurs in the first 6 months after injury. The deformity is not progressive. The cause of this can be poor reduction, but it is seen even in children with an anatomically correct reduction. Other theories to explain this are injury to the pes anserinus tendon, with loss of its normal tethering effect upon medial growth of the tibia; enchondral bone overgrowth due to increased vascularity of the medial tibia; relative overgrowth of the tibia to the fibula, leading to a lateral tethering; and valgus angulation. Spontaneous correction of the deformity has been reported. The deformity can recur after osteotomy of the tibia, and early correction is not recommended.

5. **What vascular and neurologic complications can be seen with tibial fractures in children?**

Vascular and neurologic injuries are uncommon in children, but the anterior tibial artery may be injured proximally as it passes through the interosseous membrane or distally if there is posterior displacement of the distal fragment. Displaced metaphyseal tibial fractures will require closed reduction, usually under general anesthesia. If there is clinical evidence of a dysvascular foot after reduction, arteriography should be considered. The peroneal nerve can be injured with proximal fibular injuries.

Compartment syndrome can and does occur in children with tibial injuries. The exact incidence is unknown. The assessment of pain and clinical detection of muscle compartment swelling in young children can be very difficult, making early detection of compartment syndrome difficult. Distal swelling may be an early finding.

6. **Does overgrowth of tibial fractures occur in children?**

Overgrowth of the tibia does occur in children younger than the age of 10 years but is not as predictable or as well documented as fractures of the femur. Shortening greater than 1 cm is not likely to resolve. Tibial overgrowth can be observed following femur fractures, even in the absence of a tibial fracture.

7. **How much spontaneous correction of angular deformity will occur following tibial shaft fractures?**

The cumulative experience of several large series suggests that angular correction can occur up to 18 months after fracture, with the range of improvement being 13–100%. Deformities greater than 10 degrees should not be expected to correct fully. Children under the age of 10 years have the best chance of some correction. Varus malalignment will generally correct better than valgus malalignment. Rotational deformities do not spontaneously correct. The degree of malunion that can be accepted without long-term morbidity has not been defined.

8. **What factors affect fracture healing in children with tibia fractures?**

The age of the child, the degree of soft tissue injury, and the presence of deep infection have the greatest impact on healing of tibial fractures in children. The time required for osseous union of a closed diaphyseal fracture is 2–3 weeks in a neonate, is 4–6 weeks for a toddler and younger child, and approaches the average 16 weeks seen in adults by the age of 14 years. The time required for osseous union increases for open fractures and parallels the grade of injury, with average healing times of 6 months for adolescents and 5 months for preadolescents with Gustillo grade III injuries. Nonunions and delayed unions are rare in children under the age of 11 years, but in adolescents these complications approach the incidence seen in adults. The presence of infection also greatly delays healing but is uncommon in younger children, even with open fractures, if adequate soft tissue debridement is done. The use of external fixation is associated with longer healing times. Location and fracture pattern will also affect healing times. Metaphyseal and spiral or long oblique fractures will heal more quickly than transverse diaphyseal fractures. Loss of periosteum (as in penetrating trauma with segmental bone loss) can also lead to delayed union or nonunion.

9. **What are the operative stabilization options that can be used in children with tibial fractures?**

Monolateral external fixators with pins more than 1 cm from the growth plates, plate fixation with open reduction, limited internal fixation with wires or screws, and flexible intramedullary nails can be used in a child of any age and are preferred for children with more than 1 year of growth remaining if surgical stabilization is needed. Children who are within 1 year of skeletal maturity can be treated with reamed or unreamed tibial nails.

10. **When is operative stabilization of tibial fractures indicated for children?**
Open fractures require operative debridement and aggressive soft tissue management, just as in adults. Only 9% of tibial fractures in children are open, and many Gustillo grade I or II injuries can be managed with a cast or splint. Severe soft tissue injuries, complex or unstable fractures, fractures involving the articular surface, polytrauma for which fracture stabilization facilitates care, and vascular injury needing repair require bone stabilization with internal or external fixation.

KEY POINTS: TIBIAL INJURIES

1. Proximal tibial fractures in younger children will often temporarily grow into valgus.

2. The capacity for remodeling malunion or overgrowth of shortening due to tibial shaft fractures is age-dependent.

3. Compartmental syndrome does occur in children following tibial fractures and is more common after high-energy and proximal tibial injuries.

11. **What is a toddler's fracture?**
A toddler's fracture is a fracture of the tibia in a child 9 months to 3 years of age due to low-energy forces, which may lead to a limp and fracture of the tibia. This injury may be a stress fracture of the tibia. There is generally not an associated fracture of the fibula. The fracture, if visible, is a spiral fracture of the distal diaphysis and metaphysis.

12. **What are the clinical and radiographic findings for a toddler's fracture?**
The child suddenly refuses to bear weight, with no observable trauma. There may be localized redness, warmth, and tenderness. The child will usually crawl but not walk, which is important in differentiating this from problems at the hip.
   The initial evaluation should include a complete blood count with differential and an analysis of the erythrocyte sedimentation rate and C-reactive protein. Oblique radiographs can help visualize the fracture line. Technetium bone scanning can be helpful if x-ray findings are normal. Immobilization and repeat radiographs in 10 days to 2 weeks will show periosteal reaction and sclerosis.

13. **What is the most common location of a stress fracture in an older child? What is the management of this problem?**
The proximal third of the tibia is the most common site of stress fractures in children. The peak incidence is 10–15 years of age. Fibular stress fractures are less common and occur from 2–8 years of age. The management of tibial stress fractures is rest and immobilization for 4–6 weeks. Fibular stress fractures may be managed with activity modification and immobilization as needed for comfort.

14. **What is a floating knee? How is it treated?**
A floating knee is characterized by both a distal femoral and an ipsilateral tibial fracture. These are high-energy injuries and will be seen primarily in adolescents. Coincidental ligamentous injury of the knee is seen in 10% of cases. Operative stabilization of at least one of the bones

is recommended because closed management of both injuries is associated with at least a 30% incidence of postfracture complications.

BIBLIOGRAPHY

1. Buckley SL, Smith G, Sponseller PD, et al: Open fractures of the tibia in children. J Bone Joint Surg 72A:1462–1469, 1990.

2. Buckley SL, Smith GR, Sponseller PD, et al: Severe (type III) open fractures of the tibia in children. J Pediatr Orthop 16:627–634, 1996.

3. Hansen BA, Greiff J, Bergmann F: Fractures of the tibia in children. Acta Orthop Scand 47:448–453, 1976.

4. Heinrich SD: Fractures of the shaft of the tibia and fibula. In Rockwood CA, Wilkins KE, Beaty JH (eds): Fractures in Children, 4th ed. Vol. 3. Philadelphia, Lippincott-Raven, 1996.

5. King J, Diefendorf D, Apthorp J, et al: Analysis of 429 fractures in 189 battered children. J Pediatr Orthop 8:585–589, 1988.

6. Letts M, Vincent M, Gouw G: The "floating knee" in children. J Bone Joint Surg 68B:442–446, 1986.

7. Ogden JA: Subluxation and dislocation of the proximal tibiofibular joint. J Bone Joint Surg 56A:145–154, 1974.

8. Oudjhane K, Newman B, Oh KS, et al: Occult fractures in preschool children. J Trauma 28:858–860, 1988.

9. Salter RB, Best TN: Pathogenesis of progressive valgus deformity following fractures of the proximal metaphyseal region of the tibia in young children. Instr Course Lect 41:409–411, 1992.

10. Shannak AO: Tibial fractures in children: Follow-up study. J Pediatr Orthop 8:306–310, 1988.

11. Song KM, Sangorzan B, Benirschke S, Browne R: Open fractures of the tibia in children. J Pediatr Orthop 16:635–639, 1996.

12. Zionts LE, MacEwen GD: Spontaneous improvement of post-traumatic tibia valga. J Bone Joint Surg 68A:680–687, 1986.

CHAPTER 27

FEMUR FRACTURES

Wesley Bevan, MBChB, FRACS, and Deborah Stanitski, MD

1. **How common are fractures of the femoral shaft in children?**
   Various studies have estimated the incidence of femoral shaft fracture at approximately 1% of children under the age of 12. They make up 1.6% of pediatric fractures.

2. **In children between the onset of walking and 3 years of age, what is the most common mechanism of injury?**
   A fall.

3. **In what age range is the maximum incidence of femur fractures?**
   There is a bimodal distribution, with peak incidences at 2 years and 12 years of age.

4. **How are femoral fractures classified?**
   Like other fractures, femoral fractures are classified according to the following:
   - **Location:** Proximal, middle, distal third diaphyseal, and subtrochanteric or supracondylar
   - **Position:** Angulation, displacement, or shortening
   - **Fracture pattern:** Transverse, oblique, spiral, segmental, or comminuted
   - **Injury type:** Open, closed, or soft tissue injury, and the neurologic and vascular state of the limb
   - **Other injuries:** Isolated injury or other associated injuries
   - **Bone quality:** Normal, osteoporotic (i.e., cerebral palsy or myelomeningocele), or abnormal (i.e., a benign or malignant bone lesion or osteogenesis imperfecta)

5. **What is the most common location for femoral shaft fracture?**
   Approximately 70% of these fractures occur in the middle third, 22% in the proximal third, and 8% in the distal third of the diaphysis.

6. **What is Waddell's triad of injury when a child is struck by a car while crossing the street?**
   A fractured femur, a head injury, and an intra-abdominal or intrathoracic injury.

7. **What is the most important cause to exclude in children less than 1 year of age who sustain a femoral fracture?**
   Child abuse is the most common cause of femoral fractures in children who have not yet begun walking. It is reported that up to 80% of fractures in this age group may be secondary to abuse. Child abuse needs to also be considered in toddlers, with 30% of fractures in this age group thought to be secondary to abuse.

8. **What is the first consideration in treatment of a femoral fracture?**
   Diminution of pain. A femoral fracture is very painful because it produces strong muscle spasms in the thigh, which has the largest muscle mass in the body. Splinting or skin traction (at a maximum of 5 lbs) is recommended to improve patient comfort.

9. **Identify the two basic types of traction.**
Skin traction and skeletal traction. The latter involves drilling a traction pin through the distal femur, from which the patient's limb is suspended. The traction pin is placed in the distal femur, proximal to the physis.

10. **When can Bryant's overhead skin traction be used?**
Patients weighing less than 20 lbs or younger than 2 years of age can be treated with overhead traction. Heavier patients risk neurovascular complications.

11. **When is skeletal traction necessary?**
Skeletal traction is only necessary for those fractures for which alignment can not be controlled by skin traction treatment. This may include subtrochanteric fractures, which tend to flex and abduct excessively unless treated in 90-degree–to–90-degree skeletal traction.

12. **How long is traction required prior to cast application?**
The answer depends on the patient's age and the fracture pattern. There must be adequate provisional callus to avoid excessive shortening once traction is removed. This varies from 7–10 days in the young child to as much as 3–4 weeks in the adolescent. A spica cast is then applied.

13. **What general treatment methods can be used for femoral shaft fractures?**
   - **Nonsurgical:** A Pavlik harness, traction with delayed cast immobilization, immediate spica cast, or traction
   - **Surgical:** Flexible intermedullary nails (stainless steel vs. titanium), external fixation, compression plating, submuscular plate, or a rigid locked intermedullary nail
   More recently, there has been a trend away from inpatient traction and delayed casting toward more-immediate spica casting or operative fixation and mobilization, depending on the age, weight, and fracture type. This has led to significant decrease in the inpatient stay time. In older children and adolescents, this may lead to a faster recovery with regard joint mobilization and maintenance of muscle strength, as well as improvement in psychologic well being. There are, however, risks associated with any operative procedure that need to be anticipated and should be able to be managed by the treating physician. Traction with a delayed cast and traction alone still remain valuable and successful treatment approaches.

14. **How should the newborn or young infant be treated?**
With a Pavlik harness, a splint, or both.

15. **Who are the best candidates for spica treatment?**
Patients weighing less than 40–50 lbs with a stable fracture pattern, less than 2 cm of initial shortening, and no associated injuries. Generally, these patients are under the age of 6, but weight is a more important consideration. When a child is over this weight, then management by a single caregiver becomes difficult. In this situation, other assistive devices need to be made available to help with transferring and care of the patient.
   The use of a spica cast for an unstable fracture pattern or a significant initial shortening is most likely to go on to loss of reduction over the first week . Given this, one needs to have a low threshold to wedge or adjust the spica to improve reduction before there is significant callus formation.

16. **In what position should the broken leg be placed?**
The leg needs to be in the position that best reduces the fracture. This usually involves 30–45 degrees of hip and knee flexion. The leg should be abducted or adducted to align the fracture. The anterosuperior iliac spine, the patella (i.e., the tibial tubercle), and the foot (between the second and third toe) should be aligned to minimize the risk of rotational malunion. A spica cast with the hip at 90 degrees and the knee at 90 degrees has been shown to decrease the incidence

of shortening that occurs. With treatment in a spica cast, the femoral fracture will tend to drift into varus and flexion until sufficient callus is present. To account for this loss of position over the first week in the spica, it is advisable to leave a diaphyseal femur fracture in slight valgus and slight extension, as seen on the operative x-rays.

17. **What is the best treatment for closed femoral shaft fractures in children between the age of 5 years (or 50 lbs) and adolescence?**
There are several treatment methods that are acceptable. Each method has advantages and disadvantages from fracture to fracture.

- **Flexible intermedullary nails:** The ideal fracture for this implant is a transverse mid-diaphyseal fracture. They are most appropriate for fractures in the middle 60% of the bone. They can be inserted in an antegrade or retrograde fashion, although using two retrograde nails is most common. They control fractures with significant comminution or fractures in the heavier patient less well. The use of stainless steel Enders nails is more stable, and the addition of a third wire inserted through the greater trochanter also improves stability. The addition of a knee immobilizer or gunslinger cast can also improve control in these situations. The most common complication is skin irritation about the knee when these are inserted in a retrograde fashion. Correct technique will decrease the incidence of this complication. Flexible intermedullary nails are the preferred option in this age group.
- **External fixation:** Fractures with significant comminution are well controlled with this treatment. The fixation can be applied quickly and with minimal incisions. It is ideal for treatment in an unstable patient. The pin tracts are prone to infection and unsightly scars. There are reports of fracture after removal, particularly in transverse fractures. Open fractures, multiple injuries, vascular injury, and floating knee are all indications for external fixation.
- **Plate fixation:** Traditionally, this has required a big incision with increased blood loss and a second operation to remove the plate, with risk of fracture after its removal, but fixation is stable, allowing immediate mobilization. Recently, there has been a move by some surgeons to minimally invasive submuscular plating.
- **Traction and delayed spica casting:** This requires a prolonged hospital stay prior to cast application. With immobilization, there is stiffness of the knee and significant muscle wasting. However, it remains a reliable alternative.

18. **Who are the candidates for reamed intramedullary nailing?**
The skeletally mature patient with closed physes. These patients should be treated like adults. Patients over the age of 8 years have been treated by rigid intermedullary nails, but this treatment is commonly reserved for patients over the age of 12 years. A solid nail has the advantage of providing stable fixation with maintenance of position. They are, thus, very good for comminuted fractures and allow early motion without the need for further support.

19. **What is the most significant complication associated with reamed intermedullary nailing?**
The significant disadvantage is an association with avascular necrosis of the femoral head in the skeletally immature patient. The traditional entry site for a reamed femoral nail is the piriformis fossa. Insertion through the tip of the trochanter has been advocated, and this appears to lessen the risk of avascular necrosis. However, there has also been one report of necrosis using this entry site. In addition, entry through the greater trochanter and the piriformis fossa may effect the growth of the neck of the femur, which leads to narrowing of the neck or a valgus deformity. There are other reports of the use of a modified nail inserted very lateral through the greater trochanter, which lessens the risks even more.

The greater trochanter grows by appositional growth from the age of 8 years, so disruption of the greater trochanter after this age is felt not to affect its growth. The proximal femoral growth plate is a block to blood supply directly from the adjacent metaphysis. This creates dependency on the medial femoral circumflex artery for vascularity, and entry through the piriformis fossa can damage this vessel. Until approximately age 12, the physes of the greater trochanter and the proximal femur are continuous, connected by cartilage; thus, injury to the greater trochanter at the appropriate place may also affect the growth of the neck of the femur.

KEY POINTS: FEMUR FRACTURES

1. Consider child abuse as a cause of femoral fracture in the child who is not yet walking; consider this cause also in the toddler, although child abuse is less frequently the cause at that age.

2. The treatment of femur fractures should be individualized. Options for treatment are varied and depend on patient, fracture type, and surgeon experience.

3. Although remodeling does occur, aim for an anatomic reduction. Be prepared to revise the position early if not satisfied.

20. **How should a femoral fracture with a coexisting severe closed head injury be treated?**
    With operative stabilization followed by either internal or external fixation. This approach facilitates nursing care (e.g., head position and moving the patient), accommodates computed tomography (CT) and magnetic resonance imaging (MRI) scans with ease, and promotes early rehabilitation. Operative fixation is also indicated when there is associated vascular injury, compartment syndrome, or multiple injuries.

21. **Should implants be removed?**
    This is controversial. If an implant causes pain, affects motion, is prominent, or has the potential to interfere with growth, it should be removed as soon as it has served its purpose, in other words, once the fracture has healed. Flexible intermedullary nails can affect the growth of the distal femur, and because they are not fixed distally, they can end up inside the medullary canal, becoming very difficult to remove. Plates left *in situ* can act as a stress riser, leading to fracture at the end of the plate and so should be removed. Upon removal of a plate, there is also increased risk of fracture, so activity should be restricted for at least a 6-week period.

22. **What is the most common complication following a femoral fracture?**
    Leg length discrepancy. Longitudinal growth may be accelerated in patients 2–11 years old, but this is most common in those younger than 8 years. This phenomenon, when it occurs, is limited to the first 18 months postinjury. Many authors have documented that this growth most often accounts for no more than 1 cm of difference and is therefore insignificant.

23. **What is the acceptable amount of angulation during healing?**
    This is somewhat controversial and is age- and direction-dependent. Anterior and posterior angulation in the plane of the knee joint will remodel more readily than varus and valgus angulation. Generally, guidelines should be 20 degrees of anterior angulation and 10 degrees of varus/valgus angulation in the preadolescent child. With increased age, less malreduction is tolerated. One should aim for anatomic reduction. Rotation is the deformity that remodels the least.

24. **How much shortening or over-riding can be accepted?**
    Ideally, no more than 1–2 cm should be accepted. The principle of overgrowth in children between 2 and 11 years of age is hotly contested. Thus, you should not assume that initial

shortening of 2 cm will ultimately resolve. Knee flexion of less than 50 degrees in spica cast leads to a 20% incidence of loss of reduction. This risk doubles with each centimeter of initial shortening.

BIBLIOGRAPHY

1. Anglen JO, Choi L: Treatment options in pediatric femoral shaft fractures. J Pediatr Orthop 19:592–595, 2005.

2. Aronson DD, Singer RM, Higgins RF: Skeletal traction for fractures of the femoral shaft in children: A long-term study. J Bone Joint Surg 69A:1435–1439, 1987.

3. Aronson J, Tursky EA: External fixation of femur fractures in children. J Pediatr Orthop 12:157–163, 1992.

4. Bohn WW, Durbin RA: Ipsilateral fractures of the femur and tibia in children and adolescents. J Bone Joint Surg 73A:429–439, 1991.

5. Buehler K, Thompson J, Sponseller P, et al: A prospective study of early spica casting outcomes in the treatment of femoral shaft fractures in children. J Pediatr Orthop 15:30–35, 1995.

6. Canale ST, Tolo VT: Fractures of the femur in children. J Bone Joint Surg 77A:294–315, 1995.

7. Gordon JE, Khanna N, Luhmann SJ, et al: Intramedullary nailing of femoral fractures in children through the lateral aspect of the greater trochanter using a modified rigid humeral intermedullary nail. J Pediatr Orthop 18:416–422, 2004.

8. Herndon WA, Mahnken RF, Yngve DA, et al: Management of femoral shaft fractures in the adolescent. J Pediatr Orthop 9:29–32, 1989.

9. McCartney D, Hinton A, Heinrich SD: Operative stabilization of pediatric femur fractures. Orthop Clin North Am 25:635–650, 1994.

10. Reeves RD, Ballard RI, Hughes JL: Internal fixation versus traction and casting of adolescent femoral shaft fractures. J Pediatr Orthop 10:592–595, 1990.

11. Sanders J, Browne R, Mooney J, et al: Treatment of femoral fractures in children by pediatric orthopedists: Results of a 1998 survey. J Pediatr Orthop 21:436–441, 2001.

12. Shapiro F: Fractures of the femoral shaft in children: The overgrowth phenomenon. Acta Orthop Scand 52:649–655, 1981.

13. Wilkens KE: Principles of fracture remodeling in children. Injury 36:SA3–SA11, 2004.

CHAPTER 28

HIP AND PELVIC FRACTURES

James H. Beaty, MD

1. **Are hip fractures as common in children as in adults?**
   No. Fractures about the hip account for fewer than 1% of all pediatric fractures, and the prevalence of fractures of the hip in children is less than 1% of that in adults.

2. **Why are fractures of the hip in children different from those in adults?**
   The anatomy of the proximal femur. In children, injuries can occur through the proximal femoral physis. Because the orientation of the trabeculae in the femoral neck in children is not along stress lines, fracture surfaces are smooth, with very little interlocking impaction, making closed reduction less stable in children.

3. **How are hip fractures in children classified?**
   The most widely accepted classification is that proposed by Delbet (Fig. 28-1):
   - **Type I fractures:** Transepiphyseal, with or without dislocation from the acetabulum
   - **Type II fractures:** Transcervical

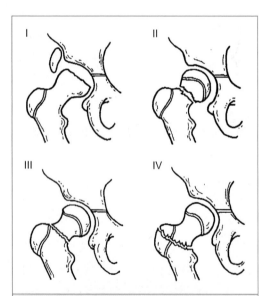

Figure 28-1. Classification of hip fractures in children. Type I, transepiphyseal with or without dislocation from the acetabulum. Type II, transcervical. Type III, cervicotrochanteric. Type IV, intertrochanteric. (From Canale ST, Beaty JH: Pelvic and hip fractures. In Rockwood CA Jr, Wilkins KE, Beaty JH (eds): Fractures in Children, 4th ed. Philadelphia, Lippincott-Raven, 1996, p 1151.)

- **Type III fractures:** Cervicotrochanteric
- **Type IV fractures:** Intertrochanteric

4. **What is the mechanism of injury?**
   Most hip fractures in children (75%) are caused by severe trauma and high-velocity forces, including motor vehicle accidents and falls. Other fractures can occur through pathologic bone, such as unicameral bone cysts, aneurysmal bone cysts, and fibrous dysplasia. In toddlers and infants, hip fractures can occur because of child abuse.

5. **How are hip fractures in children treated?**
   Treatment is based on fracture classification and the degree of displacement:
   - **Type 1 fractures:** Occasionally in infants, closed reduction and spica casting can be used for minimally displaced type I injuries. For type I injuries in most children, however, closed or open reduction should be followed by internal fixation. Smooth pins can be used in children younger than 6–8 years of age, and cannulated screw fixation can be used in children older than 8 years of age. If the femoral head is dislocated from the acetabulum, closed reduction can be attempted once, but usually open reduction is required. If open reduction is performed, the surgical approach should be in the direction of the dislocated femoral head (i.e., a posterior approach for posterior dislocation of the femoral head and an anterior approach for anterior dislocation).
   - **Type II fractures:** For type II transcervical fractures, closed or open reduction and pin or screw fixation are indicated (Fig. 28-2).

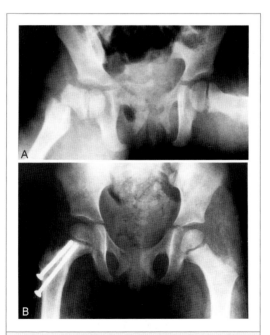

Figure 28-2. *A,* Type II (i.e., transcervical) displaced femoral neck fracture. *B,* After open reduction and internal fixation with 4.0-mm cannulated screws. (From Hughes LO, Beaty JH: Current concepts review. Fractures of the head and neck of the femur in children. J Bone Joint Surg 76A:283–292.)

- **Type III fractures:** These cervicotrochanteric fractures should be treated by reduction and internal fixation. Occasionally, with a completely nondisplaced fracture in a child younger than 8 years, spica cast immobilization is adequate; however, late displacement or coxa vara can occur, and close supervision and observation of the fracture are necessary during the initial week after injury. Any question of fracture stability should be an indication for reduction and internal fixation.
- **Type IV fractures:** These intertrochanteric fractures can be treated by traction and casting in young children or by open reduction and internal fixation with a pediatric hip compression screw, especially in an older adolescent with multiple injuries.

6. **What operative treatment is of benefit in hip fractures in children?**
   Surgery is most frequently indicated for placement of smooth pins or cannulated screw fixation after closed reduction of type II and type III fractures. Open reduction through an anterolateral Watson-Jones approach frequently is required in children in whom adequate closed reduction cannot be obtained.

7. **What surgical technique tips are helpful in the management of hip fractures in children?**
   The most important consideration is the choice of internal fixation, which is based on the child's age and the injury. In general, for type II and type III fractures, I prefer smooth pins in children younger than 3 years of age, cannulated 4.0-mm screws in children aged 3–8 years, and 6.5-mm cannulated screws in children older than 8 years. I use a pediatric hip compression screw in young children and an adult hip compression screw in older adolescents. The femoral neck in children is of harder consistency than the osteoporotic bone in elderly patients, so predrilling and pretapping may be necessary before the insertion of all screws. Spica casting after internal fixation of hip fractures frequently is required to support the internal fixation in children younger than 10 years. *The most important surgical goal is stable fixation of the fracture. Preservation of the physis of the proximal femur is a secondary goal!* (Fig. 28-3).

   The physis of the proximal femur grows only 3–4 mm a year, so fear of limb-length discrepancy should not compromise fracture fixation. If stability is questionable, the internal

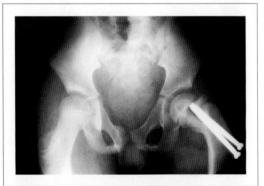

Figure 28-3. Unstable fixation of type II (i.e., transcervical) fracture with loss of reduction and nonunion. If fracture stability is questionable, fixation should extend into the femoral head, regardless of the type of fracture or the age of the child. (From Canale ST, Beaty JH: Pelvic and hip fractures. In Rockwood CA Jr, Wilkins KE, Beaty JH (eds): Fractures in Children, 4th ed. Philadelphia, Lippincott-Raven, 1996, p 1163.)

fixation device should extend into the femoral head for rigid stable fixation, regardless of the type of fracture or the child's age.

8. **What are the major complications after hip fractures in children?**
The most frequent complication is avascular necrosis of the femoral head, with an incidence of approximately 40%. I believe that avascular necrosis is related to the initial displacement of the fracture. About half of all displaced type II and type III fractures and almost all type I fractures with dislocation of the femoral head result in avascular necrosis.

Coxa vara deformity occurs after hip fractures in children owing to growth arrest of the proximal femoral physis or the fracture healing in a varus position. If the femoral neck-shaft angle decreases to 110 degrees or less, subtrochanteric valgus osteotomy and fixation yield satisfactory results.

Nonunion after femoral neck fractures occurs in approximately 5% and can occur after the injury itself or, if loss of reduction occurs, after closed management or internal fixation. Treatment is early subtrochanteric valgus osteotomy, fixation, and bone grafting.

9. **What is the prognosis for hip fractures in children?**
Unfortunately, because of the high complication rate, the prognosis may be fair or guarded, especially if complications have occurred. If the fracture heals without avascular necrosis, coxa vara, or nonunion, the child should be followed to skeletal maturity to evaluate growth of the hip and extremity.

10. **Are acetabular fractures in children different from those in adults?**
Acetabular fractures are relatively uncommon in children, accounting for 1–15% of pelvic fractures in published series. Most acetabular fractures occur in adolescents, and most are caused by high-energy trauma. Damage to the triradiate cartilage in a child may cause growth arrest and a shallow, dysplastic acetabulum. Acetabular fractures in children generally are classified as follows:
- **Type 1:** Small fragments, usually associated with hip dislocation
- **Type 2:** Nondisplaced linear fractures, associated with pelvic fractures
- **Type 3:** Large linear fractures with hip joint instability
- **Type 4:** Central fracture-dislocations

Acetabular fractures that occur with hip dislocation usually can be treated conservatively. Linear nondisplaced fractures have an excellent prognosis, and treatment should be guided by the type of associated pelvic fractures. Displaced linear fractures in the weight-bearing area that produce hip joint instability require accurate reduction to restore the weight-bearing area; this injury usually occurs in older adolescents and should be treated as in an adult, with open reduction and internal fixation with threaded Kirschner wires, 3.5- or 4-mm cannulated screws, or adult-sized implants.

Treatment of central fracture-dislocations is still controversial. Surgical treatment has been implicated in the development of avascular necrosis and heterotopic bone formation; conservative treatment may not obtain a congruent reduction, which can lead to degenerative changes. Generally, noncomminuted central fracture-dislocations, especially in older children and adolescents, should be treated surgically, but good results are not predictably obtained by either method.

11. **How are pelvic fractures in children different from those in adults?**
Pelvic fractures can occur in children (as in adults) as a result of high-velocity trauma. In children, however, because of the uniqueness of the skeletally immature pelvis, pelvic avulsion from muscle origins and insertions also can be caused by less-severe trauma and sports injuries. The other difference is the triradiate cartilage of the acetabulum, which, when injured, can cause acetabular dysplasia or growth disturbance in children. A child's pelvis is more flexible than an adult's, so single breaks in the pelvic ring are more common.

Because significant pelvic-ring disruption is less frequent in children than in adults, the mortality rate in children (2–5%) with pelvic fractures is much lower than that in adults (17–20%).

12. **What are the clinical signs of pelvic fracture?**
    - Large hematoma superficially beneath the inguinal ligament or in the sacrum
    - Decrease in the distance from the greater trochanter to the pubic spine on the affected side in lateral compression fractures (i.e., Roux's sign)
    - Bony prominence or a large hematoma and tenderness on rectal examination, indicative of a severe pelvic fracture (i.e., Earle's sign)
    - Posterior pressure on the iliac crest causes pain at the fracture site as the pelvic ring is opened, and compression of the pelvic ring at the iliac crest from lateral to medial causes pain and possibly crepitation
    - Downward pressure on the symphysis pubis and posteriorly on the sacroiliac joints causes pain and motion if there is a break in the pelvic ring
    - Flexion and extension of the hips may cause pain in the inguinal area

13. **Is radiographic examination always necessary in the evaluation of a child with a pelvic fracture?**
    Yes, although imaging studies may not always be necessary for the diagnosis of pelvic fracture in a child. One study found that pelvic examination alone had both high specificity and a negative predictive value. In a study of 174 children with pelvic fractures, pelvic examination alone was found to have a 92% sensitivity and a 79% specificity; however, pelvic radiographs were recommended in severely injured blunt-trauma patients. Another series of 347 children who had screening pelvic radiographs in a pediatric trauma center found that only 1 child had a pelvic fracture, which was clinically apparent, and the authors concluded that routine screening for pelvic fracture in unnecessary. However, to determine the location, type, and severity of fracture, radiographic examination is mandatory. We prefer to do a full-trauma series, including pelvic radiographs, in any child with a femoral fracture, spinal fracture, or hip fracture, as well as in unconscious or unresponsive patients, especially those with multitrauma, and patients in whom pelvic fractures are indicated by clinical examination.

KEY POINTS: HIP AND PELVIC FRACTURES

1. Most hip fractures in children are the result of high-energy forces from severe trauma. A careful search for associated injuries should be a part of the evaluation of these injuries.

2. Displaced hip and acetabular fractures should be reduced and fixed with age- and size-appropriate devices.

3. Most isolated pelvic fractures in younger children can be treated nonoperatively.

4. For children with hip fractures, avascular necrosis and nonunion of the fracture are the most common complications.

14. **What type of imaging is useful?**
    In addition to anteroposterior and inlet and outlet radiographs of the pelvis, computed tomography is useful for complex injuries to assess possible articular surface involvement of the acetabulum and to evaluate injuries of the sacrum or sacroiliac joint. For most pelvic fractures, however, plain radiographs are sufficient to determine fracture severity and the need for surgical treatment.

15. **What classification system is used to describe pelvic fractures in children?**
    A number of classification systems have been devised for pelvic fractures in children. Torode and Zieg proposed a four-part classification, Quinby and Rang described a three-part classification that emphasizes soft tissue injuries, and Moreno et al described four types of fracture geometry used to identify patients at risk for hemorrhage. Classifications by Young and Burgess, Letournel, Judet, Pennal, Tile, Ogden, and the Arbeitsgemeinschaft für Osteosynthesefragen/Association for Study of Internal Fixation (OA/ASIF) group are more commonly used in adolescents and adults. Key and Conwell's classification of pelvic fractures (including acetabular fractures) in adults is based on the number of breaks in the pelvic ring and also is applicable in children. For children, regardless of the classification used, the most useful information is whether the fracture is stable or unstable. Most pelvic fractures in children are stable (70% or more in most studies).

16. **What other injuries occur with pelvic fractures in children?**
    In a series of 166 children with pelvic fractures, 60% had multisystem injuries and 50% had additional skeletal injuries. In a polytrauma setting, I frequently see children who have head, neck, chest, and abdominal injuries. Related or local injuries include vascular, urologic, and neurologic injuries. The greatest rates of morbidity and mortality occur in children with more severe Malgaigne-type injuries. Hemorrhage is treated as in adults, including the use of antishock trousers and arterial embolization. Frequently, simple placement of an external fixator in an unstable pelvis will decrease the number of raw bony surfaces and will help control hemorrhage. Urethral or bladder lacerations occur in about 5% of children with pelvic fractures and can be diagnosed by insertion of a Foley catheter, followed by examination of the urine for gross or occult blood. With any signs of urinary tract disruption, a cystoureterogram should be obtained, followed by an intravenous pyelogram. Neurologic injury of the lower extremity is uncommon after pelvic fractures in children, occurring in about 1.5%.

17. **Are pelvic fractures in children treated differently from those in adults?**
    Compared with pelvic fractures in adults, many of which are severe injuries that require surgical intervention, most pelvic fractures in children involve a single injury of the pelvis and can be treated nonoperatively with bed rest, with or without traction and protected ambulation. For unstable Malgaigne-type injuries, either reduction with external fixation or a combination of external and internal fixation, especially of the sacroiliac joint, can be used. Malgaigne fractures in children younger than 4 or 5 years may remodel with conservative treatment, but in juveniles and adolescents, treatment should be similar to that in adults.

18. **How are avulsion fractures of the pelvis treated in children?**
    Conservative treatment (i.e., bed rest and protected ambulation) is sufficient for these injuries, and almost all patients return to their previous level of sports participation. Most pelvic avulsion fractures occur as a result of overpull of muscles in those participating in sports activities, especially gymnastics, football, and track.

19. **What complications should be anticipated after pelvic fractures in children?**
    Complications are rare but can include nonunion, triradiate cartilage closure, avascular necrosis, sciatic nerve palsy, or myositis ossificans.

BIBLIOGRAPHY

1. Canale ST: Fractures of the hip in children and adolescents. Orthop Clin North Am 21:341–351, 1990.
2. Davison BL, Weinstein SL: Hip fractures in children: A long-term follow-up study. J Pediatr Orthop 12:355–388, 1992.

3. Flynn JM, Wong KL, Yeg GL, et al: Displaced fractures of the hip in children: Management by early operation and immobilisation in a hip spica cast. J Bone Joint Surg Br 84:108–112, 2002.

4. Heeg M, de Ridder VA, Tornetta P III, et al: Acetabular fractures in children and adolescents. Clin Orthop 376:80–86, 2000.

5. Ismail N, Bellemare JF, Mollitt DL, et al: Death from pelvic fracture: Children are different. J Pediatr Surg 31:82–85, 1996.

6. Jeng C, Sponseller PD, Yates A, Paletta G: Subtrochanteric femoral fractures in children: Alignment after 90 degrees-90 degrees traction and cast application. Clin Orthop 341:170–174, 1997.

7. Rees MJ, Aickin R, Kilbe A, Teele RL: The screening pelvic radiograph in pediatric trauma. Pediatr Radiol 31:497–500, 2001.

8. Segal LS: Custom 95-degree condylar blade plate for pediatric subtrochanteric femur fractures. Orthopedics 23:103–107, 2000.

9. Silber JS, Flynn JM, Koffler KM, et al: Analysis of the cause, classification, and associated injuries of 166 consecutive pediatric pelvic fractures. J Pediatr Orthop 21:446–450, 2001.

10. Theologis TN, Cole WG: Management of subtrochanteric fractures of the femur in children. J Pediatr Orthop 18:22–25, 1998.

CHAPTER 29

SPINE FRACTURES IN CHILDREN

Joseph G. Khoury, MD

1. **Why do younger children tend to get more upper cervical spine injuries than subaxial?**
   Younger children have disproportionately larger heads than adults, poor development of neck musculature, and relatively horizontal facet orientation. The facets become more vertically oriented with age and in the lower cervical spine. Children under 8 years old tend to sustain injury between the occiput and C3, whereas those older than 8 years approximate the subaxial injury pattern of adults.

2. **How common is cervical spine injury in children, compared to adults?**
   Cervical spine injury is much less common in children. Children only represent 1.9% of all cervical spine trauma. The incidence gradually increases from ages 6 through 15 until it reaches adult frequency. However, children have double the fatality rates of adults. Fatality is usually due to associated injury to the head, chest, or abdomen.

3. **What is the most common cervical fracture under age 8 years?**
   Odontoid fracture.

4. **What are the most common mechanisms of injury?**
   Motor vehicle accident is the most common mechanism in all age groups. Injuries related to falls and dives increase in older children. Sports-related injuries occur in adolescents, with American football accounting for 38% of the injuries. The primary mechanism of injury is by axial loading; therefore, the rate of quadriplegia was dramatically reduced when spearing rules were introduced in the early 1980s.

5. **What is the proper way to immobilize the cervical spine in children?**
   You must avoid flexion. Because of the relatively larger head size in children, immobilization on a flat spine board places the C-spine in relative flexion. There are special spine boards for children, with a recess for the occiput. If a special board is not available, a small bump placed under the upper thoracic spine can alleviate this problem. Most upper cervical spine injuries displace more in flexion and often reduce by simply obtaining neutral alignment or slight extension.

6. **What are the initial radiographs that are required?**
   In a child who is alert, conversant, has no neurologic deficits, no cervical tenderness, no painful distracting injury, and is not intoxicated, cervical spine x-rays are not necessary to exclude an injury. Otherwise, the anteroposterior (AP) and lateral views are all that are required. The odontoid view does not aid in making the diagnosis under age 8 and is very difficult to obtain. Flexion-extension radiographs add no useful information in the acute setting if the static exam is normal. The oblique radiograph does not add to the diagnostic accuracy of the standard AP and lateral radiograph in detecting cervical spine injury in children.

7. **How should a lateral cervical spine radiograph be evaluated?**
   A routine in reviewing of films will help prevent missing injuries. First, be sure it is an adequate radiograph that visualizes to the top of T1. Next, evaluate the soft tissues for subcutaneous air

(which is always abnormal) and soft tissue swelling. The "2 at 6 and 6 at 2" rule is a helpful mnemonic (i.e., 2 cm of soft tissue shadow anterior to C6 and 6 mm of shadow in front of C2) to help you remember the maximal allowable soft tissue swelling. Trace the anterior and posterior vertebral body line and the interlaminar line and look for fractures. If a craniovertebral junction injury is suspected, refer to the Powers ratio, the Kaufman method, and the Harris method to evaluate this region radiographically (Fig. 29-1).

8. **What are some other common radiographic findings unique to the pediatric spine that can cause some confusion when evaluating radiographs?**
The anterior arch of C1 is ossified in only 20% of newborns and may not appear until 1 year of age. The posterior arch fuses at 3–4 years of age. The axis has five primary and seven secondary ossification centers that can cause confusion as they appear and fuse at various ages. The dentocentral synchondrosis can resemble a fracture and closes between 3 and 6 years of age (Fig. 29-2). The ossiculum terminale appears at 3 years of age and fuses at 12 years. In addition, each subaxial vertebra has two neurocentral synchondroses, a posterior synchondrosis, and several small vertebral-body secondary ossification centers that can resemble fractures.

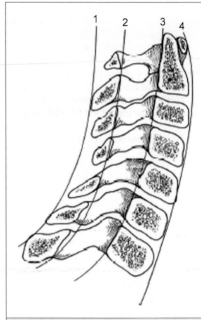

Figure 29-1. Craniovertebral junction injury.

9. **What is pseudosubluxation? How can it be differentiated from true subluxation?**
Pseudosubluxation is the apparent anterior subluxation of C2 on C3 and, less commonly, of C3 on C4. This is a normal finding in children. To help distinguish pseudosubluxation from true subluxation, draw Swischuk's line, a straight line between the interlaminar line of C1 and C3; this should pass no more than 1.5 mm anterior to the interlaminar line of C2.

10. **What is the upper limit of normal for the atlantodens interval (ADI)?**
4 mm.

11. **What is an os odontoideum?**
A defect in the dens cranial to the dentocentral synchondrosis. It probably represents unrecognized previous trauma. The borders of the tip of the dens are smooth, and it can either be in an orthotopic (i.e., normal) or dystrophic (i.e., too high) position. The key issue is instability. Flexion-extension radiographs in the awake, alert child are required. Instability >10 mm or any neurologic symptoms warrant stabilization (i.e., C1–C2 fusion).

12. **When are advanced imaging studies (i.e., a computed tomography [CT] scan or magnetic resonance imaging [MRI]) indicated?**
If an upper cervical spine injury is suspected on the standard AP and lateral radiographs, a CT scan should be obtained. On the other hand, a CT scan in the presence of normal radiographs is

unlikely to yield positive results. If an injury is suspected but not seen, the neck should be stabilized until you can perform an adequate physical examination. However, MRI can be used to directly visualize soft tissue injuries. The tectorial membrane is the critical structure that must be disrupted before significant instability occurs between the occiput and C1. MRI has a sensitivity of 87% and a specificity of 100% for predicting instability at this level. MRI can be very helpful in clearing the C-spine in obtunded children who are unable to cooperate with the physical exam. Concomitant injury is very common in this population and often warrants advanced imaging for a head, chest, or abdominal injury. In this setting, the cervical spine is often routinely added and can substitute for plain radiographs.

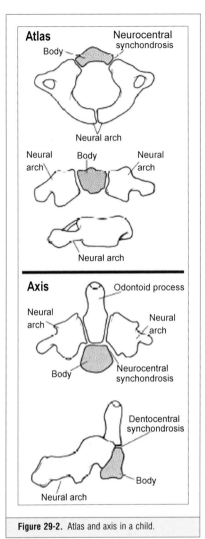

Figure 29-2. Atlas and axis in a child.

13. **What is SCIWORA?**
The acronym stands for **s**pinal **c**ord **i**njury **w**ithout **r**adiographic **a**bnormality. Typically, the injury is apparent on MRI, with spinal cord and surrounding soft tissue edema at the level of injury. The spinal column can elongate several centimeters in children without damage to the osseous structures. SCIWORA is more common in children under 8 years old. The prognosis hinges on the severity of neurologic involvement at presentation.

14. **Which type of cervical spine injury is most often fatal at the scene?**
Occipitoatlantal dislocation is a severe injury often due to a distraction moment. Survival is predicated on rapid cardiopulmonary resuscitation (CPR) and ventilatory support because the respiratory system is often involved. Avoid traction during immobilization and treatment. The mainstay of treatment is early fusion and mobilization to facilitate respiratory support.

15. **What structure damage results in atlantoaxial instability?**
The transverse atlantal ligament. Suspect this injury if there is more than 5 mm of space at the atlanto-dens interval. Treatment is controversial, with some advocating immediate fusion, versus 8–12 weeks of immobilization. If instability remains after nonoperative treatment, surgery is required.

KEY POINTS: SPINE FRACTURES IN CHILDREN

1. Children tend to get more upper cervical spine injury due to their increased head size and more horizontally oriented facet joints.

2. Almost all cervical spine injuries in children tend to displace on a standard spine board because of the relatively larger size of a child's head.

3. There are many normal variations and developmental stages that must be considered when evaluating cervical spine radiographs in children; many of these differences may be interpreted as injury.

16. **How much room does the spinal cord need?**
    The space within the atlas is made up of three structures in roughly equal proportions (Steel's rule of thirds). The anterior third is occupied by the dens. The central third is occupied by the spinal cord, and the posterior third by empty lymphatic space. In general, 14 mm is considered the minimum necessary space available for the cord between the dens and the interlaminar line of the atlas.

17. **How do odontoid fractures in children differ from those in adults?**
    In children, the fracture usually occurs through the synchondrosis. This is below the base of the dens (where adults typically fracture) and the level of the facets. Displacement is generally anterior and, therefore, immobilized and treated in extension. The goal is to obtain at least 50% apposition and hold in a Minerva cast or brace or a halo for 6–8 weeks.

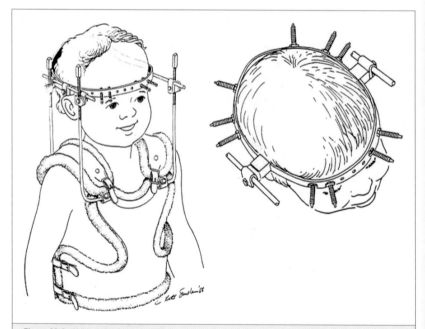

Figure 29-3. Halo application in a child.

18. **How is halo application different in children?**
Special considerations (Fig. 29-3) include the following:
- **The size of the halo:** This is often a special-order item.
- **The locations of the cranial sutures:** If the skull is considered as a clock from above the cranial sutures are at 4:30 and 7:30.
- **The number of pins:** The number of pins is inversely proportional to the age of the child. Up to 10 pins may be used in very young children.
- **Torque on the pins:** Less torque is used as age decreases and the number of pins increases. Typical torque is 2–3 lbs per pin in young children, gradually increasing to 8 lbs on 4 pins in adolescents.
- **Preparation:** A pre-halo CT may be helpful to aid in halo pin placement.

BIBLIOGRAPHY

1. Bush C, Cullen M, Klein M, Farmer D: The pediatric trauma C-spine: Is the "odontoid" view necessary? J Pediatr Surg 35:994–997, 2000.
2. Cattell HS, Filtzer DL: Pseudosubluxation and other normal variations in the cervical spine in children. A study of one hundred and sixty children. J Bone Joint Surg 47A:1295–1309, 1965.
3. Dormans JP, Closkey R, Flynn JM, Mahboubi S: The role of MRI in the assessment of pediatric cervical spine injuries. In Proceeding of the Pediatric Orthopaedic Society of North America, Annual Meeting. Lake Buena Vista, FL, May 15–19, 1999, p 70.
4. Hernandez JA, Chupik C, Swischuk LE: Cervical spine trauma in children under 5 years: Productivity of CT. Emerg Radiol 10(4):176–178, 2004.
5. Herzenberg JE, Hensinger RN, Dedrick DK, Phillips WA: Emergency transport and positioning of young children who have an injury of the cervical spine. The standard backboard may be hazardous. J Bone Joint Surg 71A:12–22, 1989.
6. Leventhal HR: Birth injuries of the spinal cord. J Pediatr 56:447–453, 1960.
7. Mabarak SJ, Camp JF, Vuletich W, et al: Halo application in the infant. J Pediatr Orthop 9:612–614, 1989.
8. Pang D, Pollack IF: Spinal cord injury without radiographic abnormality in children—The SCIWORA syndrome. J Trauma 29:654–664, 1989.
9. Swischuk LE: Anterior displacement of C2 in children: Physiologic or pathologic. Radiology 122:759–763, 1977.

CHAPTER 30

SHOULDER INJURIES

Shyam Kishan, MD, and James O. Sanders, MD

1. **How is the clavicle embryologically different from other long bones?**
   It is the first long bone to ossify *in utero,* with two primary centers, medial and lateral. The site of fusion of these two centers is at the junction of the mid and lateral thirds of the bone. It is the only long bone to undergo membranous ossification; hence, it is affected in disorders of membranous ossifications (e.g., cleidocranial dysostosis).

2. **How are medial sternoclavicular injuries in the child different from those in an adult?**
   Because the medial end closes very late (at 22 years of age or later), you must have a high index of suspicion for medial physeal separation in patients with an apparent sternoclavicular dislocation. Anterior displacement is more common and is unstable. Posterior displacement has potential for vascular or airway injury. An apical lordotic view or a computed tomography (CT) scan is necessary for the diagnosis. A thoracic surgeon should be available during the reduction. A closed reduction can sometimes be accomplished with a towel clip.

3. **What is different about lateral clavicular injuries in the child, compared with the adult?**
   The acromioclavicular and coracoclavicular ligaments insert into the periosteum and help preserve the periosteal tube in lateral clavicular fractures and acromioclavicular dislocations, often resulting in a temporary double or Y-shaped clavicle. The remodeling potential is excellent.

4. **How common are clavicular fractures?**
   It is the most common birth fracture (with 2.8–7.2 per 1000 births incidence). Of obstetric fractures, 84–92% are clavicular. About half of all closed fractures occur under the age of 10 years. Displacement is more common in adolescents.

5. **What is the differential diagnosis of a clavicle fracture at birth?**
   Proximal humerus fracture, septic arthritis, brachial plexus palsy, osteomyelitis (as in congenital syphilis), congenital pseudarthrosis, and cleidocranial dysplasia are some of the differential diagnoses. A careful physical examination and imaging studies can usually separate these conditions.

6. **Describe the typical displacement of a clavicle fracture.**
   The medial (i.e., proximal) end is displaced upward by the pull of the sternocleidomastoid. The lateral end is depressed by the weight of the arm, as well as by the pull of the pectoralis. The fracture is shortened by the pectoralis and the subclavius. A distal clavicle fracture resembles a peeled banana (Fig. 30-1).

7. **How are clavicle fractures treated?**
   The two commonly described methods of treatment are the sling and the figure-of-eight bandage. There is little difference in outcomes between those two. The sling is usually more comfortable.

8. **What are the indications for surgery in clavicle fractures?**
   Potential operative indications in children are very rare and include irreducible fractures, vascular injury, severe skin damage in open fractures, marked displacement with potential skin ulceration,

brachial plexus palsy from clavicle compression, impingement of the clavicle upon the great vessels, and established symptomatic pseudarthrosis. Complications of internal fixation include nonunion, implant failure, migration of pins, refracture after removal, infection, and unsightly, symptomatic scars.

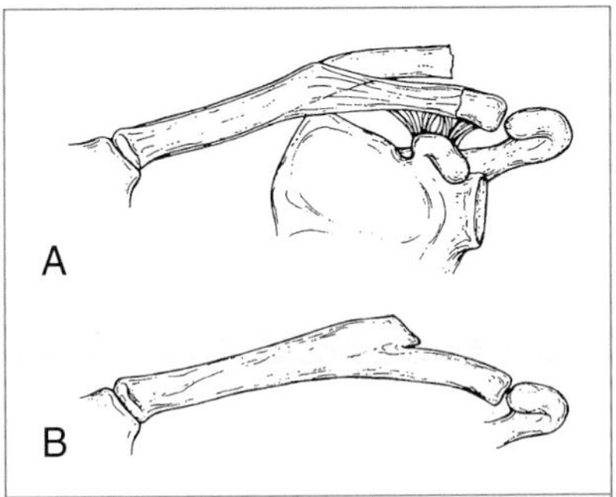

9. **What are the complications of clavicle fractures?**
Malunion is perhaps the most common complication, noticeable as a bump. Remodeling is excellent in the young child, and the malunion usually presents no long-term problem. Other complications are usually the result of the injury rather than the fracture and include vascular injury, brachial plexopathy, and pneumothorax. Supraclavicular nerve damage and skin ulceration from extreme angulation have been reported. More important, typically, than the clavicle fracture are associated injuries. Always look for other injuries, including rib fractures, mediastinal widening, and scapulothoracic dissociation in patients with high-energy trauma or with ipsilateral decreased or absent upper-extremity pulses.

Figure 30-1. *A*, Distal clavicle fracture in a child. A banana peeled from its skin. *B*, Healing within the intact periosteal tube. (From Webb LX: Fractures and dislocations about the shoulder. In Green NE, Swionkowski MF [eds]: Skeletal Trauma in Children. Philadelphia, W.B. Saunders, 1993, p 327.)

10. **What are the features of congenital pseudarthrosis of the clavicle?**
This peculiar condition is almost always seen on the right side. In the rare instance of being left sided, it is associated with dextrocardia. It may be distinguished from a fracture because the ends are atrophic and tapered. The etiology is enigmatic, effects of the developing branchial vasculature and failure of fusion of the two primary ossific nuclei being two popular theories. Surgery is indicated primarily for pain and cosmesis.

11. **What is an os acromiale?**
It is a normal anatomic variant, with one of the ossification centers of the acromion failing to unite with the rest of the scapula. The borders are rounded, and it is bilateral in about 60% of cases. The differential is an acromial fracture, and often it can be differentiated by the lack of pain and the radiographic features. A bone scan may also be helpful.

12. **How is the acromioclavicular separation treated in a child?**
This is a fairly rare injury, seen occasionally in the older adolescent. One cannot overemphasize that, in the younger child, it is almost always a periosteal sleeve disruption and is quite benign. The treatment is nonoperative, with a sling or shoulder immobilizer.

13. **What percentage of growth of the humerus is from the proximal physis?**
The proximal humeral physis accounts for 80% of the growth of the humerus overall; however, this percentage varies with age. Before the age of 2 years, less than 75% of growth occurs at the proximal physis, increasing to 85% at age 8, and remaining constant at 90% after age 11.

14. **How much displacement is acceptable in a proximal humerus physeal fracture, and why?**
Up to 70 degrees of angulation and 100% displacement is acceptable under the age of 5 years; 40–70 degrees of angulation and 50–100% displacement for ages 5–12 years; and up to 40 degrees of angulation and 50% displacement for children >12 years of age. Remodeling potential

is superb because of the large amount of growth from the proximal humeral physis. Although proximal humeral physeal fractures typically propagate through the zone of hypertrophy adjacent to the zone of provisional calcification, undulations do occur through other zones. Fractures rarely disturb the physeal growth because these zones are distal to the proliferating cells.

15. **What is the typical deformity of the displaced proximal humeral fracture?**
The tough posteromedial periosteum is the hinge for these fractures. The distal fragment displaces anterolaterally. In fully displaced fractures, the proximal fragment is quite abducted and externally rotated by the pull of the rotator cuff, and the distal fragment is adducted by the pectoralis major and shortened by the deltoid. Remembering this anatomy aids in the reduction of these fractures. Occasionally, the periosteum or biceps tendon is interposed, preventing reduction.

16. **What are the indications for surgery in proximal humeral fractures?**
Since the results of nonoperative care are excellent, surgery is rarely indicated. An older child (nearing skeletal maturity) with a displaced fracture may be considered for surgery. Polytrauma with other fractures is another potential indication to help mobilize the patient quickly. Obviously, an open fracture is a surgical indication.

17. **What is the *vanishing epiphysis* sign?**
Salter-Harris I fractures of the proximal humerus may appear to have the epiphysis vanish as it rolls behind the proximal shaft. Comparison views should be obtained of the contralateral shoulder.

18. **How may one confirm the diagnosis of a displaced transphyseal fracture of the proximal humerus in the neonate?**
Although an arthrogram or magnetic resonance imaging (MRI) can identify proximal humeral physeal separations, ultrasound is noninvasive, diagnostic, and easily done at the bedside, if needed.

19. **A 2-week-old child is brought to the hospital and is diagnosed with a proximal humerus fracture. Little callus is evident on the plain radiographs. How would you approach this injury?**
Birth injuries heal rapidly. At 2 weeks, abundant callus would be seen in a birth injury. Abuse should be high on the differential. The fracture should be treated appropriately, but child protection services should be informed.

20. **Is there a condition such as a slipped proximal humeral epiphysis?**
A chronic slipped proximal humeral epiphysis is a rare disorder that is reported from gymnastics, radiotherapy, and hyperpituitarism. The proximal physis slips into varus and usually responds well to nonoperative treatment.

21. **What is the little leaguer's shoulder?**
This is a stress injury of the proximal humeral physis. The physis widens and is symptomatic. Repetitive stress is the etiology. Rest for 3–4 weeks from pitching usually resolves the condition. Occasionally, premature growth arrest occurs. Enforcement of strict pitching restrictions has decreased the incidence.

22. **What is Sprengel's deformity?**
The scapula first appears at the C4–C5 level in the fifth gestational week. During the sixth and seventh gestational weeks, it enlarges to extend from C4–C7. During the seventh week, the shoulder joint forms, and the scapula descends from the cervical area to its position overlying the first through fifth ribs. Failure of the scapula to descend, usually from a fibrous or osseous tether (i.e., omovertebral bone), results in Sprengel's deformity. It is often associated with

congenital cervical spine anomalies (i.e., Klippel-Feil syndrome). Surgery is indicated for significant impairment of function or cosmetic deformity.

23. **What is a floating shoulder?**
A scapular neck fracture in combination with clavicular fractures or acromioclavicular separation is called a floating shoulder.

KEY POINTS: SHOULDER INJURIES

1. The clavicle is the first long bone to ossify *in utero,* with two primary centers, medial and lateral.

2. Because the medial end closes very late (at 22 years of age or later), you must have a high index of suspicion for medial physeal separation in patients with an apparent sternoclavicular dislocation.

3. Fracture of the clavicle is the most common birth fracture (2.8–7.2 per 1000 births incidence). Of obstetric fractures, 84–92% are clavicular.

4. The two commonly described methods of treatment are the sling and the figure-of-eight bandage. There is little difference in outcomes between those two, but the sling is usually more comfortable.

5. Since the scapula is well padded and protected by muscles, a scapular body fracture requires rather high-energy trauma. In the child, abuse must be considered high on the differential in the absence of history of other accidental high-energy trauma.

24. **What is the significance of scapular body fractures?**
Since the scapula is well padded and protected by muscles, a scapular body fracture requires rather high-energy trauma. In the child, abuse must be considered high on the differential in the absence of history of other accidental high-energy trauma. As over 75% of all patients with scapula fractures have other injuries, it is wise to have the trauma service consulted in the care of these patients.

25. **What x-ray views are ordered for scapular fractures?**
Standard anteroposterior and lateral views (i.e., scapular Y views) should be ordered. In addition, an axillary view for glenoid or coracoid fractures or a Stryker's notch view for coracoid fractures may be ordered, according to the fracture pattern.

26. **How does one treat scapular fractures?**
In general, most scapular fractures are treated nonoperatively with a sling. The associated injuries are typically far more important. Intra-articular fractures with displacement, fractures creating shoulder instability, and open injuries requiring debridement are some of the indications for operative treatment.

27. **What is scapulothoracic dissociation?**
This is a serious injury resulting from high-energy trauma, essentially amounting to a closed forequarter amputation. Vascular and neurologic damage is common, as are other associated bony and visceral injuries.

28. **Why are glenohumeral shoulder dislocations more common in the adolescent than in the younger child?**
    The bone fails through the metaphyseal area in the younger child, whereas the bone has become stronger in the older child and the ligaments fail first with typical loadings.

29. **What is the prognosis for traumatic glenohumeral dislocation in the adolescent?**
    The risk of recurrence requiring operative treatment is very high. Recurrence rates as high as 90% have been described in patients between 10 and 20 years of age.

BIBLIOGRAPHY

1. Allman FL: Fractures and ligamentous injuries of the clavicle and its articulations. J Bone Joint Surg 49A:774–784, 1967.
2. Asher MA: Dislocations of the upper extremity in children. Orthop Clin North Am 7:583–591, 1976.
3. Beaty JH: Fractures of the proximal humerus and shaft in children. Instr Course Lect 41:369–372, 1992.
4. Gardner E: The embryology of the clavicle. Clin Orthop Rel Res 58:9–16, 1968.
5. Gomez-Brouchet A, Sales de Gauzy J, Accadbled F, et al: Congenital pseudarthrosis of the clavicle: A histopathological study in five patients. J Pediatr Orthop 13:399–401, 2004.
6. Sarwark JF, King EC, Luhmann SJ: Proximal humerus, scapula, and clavicle. In Beaty JH, Kasser JR (eds): Rockwood and Wilkins's Fractures in Children, 6th ed. Philadelphia, Lippincott Williams & Wilkins, 2006, pp 703–771.
7. Webb LX, Mooney JF III: Fractures and dislocations about the shoulder. In Green NE, Siontkowski MF (eds): Skeletal Trauma in Children, 3rd ed. Philadelphia, W.B. Saunders, 2003, pp 322–343.
8. Webb PA, Suchey JM: Epiphyseal union of the anterior iliac crest and medial clavicle in a modern multiracial sample of American males and females. Am J Phys Anthropol 68:457–466, 1985.

CHAPTER 31

FRACTURES IN THE ELBOW REGION

Kaye E. Wilkins, DVM, MD

1. **What is the order of appearance of the secondary ossification centers of the distal humerus in the immature skeleton?**

   To evaluate radiographs of the immature distal humerus, it is important to know the sequence of the appearance of the ossification centers of the distal humerus (Fig. 31-1). The first center, that of the lateral condyle (B), appears at some time after the first year. This is followed by the medial epicondyle (D), which appears around the 6th year. The third center to appear is the medial condyle (C), at some time after the 9th year. The final center is that of the lateral epicondyle (A), appearing around the 14th year. The centers tend to appear earlier in females.

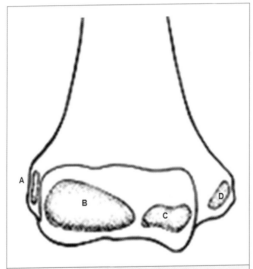

Figure 31-1. Secondary ossification centers. *A*, Lateral epicondyle. *B*, Lateral condyle. *C*, Trochlea or medial condyle. *D*, Medial epicondyle.

2. **What are the bones most commonly injured around the elbow in children?**

   About 86% of fractures in the elbow region occur in the distal humerus. Of these, 79.8% are supracondylar fractures, 16.9% involve the lateral condyle, and 12.5% involve the medial epicondyle. Medial condyle, T-condylar, and lateral epicondyle fractures combined occur less than 1% of the time.

   Chambers H, Stanley EA, De La Graza JF, et al: Fractures of the elbow region. In Beatty JH, Kasser JR (eds): Rockwood and Wilkin's Fractures in Children, 5th ed. Philadelphia, Lippincott Williams & Wilkins, 2001, pp 483–740.

3. **The forearm normally is angulated away from the body at the elbow. Is there a term for this?**

   This outward angulation of the forearm in relationship to the humeral shaft at the elbow is called the *carrying angle*. It has been said that this term comes from the fact that this normal valgus angulation allows the person to carry a bucket of water at the side without hitting the legs. This normal valgus angulation is about 15 degrees in most children.

   Beals BK: The normal carrying angle of the elbow. Clin Orthop 19:194–196, 1976.

4. **Occasionally, following a supracondylar fracture, the patient is described as having *cubitus varus*. What is meant by that term?**

   When the angulation of the forearm in relationship to the humeral shaft is away from the midline, it is referred to as *cubitus valgus*. When the angulation is toward the midline or body, the term used for this deformity is *cubitus varus*.

5. **What is a supracondylar fracture of the humerus?**

   It is a fracture through the distal metaphysis, proximal to the distal physis (i.e., the growth plate). The fracture is usually transverse in the coronal (i.e., medial to lateral) plane. In the saggital (i.e., anterior to posterior) plane, the fracture line is often oblique, from anterior distal to posterior proximal.

6. **What are the two major types of supracondylar fractures?**

   The types of supracondylar fractures are determined by whether the failure occurs when the elbow is forced into either hyperextension or hyperflexion:

   - **Extension type:** More common, being observed in 90–95% of all supracondylar fractures. This type is caused by a hyperextension mechanism in which the distal fragment (i.e., the distal metaphysis and humeral condyles) is displaced posterior to the proximal fragment.
   - **Flexion type:** The distal fragment is flexed forward and lies anterior to the distal fragment. It is less common, accounting for only 5–10% of all supracondylar fractures.

   Chambers H, Stanley EA, De La Graza JF, et al: Fractures of the elbow region. In Beatty JH, Kasser JR (eds): Rockwood and Wilkin's Fractures in Children, 5th ed. Philadelphia, Lippincott Williams & Wilkins, 2001, pp 483–740.

7. **Extension supracondylar fractures are commonly seen in the last half of the first decade (i.e., 6–7 years of age.) Is there a biologic reason for this?**

   Around the age of 6 or 7 years, the child achieves maximum ligamentous laxity. Thus, when the child falls on the outstretched upper extremity, the elbow is directed into a hyperextended position. This forces the tip of the olecranon into its fossa. As a result, all the linear force originally directed proximally up the upper extremity when the hand hits the ground is converted to a bending force in the supracondylar area of the distal humerus. Since this is a new and relatively immature metaphyseal bone, it fails quite easily. The degree of completeness of the fracture depends on the combination of the bending moment and the severity of the force applied.

8. **Extension supracondylar fractures are classified into three subtypes. How is this classification used in determining the method of treatment?**

   The original description of the subtypes of extension supracondylar fractures was proposed by Garland in 1950. Various authors have subsequently modified this classification. I believe that the original classification into three types is still the simplest and most useful. It is based on the degree of displacement and the amount of intrinsic stability, which guide the appropriate treatment:

   - **Type I displaced fractures:** These are essentially undisplaced and can be treated with simple immobilization, using either a long-arm cast or a posterior splint.
   - **Type II fractures:** Usually have enough intrinsic stability, because of the intact posterior cortex, that when the elbow is flexed up to the safe limit of 120 degrees, the distal

fragment does not rotate when the upper extremity is fully internally or externally rotated. Thus, this type of fracture pattern can be treated with a long-arm cast in which the elbow is flexed up to around 120 degrees. If there is so much swelling about the elbow that there is evidence of vascular compromise distal to the extremity at 120 degrees of elbow flexion, then this type II fracture must be surgically stabilized, as for type III fractures, so that the elbow can be placed in less flexion.

- **Type III fractures:** Completely displaced, and, thus, there is no intrinsic stability. In addition, because of the more severe nature of this injury, there is usually a much greater degree of swelling of the soft tissues around the elbow. As a result, once a closed reduction is achieved, the fragments are usually stabilized by pins placed percutaneously across the fracture fragments. Once stabilized by these pins, the elbow is protected with a splint or cast. Because the fragments are stabilized internally, the elbow can then be immobilized at the safer angle of 90 degrees of flexion.

Garland JJ: Management of supracondylar fractures of the humerus in children. Surg Gynecol Obstet 109:145–154, 1959.

Green NE: Fractures and dislocations about the elbow. In Green NE, Swinotkowski MF (eds): Skeletal Trauma in Children, Vol. 3, 2nd ed. Philadelphia, W.B. Saunders, 1998, pp 259–318.

9. **Since type III supracondylar fractures need to be stabilized, what is the best technique to achieve this?**

Once the reduction has been achieved, there is too much swelling to stabilize the fracture fragments with a cast alone. The currently accepted method is to secure the fracture fragments with smooth pins placed percutaneously. These can be inserted in various patterns. The strongest construct is medial-lateral pins, which cross above the fracture site. The fracture can also be stabilized with two pins inserted laterally. This construct is less stable to prevent rotation in the horizontal plane, which does not seem to be of any significance clinically. The original studies by Zionts and associates have shown that three pins placed laterally can provide rotational stability almost equal to that provided by medial-lateral pins, without the danger of ulnar nerve injury.

More recent reports by Cheng and Skaggs and their associates have found that, in the clinical setting, the results with two diverging lateral pins were equal to those with medial-lateral cross pins.

Cheng JC, Lam TP, Shen WY: Closed reduction and percutaneous pinning for Type III displaced supracondylar fractures in children. J Orthop Trauma 9:511–515, 1995.

Garland JJ: Management of supracondylar fractures of the humerus in children. Surg Gynecol Obstet 109:145–154, 1959.

Skaggs DL, Cluck MW, Mostifi A, et al: Lateral entry pin fixation in the management of supracondylar fractures in children. J Bone Joint Surg. 86A:702–707, 2004.

Zionts LE, McKellop HA, Hathaway R: Torsional strength of pin configurations used to fix supracondylar fractures of the humerus in children. J Bone Joint Surg 76A:253–256, 1994.

10. **What is the most common risk associated with the insertion of a pin medially in the distal supracondylar fragment to stabilize the fracture after the reduction has been obtained?**

To insert the medial pin, it should go directly through the center or anterior cortical surface of the medial epicondyle. The location of the ulnar nerve in its groove just posterior to the medial epicondyle makes it vulnerable to injury if the pin inadvertently courses in a more posterior direction. In some patients, the nerve is very mobile and can course anterior to the epicondyle. In these patients, placing the medial pin with the elbow flexed can greatly increase the risk of injury to the ulnar nerve. When a medial pin is used, the rate of ulnar nerve injury can be as high as 5%. This is one reason that many surgeons use stabilization techniques that avoid the need for a medial pin.

Ikram MA: Ulnar nerve palsy: A complication following percutaneous fixation of supracondylar fractures of the humerus in children. Injury 27:303–305,1996.

11. **Extension supracondylar fractures have a higher incidence of associated complicating injuries. What are some of these?**
    - **Nerve injuries:** Any of the three major nerves (i.e., the median, radial, and ulnar nerves) can be injured with supracondylar fractures. Originally, it was believed that the radial nerve was the most commonly injured nerve in extension supracondylar fractures. Recent studies by Cramer and associates have shown, however, that if a very careful neurologic examination is performed, you will find that the anterior interosseous nerve is probably the most commonly injured. This branch of the median nerve stimulates the muscles that flex the interphalangeal joints of the index finger and thumb. There is no sensory deficit. Fortunately, at least 95% of the nerve injuries resolve spontaneously. The ulnar nerve is most commonly injured with flexion supracondylar fractures.
    - **Vascular injuries:** The brachial artery can be injured by the sharp edge of the distal portion of the proximal fragment. This more commonly occurs if the distal fragment is displaced both posteriorly and laterally. The range of injuries varies from temporary compression to partial or complete obstruction due to interval tears to complete rupture of the artery. Fortunately, in most cases, there is sufficient collateral circulation to maintain the viability of the extremity.
    - **Compartment syndrome:** In some cases, injury to the brachial artery produces vasospasm at the meta-arteriole level, producing ischemia of the forearm muscles, especially the flexors. This ischemia causes a dysfunction of the muscle cell, resulting in severe swelling of the compartment, which in turn produces more ischemia.

12. **What are the classic clinical findings for an impending forearm compartment syndrome associated with a supracondylar fracture?**
    Remember the 5 Ps:
    - The extremity can be **p**ulseless. (In some cases, however, the pulse may be present.)
    - There is severe **p**ain in the forearm due to ischemia of the muscles.
    - There is dysfunction of the muscles, manifest by **p**aralysis.
    - The compromise of the arterial supply produces **p**allor.
    - Compression of the nerves produces **p**aresthesias and, in some cases, even anesthesia.

    Flynn JC, Zink WP: Fractures and dislocations of the elbow. In MacEwen GD, Kasser JR, Heinrich SD (eds): Pediatric Fractures: A Practical Approach to Assessment and Treatment. Baltimore, Williams & Wilkins, 1993.

13. **Volkman's ischemic contracture is the most feared complication associated with supracondylar fractures. What is it? How is it manifested?**
    If a compartment syndrome is not recognized early, the muscle cells become fibrotic, producing the characteristic Volkmann's ischemic contracture. Patients with this condition develop rigid fibrotic contractures of the forearm muscles. This makes movement in the hand extremely restricted and creates a very significant disability. Fortunately, this complication occurs in less than 1% of cases.

    Blount WP: Volkmann's ischemic contracture. Surg Gynecol Obstet 90:244–246, 1950.

14. **What is the most common complication with supracondylar fractures?**
    The most common problem associated with inadequate treatment of extension supracondylar fractures is a deformity termed *cubitus varus*. This occurs because the distal fragment can tilt into a varus alignment in relationship to the shaft (Figs. 31-2 and 31-3).

    DePablos J, Tejero A: Fractures of the shoulder, upper limb and hand. In Benson MKD, Fixsen JA, Macnicol MF, Parsh K (eds): Children's Orthopedics and Fractures. London, Churchill Livingstone, 2002, pp 613–624.

15. **Cubitus varus is termed an *iatrogenic* problem. Why?**
Cubitus varus occurs when the fracture is not managed appropriately. It can be the result of either not achieving an adequate reduction in the first place or not maintaining it with adequate stabilization.

Sharrand WJW: Paediatric Orthopaedics and Fractures. Oxford, Blackwell Scientific, 1971.

16. **Does a cubitus varus deformity produce any significant disability or functional impairment?**
Usually, cubitus varus represents primarily a cosmetic deformity. The unsightly aspect of cubitus varus is manifested mainly by the marked prominence of the lateral condyle. This is accentuated by the forearm being angulated in a varus direction in relationship to the arm. Often there is an associated hyperextension deformity of the distal femur, which can accentuate the uncosmetic aspect of the varus angulation.

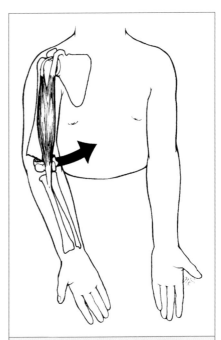

Figure 31-2. Cubitus varus. The eccentric pull of the biceps tilts the distal fragment into varus position *(arrow)*, producing the gunstock deformity of cubitus varus.

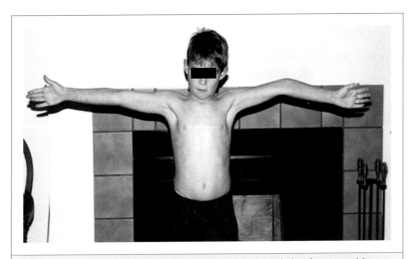

Figure 31-3. Clinical photo of a patient with cubitus varus following malunion of a supracondylar fracture.

There is rarely any significant functional deficit associated with this malalignment of the distal fragment. The varus deformity does, however, predispose the distal humerus to sustain subsequent fractures of the lateral condyle.

McIntyre W, Gruel GR, Sullivan JA, et al: Fractures of the elbow. In Letts RM (eds): Management of Pediatric Fractures. New York, Churchill Livingstone, 1994, pp 167–322.

17. **How long does it take for a supracondylar fracture to heal?**
Since this is an area of actively growing bone, healing is rapid. There is usually adequate fracture callus to remove all forms of stability (i.e., pins and casts) at 3 weeks to permit active motion.

18. **Supracondylar fractures can have a high rate of complications acutely. Are there any long-term effects?**
If an adequate reduction is achieved and stabilization is appropriate, a full return of motion can usually be expected in almost all cases. Because of the magnitude of soft tissue injury, it may be 2–3 months after cast removal before full elbow motion has returned. By and large, the patient can expect a full recovery from this injury.

19. **Supracondylar fracture represents a major injury to the elbow. When should physical therapy be initiated?**
Postfracture physical therapy usually is not indicated. In fact, it may lead to a delay in resumption of motion. Almost all the patients regain a full range of motion on their own.

20. **How do flexion-type supracondylar fractures differ from the extension type?**
The flexion fractures differ from the extension fractures in many ways. First, in the structural pattern of the fracture, the distal fragment is flexed anteriorly. Second, these fractures are reduced by extending the fragments instead of flexing these fragments, as in the extension types. Third, with those fractures that are completely displaced, there is an increased incidence of the need to perform an open reduction because of the inability to obtain a satisfactory reduction by manipulation alone. Finally, because of posterior displacement of the proximal fragment, the ulnar nerve is the nerve most commonly injured with these fractures.

21. **What is the most common iatrogenic complication of a flexion supracondylar fracture?**
Flexion injuries, if not adequately reduced, may result in a loss of elbow extension. The cosmetic deformity associated with this fracture pattern is most commonly a cubitus valgus deformity.

22. **What is a fracture of the lateral condyle?**
Characteristically, this is an injury in which, instead of being completely transverse, the fracture line goes obliquely from the articular surface of the distal humerus and exits laterally in the lateral distal humeral metaphysis. The fracture can originate in either the radiocapitellar groove (in which case it is termed a *Milch type I injury*) or the trochlea (these are termed *Milch type II injuries*).

23. **How does the mechanism of injury in this fracture differ from that of a supracondylar fracture?**
Characteristically, failure of the lateral condyle of the distal humerus occurs when the elbow is forced into varus position. The fragment is either pulled off by the extensor muscles or pushed off by the radial head or semilunar notch of the olecranon.

24. **Patients with supracondylar fractures can have neurovascular complications but usually regain full elbow motion. Can the same be said of patients with lateral condyle fractures?**

Since the elbow is an exact-fitting joint, if the articular surface of the distal humerus is not reduced anatomically, incongruity may result, producing a loss of motion and subsequent degenerative arthritis. In addition, since the fracture line traverses the physeal plate, growth abnormalities can occur, which also can create functional difficulties. Rarely does this type of fracture produce any type of injury to the neurovascular structures.

25. **A lateral condyle fracture is often referred to as having a *stage III displacement*. What is the difference between a stage III and a stage I or II displacement?**

See Fig. 31-4 for illustrations of the following stages:

- **Stage I:** The fracture fragment is essentially undisplaced. The fracture gap is 2 mm or less.
- **Stage II:** There is greater than 2 mm of gap between the fragments, but the condylar fragment is still in close proximity to the distal humerus and is usually laterally rotated only minimally. In many cases, the articular surface is still intact.
- **Stage III:** There is wide displacement, and the condylar fragment is markedly rotated, in some cases as much as 180 degrees, so that the articular surface may be facing the fracture surface of the distal humerus.

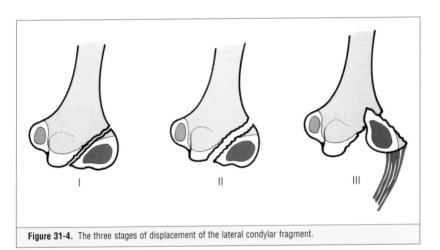

Figure 31-4. The three stages of displacement of the lateral condylar fragment.

26. **Clinically, do lateral condylar fractures differ in appearance from supracondylar fractures?**

With lateral condylar fractures, usually there is little displacement in the sagittal plane so that the elbow does not appear hyperextended. Since the fracture line involves only the lateral articular surface, hematoma formation is usually localized laterally over the condyle. Because of the lesser displacement, the degree of pain is often less with lateral condyle fractures.

27. **Does the stage of displacement affect the usual treatment of these injuries?**

- **Stage I:** These injuries usually require only immobilization with a cast or splint until sufficient fracture callus is seen on the follow-up radiographs.
- **Stage II:** These injuries require reduction of the condylar fragment and stabilization with smooth pins placed across the fracture site. In some cases, if the fracture hematoma is still fresh and the displacement is minimal, the reduction can be achieved by closed manipulation

and the pins placed across the fracture site by percutaneous techniques using an image intensifier.

- **Stage III:** In these fractures, as well as in many stage II fractures, the fracture fragment cannot be reduced adequately by closed manipulative techniques. In these cases, the fracture site must be approached surgically first to achieve a reduction. Once the fracture fragments are adequately reduced, they must then be stabilized with two pins, usually placed laterally across the fracture site.

Jakob R, Fowles JV: Observations concerning fractures of the lateral humeral condyles in children. J Bone Joint Surg 40B:430–436, 1975.

28. **Since stage I fractures are said to require only simple cast immobilization, is any special follow-up needed?**
The lateral condylar fragment contains the origin of the forearm extensor muscles. Even if the arm is immobilized in a cast, these muscles can still contract and cause a late displacement of the condyle fragments. Thus, if this type of lateral condyle fracture is immobilized only with a cast or splint, it needs to be followed and radiographs must be taken again in 5–7 days to be sure that there is no late displacement. Fractures stabilized with pins usually do not displace late.

29. **How long is immobilization required for lateral condyle fractures?**
Casts and pins can usually be safely removed in 3–4 weeks to allow early active motion.

30. **What are the consequences of inadequate treatment of a lateral condyle fracture?**
If the fragments are not adequately reduced and stabilized, there is a high incidence of the development on a nonunion (Fig. 31-5). Because of the instability of the condylar fragment, it tends to migrate proximally, creating a valgus angulation at the elbow (Fig. 31-6). With time (usually many years later), this valgus alignment produces a chronic irritation to the ulnar nerve, causing it to become nonfunctional. This delayed paralysis is termed *tardy ulnar nerve paralysis*.

31. **What is the more common injury involving the distal humerus in infants and small children?**
The *entire distal humeral physis* can become separated from the distal humeral metaphysis. This distal fragment involves both the lateral and the medial condyles. Although they do occur, lateral condylar and supracondylar fractures are very rare in this age group.

DeLee JC, Wilkins RE, Rogers LF, Rockwood CA Jr: Fracture separation of the distal humerus epiphysis. J Bone Joint Surg 62A:46–51, 1980.

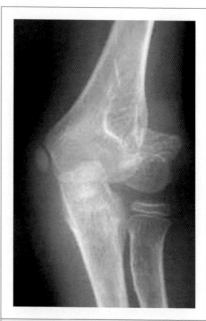

Figure 31-5. Inadequate stabilization of this lateral condyle fracture caused it to develop a nonunion.

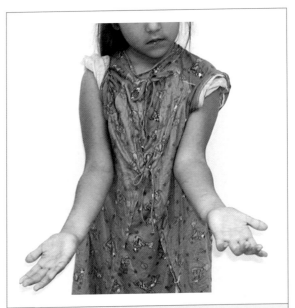

Figure 31-6. Clinically, the nonunion caused the elbow to drift into valgus alignment. This child had not yet developed a tardy ulnar nerve palsy.

32. **The secondary ossification centers are not present in infants. Does this present a problem in recognizing distal humeral physeal injuries in this age group?**
Yes. In some patients, especially very young infants, the secondary centers have not ossified. The diagnosis is correlated with the clinical finding of severe elbow swelling and so-called muffled crepitus (named because the raw fracture edge of the distal metaphysis is rubbing against the softer physeal cartilage of the distal fragment). On radiographs, the proximal forearm ossification centers lie posterior and medial to the ossification of the distal humeral metaphysis. The exact location of the unossified epiphyseal fragment can be confirmed with either an elbow arthrogram or an ultrasonogram.

33. **For the child in whom the secondary centers are ossified, are there specific findings on the radiographs that help to establish the diagnosis of a fracture of the entire distal humeral physis?**
In the older child in whom the lateral condyle has ossified, this secondary ossification center always remains directly aligned with the proximal radial metaphysis. The distal epiphyseal fragment is almost always posterior and medial to the distal humeral metaphysis.

34. **What is the most common mechanism for fractures of the entire distal humeral physis in infants?**
In the small infant, this is usually the result of a twisting force. Children of this age do not run and thus do not fall on their outstretched extremities. Therefore, many of these injuries in this age group are the result of child abuse.

35. **Because this injury involves the physis, do most of these completely displaced fractures of the entire distal humeral physis require an open reduction, as do stage III lateral condyle fractures?**

No. Usually, these fractures are easily reduced with manipulative closed reduction. Because the extremity in a small child is short and fat, however, cast immobilization is usually inadequate. These fractures almost universally require stabilization with pins placed percutaneously. At the time of the reduction, an arthrogram is usually performed to confirm the adequacy of the reduction.

KEY POINTS: FRACTURES IN THE ELBOW REGION

1. About 86% of fractures in the elbow region occur in the distal humerus. Of these, 79.8% are supracondylar fractures, 16.9% involve the lateral condyle, and 12.5% involve the medial epicondyle.

2. When the angulation of the forearm in relationship to the humeral shaft is away from the midline, it is referred to as *cubitus valgus*. When the angulation is toward the midline or body, the term used for this deformity is *cubitus varus*.

3. The two types of supracondylar fractures are determined by whether the failure occurs when the elbow is forced into hyperextension or hyperflexion. The extension type is more common (causing 90–95% of cases). In the flexion type (5–10% of cases), the distal fragment is flexed forward and lies anterior to the distal fragment.

4. Extension supracondylar fractures have a higher incidence of complications, including nerve injuries, vascular injuries, and compartment syndrome. The most common problem associated with inadequate treatment of extension supracondylar fractures is a cubitus varus deformity.

5. Inadequate treatment of a lateral condyle fracture is associated with a high incidence of nonunion, which may result in valgus angulation at the elbow and chronic irritation to the ulnar nerve, causing it to become nonfunctional. This delayed paralysis is termed *tardy ulnar nerve paralysis*.

36. **What are the most common complications associated with fractures of the entire distal humeral physis?**

Often these are unrecognized or neglected, especially if the injury is the result of child abuse. Fortunately, these fractures heal quite rapidly, with considerable remodeling. Potential complications include the following:

- **Cubitus varus:** If the distal epiphyseal fragment remains tilted, some degree of cubitus varus may remain. Rarely is the cubitus varus following this injury of significant magnitude to require surgical correction.
- **Neurovascular complications:** These have only rarely been reported following this injury.
- **Avascular necrosis:** In some cases, the vessels supplying the secondary ossification centers of the trochlea (i.e., the medial condyle) can be injured. This may result in avascular necrosis developing in this area, which can produce a secondary disruption of the articular surface, with subsequent loss of elbow motion.

37. **How common is injury to the medial condyle in children?**

In comparison to fractures of the lateral condyle, injuries to the medial condyle (Fig. 31-7) are very rare, accounting for less than 0.5% of the fractures of the distal humerus.

38. **Are there biologic factors that contribute to a failure to correctly diagnose fractures of the medial condyle?**

The secondary ossification centers of the medial condyle often do not appear until the patient is 9 or 10 years of age. Because the medial condyle is unossified, the displacement of the fragment may not be apparent on the routine radiographs. Special imaging studies such as sonography or arthrography may be required to make the diagnosis. Probably the greatest error related to its rarity is a failure to even think of this fracture occurring in this age group.

39. **What is the result of not recognizing or treating correctly a fracture of the medial condyle?**

The distal fragment can produce a disabling nonunion, with the elbow drifting into a progressive cubitus varus (Figs. 31-8 and 31-9). In addition, there may be the biologic effects of the disruption of the

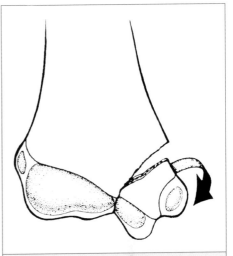

Figure 31-7. Fracture of the medial condyle. This includes the medial epicondyle and the ossification center of the medial aspect of the trochlea. This fragment may be displaced anteriorly and medially by the origin of the forearm flexor muscles *(arrow)*.

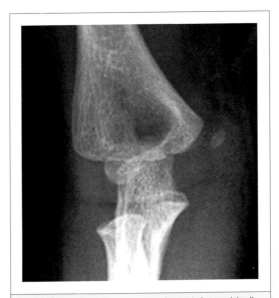

Figure 31-8. Initially, this fracture was interpreted as a minimally displaced fracture of the medial epicondyle and was treated conservatively.

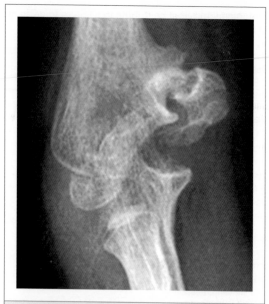

Figure 31-9. Radiographs of the fracture in Fig. 31-8, taken 18 months later, demonstrated that it was an unrecognized fracture of the medial condyle with a resultant nonunion and varus deformity.

vascular supply to the medial condyle, resulting in avascular necrosis.

40. **We have been discussing injuries to the condyles. How do injuries to the epicondyles differ?**

An epicondyle is an apophysis; that is, it is a secondary ossification center for the bony prominence that serves as the origin of muscles. It is also extra-articular. The medial epicondyle is a separate prominence that serves as the origin of the forearm muscles. In the distal humerus, the medial epicondyle ossifies at about 5–7 years of age. The lateral epicondyle serves as the origin of the muscles for the forearm extensors. This secondary ossification center appears around the age of 9–11 years. Injuries to the epicondyles usually are the result of an avulsion force exerted by either the muscle origins or the collateral ligaments.

41. **What is the most commonly injured epicondyle around the elbow?**

Avulsion of the medial humeral epicondyle (Fig. 31-10) accounts for about 14% of all

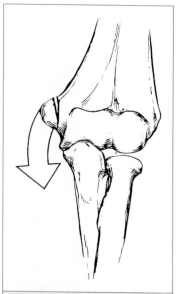

Figure 31-10. The medial epicondyle is often avulsed by the ulnar collateral ligaments or the flexor muscles of the forearm (*arrow*).

injuries involving the distal humerus in the child. Isolated fractures of the lateral humeral epicondyle are extremely rare.

42. **Since these injuries are the result of avulsion forces, is a fracture of the medial epicondyle usually an isolated fracture?**

No. This has an anatomic basis. The medial (i.e., ulnar) collateral ligaments all arise from the medial epicondyle. When the elbow sustains a traumatic dislocation in the adult patient, the collateral ligaments are often ruptured. In the pediatric patient, however, the collateral ligaments are stronger than the apophyseal plate of the medial epicondyle. Thus, failure occurs through the relatively weaker apophyseal plate of the epicondyle. In more than 50% of acute traumatic elbow dislocations in pediatric patients, the medial epicondyle may be avulsed from its attachment to the distal humerus.

Other mechanisms of injury, such as direct blows to the epicondyle, sudden forceful flexure muscle forces (as seen with arm wrestling or throwing), or simply a severe valgus stress to the elbow, can also cause the epicondyle to become avulsed from the distal humerus.

43. **What is the most severe complication associated with avulsions of the medial epicondyle?**

When the elbow is dislocated, the epicondylar fragment can become interposed between the articular surfaces of the distal humerus and the olecranon. When the elbow is reduced, this epicondylar fragment usually is extruded to return to close to its original attachment to the distal humerus. However, it may remain within the joint. If unrecognized, this interposed epicondyle can produce severe damage to the articular surface of the elbow.

In addition, the incarcerated epicondyle and the adjacent flexor mass may become wrapped around the ulnar nerve to produce a compression neuropathy.

Thus, after reducing a traumatic elbow dislocation, it is very important to be sure that the medial epicondyle has not become incarcerated within the joint and that the ulnar nerve is functioning fully.

44. **How are avulsion fractures of the medial epicondyle usually treated?**

Treatment usually is by nonoperative methods. The key is to reestablish elbow motion with encouragement of early active motion exercises. Even if the epicondylar fragment remains displaced and forms a fibrous nonunion, there is rarely any significant disability in elbow function.

Bernstein SM, King JD, Sanderson RA: Fractures of the medial epicondyle of the humerus. Contemp Orthop 23:637–641, 1981.

45. **What are the indications for surgical fixation of the medial epicondyle?**

First and foremost, an absolute indication for surgical intervention is if the epicondylar fragment is incarcerated within the joint. It must be removed surgically.

The other indications for surgical intervention remain controversial. Some practitioners believe that, in high-performance athletes who use their upper extremities extensively and apply strong valgus stresses to them, the elbow must be extremely stable. There is some evidence that an ununited medial epicondyle may produce sufficient elbow instability as to interfere with high athletic performance. Thus, in these individuals, open reduction with internal fixation of the fragment may be indicated. The fixation technique must allow the patient to begin early motion.

The presence of ulnar nerve dysfunction is relative. Certainly, if both motor and sensory functions are lacking, the epicondyle and nerve should be explored. If there is only a mild paresthesia or motor weakness, then simple observation may be all that is necessary.

46. **What is the most common complication associated with avulsion of the medial epicondyle?**

Although incarceration of the epicondyle within the elbow joint can produce severe elbow dysfunction, it is a relatively rare complication. The most common sequela following this injury is loss of elbow motion. This is especially true if it is associated with an elbow dislocation.

Because stiffness can occur with a fracture of the medial epicondyle, it is important that motion be initiated early with patients treated both operatively and nonoperatively.

47. **In the pediatric patient, what portion of the proximal radius is especially vulnerable to injury? Why?**

The radial neck is the area of the proximal radius most commonly injured. This is because it is a metaphyseal structure, composed of a high percentage of weak cancellous bone. In addition, the radial head is relatively protected from injury because it consists of a greater amount of cartilage than that in the adult.

48. **Where may the pain associated with a fracture of the radial neck manifest?**

Often, in the child, pain associated with a fracture of the radial neck is referred to the area of the wrist. The key to differentiating an injury of the radial neck from an injury of the distal radius is that there is usually no swelling or local tenderness over the distal radius with a fracture of the radial neck. The tenderness and swelling are localized proximally at the elbow over the proximal radius. In addition, the pain of a fracture of the radial neck is accentuated when the forearm is supinated and pronated.

49. **The radial neck in a child is relatively well protected by the overlying muscles. What forces need to be applied to this area to cause the neck to fail?**

The most common mechanism of injury is a **valgus force** applied to the elbow. When the elbow is forced into valgus, a compressive force is applied against the radial head by the lateral condyle. Failure occurs at the weaker area of the radial neck. In this type of fracture, the radial head is forced into varying degrees of lateral angulation and translocation in relationship to the distal shaft.

A second, but rarer, mechanism occurs when the elbow becomes **dislocated**. The lateral condyle can force the radial head off during either the dislocation or the reduction process. In this rarer mechanism, the radial head is usually completely displaced from the radial shaft.

The radial neck can also undergo **stress fractures**, which are very rare.

Torsional injuries can force the neck and shaft away from the head. The shaft is primarily displaced, and the head remains within the confines of the orbicular ligament.

50. **What warning should the parents of a child with a fracture of the radial neck be given prior to initiating treatment?**

In this injury, the bone is small, and, to the uneducated eye of the parents, the fracture displacement often appears minimal. The parents need to understand that, in addition to the fracture, there is often a considerable amount of soft tissue injury, especially if the head fragment is displaced. Because of this soft tissue injury, there may be postreduction stiffness, especially with loss of supination and pronation, even if an anatomic reduction is achieved. This is especially true if the reduction has to be achieved by open operative techniques.

51. **What are the usually accepted methods of treatment for fractures of the radial neck?**

In the more common valgus injuries, the treatment is usually dictated by the degree of angulation with the radial neck. Angulation of 30 degrees probably does not need manipulation. Greater than 30 degrees but less than 60 degrees of angulation can usually be reduced to an acceptable limit of less than 30 degrees by one of the closed manipulative techniques. Greater than 60 degrees of angulation usually requires some type of operative technique to obtain an adequate reduction.

In completely displaced fractures associated with elbow dislocations, an open operative procedure is almost always required.

52. **Since fractures of the radial neck often result from a strong valgus force applied to the elbow, might not other injuries in the elbow area occur at the same time?**
Yes, as a result of the valgus stress applied to the elbow, the medial epicondyle may be avulsed. This valgus stress can also produce a greenstick fracture of the olecranon.

53. **Even though it is a small fracture, certainly there are complications associated with fractures of the radial neck, correct?**
Correct. The most common complication is a loss of range of forearm motion, usually pronation. Other complications, such as radial head overgrowth, nonunion, avascular necrosis of the radial head, and proximal radioulnar synostosis, can also produce a loss of elbow or forearm motion.

54. **The olecranon is structurally an apophysis. Because of this anatomic fact, does it have a unique secondary ossification process?**
Yes. The olecranon is structurally an apophysis that serves primarily as the insertion for the triceps tendon. This apophysis contributes very little to the length of the ulna.

    The apophysis may have more than one ossification center. Initially, the unossified portion of the olecranon apophysis supports greater than 50% of the articular surface of the olecranon. As it matures, the ossification front of the proximal metaphysis of the olecranon migrates proximally so that it supports only 25% or less of the articular surface (Fig. 31-11).

55. **What are the common mechanisms responsible for fractures of the olecranon in children?**
The most common mechanism is probably an injury that occurs with the elbow locked in extension (i.e., extension injury). In this position, the forearm is subjected to varus or valgus forces, causing the metaphyseal portion of the olecranon to undergo a greenstick type of failure. If a valgus force is applied, there is usually an associated fracture of the radial neck laterally or avulsion of the medial epicondyle medially. If a varus force is applied, the radial head may dislocate. This combination of a lateral dislocation of the radial head associated with a greenstick valgus angulated fracture of the olecranon is termed a *Monteggia's type III lesion.*

    If the elbow is forced into hyperextension, a type of failure may occur in which the anterior articular surface becomes disrupted, whereas the posterior cortex or periosteum of the olecranon remains intact.

    If the elbow is stressed while it is flexed (i.e., flexion injury), failure of the olecranon

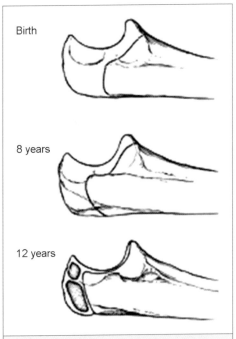

Birth

8 years

12 years

Figure 31-11. Olecranon ossification. The ossification front of the metaphysic migrates proximally as the olecranon matures. Note the two separate centers that develop close to maturity. These separate centers can be misinterpreted as fracture lines.

metaphysis occurs on the posterior cortex, producing a resultant separation of the fragments with a loss of the extension mechanism of the elbow.

56. **How are extension fractures of the olecranon commonly treated in children?**
In varus and valgus injuries, the elbow is manipulated into extension, and the deformity is corrected by applying the reverse force (e.g., a varus force applied to a valgus deformity). In hyperextension injuries, if the posterior extension mechanism remains intact, simply hyperflexing the elbow can reduce the fracture.

57. **In the flexion injuries, what biomechanical function must be reestablished?**
With these injuries, the posterior extensor mechanism of the olecranon is usually completely disrupted. If there is only a slight displacement (i.e., 2 mm of separation of the fragments or less), the elbow can be forced into extension and immobilized in this position until an adequate callus is produced. Usually, there is greater than 2 mm of disruption, and, thus, the fracture fragments need to be reduced by operative methods. Because of the deforming effect of the extensor forces on the muscles, this reduction needs to be secured with some type of internal fixation device.

58. **The term _Monteggia_ is often used to describe a type of fracture complex in the forearm. Where did this term originate? What type of injury does it describe?**
This term has been around for almost 2 centuries. In 1814, Giovanni Monteggia described an injury complex that included a fracture of the proximal ulna and an accompanying dislocation of the radial head. This injury complex has carried his name ever since.

59. **Does Monteggia's fracture-dislocation injury occur only as a single pattern?**
No. It consists of four types, based on the direction of displacement of the radial head and the fracture pattern of the proximal ulna (Fig. 31-12). José Luis Bado of Montevideo, Uraguay, proposed this classification scheme in the late 1950s:

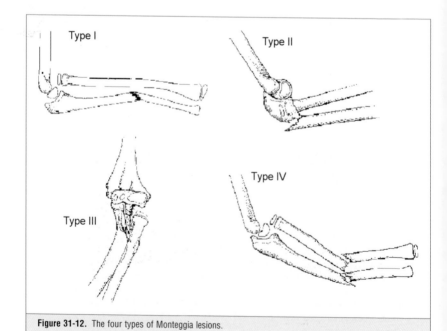

Figure 31-12. The four types of Monteggia lesions.

- **Type I:** In this type, the radial head is displaced anteriorly and there is an oblique fracture of the proximal shaft of the ulna. This type usually occurs as the result of a hyperextension force to the forearm and elbow.
- **Type II:** This type is extremely rare in children. The fracture pattern is a flexion type of injury to the proximal ulnar metaphysis. The radial head dislocates posteriorly. The mechanism is usually the same as for traumatic dislocation of the elbow, in which a linear force is applied proximally up the forearm to a semiflexed elbow.
- **Type III:** This is the result of application of a varus force to the extended elbow. There is a greenstick varus fracture of the proximal ulna or olecranon and a lateral dislocation of the radial head.
- **Type IV:** This is a fracture involving the shafts of both the radius and the ulna (usually at different levels) and an associated dislocation of the radial head, which is usually either anterior or lateral.

Bado JL: The Monteggia lesion. Clin Orthop 50:71–86, 1967.

60. **What are Monteggia equivalents?**

These are injuries involving the proximal radius or ulna, for which Bado believed the mechanism of injury was similar to that of a classic Monteggia lesion. With the exception of the type IV lesion, equivalents have been described for each of the major types of lesions. For example, an isolated traumatic dislocation of the radial head is classified as a type I equivalent.

61. **What is probably the most frequent iatrogenic complication associated with Monteggia's fracture?**

Often, the fracture of the ulna is quite obvious, both clinically and radiographically. The dislocation of the radial head may be subtle and may not be appreciated (Fig. 31-13). If left untreated, this chronically dislocated radial head can produce a significant disability in elbow function.

Thus, it is extremely important in all cases in which the ulnar shaft is fractured to inspect the relationship of the radial head to the ossification center of the lateral condyle carefully to be sure that there is not a coexistent disruption of this joint. A line drawn proximally up the long axis of the proximal radius through the radial head should always pass proximally through the center of the ossification center of the lateral condyle, regardless of the radiographic position.

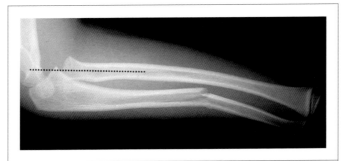

Figure 31-13. Missed Monteggia. With this injury, the fracture of the ulnar shaft is readily apparent. However, the associated dislocation of the radial head may not be appreciated as easily. The line drawn proximally up the proximal radius courses above the center of the capitellum.

62. **Monteggia's type I lesion consists of two separate disruptions. Is there a specific order in which these injuries should be treated?**
Yes. Treatment of the type I lesion requires two steps. First, the length of the ulnar shaft, which is usually angulated anteriorly, must be reestablished by reducing the fracture. Once the ulnar length has been reestablished, the second step is to reduce the radial head. This is usually easily performed by applying a force directly over the head in a posterior direction while hyperflexing the elbow. If the ulnar fracture is unstable, it may need to be stabilized with an intramedullary pin. After reduction, the elbow is immobilized in some degree of hyperflexion to decrease the deforming force on the biceps muscle.

On rare occasions, the orbicular ligament may become interposed, preventing a closed reduction of the radial head. In this case, open reduction may be necessary.

63. **Because the type II Monteggia's lesion is a flexion injury, how does the treatment procedure differ from that of the type I lesion?**
The reduction mechanism is usually the opposite. The olecranon fracture and radial head are usually both reduced by extending, rather than flexing, the elbow and immobilizing it in extension rather than in flexion.

64. **Since Monteggia's type III lesion involves a varus force in its causation, is a valgus force needed in the reduction process?**
Yes. These are essentially extension varus greenstick fractures of the olecranon. The olecranon fracture is first reduced by extending and applying a valgus force to the elbow. This usually simultaneously reduces the radial head. Sometimes direct pressure over the radial head may be necessary to achieve the final reduction. Occasionally, as with type I lesions, the orbicular ligament becomes interposed and may require surgical extraction.

65. **The type IV Monteggia's lesion produces a condition in which the proximal radius is said to be floating freely. How does this affect the treatment process?**
Because the radius is a free segment, it is difficult to reduce it by manipulation alone. Thus, the type IV lesion is first converted to a type I lesion by surgically stabilizing the shafts of the radius and generally the ulna as well with either intramedullary fixation or plates and screws. Once the shafts have been stabilized, the radial head usually is easier to reduce by manipulation in the same manner as for a type I lesion.

66. **Are nerve injuries common with Monteggia lesions?**
Nerve lesions occur primarily with type III lesions. They are extremely rare in type I and II lesions. The anterolateral displacement of the radial head may produce compression of the posterior interosseous branch of the radial nerve. This results in a loss of wrist and finger extension. Almost all of these nerve injuries resolve following reduction of the radial head.

67. **How does the incidence per age group of elbow dislocations differ from that of supracondylar fractures?**
The peak age incidence for supracondylar fractures is 7 years, which is the period of maximal ligamentous laxity. Elbow dislocations tend to be more of a second-decade injury, with the peak occurring at around 12 or 13 years of age.

68. **In what direction does the proximal radioulnar segment displace in elbow dislocations in children?**
In traumatic elbow dislocations, the proximal radioulnar complex can displace in one of four directions. The proximal radioulnar complex can displace in either a posterior or an anterior direction to the distal humerus. Both the posterior and the anterior types have subtypes, in which the radioulnar segment is either medial or lateral. Most often, the radioulnar segment displaces in a posterolateral direction.

69. **There is some confusion about a common condition that occurs when acute traction is applied to a young child's upper extremity. This is called either a *pulled elbow* or a *nursemaid's elbow*. Does this represent a true dislocation of the proximal radioulnar joint?**

No. The so-called nursemaid's or pulled elbow is actually a displacement of the orbicular ligament into the radioulnar joint. The condition usually occurs before the age of 5 years. It occurs when the forearm is pulled into hyperpronation as the elbow is forced simultaneously into extension. Because of the weakness of the distal portion, the orbicular ligament slips proximally over the radial head to become interposed between the lateral condyle and the radial head. With the orbicular ligament interposed between the articular surfaces, the child becomes reluctant to flex the elbow and holds it in an extended position at the side of the body.

Reduction is easily achieved by reversing the inciting mechanism—that is, forceful forearm pronation coupled with elbow extension. To reverse this injury, the forearm is supinated while the elbow is forced into hyperflexion. If the surgeon's thumb is placed over the lateral edge of the radial head as this maneuver is performed, the orbicular ligament can be palpated as it is extended out of the elbow joint. If the ligament is successfully extruded from the joint, the elbow pain is soon relieved and the patient promptly resumes active flexion.

70. **You are often asked to evaluate the lateral projection of a radiograph of an injured elbow to see whether there is a positive fat pad sign. What does this term mean?**

There are two fat pads in the region of the elbow that lie extra-articularly. The largest one lies on the capsule on its posterior aspect. This posterior fat pad and its underlying capsule in the normal uninjured hand lie totally within the olecranon fossa of the distal humerus. Because of this fact, this fat pad is not visualized on the lateral radiograph. A smaller fat pad overlies the anterior capsule. This fat pad also lies in the depths of the anterior coronoid fossa. A very small portion of this fat pad may be visible on the lateral radiograph because the coronoid fossa is fairly shallow.

Injury to one of the bones making up the elbow joint produces an effusion composed primarily of blood (i.e., hemarthrosis), which distends the capsule (Fig. 31-14). This in turn extracts the anterior and posterior fat pads from their respective fossae, making them now visible (i.e., a positive fat pad sign) on the lateral radiographs of the elbow (Fig. 31-15). The most common cause of a positive elbow fat pad sign is an undisplaced fracture of the distal humerus. An elbow also may demonstrate a positive fat pad sign in nontraumatic conditions, such as septic arthritis or a primary arthritic process. Thus, the significance of this radiographic finding must be correlated with the patient's history and clinical examination.

Murphy WA, Siegel MJ: Elbow fat pad with new signs and extended differential diagnosis. Radiology 124:659–665, 1977.

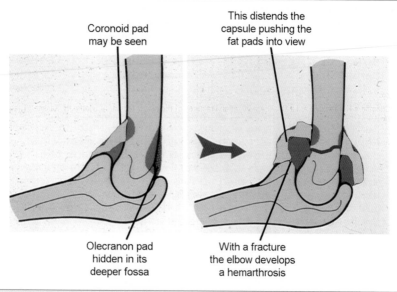

Coronoid pad
may be seen

This distends the
capsule pushing the
fat pads into view

Olecranon pad
hidden in its
deeper fossa

With a fracture
the elbow develops
a hemarthrosis

Figure 31-14. *Left,* Normally, there are fat pads lying in the coronoid and olecranon fossae. The posterior olecranon fat pad lies completely within its respective fossa and thus is not seen on the lateral radiograph. Since the coronoid fossa anteriorly is shallow, some of its fat pad may normally be visualized. *Right,* With the development of a hemarthrosis associated with a fracture, the joint capsule is distended, which in turn displaces these fat pads so that they become visible on lateral radiographs.

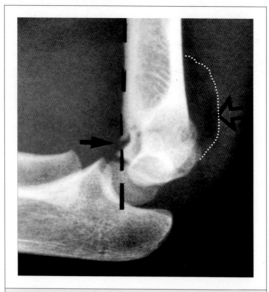

Figure 31-15. Lateral radiograph of an undisplaced fracture *(solid arrow)* with displacement of the olecranon fat pad *(open arrow and solid line)*.

BIBLIOGRAPHY

1. Bado JL: The Monteggia lesion. Clin Orthop 50:71–86, 1967.

2. Beals BK: The normal carrying angle of the elbow. Clin Orthop 19:194–196, 1976.

3. Bernstein SM, King JD, Sanderson RA: Fractures of the medial epicondyle of the humerus. Contemp Orthop 23:637–641, 1981.

4. Blount WP: Volkmann's ischemic contracture. Surg Gynecol Obstet 90:244–246, 1950.

5. Chambers H, Stanley EA, La De, Graza JF, et al: Fractures of the elbow region. In Beatty JH, Kasser JR (eds): Rockwood and Wilkin's Fractures in Children, 5th ed. Philadelphia, Lippincott Williams & Wilkins, 2001, pp 483–740.

6. Cheng JC, Lam TP, Shen WY: Closed reduction and percutaneous pinning for Type III displaced supracondylar fractures in children. J Orthop Trauma 9:511–515, 1995.

7. Cramer KE, Green NE, Devito DP: Incidence of interosseous nerve palsy in supracondylar humerus fractures in children. J Pediatr Orthhop 13:502–505, 1993.

8. DeLee JC, Wilkins RE, Rogers LF, Rockwood CA Jr: Fracture separation of the distal humerus epiphysis. J Bone Joint Surg 62A:46–51, 1980.

9. DePablos J, Tejero A: Fractures of the shoulder, upper limb and hand. In Benson MKD, Fixsen JA, Macnicol MF, Parsh K (eds): Children's Orthopedics and Fractures. London, Churchill Livingstone, 2002, pp 613–624.

10. Flynn JC, Zink WP: Fractures and dislocations of the elbow. In MacEwen GD, Kasser JR, Heinrich SD (eds): Pediatric Fractures: A Practical Approach to Assessment and Treatment. Baltimore, Williams & Wilkins, 1993.

11. Fowles JV, Kassab MT: Observations concerning radial neck fractures in children. J Pediatr Orthop 6:51–57, 1986.

12. Garland JJ: Management of supracondylar fractures of the humerus in children. Surg Gynecol Obstet 109:145–154, 1959.

13. Green NE: Fractures and dislocations about the elbow. In Green NE, Swinotkowski MF (eds): Skeletal Trauma in Children, Vol. 3, 2nd ed. Philadelphia, W.B. Saunders, 1998, pp 259–318.

14. Ikram MA: Ulnar nerve palsy: A complication following percutaneous fixation of supracondylar fractures of the humerus in children. Injury 27:303–305, 1996.

15. Jakob R, Fowles JV: Observations concerning fractures of the lateral humeral condyles in children. J Bone Joint Surg 40B:430–436, 1975.

16. McIntyre W, Gruel GR, Sullivan JA, et al: Fractures of the elbow. In Letts RM (ed): Management of Pediatric Fractures. New York, Churchill Livingstone, 1994, pp 167–322.

17. Murphy WA, Siegel MJ: Elbow fat pad with new signs and extended differential diagnosis. Radiology 124:659–665, 1977.

18. Sharrand WJW: Paediatric Orthopaedics and Fractures. Oxford, Blackwell Scientific, 1971.

19. Skaggs DL, Cluck MW, Mostifi A, et al: Lateral entry pin fixation in the management of supracondylar fractures in children. J Bone Joint Surg 86A:702–707, 2004.

20. Wood CW, Tullos HS, King JW: The throwing arm: Elbow joint injuries. J Sports Med 1:43–47, 1973.

21. Zionts LE, McKellop HA, Hathaway R: Torsional strength of pin configurations used to fix supracondylar fractures of the humerus in children. J Bone Joint Surg 76A:253–256, 1994.

CHAPTER 32

WRIST AND FOREARM FRACTURES

J. Eric Gordon, MD

1. **How can a fracture of the wrist or forearm be differentiated from a sprain by history or physical examination in children?**

   History or physical examination can be helpful in differentiating fractures from sprains but cannot be definitive. Fractures or sprains can occur with either a significant or a trivial mechanism of injury. Fractures have point tenderness over a specific area of bone, whereas wrist sprains tend to have more diffuse tenderness over the ligamentous areas of the wrist, such as the ulnar collateral ligament. A child may be able to move the wrist or not move the wrist, regardless of the presence of a fracture. A radiograph should be obtained to differentiate these diagnoses.

2. **What radiographs should be obtained if a wrist or forearm fracture is suspected?**

   Anteroposterior and lateral radiographs of the forearm that include both the wrist and the elbow should be obtained. These should be positioned so that the entire forearm is rotated between views to obtain the anteroposterior and lateral views, not just pronating and supinating the wrist. This should allow visualization of anteroposterior and lateral views of both the wrist and the forearm.

3. **What special types of fractures occur in the wrist or forearm in children that do not occur in adults?**

   Physeal fractures, buckle or torus fractures, greenstick fractures, and plastic deformation all occur in children but not in adults.

4. **What should be done if there is point tenderness over the forearm or wrist but no fracture visible on the radiographs?**

   When no fracture is visible but tenderness is present, there may be a nondisplaced fracture, either through the growth plate or the bone. Frequently these fractures can be seen 10–14 days later if new radiographs are obtained. This occurs because the first stage in fracture healing involves resorption of the bone along the fracture site, thus making it more visible. The best practice is to place a short-arm cast or splint over the wrist, or a long-arm cast or splint for more proximal injuries, and to obtain new radiographs and examine the patient out of immobilization after 10–14 days.

5. **What is a physeal (or epiphyseal) fracture?**

   Physeal fractures occur through the physis or growth plate in children. The distal radius is the most common area in which these happen in the forearm.

6. **What is a buckle or torus fracture?**

   Buckle or torus fractures occur particularly around the wrist in children. These represent fractures in which the bone is soft and compresses or buckles in the metaphysis, especially in the distal radius.

7. **What is a greenstick fracture?**

   Greenstick fractures occur in the diaphysis or midshaft area of the radius and ulna and represent an incomplete fracture.

8. **What is plastic deformation?**

   Plastic deformation occurs when the bone in the midshaft area bends rather than breaks, resulting in a bone that has no obvious fracture but is bent out of alignment.

9. **Are wrist sprains common in children?**

   No, wrist sprains tend to be relatively less common than fractures. Tenderness around the wrist after trauma often represents a mild buckle or torus fracture, rather than a sprain.

10. **How should a fracture be described?**

    The fracture should be characterized by describing the location of the fracture and any classification of type (such as the Salter classification for physeal fractures), and then describing the direction of displacement of the distal fragment with respect to the proximal fragment. Further, angulation should be communicated by describing the direction of the apex of the fracture, with the amount of angulation in degrees. A typical distal radius physeal fracture would be described as a distal radius Salter II fracture with dorsal displacement and 30-degree apex volar angulation.

11. **In what radiographic views should the radius be aligned with the capitellum?**

    All views. If the proximal radius is not aligned with the capitellum in any view, then it is most likely dislocated.

12. **What should be suspected if an isolated ulnar shaft fracture is seen on radiographs of a child's forearm?**

    Whenever a fracture of the ulna occurs without a fracture of the radius, Monteggia's fracture-dislocation should be suspected.

13. **What is Monteggia's fracture?**

    Monteggia's fracture or Monteggia's fracture-dislocation involves a fracture of the ulna with an associated radial head dislocation (at the elbow).

14. **What carpal bone fracture can also occur in older children and adolescents?**

    Fractures of the scaphoid can occur and are concerning. They are often difficult to identify radiographically and heal slowly. Tenderness over the snuffbox area of the wrist is indicative of a scaphoid fracture.

15. **What radiographs should be obtained for you to look for evidence of a scaphoid fracture?**

    The usual anteroposterior (or posteroanterior) and lateral views of the wrist should be obtained, along with a scaphoid or ulnar deviation posteroanterior view of the wrist. This view will profile the scaphoid and make it easier to identify fractures.

16. **What should be done if there is snuffbox tenderness but no evidence radiographically of a scaphoid fracture?**

    A thumb spica cast should be placed, incorporating the thumb distal to the interphalangeal joint and extending up to the elbow.

17. **What fractures require reduction?**

    Fractures require reduction if the displaced position of the fracture will not remodel into anatomic position, allowing normal forearm motion given the location of the fracture, the amount of displacement and angulation, and the age of the child.

18. **What motion associated with the forearm is most likely to be lost if good alignment of the radius and ulna is not present after fracture healing and remodeling?**
Pronation and supination is most sensitive to forearm malalignment, including angulation and malrotation.

19. **What is remodeling?**
Remodeling is the progressive, spontaneous realignment of fractured bones during the healing process (Fig. 32-1).

20. **What factors are most important in predicting which fractures will remodel the most?**
Fractures in younger patients and more-distal fractures tend to remodel more. Fractures will remodel more in the plane of motion of the adjacent joint.

21. **What is bayonet apposition?**
Bayonet apposition occurs when the two bones are aligned side by side.

22. **For what age does it become necessary to reduce bayonet apposition and to achieve a more anatomic end-to-end apposition?**
At approximately age 10 there is insufficient remodeling capacity in the radius and ulna to remodel bayonet apposition into acceptable alignment, leaving children with unacceptable motion. Prior to age 10, fractures left in bayonet apposition but with good alignment will remodel, leaving the child with well-formed bones and good motion. Like most rules involving children's age, this is a relative age that is influenced by growth potential and relative maturity.

23. **How should one go about reducing (or setting) a fracture?**
Reproducing the mechanism of injury should reduce the fracture. Typically, hyperextending the wrist, applying traction to bring the fracture out to length, and then pushing the distal fragment volarly as the wrist is flexed can reduce dorsally displaced fractures.

24. **What anesthesia is necessary when reducing a fracture?**
In the past, little or no anesthesia or analgesia was used. Reduction is much easier and more comfortable for the child if conscious sedation (using intravenous [IV] medications) or nitrous oxide and a hematoma block is utilized.

25. **Should a long-arm or a short-arm cast or splint be placed?**
Buckle and nondisplaced fractures of the wrist can be immobilized in a short-arm cast or splint (extending from the metacarpal heads to just below the elbow). The cast should always extend above the middle of the forearm in order to adequately immobilize the wrist. Fractures that require reduction and fractures of the mid to proximal forearm have traditionally been immobilized in long-arm casts. Most recently, however, two papers have indicated that distal-third fractures can be safely immobilized in short casts.

26. **Should the forearm be placed in pronation, in a neutral position, or in supination in the cast or splint?**
The forearm position is a matter of great debate. Advocates for placing the forearm in pronation, neutral position, and supination for various fractures can be found. Most often, we have placed the forearm in a position of neutral rotation and checked the reduction using a portable fluoroscanner prior to cast application. If the position is unstable or unacceptable, the reduction can be evaluated in supination and pronation. The position in which the fracture is best reduced is selected for the position in the cast.

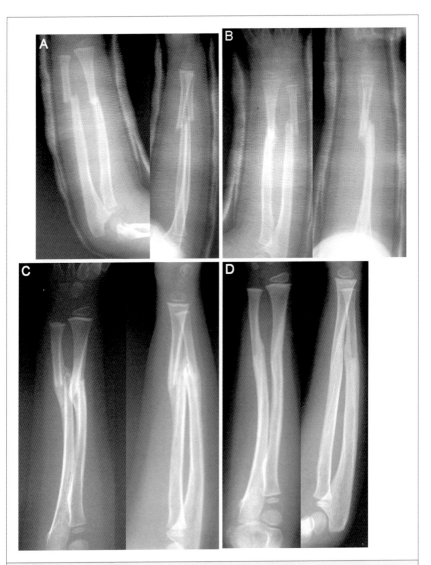

Figure 32-1. *A,* Anteroposterior and lateral radiographs of a 5-year-old child after reduction of a midshaft radius and ulna fracture, showing bayonet apposition of both the radius and the ulna. *B,* Anteroposterior and lateral radiographs of the same patient in the cast 2 weeks after the fracture. The bones still have bayonet apposition. *C,* Anteroposterior and lateral radiographs of the same patient at the time of cast removal 6 weeks after the fracture, with abundant bone healing. *D,* Anteroposterior and lateral radiographs of the same patient 6 months after the fracture, showing remodeling and restitution of normal bone alignment. The patient had normal motion at this time.

27. **Should a cast or a splint be used to immobilize the wrist or forearm fracture?**
    A splint is always the safest option, allowing swelling of the forearm without being restrictive. A cast is usually better at controlling the fracture position after reduction. A good compromise is to place a cast and then to bivalve the cast, splitting the cast volarly and dorsally with a cast saw down to the cast padding after it has hardened. This provides good control of the fracture, with some ability to accommodate swelling. Whenever a cast or a splint is placed, instructions should be given to the family to keep the forearm elevated above the level of the heart (the forearm in a sling is below the level of the heart) for 2–4 days after the fracture. The family should also be instructed to return for pain not controlled easily with oral analgesics. If increased pain does occur, the cast or splint should be released circumferentially, and if the pain is not relieved, the presence of a compartment syndrome should be considered.

28. **How often should you obtain radiographs?**
    For fractures that are nondisplaced, radiographs should be obtained at the time of cast removal, or earlier if pain increases, indicating that the fragments may have shifted. For displaced fractures, radiographs should be obtained after a reduction to assess alignment, again in 1–2 weeks to assess alignment, and, in older patients with more unstable fractures, at 3 weeks after reduction. Most fractures should have radiographs at the time of cast removal. Displaced fractures should have a final radiograph 4–6 weeks after cast removal. Physeal fractures should be followed with radiographs every 3–6 months until evidence of normal continued growth or evidence of a growth arrest is identified.

29. **How long does it take for a child's wrist or forearm fracture to heal?**
    Healing time depends on the age of the child, the location and type of the fracture, and what one means when one says "healing." The time necessary for the cast to remain on varies from 3 weeks for very young children and for children under the age of 12 with metaphyseal buckle fractures to 8–10 weeks for adolescents with midshaft forearm fractures. Usually, children aged 4–12 years require 4–6 weeks of casting to heal metaphyseal and physeal fractures and 6–8 weeks of casting to heal midshaft fractures.

KEY POINTS: WRIST AND FOREARM FRACTURES

1. If a child is suspected of having a wrist or forearm fracture, a careful physical examination should be performed and radiographs that include the area of tenderness should be obtained.

2. If a fracture is identified, images of the entire forearm, including the elbow in both anteroposterior and lateral images, should be obtained to ensure that another fracture or dislocation is not present.

3. A cast or splint should be applied out so that swelling is not restricted, which would produce a compartment syndrome.

30. **What should be done after cast removal for a child's wrist or forearm fracture?**
    Most children with distal or midshaft fractures benefit from wearing a removable Velcro wrist splint for 4–6 weeks after cast removal. The splint can be removed while the child is sleeping and during quiet activities, and it can be worn during more vigorous activities, allowing the child to regain motion and yet have protection for the fracture during healing.

31. **Is physical therapy necessary for children to regain motion lost during healing in a cast after a fracture?**

    Physical therapy is rarely needed for children after wrist and forearm fractures. Most children regain motion while working into normal activities of daily living. Physical therapy is occasionally indicated after fractures with severe soft tissue injuries or if motion is not well on its way to becoming normal 1–2 months after cast removal.

32. **When should pins or other internal fixation be used to treat a wrist or forearm fracture?**

    Pins or other internal fixation should be used when a cast is inadequate to maintain the fracture with adequate alignment until healing occurs.

33. **Should a cast always be tried before proceeding with internal fixation of a fracture?**

    Casting alone cannot reliably stabilize some fractures. Adolescents over the age of 12 years with completely displaced midshaft radius and ulna fractures nearly universally require internal fixation to obtain good results. Similarly, fractures that require an open reduction to obtain adequate alignment should almost always be stabilized with some sort of internal fixation.

34. **What type of internal fixation can be used in wrist and forearm fractures?**

    Wrist and forearm fractures can be stabilized by a wide variety of devices. Most often for fractures in the physis or metaphysis, Kirschner wires can be used, often placed percutaneously, to pin the fracture in place. Plates can be used for the occasional older patients with unstable metaphyseal fractures or for patients with displaced midshaft fractures. Titanium elastic nails have gained popularity lately for treating midshaft fractures. These nails can be placed into the ulna through the proximal ulnar metaphysis or olecranon and into the radius through the distal radial metaphysis.

35. **Can the bones refracture after healing?**

    Yes. In fractures of the diaphysis, the refracture rate is 5–7%, and refracture can occur up to 1 year after the original injury. These fractures most often, but not always, occur through the site of the original fracture. Fractured metaphyses and physes rarely refracture. To avoid refracture, a child should be restricted from contact sports after cast removal for at least as long as the child was casted.

BIBLIOGRAPHY

1. Bohm ER, Bubbar V, Hing KY, Dzus A: Above and below-the-elbow plaster casts for distal forearm fractures in children. A randomized controlled trial. J Bone Joint Surg 88A:1–8, 2006.

2. Luhman SJ, Gordon JE, Schoenecker PL: Intramedullary fixation of unstable both-bone forearm fractures in children. J Pediatr Orthop 18:451–456, 1998.

3. Zionts LE, Zalavras CG, Gerhardt MB: Closed treatment of displaced diaphyseal both-bone forearm fractures in older children and adolescents. J Pediatr Orthop 25:507–512, 2005.

CHAPTER 33

PEDIATRIC HAND INJURIES

Donald S. Bae, MD, and Peter M. Waters, MD

1. **How common are pediatric hand fractures?**

   The most commonly fractured bones in children and adolescents are the phalanges of the fingers, representing approximately 30–40% of all skeletal injuries in skeletally immature patients. Approximately 15–30% of these involve the physes.

   Overall, there is a bimodal distribution of hand injuries with respect to age. Infants and toddlers typically sustain fingertip or distal phalangeal injuries, or both, usually from crushing mechanisms. Older children and adolescents are also susceptible to hand fractures, particularly during sports participation.

2. **Do all pediatric hand fractures heal and remodel with nonoperative treatment?**

   The vast majority of pediatric hand fractures may be treated nonoperatively. However, there are some characteristic pediatric hand injuries that require surgical care (e.g., Seymour's fractures, phalangeal neck fractures, and intra-articular injuries). Early identification and prompt treatment is imperative for full functional return. Risk factors for poor outcomes include a failure to obtain adequate anteroposterior and lateral radiographs, a failure to obtain postreduction radiographs following treatment of displaced fractures, and false assumptions on the remodeling potential. In general, skeletal injuries in young children that are located close to the physis, with deformity in the plane of adjacent joint motion, have the greatest remodeling potential.

3. **What is a Seymour's fracture?**

   A Seymour's fracture is an open physeal fracture of the distal phalanx (Fig. 33-1). Typically seen in infants and toddlers after crushing injuries to the fingertip, these fractures are associated with a nail bed laceration. Often, the germinal or sterile matrix will be incarcerated within the fracture site. Closed reduction may be blocked by interposition of the nail fold in the fracture

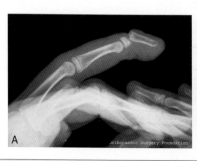 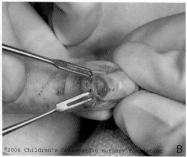

Figure 33-1. *A,* Lateral radiograph of a Seymour's fracture. *B,* Intraoperative photo of a Seymour's fracture. The nail plate has been removed, revealing a nailbed laceration and an open physeal fracture of the distal phalanx.

site, deep to the nail plate. Functional outcomes are poor in unrecognized or inappropriately treated cases. The nail plate must be removed to identify the open fracture, nail bed laceration, and germinal or sterile matrix displacement. Prompt irrigation and debridement of the open fracture, followed by nail-bed repair and fracture stabilization with appropriate splinting or internal fixation with longitudinal Kirschner (K) wires, is recommended.

4. **How are phalangeal neck fractures treated?**
    Phalangeal neck fractures are characteristic injuries of childhood. Typically, these injuries occur when the digit is crushed in a closing door or a swing. The distal fragment is often rotated and displaced as the patient attempts to withdraw the hand. The middle phalanx is more commonly affected than the proximal phalanx, and the border digits are most frequently involved. As the phalangeal condyles are incompletely ossified in the younger patient, these injuries often present with innocuous-appearing radiographs, depicting only a small fleck or cap of avulsed bone. Displaced injuries have little remodeling potential, are prone to nonunion, and are at high risk for secondary displacement following closed reduction alone. For this reason, acute displaced phalangeal neck fractures should be treated with closed reduction and percutaneous pin fixation (Fig. 33-2). In chronic cases, dorsal malunion and bony formation within the subcondylar fossa will result in a loss of flexion (Fig. 33-3). These patients may require subcondylar fossa reconstruction or corrective osteotomy to regain interphalangeal flexion.

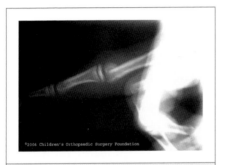

Figure 33-2. Lateral radiograph depicting a displaced phalangeal neck fracture.

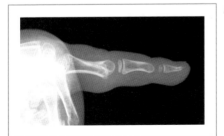

Figure 33-3. Lateral radiograph of a phalangeal neck fracture malunion with obliteration of the subcondylar fossa.

5. **What is an extra-octave fracture?**

   An *extra-octave fracture* refers to a displaced physeal fracture of the small finger phalanx with apex radial angulation (Fig. 33-4). This results in malrotation and ulnar deviation of the small finger. As with other displaced physeal fractures of the phalanges with malrotation or angulation of greater than 10 degrees, treatment consists of closed reduction and immobilization.

6. **What is the pediatric equivalent of the adult gamekeeper's thumb?**

   Salter-Harris III fractures of the base of the thumb's proximal phalanx are the pediatric equivalent of the adult gamekeeper's injury. In these cases, the ulnar collateral ligament of the metacarpophalangeal joint remains attached to its insertion at the ulnar base of the proximal phalanx. Given that this represents a displaced intra-articular fracture with joint instability, open reduction and internal fixation are recommended.

7. **How can one assess for a flexor tendon laceration in a young or uncooperative child?**

   In the very young or uncooperative child, a number of physical examination maneuvers may aid in assessing for a possible flexor tendon injury. These include the following:

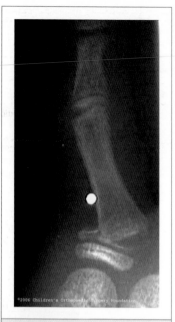

Figure 33-4. A displaced physeal fracture of the small finger's proximal phalanx, the so-called *extra-octave fracture*.

   - Gently palpate or compress the digital flexor muscles in the forearm, looking for the presence or absence of passive finger flexion.
   - Carefully observe the digital cascade in the resting position. In cases of flexor tendon laceration, the affected digit will assume a position of increased extension (Fig. 33-5).
   - Observe passive digital flexion with passive wrist extension—the so-called tenodesis effect. Flexor tendon injuries will result in persistent digital extension with passive wrist extension.

8. **How can one assess for a digital nerve laceration in a pediatric patient?**

   In patients older than 5 years, sensibility may typically be assessed by testing for light touch or two-point discrimination, similar to adults. Younger patients, however, will not be able to perform two-point discriminatory testing. A warm-water-immersion test may be performed in these cases (Fig. 33-6). Following prolonged immersion in warm water, normally innervated skin will wrinkle; absence of wrinkling connotes nerve injury.

9. **What is the most appropriate postoperative program for a young child following flexor tendon repair?**

   Although early controlled motion exercises have been advocated following flexor tendon repairs in adults, cast immobilization for 4 weeks postoperatively results in equal or superior results in children under the age of 16 years.

KEY POINTS: PEDIATRIC HAND INJURIES

1. The principle of tenodesis is helpful in assessing for possible flexor tendon injury or digital malrotation in the young or uncooperative child.

2. Flexor tendon repairs in children are best treated postoperatively with cast immobilization.

3. Risk factors for a poor outcome of pediatric hand fractures include inadequate radiographs, a failure to obtain postreduction radiographs, and false assumptions on the remodeling potential.

4. In general, replantation should be considered in digital amputations in children.

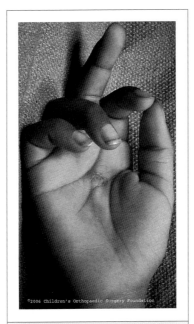

Figure 33-5. Flexor tendon laceration of the long finger, which assumes an extended position due to loss of the tenodesis effect.

10. **What are the indications for digital replantation in pediatric patients?**
In general, any digital amputation in a child is considered an indication for replantation. Factors favoring digital survival following replantation include the following:
- Sharp amputations
- Body weight greater than 11 kg
- Repair of more than one vein
- Bone shortening
- Rigid internal fixation
- Prompt reperfusion after arterial repair

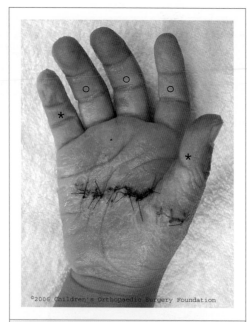

©2006 Children's Orthopaedic Surgery Foundation

Figure 33-6. Warm water immersion test performed in a young child with lacerations of the common digital nerves to the index, long, and ring fingers. Note the lack of skin wrinkling in the index, long, and ring fingers *(circles)* compared to the normal wrinkling of the small finger and thumb *(asterisks)*.

BIBLIOGRAPHY

1. Al-Qattan MM: Extra-articular transverse fractures of the base of the distal phalanx (Seymour's fracture) in children and adults. J Hand Surg 26B:201–206, 2001.

2. Baker GL, Kleinert JM: Digit replantation in infants and young children: Determinants of survival. Plast Reconstr Surg 94:139–145, 1994.

3. Fischer MD, McElfresh EC: Physeal and periphyseal injuries of the hand: Patterns of injury and results of treatment. Hand Clin 10:287–301, 1994.

4. Hastings H, Simmons BP: Hand fractures in children: A statistical analysis. Clin Orthop 188:120–130, 1984.

5. O'Connell SJ, Moore MM, Strickland JW, et al: Results of zone I and zone II flexor tendon repairs in children. J Hand Surg 19A:48–52, 1994.

6. Peterson HA, Madhok MS, Benson JT, et al: Physeal fractures: Part I. Epidemiology in Olmsted County, Minnesota, 1979–1988. J Pediatr Orthop 14:423–430, 1994.

7. Simmons BP, Peters TT: Subcondylar fossa reconstruction for malunion of fractures of the proximal phalanx in children. J Hand Surg 12A:1079–1082, 1997.

V. SPORTS-RELATED INJURIES

YOUTH SPORTS AND RELATED INJURIES

Kevin Shea, MD, and Kurt Nilsson, MD

CHAPTER 34

1. **What portion of youth sports injuries occurs in organized sports?**
   Approximately one-third. The remainder occurs during physical education classes and nonorganized sports.

2. **In the United States, what sports produce the highest rates of injuries?**
   When injury data are adjusted for the number of participant hours, the trend is for American football to be the highest-risk sport, followed by basketball, gymnastics, soccer, and baseball. Approximately one third of these injuries occur in youths between the ages of 5 and 14 years, with two thirds occurring in those 15 years or older. American football produces the highest rate of injury, with varsity high school athletes having an injury rate between 20% and 40%; however, 75% of these injuries are minor, resulting in minimal loss of participation. Up to 10% can require hospitalization, and 2% need reconstructive procedures.

3. **In the United States, fatal injuries occur most often in which sport?**
   Baseball. Fatal injuries are usually related to bat or ball blows to the chest or head. Proper equipment, good supervision, and appropriate rules are important in reducing these injuries. Football has the highest rate of fatal injuries per player-hour.

4. **Should children avoid participation in certain sports?**
   The American Academy of Pediatrics (AAP) has recommended that children not be involved with boxing.

5. **What is the most common cause of sudden cardiac death in young athletes?**
   Hypertrophic cardiomyopathy (HCM). HCM is a genetically determined disorder leading to abnormal enlargement of the left ventricle, which, when under exercise stress, may cause relative cardiac ischemia or conduction anomalies, leading to cardiac arrhythmias and possibly death. Other potentially fatal disorders include anomalous coronary arteries, a ruptured aorta, and myocarditis. Any family history of sudden death or personal history of presyncope or syncope during exertion should prompt a medical evaluation for cardiac causes.

6. **In preparticipation screening evaluations, what component is the most sensitive for identifying individuals at significant risk for injury from sports participation?**
   The medical history is the most cost-effective component of the screening evaluation. Episodes of prior musculoskeletal injury, neurologic injury, and cardiopulmonary problems should be noted. Questions related to general health, immunizations, hospitalizations, and limitations of function are helpful as well. Specifically, athletes should be asked about their prior history of concussion, unconsciousness, paresthesias, heat-related illness, and previous musculoskeletal treatments or problems. Syncope is an important clue to undetected heart disease. Unfortunately, even with conscientious screening, identifying all individuals at high risk for sudden death (usually cardiac in origin) is not possible. Athletes and parents should always be informed that screening cannot ensure protection from and prevention of all injuries.

7. **What specific factors significantly increase the risk for heat illness during sports participation?**
   - Obesity
   - Recent viral illness (especially gastroenteritis)
   - History of previous heat illness
   - Prepubescence
   - Mental retardation
   - Lack of recent conditioning in the heat
   - Failure to replenish the previous day's water loss
   - Chronic illness such as cystic fibrosis and inflammatory bowel disease

8. **What situational factors place all participating youths at increased risk of heat illness?**
   - High heat
   - High humidity
   - Direct sunlight
   - No breeze
   - Dark or heavy clothing (e.g., football pads, helmets, and uniforms)
   - First practice of the season
   - Artificial turf
   - A long event
   - Multiple competitions in a day or on consecutive days
   - Recent fluid restrictions

9. **What guidelines can be used to reduce the incidence of heat illness?**
   - Athletes should be acclimatized prior to the start of a sports season.
   - Weather conditions should be evaluated for the combination of temperature, humidity, sunlight, and wind.
   - Rest breaks in the shade should be scheduled and followed.
   - Individuals at risk should be identified.
   - Chilled fluids should be readily available.
   - Periodic drinking breaks should be enforced.
   - Water restrictions should never be used as discipline.
   - Deliberate dehydration for weight loss must be discouraged.
   - Clothing should be lightweight and of light color.
   - Events should not be scheduled during peak hours of heat and sun.
   - Players, parents, and coaches all need to be educated about the potential risks of heat illness and how they are avoided.
   - Athletes at significant risk should have daily weights recorded to assure adequate rehydration after the previous day's practice.

10. **How much salt replacement is needed in fluids?**
    Sweat is hypotonic to body fluids, containing 40–80 mEq/L of sodium and less than 5 mEq/L of potassium. Initially, plain water adequately replaces these losses. Electrolyte solutions are needed only after 1–2 hours of continuous rigorous activity. Salt tablets and hypertonic solutions are dangerous because they can produce intracellular dehydration owing to their osmotic effect in the serum.

    Ideally, water should be cooled to stimulate thirst. Although sugar added to the solution may improve palatability, a high sugar concentration slows gastrointestinal motility and can cause bloated feelings and nausea.

11. **What is the difference between weight lifting and weight training?**
Weight training refers to the use of free weights or weight and resistance machines to enhance strength and endurance. Submaximal weights are lifted repeatedly until the muscles fatigue. The object is to enhance performance for other sporting activities. In weight lifting, the object is to perform a one-repetition maximal lift.

12. **Before puberty, can children gain strength from weight training?**
Prepubescent children can increase strength by 20–40% in a well-supervised program. Although these children lack the higher level of androgens that facilitates hypertrophy of muscles, strength gains do occur owing to a combination of enhanced recruitment of motor units, synchronization, and some degree of muscle hypertrophy.

13. **For children, does the risk of using weights outweigh any potential benefits?**
With proper instruction and supervision, weight-training programs can be relatively safe, even for children. A proper strength conditioning program should be a prerequisite for youths participating in contact sports. Strength, particularly of the cervical spine, can reduce the incidence of injuries. For a program to be safe, proper technique needs to be emphasized. The equipment must be in good repair. An attentive partner is important whenever free weights are used. Strengthening should be balanced with a consistent stretching program. Most authorities recommend avoiding maximal weight lifting in children.

14. **Should performance-enhancing substances be used in young athletes?**
The American Academy of Pediatrics strongly condemns the use of performance-enhancing substances and vigorously endorses efforts to eliminate their use among children and adolescents. There has been little, if any, research on the efficacy or safety of these substances in children.

15. **What are the two most common anatomic sites of injury for high school basketball players?**
Injuries of the ankle are by far the most common, followed by injuries of the knee. Up to 70% of all high school varsity basketball players will sustain an ankle sprain during their careers. Up to one third of these are recurrent. The occurrence rate of ankle sprains is similar in both boys and girls. Girls, however, are at an increased risk for knee injuries, particularly rupture of the anterior cruciate ligament (ACL).

KEY POINTS: YOUTH SPORTS AND RELATED INJURIES

1. When injury data are adjusted for the number of participant-hours, the trend is for American football to be the highest-risk sport, followed by basketball, gymnastics, soccer, and baseball.

2. Fatal injuries are most common in baseball. They are usually related to bat or ball blows to the chest or head. Football has the highest rate of fatal injuries per player-hour.

3. Hypertrophic cardiomyopathy is the most common cause of sudden cardiac death in young athletes.

4. The medical history is the most cost-effective component of the preparticipation screening evaluation.

5. The American Academy of Pediatrics strongly condemns the use of performance-enhancing substances and vigorously endorses efforts to eliminate their use among children and adolescents.

16. **Do high-top shoes prevent ankle sprains in basketball players?**

    Probably not. Most data suggest no statistical reduction in ankle injury rates with the use of high-top shoes. Taping and the use of lace-up braces do support the ankle and reduce injuries, compared with shoes alone.

17. **How effective are modern American football helmets in preventing cervical spine injury?**

    Helmets do not prevent cervical spine injury, and, to the extent that they encourage using the head to strike opponents (i.e., spearing), they increase the risk of neck injury and paralysis.

    Since their introduction, helmets (and face guards) have significantly reduced the incidence of closed head injuries and facial injuries. Quadriplegia is now more common than fatal head injuries. Among high school participants in American football, the rate of quadriplegia is approximately 0.7 per 100,000 players (compared with 2.7 per 100,000 players at the collegiate level).

18. **What is the most common scenario associated with catastrophic head or neck injury in American football players?**

    Defensive players sustain 70% or more of all catastrophic injuries, with 75% occurring while tackling. A direct axial load to the straight or flexed cervical spine (i.e., spearing) is the most common mechanism.

19. **What can be done to minimize the risk of these catastrophic injuries in American football?**

    In 1976, the National Collegiate Athletic Association (NCAA) and the National Federation of State High School Associations made rule changes to prohibit spearing (i.e., using the head as a battering ram) as the initial point of contact when blocking or tackling. This has greatly reduced the incidence of quadriplegia but has not eliminated it. Players must be repeatedly instructed about the dangers (and, therefore, the illegal nature) of spearing. Parents, coaches, and health professionals must be sure that proper techniques are being taught and used. Rules must be enforced. Helmets and pads should fit properly. A weight-training program to strengthen the neck muscles should be a requirement for all athletes involved in contact sports, particularly American football.

20. **What two sports have the highest rate of quadriceps contusion? What are its causes and complications?**

    Soccer and American football. This injury usually results from a direct blow to the anterior aspect of the thigh. Although pads have been developed for American football to try to prevent this injury, contact from an opponent's knee, shoulder pad, or helmet can occur on the margins of the pad and produce this injury. Untreated, this injury can easily be exacerbated with recurrent bleeding, leading to prolonged loss of time from sports. Occasionally, myositis ossificans can result as well. This injury should not be underestimated.

21. **How do hip pointers occur?**

    Commonly occurring in contact or collision sports such as American football and soccer, this injury results from a direct blow to the iliac crest apophysis. These heal with rest and time but are notoriously painful, debilitating in the short run, and slow to resolve (taking up to 8–10 weeks). American football waist pads are designed to reduce the occurrence of this injury but must be fitted properly.

22. **How do stingers and burners occur?**

    These terms refer to an injury of the brachial plexus that is typically transient. It usually results from a stretching mechanism, often occurring in American football from a direct blow that depresses the shoulder and simultaneously bends the neck in the opposite direction. The result is paresthesias and paralysis, which can take moments to weeks to resolve. Recurrent injury often results from a premature return to contact sports. This can lead to progressive fibrosis of the brachial plexus and occasionally results in persistent symptoms or permanent disability. Recurrent stingers or burners can be related to relative stenosis of the cervical canal, as measured by the Pavlov ratio. Unless this is accompanied by other changes in the radiographic appearance of the cervical spine, these individuals do not seem to be at significantly increased risk for development of subsequent cervical spinal cord injury.

23. **What are the most common causes of wrist pain in gymnasts?**
An overuse syndrome of the distal radial physis is a fairly common cause of gradual-onset wrist pain in a gymnast. The process is termed a physiolysis and appears to be analogous to a stress fracture involving the physeal (i.e., growth) plate. With rest, this usually resolves without complication; however, occasionally, premature closure of the distal radial physis can occur, with subsequent relative overgrowth of the ulna. This positive ulnar variance can result in excessive pressure on the lateral carpus and subsequent triangular fibrocartilage complex (TFCC) tears and ongoing wrist pain.

Other considerations include Kienböck's disease (i.e., osteonecrosis of the lunate), impingement of the dorsal interosseous nerve at the wrist, synovial or capsular impingement of the wrist joint, and tears or inflammation of the TFCC.

24. **What tests should be performed in the evaluation of a prepubescent female gymnast with an injury to the proximal hamstring area?**
Anteroposterior (AP) radiograph of the pelvis. Although the mechanism described is consistent with the common hamstring strain, most of these injuries occur at the musculotendinous junction and are usually at the mid-portion of the distal thigh. In the skeletally immature gymnast, proximal injuries are often due to ischial avulsion fractures, resulting from a pike position stretch. After appropriate history and physical examination, a single AP pelvic radiograph will most often demonstrate widening irregularity and, occasionally, displacement of the affected apophysis. Typically, the other ischium provides a normal study for comparison.

25. **What should be considered in the differential diagnosis of low back pain in a gymnast?**
One of the most common problems is spondylolysis, which is most likely induced by recurrent hypertension stresses, which are very common to many gymnastic positions and stunts. Although typically associated with very minimal grades of slippage, a substantial amount of spondylolisthesis can result. Initially, a lower back with spondylolysis may be radiographically normal, and the condition may be detectable only by bone scan (i.e., single photon emission computed tomography [SPECT] imaging) or a computed tomography (CT) scan.

Many times, the cause of back pain in gymnasts cannot be specifically identified. Impingement of the posterior elements and the facets is often suspected. Disk injury or herniation should be considered. Significant trauma, fracture, and displacement of the ring apophysis can occur as well.

Night pain and subtle neurologic findings should suggest the possibility of a more serious source of the back pain, such as a tumor, an infection, a tethered cord, an intradural lipoma, or another spinal anomaly. Occasionally, osteoid osteoma occurs in the lumbar spine of youths. Injury and apophysitis of the spinous process apophyses also occur.

26. **What are the most common injuries in the immature skeleton in young runners?**
Most young runners participate, at least initially, with relatively few injuries. With time, they can develop overuse syndromes similar to their adult counterparts. Apophyseal problems such as Sever's disease (i.e., calcaneal apophysitis), Osgood-Schlatter disease, and avulsion fractures of the apophyses about the hip and pelvis are common in young runners. Stress fractures of the metatarsals, the tibia, the fibula, and the femoral neck can occur as well.

27. **What is the most common source of injuries in young runners?**
    As with adults, training errors are by far the most common cause of injury. A sudden increase in training distance and intensity is the most common error. Excessive mileage, a lack of rest, running on hard surfaces, inadequate shoe wear, and lack of a concurrent stretching program are other common mistakes.

28. **What is fair-play youth hockey scoring?**
    Fair-play scoring is an innovative strategy used to score youth hockey games and tournaments in which teams are rewarded for fewer penalties and are punished for larger numbers of penalties. Fair-play scoring has been shown to significantly decrease the number of injuries sustained in youth ice hockey leagues compared to when the scoring system was suspended.

29. **What is the age of onset of ACL tears for young soccer players?**
    A recent study demonstrated that young soccer athletes begin to sustain ACL injury at about 12 years of age. Females sustain more ACL tears at a younger age than males, and the incidence of ACL tears in females is also higher in young age groups.

30. **What is the female athlete triad?**
    The female athlete triad refers to disordered eating, amenorrhea, and osteoporosis in female athletes. The exact incidence is unknown and varies according to sport participation. Those sports that emphasize leanness, such as distance running and gymnastics, seem to be at the highest risk. Disordered eating, including anorexia nervosa and bulimia, lead to a caloric deficit that may impair normal luteinizing hormone (LH) pulsatility, thereby leading to disordered menses, decreased estrogen release, and osteoporosis. Identification of disordered eating by friends, family, athletic trainers, coaches, and team physicians is essential for preventing long-term complications of decreased bone mineral density.

31. **Why do female athletes, both pediatric and adolescent, and adults have a higher incidence of knee injury with sports that involve planting a directional change activity?**
    Numerous factors have been proposed to explain this phenomenon. The factors include the narrow intercondylar notch width, hormonal effects on soft tissues, overall joint laxity, relative weakness of the muscles of the lower extremity, and differences in landing mechanics. Ongoing research is focusing on all of these factors, although, at this time, none of the factors has been demonstrated to be the single most important cause of knee injury in female athletes.

32. **Can children with a solitary kidney participate in sports?**
    The absence of a kidney does not preclude participation in sports. The athlete may need individual assessment for contact, collision, and limited-contact sports. Special protective padding may be required.

33. **Which skin disorders would prevent an athlete from participating in sports?**
    Boils, herpes simplex, impetigo, scabies, and molluscum contagiosum are contagious conditions. While the patient is contagious, participation in gymnastics with mats, martial arts, wrestling, or other collision, contact, or limited-contact sports should not be allowed.

34. **Can one-eyed athletes participate in sports?**
    The AAP recommends that all youths involved in organized sports be encouraged to wear appropriate eye protection. All functionally one-eyed athletes should wear appropriate eye protection for all sports. Functionally one-eyed athletes and those who have had an eye injury or surgery must not participate in boxing or full-contact martial arts.

BIBLIOGRAPHY

1. American Academy of Pediatrics: Medical conditions affecting sports participation. Pediatrics 107:1205–1209, 2001.
2. Busch M: Sports medicine. In Morrissy RT (ed): Lovell and Winter's Pediatric Orthopaedics, 5th ed. Philadelphia, Lippincott Williams & Wilkins, 2001, p 1273.
3. Caine D, Roy S, Singer K, Broekhoff J: Stress changes of the distal radial growth plate. Am J Sports Med 20:290–298, 1992.
4. Cantu R, Mueller FO: Catastrophic football injuries: 1977–1998. Neurosurgery 47:673–677, 2000.
5. Committee on Sports Medicine and Fitness: Protective eyewear for young athletes. Pediatrics 113:619–622, 2004.
6. Gomez J, for the American Academy of Pediatrics Committee on Sports Medicine and Fitness: Use of performance-enhancing substances. Pediatrics 115:1103–1106, 2005.
7. Lysholm J, Wiklander J: Injuries in runners. Am J Sports Med 15:168–171, 1987.
8. Maffulli N: Intensive training in young athletes. The orthopaedic surgeon's viewpoint. Sports Med 9:229–243, 1990.
9. Maron BJ: Sudden death in young athletes. N Engl J Med 349:1064–1075, 2003.
10. Patel DR, Pratt HD, Greydanus DE: Pediatric neurodevelopment and sports participation. When are children ready to play sports? Pediatr Clin North Am 49:505–531, v–vi, 2002.
11. Purvis J, Burke R: Recreational injuries in children: Incidence and prevention. J Am Acad Orthop Surg 9:365–374, 2001.
12. Roberts WO, Brust JD, Leonard B, Hebert BJ: Fair-play rules and injury reduction in ice hockey. Arch Pediatr Adolesc Med 150:140–145, 1996.
13. Sallis RE, Jones K, Sunshine S, et al: Comparing sports injuries in men and women. Int J Sports Med 22:420–423, 2001.
14. Shea KG, Pfeiffer RP, Wang J, Curtin ML: ACL injury in pediatric and adolescent soccer players: An analysis of insurance data. J Pediatr Orthop 24:623–628, 2004.
15. Smith NJ, et al: The prevention of heat disorders in sports. Am J Dis Child 138:786–790, 1984.
16. Torg JS, Guille JT, Jaffe S: Injuries to the cervical spine in American football players. J Bone Joint Surg Am 84:112–122, 2002.
17. Yeager KK, Agostini R, Nattiv A, Drinkwater B: The female athlete triad: Disordered eating, amenorrhea, osteoporosis. Med Sci Sports Exerc 25:775–777, 1993.
18. Zillmer D, Powell J, Albright J: Gender-specific injury patterns in high school varsity basketball. J Womens Health 1:69, 1992.

CHAPTER 35

STRESS FRACTURES

Jeffrey S. Shilt, MD, and Neil E. Green, MD

1. Name the two types of stress fractures.
Two subtypes are generally recognized:
- **Fatigue fractures:** These occur in normal bones that are injured through continual excessive loads in otherwise healthy, active patients.
- **Insufficiency fractures:** These occur as a result of more-normal loads on weak bones in patients with underlying chronic disorders.

2. What are the two sites of stress fractures?
The **compression** side of a bone is the most common site. Stress fractures here are the result of axial loading of an extremity. For example, a stress fracture of a metatarsal is the result of increased axial bone stress. Stress fracture of the posterior medial cortex of the proximal tibia is also the result of increased axial stress.

The second site of stress fracture is on the **tension** side of a bone. This is the result of a combination of bending forces and muscle forces acting to increase the bending of a bone. As mentioned, if the tibia has an increase in its anterior bow, excessive stress will result in a stress fracture of the anterior cortex of the tibia (i.e., the tension side of the bone).

3. Do stress fractures occur in the upper extremity?
Although lower-extremity stress fractures occur much more frequently than stress fractures in the axial skeleton and the upper extremity, certain individuals who participate in activities that induce higher biomechanical loads in the upper extremity and axial skeleton will present with a predilection for stress lesions in these areas.

4. What type of stress fractures occur in the femoral neck? What is their management?
Although less common than stress fractures in the lower leg and foot, stress fractures do occur in the neck of the femur in children. If the fracture is not adequately treated, a complete fracture with displacement may occur, which places at risk the blood supply of the femoral head.

The compression-side stress fracture usually heals with reduction of the stress (i.e., crutch ambulation with a lack of weight-bearing on the injured extremity). On the other hand, a stress fracture that occurs on the tension side of the femoral neck heals with more difficulty, and it may not heal with simple crutch ambulation. These types are the most likely to result in a complete fracture. Therefore, if this fracture does not heal with conservative measures, internal fixation with screws in the femoral neck may be required.

5. Which type of femoral neck fracture—compression or tension—is more common in individuals with an open femoral capital physis?
Although both tensile and compression fractures occur in adults, all cases in skeletally immature patients reported in the literature occurred on the compression side.

6. What is the implication of having a compression-type femoral neck fracture?
In distinction from those occurring on the tensile surface, compression-type fractures can likely be treated nonoperatively.

7. **What is the triggering event that disrupts normal bone remodeling and results in stress fractures?**

Stress fractures are classically depicted as high-activity-volume injuries, but the rate of the increase in exercise volume is more likely the etiology of these injuries.

8. **What location can be a cause of low back pain (LBP) or buttock pain as a result of a stress fracture?**

The differential diagnosis of persistent LBP or buttock pain with activity relieved by rest should include a sacral stress fracture.

9. **What volume of training is considered the breakpoint for moderate or vigorous training?**

More than 16 hours per week.

10. **What duration of symptoms requires a more extensive work-up than just activity reduction?**

Persistent pain for >3 weeks is correlated with a worse prognosis in these patients with stress fractures, despite activity reduction.

11. **What is the female athlete triad?**

Disordered eating, amenorrhea, and osteoporosis.

12. **Which female athletes are at greatest risk for the female athlete triad?**

Athletes most at risk are figure skaters, gymnasts, dancers, and long-distance runners. These activities stress physical appearance in competition, and a low body-mass index is the norm.

13. **What are the cause and natural history of stress fractures?**

Stress fractures are the result of repetitive stress to bones that do not have the ability to recover. Repetitive activities produce nonpainful microfractures of bone trabeculae. If the trauma is minimal or if the child rests between episodes of trauma, the microfractures will heal. On the other hand, if the child continues with the offending activity, such as running and playing, the microfractures will increase to the point that pain will occur with activity. This is the first symptom of a stress fracture in most patients, although some young children may limp without complaining of pain. If the child heeds the pain and reduces the stress at this point, the fracture should heal without other treatment. If the child continues with the activity, the stress fracture will become more evident, clinically and radiographically.

14. **What are the symptoms of a stress fracture?**

Children with a stress fracture will complain of pain with activity but will not have pain when they are sedentary. Young children may not complain of pain, but their parents will notice that they limp during activity. Because children will usually continue to be active in spite of pain, the child's limp will worsen with increasing activity. Older children will be able to pinpoint the site of the pain; however, young children will usually not be able to tell their parents or the physician where they hurt.

15. **How does one make the diagnosis of a stress fracture?**

In children whose symptoms suggest a stress fracture, the clinical examination will reveal point tenderness of the bone at the point of the stress fracture. Adults or teenagers with stress fractures may present for diagnosis and treatment before the radiographs are abnormal because radiographic changes frequently lag behind clinical symptoms by weeks. In individuals with symptoms of a stress fracture with normal radiographs, a bone scan may be helpful. Since young children complain about pain less frequently than the older individual, however, radiographic changes are usually present by the time they present for diagnosis and treatment.

16. **What are the radiographic findings with a stress fracture?**
   Stress fractures of long bones are usually cortical. There will be periosteal reactive bone proximal and distal to the lesion. The cortex of the bone is thickened as a result of the increased bone density, resulting from the healing of the fracture. If the fracture persists, the fracture line may become evident, beginning at the cortex and progressing centrally. The longer the patient is symptomatic, the more evident the fracture becomes.

17. **What is the differential diagnosis of a stress fracture?**
   The most common lesion that one may mistake for a stress fracture is an osteoid osteoma. The pain of an osteoid osteoma usually does not increase with activity, however. It will cause pain at both times of activity and of inactivity, especially at night. Both lesions will produce periosteal reactive bone and cortical thickening. The nidus of the osteoid osteoma can usually be identified on a computed tomography (CT) scan if the differential diagnosis is difficult. In addition, osteoid osteoma will produce a more intense and widespread reaction on a bone scan, as opposed to the more localized reaction seen with a stress fracture.

   A malignancy such as Ewing's sarcoma can be differentiated by its more widespread periosteal reaction and bone destruction, as well as soft tissue mass. Occasionally, an area of subacute or chronic bone infection may simulate a stress fracture.

18. **Do stress fractures occur only in high-performance athletes?**
   Stress fractures can and do occur in anyone. Children in particular are very prone to the development of stress fractures because of their high energy levels and the relative lower density of their bones. Most children with a stress fracture seen in an orthopaedic practice will be those who are very involved in play or in many sports and activities. Even relatively sedentary children may develop a stress fracture so long as the involved level of activity produces stress greater than the bone's ability to resist it.

19. **Are some people more prone to the development of a stress fracture than others?**
   Since stress fractures are the result of excessive stress, if one has an abnormally angulated bone or portion of an extremity, increased stress will be delivered to a bone, increasing the chance of development of a stress fracture. For example, a child with a varus deformity of the hindfoot will place more stress than normal on the base of the fifth metatarsal, which may result in the development of a stress fracture of the proximal diaphysis of the fifth metatarsal (i.e., a Jones fracture). Another example is a stress fracture of the anterior cortex of the middle third of the tibia, which is the result of an anterior bow of the tibia. This anterior bow increases the tension stress on the tibia, which may result in a stress fracture.

   Stress fractures can also be seen in children who have been immobilized. For example, the child who has sustained a traumatic fracture of the lower extremity requiring immobilization will develop osteopenia in the entire immobilized extremity. If the child returns to any activity too vigorously and too soon, he or she is prone to developing a stress fracture. Simple walking may even be sufficient to produce a stress fracture of a metatarsal.

20. **What are the most common locations of stress fractures in children?**
   Stress fractures occur most commonly in the bones of the lower leg and foot. Their most common location is in the posterior medial aspect of the proximal tibia (Fig. 35-1). One will see increased bone density with some evidence of periosteal healing. The child will have point tenderness over the stress fracture in the tibia.

   The medial aspect of the distal tibia is another common location of a stress fracture, as is the distal third of the fibula and the calcaneus. The calcaneal stress fracture is frequently not seen on the initial radiograph, but if the diagnosis is made on a clinical basis and the foot is immobilized, the stress fracture will be seen after the cast is removed. Metatarsal stress fractures are also frequently seen in children, not only in those children involved in sports, but also in children who have been immobilized.

21. **What is the treatment of a stress fracture?**

The stress fracture is treated by elimination of the offending activity. In the high-performance athlete, one may simply eliminate the activity that is the cause, such as running. In children, however, elimination of the stress is important, but immobilization of the extremity is equally important. Young children whose stress fractures are the result of normal activities must be immobilized to rest the bone adequately and to allow healing of the stress fracture. Immobilization is continued for 4–6 weeks or until there is no tenderness of the bone and radiographs show periosteal healing. The child is then allowed to walk, but with activity modification.

In the adolescent or teen who is able to comply with a more complicated regimen, one may use immobilization for a shorter period of time or may simply reduce stress with crutch ambulation. Conditioning may be maintained by changing activities—for example, by swimming or bike riding instead of running.

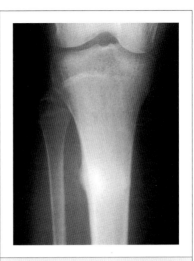

Figure 35-1. Anteroposterior radiograph of the tibia of an 11-year-old girl who had pain in her leg with activity. She played basketball during the winter and softball in the spring. The radiograph demonstrates an area of increased bone density on the anteromedial aspect of the proximal tibia. The periosteum is thickened, and there is also endosteal callus (the transverse line of internal callus). Simple reduction of her activity level allowed the fracture to heal completely.

KEY POINTS: STRESS FRACTURES

1. The incidence of stress fractures in children is on the rise as the participation in sporting activities is increasing.

2. Stress fractures must be differentiated from malignant tumors, osteoid osteoma, and osteomyelitis.

3. Magnetic resonance imaging (MRI) is the most sensitive radiographic tool for diagnosis.

4. The proximal tibia is the most common location for pediatric stress fractures.

5. The mainstay of treatment for most stress fractures involves a modification or elimination of precipitating activity.

6. Tension-type femoral neck and medial malleolus fractures are stress fractures that often require surgical treatment.

22. **Do stress fractures occur in the spine? What are some causes?**

Spondylolysis, or fracture of the pars interarticularis, is in most cases a stress fracture. The pars is part of the posterior elements of the vertebrae. Stress may be concentrated in the pars interarticularis, resulting in a stress fracture. It has been shown that certain activities will increase the risk of developing spondylolysis. Axial loading of the extended spine with the lumbar spine in lordosis increases the stress on the pars interarticularis of the lower two lumbar vertebrae, especially L5. Gymnasts are especially prone to the development of spondylolysis because they axially load their spines in extension. (Picture the gymnast's landing posture at the ending of her routine.) Interior football linemen are also uniquely susceptible to a stress fracture of the pars interarticularis. They come up from their three-point stance to block defensive linemen with the spine in lordosis.

23. How does one make the diagnosis of spondylolysis?

Clinically, children with spondylolysis will complain of back pain with activity. On examination, these children will have pain with spinal motion, especially extension. They frequently have hamstring tightness, as demonstrated by limited forward bending. The lesion may be seen on a lateral radiograph of the lumbosacral spine if the fractures are bilateral and have been present for a sufficient period of time to become evident radiographically. The oblique radiograph of the lumbosacral spine will best show the stress fracture of the pars interarticularis. If the radiographs do not demonstrate the lesion, a bone scan will usually reveal increased uptake of the nucleotide in the region of the pars. Single photon emission computed tomographic images should also be obtained to see and localize the lesion better. Finally, a CT scan of this area of the spine will demonstrate the fractures.

24. How should one treat spondylolysis?

Patients with spondylolysis will have back pain with activity. As the lesion progresses, pain may persist, even when the patient is sedentary. The pain will be more severe during periods of activity, however. Once the diagnosis has been made, reduction of stress is the main treatment, as it is for any stress fracture. The stress fracture of the pars is unlikely to heal, however. The lesion that may heal is the stress fracture that has recently occurred and is not complete. A bone scan should be performed; if there is significantly increased activity in the region of the pars interarticularis, one may assume that the stress fracture is attempting to repair itself.

Immobilization of these patients may result in complete healing of the fracture. In most patients, immobilization of the spine with a thoracolumbosacral orthosis (TLSO) allows the inflammation to subside. Most of the time, the fracture heals with a fibrous nonunion that is stable. Once the patient is comfortable, he or she is begun on an exercise program that will allow a progressive return to sports.

25. What is spondylolisthesis? How is it classified?

If a stress fracture does not heal or does not develop stable fibrous nonunion, the fracture fragments may separate. This allows the vertebral body to slide anteriorly while the posterior elements of the vertebra remain in their normal position. Once the vertebral body has slipped forward far enough that it is identifiable radiographically, spondylolysis has become spondylolisthesis.

The severity of spondylolisthesis is graded according the amount of forward slippage. If the slippage is 25% or less as measured against the next caudal vertebra or sacrum, the spondylolisthesis is classified as grade I. In grade II spondylolisthesis, the slipped vertebra has moved 25–50% forward. In grades III and IV, the slippage is 75% and 100%, respectively. In grade V spondylolisthesis, or spondyloptosis, not only has the body of L5 slipped 100% in front of the sacrum, but it has also actually slipped far enough forward that it has begun to descend caudally in front of the sacrum.

26. Do stress fractures occur in growth plates?

Stress fractures of growth plates are uncommon, but they do occur. Children with open physes may experience stress applied mainly to a growth plate (Fig. 35-2). The physeal stress fracture will have the same symptoms as the stress fracture of the ossified portion of the bone, namely, pain with activity. Gymnasts may develop stress fractures of their distal radius physis. Stress fractures of the olecranon apophysis can be seen in skeletally immature weightlifters. Another apophyseal stress injury is the stress reaction of the tibial tubercle, called Osgood-Schlatter disease. This lesion may occasionally lead to a complete fracture of the tibial tubercle if a very forceful contraction of the quadriceps muscle pulls loose an already weakened tibial tubercle.

27. **Will all stress fractures heal with reduction of stress or immobilization?**

Most stress fractures will heal with reduction of the stress, which usually requires immobilization in children. Stress fractures on the tension of a bone, as mentioned previously, are more prone to nonunion. The two most common locations for tension-side stress fractures are the superior cortex of the femoral neck and the anterior cortex of the midtibia if there is an associated anterior bow of the tibia. Both these fractures frequently require surgical treatment. In the femoral neck, if the tension-side stress fracture does not heal with avoidance of weightbearing, then internal fixation of the femoral neck will be required.

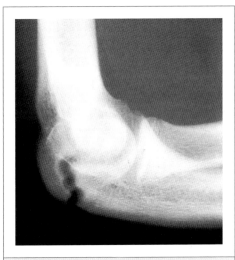

Figure 35-2. Lateral radiograph of the right elbow of a 14-year-old boy who had pain in both elbows for more than 5 months. He played football and had been lifting weights for more than a year. This radiograph demonstrates a very wide olecranon apophysis. The apophysis should be nearly closed in a male of his bone age since all the physes of the elbow are closed on this radiograph. Immobilization relieved the pain in the left elbow, but the right elbow pain persisted. Because there was no improvement with immobilization, the fracture was operated on. The fracture was mobile on exploration. It was internally fixed with an intramedullary screw, and the fracture defect was bone grafted.

BIBLIOGRAPHY

1. Devas MB: Stress fractures in children. J Bone Joint Surg 45B:528–541, 1963.
2. Green NE, Rogers RA, Lipscomb AB: Nonunion of stress fractures of the tibia. Am J Sports Med 13:171–176, 1985.
3. Loud KJ, Gordon CM, Micheli LJ, Field AE: Correlates of stress fractures among preadolescent and adolescent girls. Pediatrics 115:e399–e406, 2005.
4. Walker RN, Green NE, Spindler KP: Stress fractures in skeletally immature patients. J Pediatr Orthop 16:578–584, 1996.

CHAPTER 36

UPPER-EXTREMITY SPORTS INJURIES

Christopher K. Kim, MD, and Henry G. Chambers, MD

1. **What is an acromioclavicular (AC) joint injury?**
   Fractures of the distal clavicle represent approximately 10–12% of all clavicular fractures. A fall on the point of the shoulder that drives the scapula downward usually causes an AC dislocation in the older adolescent and adult, but fractures of the distal clavicle are much more common in children with the same mechanism. These fractures represent pseudodislocations because the distal shaft is herniated upward through a rupture of the thick periosteal tube that surrounds the distal clavicle. The coracoclavicular and AC ligaments remain intact to the periosteal tube, along with the usually apparent distal clavicular physis.

2. **What diagnostic views are necessary in an AC joint injury?**
   Adequate radiographic views need to be taken to evaluate AC joint injuries. Routine radiographs of the shoulder are often well centered on the glenohumeral joint and therefore allow too much penetration to visualize the distal clavicle and the AC joint adequately. An axillary view and a 20-degree cephalic tilt view can further demonstrate the displacement in the AC region. When injuries to the region of the distal clavicle are suspected but not well defined on routine views, stress radiographs can be requested. Radiographs of both AC joint regions are taken simultaneously on the same x-ray cassette. The first view is taken without weights, and the second stress view is taken with weights suspended from the wrists.

3. **How are AC injuries treated?**
   Most authors agree that distal clavicular injuries in children and adolescents represent fractures through the distal physis or pseudodislocations rather than true adult-like AC separations (Fig. 36-1). Most agree that, as long as there is no gross deformity or instability, this injury can be treated conservatively. Therefore, types I through III can usually be treated with a short period of immobilization followed by progressive range of motion and strengthening exercises. Most fractures will heal, and function will be regained within 4–6 weeks. Return to sports is delayed until full shoulder motion and strength are obtained. Residual bony prominence is not a contraindication to a return to sports. Types IV through VI injuries that show fixed deformity or gross displacement will generally require open reduction and internal fixation. Surgically, the joint will need to be reduced and the periosteal tube repaired. In the older patient, supplemental temporary fixation is performed with a coracoclavicular screw. This screw is removed in 6–8 weeks, when rehabilitation is begun.

4. **How are AC joint injuries classified?**
   Rockwood's classification is similar to that used in adults for AC dislocation. The classification in children is based on the position of the distal clavicle and the accompanying injury to the periosteal tube rather than on injury of the ligaments, as occurs in true dislocation.
   - **Type I:** Mild ligamentous sprain of the AC ligaments without disruption of the periosteal tube. The distal clavicle is stable on examination, and radiographic findings are normal compared with the opposite shoulder.
   - **Type II:** There is partial disruption of the dorsal periosteal tube, with some instability at the distal clavicle on examination. Radiographically, there is a slight widening of the AC joint but no change in the coracoclavicular interval.

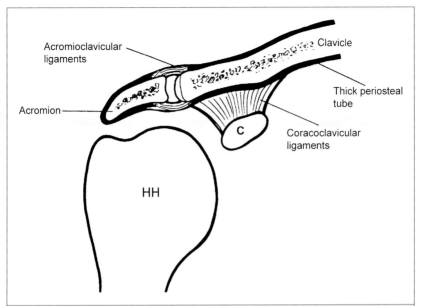

Figure 36-1. Anatomy of the distal clavicle and acromioclavicular joint in children. Note the thickened periosteal tube surrounding the distal clavicle, which is continuous with the acromioclavicular and coracoclavicular ligaments.

- **Type III:** There is a large dorsal longitudinal split in the periosteal tube, with gross instability of the distal clavicle. Radiographs reveal superior displacement of the clavicle in relation to the coracoid and acromion. The coracoclavicular interval is 25–100% greater than on the normal shoulder.
- **Type IV:** This injury is similar to type III, but the clavicle is displaced posteriorly and is buttonholed through the trapezius muscle fibers, with the distal end completely buried in muscle. On anteroposterior (AP) radiographs, there is little superior migration. The axillary radiographs show posterior displacement of the distal clavicle in relation to the acromion.
- **Type V:** There is a complete dorsal periosteal split, with superior subcutaneous displacement of the clavicle. This is often associated with a split of the deltoid and trapezius attachments. On radiographs, the coracoclavicular distance is greater than 100%, compared with the normal shoulder.
- **Type VI:** An inferior dislocation of the distal clavicle occurs, with the distal clavicle lodged beneath the coracoid process.

5. **What is a sternoclavicular (SC) joint injury?**
   The SC joint in children is much less commonly affected by injuries than the physis or medial metaphysis. True dislocations of the SC joint in children are reported but are extremely rare. Most injuries about the medial end of the clavicle involve the medial physeal plate and occur as Salter-Harris type I or II fractures. Injuries to the medial clavicle can occur in athletic events, predominantly in contact or collision sports. The most common mechanism of injury is an indirect blow to the lateral aspect of the shoulder that transmits force along the clavicle, resulting in a fracture of the physis medially. If the shoulder is compressed and rolled forward, a posterior displacement at the medial end will occur. If the shoulder is compressed and forced posteriorly, anterior displacement will occur. These injuries are best described using the

Salter-Harris classification of fractures and also using the direction of the displacement of the shaft fragment.

6. **How is shoulder instability classified?**
By degree of instability, direction of instability, and cause of the dislocation. The etiologic classification is the most important when formulating treatment options and predicting the prognosis. The degree of instability can be divided into subluxation versus dislocation. The directions of instability are anterior, posterior, inferior, and multidirectional. Anterior dislocations of the glenohumeral joint in children are the most common, accounting for more than 90% of injuries. Isolated cases of posterior dislocations in children and adolescents have been reported, but true traumatic posterior instability of the shoulder is rare. Inferior dislocations are very rare. Instability can be traumatic or atraumatic, which can be further broken down into voluntary versus involuntary, and recurrent. To be classified as a case of traumatic instability, a history of significant high-energy trauma and an appropriate mechanism should exist. Atraumatic instability of the glenohumeral joint only exists in the presence of multidirectional laxity of the shoulder. Recurrent instability can exist after either traumatic or atraumatic instability.

7. **What are the causes of traumatic instability?**
Anterior instability of the glenohumeral joint is the most common form of traumatic injury. A fall onto an outstretched hand that forces the arm into excessive abduction and external rotation is the primary mechanism of injury. The humeral head is levered anteriorly, tearing the anterior glenohumeral ligament complex and eventually dislocating, with the humeral head lodging against the anterior neck of the glenoid. Commonly, this results in a Bankart-type injury, in which the inferior glenohumeral ligament attachment is stripped off the anterior neck of the glenoid. Posterior dislocations are not commonly reported in children.

With traumatic anterior glenohumeral dislocations, patients present with obvious deformity, swelling, and (always) pain. The arm is held slightly abducted, externally rotated, and supported by the other arm. The neurologic and vascular status must be assessed. The axillary nerve is the most common nerve to be injured with anterior dislocation, but the entire brachial plexus can be involved. The sensory distribution of the axillary nerve is along the upper lateral arm and can be tested by light touch or pinprick. The motor innervation to the deltoid can be tested by having the patient voluntarily contract the deltoid in an attempt to abduct the elbow lightly.

Traumatic posterior dislocation is less apparent on clinical examination. Looking at the shoulder from above, flattening of the anterior aspect of the shoulder is noted with the hand across the abdomen. The hallmark of posterior dislocation is the lack of external rotation and an inability to supinate the forearm.

AP radiographs of the glenohumeral joint, as well as the axillary lateral view and the scapular lateral view, should be obtained. In the AP view, there will be an empty glenoid sign in which the articular surface of the humeral head does not fit into the glenoid. In the other two views, the head will be seen either anterior to or posterior to the glenoid.

In acute situations, we have performed a closed reduction by one of the standard and accepted techniques. Light sedation with either intravenous or intramuscular techniques is adequate for reduction. Any maneuver that gently and carefully reduces the joint is acceptable. X-rays should be obtained after the reduction maneuver.

Postreduction care is somewhat controversial. In the limited literature available on anterior dislocation in the child, it is inconclusive whether immobilization after reduction truly alters the prognosis. Itoi et al suggested, using magnetic resonance imaging (MRI) scans, that the best position of immobilization may be external instead of the more common internal rotation. After a period of immobilization, an aggressive rehabilitation program should be instituted, focusing on strengthening the rotator cuff and deltoid. The most common problem with anterior dislocation of the shoulder is recurrent instability. For posterior dislocations, a gentle reduction maneuver should be performed. After reduction, the arm is immobilized in a neutral position or a slight external rotation with the arm at the side. This may require a modified spica cast or a custom brace.

8. **What are the causes of atraumatic instability?**
   This is the most common type of instability in children and adolescents. A shoulder dislocation in a child without a clear-cut significant history of trauma should arouse suspicion that this may be an instance of atraumatic instability. These patients have inherent joint laxity, and the glenohumeral joint can be dislocated either voluntarily or involuntarily as a result of minimal trauma. Voluntary instability is accomplished by consciously firing certain muscles while inhibiting their antagonists. Voluntary instability can be associated with psychological instability.

   The most notable finding is the lack of pain associated with subluxation or dislocation. In most cases, reduction is not required because spontaneous reduction occurs. Clinical examination shows multiple-joint laxity, which may include hyperextensibility of the elbows, knees, and metacarpophalangeal joints. Skin hyperelasticity and striae may be present. In cases of acute trauma, the opposite shoulder should be examined for findings of multidirectional laxity because the affected shoulder may be too painful to undergo a complete examination. These signs of multidirectional laxity at the glenohumeral joint include a positive sulcus sign and significant humeral head translation on anterior and posterior drawer tests. The sulcus sign, a dimpling of the skin below the acromion when manual longitudinal traction is applied to the arm, is due to inferior subluxation of the humeral head within the glenohumeral joint. The drawer test is performed with the examiner seated at the side of the patient. The scapula is stabilized with one hand while the opposite hand manually translates the humeral head anteriorly and posteriorly. In patients with atraumatic instability, all are painless. The radiographic examination findings in these patients are usually normal.

   In treating the patient with atraumatic instability, a nonoperative approach emphasizing a vigorous rehabilitation program involving strengthening of the rotator cuff is used. Most patients without significant emotional or psychiatric problems successfully improve shoulder stability with this program. For patients with multidirectional instability who fail to improve after a thorough rehabilitation program, capsular-type reconstruction has been recommended.

9. **How frequent are recurrent dislocations? How should they be treated?**
   The literature on the natural history of glenohumeral dislocation in adolescents and young adults demonstrates recurrence rates of 25–90%. The true incidence of recurrent dislocations of the glenohumeral joint in a child is difficult to assess because of both the rarity of the injury and the variations in reports in the literature. In 1963, Rowe reported a 100% incidence of recurrence in children younger than the age of 10 years who sustained anterior dislocation. He reported a 94% incidence of recurrence in adolescents and young adults between the ages of 11 and 20 years. In 1975, Rockwood reported a recurrence rate of 50% in a series of patients between 13.8 and 15.8 years of age. Recently, Marans and associates reported on the fate of 21 children between the ages of 4 and 15 years with open physes at the time of initial dislocation. They found a 100% recurrence rate no matter what postreduction treatment program was used.

   Treatment of the patient with recurrent anterior dislocation of the shoulder should begin with an attempt to confirm the cause of the dislocation. If the cause is atraumatic, then continued nonoperative treatment is recommended. If it is determined that recurrent dislocation has a true traumatic cause, treatment is surgical.

10. **What is impingement syndrome?**
    Impingement is much less common than in adults but can be a cause of symptoms in the pediatric athlete. Classically, impingement occurs as the structures (i.e., the greater tuberosity, the supraspinatus tendon, the long head of the biceps, and the subacromial bursa) pass beneath the anterior and inferior surfaces of the coracoacromial arch, which is composed of the

coracoid, acromion, and coracoacromial ligament. This mechanical contact on a repetitive basis leads to acute and chronic inflammation and to the changes and clinical symptoms that we describe as impingement syndrome. Neer described impingement as a continuum; if left untreated, the process can progress from stage I (which includes acute inflammation and swelling) to stage II (a more chronic phase of inflammation, chronic scarring, and tendinitis) through to stage III (which is defined as a rotator cuff tear).

Most athletes in sports that require overhead repetitive shoulder function, such as swimming, baseball, and tennis, perform at a high level just below maximum stress. This repetitive microtrauma can lead to structural changes in the tendons, ligaments, and capsulae. An intrinsic overload in the rotator cuff tendons can lead to tendinitis, secondary muscle weakness, and biomechanical imbalance.

Younger patients, both pediatric and adolescent, have a higher incidence of inherent multidirectional instability. In sports activities requiring repetitive stress on the shoulder, these patients require greater dynamic stability by the rotator cuff musculature. As the rate of stress increases and the rotator cuff becomes fatigued, impingement results secondary to the multidirectional instability. Treatment is therefore directed at improving joint stability rather than primarily correcting impingement phenomena.

11. What are the symptoms of impingement syndrome?

The presenting symptom in all patients is pain. In mild cases, pain occurs only with certain activities, but as severity increases, the pain can become constant. Night pain is the hallmark symptom of rotator cuff disease. The pain is usually described as anterior or deep and can radiate down the lateral aspect of the arm to the area of the deltoid insertion. As the process becomes more severe, range of motion and strength can be diminished. Deficits in elevation and internal rotation are usually the first signs noted by the patient. The gross appearance of the shoulder is normal. In advanced cases, atrophy of the deltoid and the supraspinatus can appear. Range of motion is often normal. Strength can be affected by pain.

The impingement sign is always positive in patients with pure impingement. It is elicited by stabilizing the scapula while forcing the arm into internal rotation and forward flexion. This maneuver compresses the subacromial space and causes pain in patients with impingement. The impingement test is done to confirm the diagnosis in the absence of instability.

Substantial relief of symptoms occurring after injection of 10 mL of 1% Xylocaine (i.e., lidocaine) into the subacromial space indicates a positive test result. Great care should be taken to elicit signs of instability and generalized laxity on examination to confirm a diagnosis of secondary impingement.

12. How should impingement be treated?

Most young athletes present with mild symptoms only during specific activities. These patients may continue to participate while beginning treatment with oral nonsteroidal anti-inflammatory medications and rehabilitation. They should use moist heat-to-ice contrast treatment, along with a program of flexibility and rotator cuff strengthening exercises, on a daily basis. In moderately severe cases in which the patient has pain at rest after athletic events, the athlete is removed from the activity. Nonsteroidal anti-inflammatory medications and modality treatments such as ultrasound are initiated. When the pain at rest subsides, the athlete should begin the usual rehabilitation program, including flexibility training and strengthening. In severe cases that have persisted more than 3 months despite a supervised treatment program, further work-up with shoulder MRI is performed. If the diagnosis of impingement is confirmed, the athlete continues with the rehabilitation process. Rarely, in older adolescents, surgical treatment may be necessary. The young athlete with impingement should be made to realize that overuse is the common denominator in this problem. The overhand athlete should be pain-free and actively involved in a rehabilitation program before returning to specific sports.

13. **What are the stresses on the throwing elbow? What disorders can occur?**

In both the young throwing athlete and the mature thrower, four distinct areas are vulnerable to throwing stress:

- Tension overload of the medial elbow restraints
- Compression overload on the lateral articular surface
- Posterior medial shear forces on the posterior articular surfaces
- Extension overload on the lateral restraints

During early cocking and especially during late cocking, a significant distraction force is applied to the medial aspect of the elbow. The resultant force presents as tension on the medial epicondylar attachments, including the flexor muscle origin and the ulnar collateral ligaments. With overuse, the weakest link in the medial complex can be injured. In the young athlete, subsequent injury or avulsion of the medial epicondylar ossification center is often encountered. The ulnar collateral ligaments may be stretched, resulting in traction spurs on the coronoid process. Traction injury to the ulnar nerve and flexor muscle strain may also ensue.

Compression of the lateral articulation, in which the radial head abuts the capitellum, occurs mainly during early and late cocking. Sequelae include growth disturbances, chondral or osteochondral fractures of the capitellum, and growth disturbances and deformation of the radial head.

Posterior articular surface damage develops in two phases of throwing. During late cocking, a posterior medial shear force develops about the olecranon fossa. Throughout follow-through, hyperextension of the elbow is prominent, placing stress on the olecranon and the anterior capsule. These stresses commonly produce disease at three sites:

- The posterior medial spur
- The true posterior olecranon spurs
- The traction spurs of the coronoid process

Lateral extension overload occurs during acceleration when extreme pronation of the forearm results in a tension force applied to the lateral ligaments and the lateral epicondyle. Consequently, lateral epicondylitis may develop.

14. **What are the biomechanics of the throwing elbow in baseball?**

The pitch is divided into five stage:

- **Phase 1:** The wind-up or preparation phase, ending when the ball leaves the glove hand
- **Phase 2:** Termed *early cocking*; a period of shoulder abduction and external rotation that begins as the ball is released from the nondominant hand and terminates with contact of the forward foot on the ground
- **Phase 3:** The late cocking phase; continues until maximum external rotation is obtained
- **Phase 4:** The short propulsive phase of acceleration that starts with internal rotation of the humerus and ends with ball release
- **Phase 5:** The follow-through phase, which starts with ball release and ends when all motion is complete

15. **What is little leaguer's elbow?**

This is a group of pathologic entities in and about the elbow joint in young developing throwers. The injury includes:

- Medial epicondylar fragmentation and avulsion
- Delayed or accelerated apophyseal growth of the medial epicondyle
- Delayed closure of the medial epicondylar growth plate
- Osteochondrosis and osteochondritis of the capitellum
- Deformation and osteochondritis of the radial head
- Hypertrophy of the ulna
- Olecranon apophysitis, with or without delayed closure of the olecranon apophysis

These abnormalities are secondary to the biomechanical throwing stresses placed on the young developing elbow.

KEY POINTS: UPPER-EXTREMITY SPORTS INJURIES

1. Upper-extremity sports injuries in children have increased significantly over the past decade as participation in throwing sports has become a year-round endeavor.

2. Highly competitive pitchers are often in several leagues during one season and then on traveling all-star teams for the entirety of the year. This places a huge stress on the rapidly growing bones of young children and on immature muscles around the joints of the shoulder, elbow, wrist, and hand.

3. Although some acute injuries result from falling or being struck in a sporting event, many more injuries result from chronic overuse, usually accompanied by poor throwing mechanics.

16. **What factors should be considered in the evaluation of the elbow of a young athlete?**

A timely and accurate diagnosis is the keystone to successful treatment of the many conditions associated with little leaguer's elbow. Age, position, handedness, activity level, location of the pain, duration of the pain, radiation, trauma, the mechanism of injury, the nature of the onset, and past medical history are all salient factors in the history.

The age of young throwers can be divided into three groups, as follows:

- **Childhood:** Terminates with the appearance of secondary centers of ossification
- **Adolescence:** Terminates with the fusion of all secondary centers of ossification to their respective long bones
- **Young adulthood:** Terminates with completion of all bone growth and the achievement of final muscular form

During childhood, the most frequent complaints are sensitivity about the medial epicondyle, which is usually secondary to microinjuries at the apophysis and the ossification center. When the athlete enters adolescence, the athlete increases the valgus stresses on the elbow, and the result can be an avulsion fracture of the entire medial epicondyle. Some adolescents develop enough chronic stresses to cause delayed union, or possibly nonunion, of the medial epicondyle. By young adulthood, the medial epicondyle has fused, and injuries of the muscular attachments and ligaments of the epicondyle become more prevalent.

The position played by the thrower provides insight into the magnitude of stresses placed on the elbow and the relative incidence of elbow complaints. The usual order of prevalence of elbow complaints among players is, in order of most to least prevalent, pitchers, infielders, catchers, and outfielders.

Most throwers present with elbow problems in the dominant extremity unless direct trauma is the cause of the problem. Pain is the most common complaint. Localization, duration, character, temporal sequence, activity level, and nature of the onset are all clues to the underlying problem. Although pain is the most frequent complaint, related but less frequent problems include decreased elbow motion, mild flexion contracture, swelling, decreased performance, and local sensitivity of the elbow. It is also helpful to remember that the elbow may be the site of referred pain. Therefore, associated neck, shoulder, and wrist pain or restricted motion must be appraised.

Young throwers often have unilateral hypertrophy of the muscle and bone of the dominant extremity. Therefore, the presence of hypertrophy, valgus deformity, and flexion contracture should not be considered uncommon in young throwers.

Because of the high incidence of elbow and shoulder problems in young throwing athletes, it is recommended that no more than 75 pitches per game be thrown, with no more than 6 innings per week.

17. **What are the types and symptoms of medial complex injuries? How should they be treated?**

Most children with little leaguer's elbow present with medial elbow complaints. Medial complex injuries can be divided into three entities:

- Medial tension injuries
- Medial epicondylar fractures
- Medial ligament rupture

Patients with medial tension injuries present with a triad of symptoms including progressive medial pain, diminished throwing effectiveness, and decreased throwing distance. Repetitive valgus stresses and flexor forearm pull usually produce a subtle apophysitis or stress fracture through the medial epicondylar epiphysis. Physical manifestations include tenderness, swelling over the medial epicondyle, and an elbow flexion contracture of more than 15 degrees.

Radiographs show fragmentation and widening of the epiphyseal lines compared to the contralateral elbow. In most cases, a 4- to 6-week course of rest from throwing, along with ice and nonsteroidal anti-inflammatory medications, will result in cessation of symptoms. After 6 weeks, when the patient has no symptoms and has a pain-free range of motion, strengthening exercises are begun. A progressive throwing program is initiated at 8 weeks. Occasionally, symptoms may reappear when throwing is resumed; in these cases, throwing should be delayed until the next season.

When more substantial acute valgus stress is applied through violent muscle contraction during throwing, an avulsion fracture of the medial epicondyle may ensue. There may be a painful elbow, with point tenderness over the medial epicondyle and an elbow flexion contracture that may exceed 15 degrees. Radiographs most often show only a minimally displaced epicondylar fragment or a significant displacement, with or without displacement into the joint.

Woods and Tullos have divided these lesions into two types:

- **Type 1:** Occurs in younger children and produces a large fragment that involves the entire medial epicondyle and often displaces and rotates
- **Type 2:** Occurs in adolescents and produces a small fracture fragment

Most treatment protocols center on how much displacement is present. In minimally displaced (less than 2 mm) or nondisplaced fractures, simple posterior splint immobilization is initiated. After the acute symptoms have subsided, the patient's arm may be removed from the splint and active motion exercises may be started. Radiographic evidence of healing should be apparent by 6 weeks, and aggressive active range-of-motion exercises, as well as a progressive strengthening program, should be begun. Competitive throwing may be resumed when the patient has normal, painless range of motion, strength, and endurance while on the throwing program.

In moderately displaced (more than 2 mm) fractures with a large fragment, open reduction and internal fixation are appropriate. Two small cancellous screws may be necessary to prevent rotation. Early motion after the surgery is extremely advantageous in the adolescent. Depending on the quality of the fixation, range-of-motion exercises begin 1–2 weeks after surgery while the patient is wearing a functional orthosis.

Injuries to the ulnar collateral ligaments are not common in young throwing athletes. Most patients have tenderness about the medial aspect of the elbow for months to years before the ligament is injured. Commonly, a rupture occurs as a catastrophic event. Clinically, there will be subtle medial elbow instability, which can be demonstrated by flexing the elbow to 25 degrees to unlock the olecranon from its fossa and gently stressing the medial side of the elbow. Treatment of a complete tear of the ulnar collateral ligament in young throwers who wish to resume their activity is surgical. This can be accomplished by direct repair or reconstruction using a tendon graft.

18. **What is Panner's disease (i.e., osteochondrosis)? How is it treated?**

This entity is a disease of the growth or ossification centers in children that begins as degeneration or necrosis of the capitellum and is followed by regeneration and recalcification.

Panner's disease is a focal localized lesion of the subchondral bone of the capitellum and its overlying articular cartilage. The lesion is usually noted in the anterior central capitellum, where it is in maximal contact with the articulation of the head of the radius. Radiographs show that the capitellar ossification center is fragmented, owing to irregular patches of relative sclerosis alternating with areas of rarefaction. The natural history of Panner's disease is that as growth progresses, the capitellar epiphysis eventually assumes a normal appearance in size, contour, and subchondral architecture. Initial treatment should consist of rest, avoidance of throwing, and sometimes splinting until the pain and tenderness subside.

19. **How is osteochondritis dissecans (OCD) evaluated, classified, and treated?**
OCD is currently looked upon as a singular entity within the multiple entities encompassed by the term *little leaguer's elbow*. OCD of the capitellum appears to be secondary to compressive forces occurring between the capitellum and the radial head during throwing. Osteochondritis is a focal lesion of the capitellum occurring in the 13- to 16-year-old age group, usually characterized by elbow pain and a flexion contracture of 15 degrees or more. Onset is insidious, with a focal island of subchondral bone demarcated by a rarefied zone on radiographs. Sequelae include loose bodies, residual deformity of the capitellum, and, often, residual elbow disability. OCD must be differentiated from Panner's disease. Age, onset, loose body formation, radiographic findings, and deformity of the capitellum all aid in the differentiation. Panner's disease usually affects a younger population, and the onset is acute with fragmentation of the entire ossific nucleus.

   The cause of OCD of the elbow has not been determined. Three popular theories include ischemia, trauma, or genetic factors. Typically, the patient with OCD presents with a dull, poorly localized pain that is aggravated by use, especially throwing, and is relieved by rest. These patients commonly complain of limitation of motion. Later in the course of the disease, locking and catching with severe pain may supervene. Radiographs will usually show the typical rarefaction, irregular ossification, and a crater adjacent to the articular surface of the capitellum. Arthroscopy is an excellent method of determining the size of the lesion, its fixation, and the condition of the articular cartilage of the capitellum and the radial head.

BIBLIOGRAPHY

1. Rockwood CA Jr: Fractures and dislocations of the ends of the clavicle, scapulae and glenohumeral joint. In Rockwood CA, Wilkins KE, Beatty JH (eds): Fractures in Children, vol 3. Philadelphia, J.B. Lippincott, 1996.
2. Stanitski CL, DeLee JC, Drez D: Pediatric and Adolescent Sports Medicine. Philadelphia, W.B. Saunders, 1994.
3. Tibone JE: Shoulder problems of adolescents: How they differ from those of adults. Clin Sports Med 2:423–427, 1983.
4. Wilkins KE: Fractures and dislocations of the elbow region. In Rockwood CA, Wilkins KE, Beatty JE (eds): Fractures in Children. Philadelphia, J.B. Lippincott, 1996.

CHAPTER 37

LOWER-EXTREMITY SPORTS INJURIES

Michael T. Busch, MD

1. **What is an apophysis? What is its significance in youth sports injuries?**
   Apophyses are specialized growth centers of the immature skeleton that occur around joints. Major muscles or muscle groups have their origin at or insert into these areas. They are prone to a variety of injuries in youths participating in sports. From repetitive use, youths can develop an overuse tension near-rupture injury often referred to as an *apophysitis*. With time, exertion, or a combination of the two, these can sustain a sudden avulsion fracture.

2. **What apophyses are located about the hips and pelvis? What inserts or originates in these locations?**
   See Table 37-1 and Fig. 37-1.

TABLE 37-1.   ORIGINS AND INSERTIONS IN APOPHYSES ABOUT THE HIPS AND PELVIS

Apophysis	Origin or Insertion
Iliac crest	External oblique muscle of the abdomen
Anteriosuperior iliac spine	Sartorius
Anterioinferior spine	Direct head of the rectus femoris
Lesser trochanter	Iliopsoas
Greater trochanter	Gluteus medius
Ischium	Hamstrings

3. **How are most apophyseal avulsion fractures treated?**
   Most apophyseal avulsion fractures around the pelvis do not displace significantly. The periosteum is usually in continuity with the fragment, so with time the fracture will heal satisfactorily. Even with moderate displacement, surgical fixation is rarely indicated. Complications are rare. Crutches help to rest the area and the muscles around the hip. Sports activities should be terminated or significantly modified until healing has completed, which can take from 4 to 12 weeks. A premature return to sports is associated with a risk of recurrent injury or symptoms.

4. **Besides avulsion fractures, which two serious injuries of the hip and pelvis are most often associated with sports injuries?**
   Traumatic posterior dislocations of the hip, usually produced by an axial load applied to the adducted hip, frequently occur in football players. The dislocation is often accompanied by a fracture of the posterior wall of the iliac portion of the acetabulum. If the fragment is small, it may heal without compromising the stability of the acetabulum. If larger, open reduction and internal fixation may be necessary.

Complications include avascular necrosis (AVN), chondrolysis, and traumatic arthritis.

Occasionally, pathologic fractures of the femoral neck occur. These are typically secondary to benign lesions such as simple bone cysts, aneurysmal bone cysts, fibrous dysplasia, and, sometimes, stress fractures. Compression-side stress fractures of the medial femoral neck are treated by rest, crutches, graduated, monitored, return to activities. Tension-side failures of the superior neck are prone to complete fractures and are therefore treated by percutaneous screw fixation.

5. **What are the two most common serious complications arising from traumatic hip dislocation?**
    Small fracture fragments are sometimes difficult to visualize with plain radiography. The source of these includes the posterior margin at the acetabulum, the femoral head, and the origin of the ligamentum teres from the acetabular fossa. If trapped in the joint and left unrecognized, these can lead to chondrolysis and arthritis.

    AVN of the femoral head can occur after any traumatic hip dislocation. In youth sports, the hip will often spontaneously reduce on the field. This makes diagnosis more difficult and must, therefore, be kept in mind. The longer the hip is dislocated, the higher the rate of AVN. However, it can even occur in cases of spontaneous (immediate) reduction. Radiographic evidence of AVN is usually evident after 1 year but can take up to 2 years to present. Magnetic resonance imaging (MRI) appears to be the best way to detect AVN before collapse occurs.

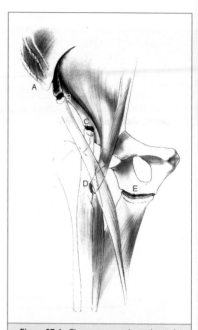

Figure 37-1. There are several apophyses in the area of the hip and pelvis. Avulsion fractures and overuse syndrome of these apophyses are fairly common in youth sports injuries. The muscle origin and insertion are illustrated. *A,* The abdominal wall muscles insert into the iliac crest apophysis. *B,* The sartorius originates from the anterosuperior iliac spine apophysis. *C,* The direct head of the rectus femoris originates from the anteroinferior iliac spine apophysis. *D,* The iliopsoas tendon inserts into the lesser trochanteric apophysis of the proximal femur. *E,* The hamstrings originate from the ischial apophysis. (From Busch MT: Sports medicine. In Morrissy RT (ed): Lovell and Winter's Pediatric Orthopaedics, 4th ed. Philadelphia, Lippincott-Raven, 1996, p 1298.)

6. **What common adolescent hip problem is often not diagnosed promptly, and what are the serious potential medical and legal consequences?**
    Slipped capital femoral epiphysis (SCFE), sometimes diagnosed as *hip strain,* is the most common adolescent hip problem, yet it is often misdiagnosed by nonmusculoskeletal specialists. Failure to recognize SCFE can lead to progression of the slip and the accompanying risks of devastating complications of AVN (i.e., ischemic necrosis) and chondrolysis.

7. **What is the clinical presentation of SCFE?**
    Patients with SCFE can present with a variable history of an insidious onset of hip, thigh, or knee pain. At times, the onset is acute and severe. Some patients will be able to walk, whereas others will be too sore to ambulate without support. The key feature on clinical exam is the outwardly rotated gait and the obligate external rotation when the affected hip is flexed.

8. **If a teenage athlete presents with pain and swelling in the anterior thigh without a clear history of significant trauma, what should be considered in the differential diagnosis?**
Quadriceps contusions sometimes result from fairly minor injuries. Interstitial muscle tears, particularly of the rectus femoris, can present as a spontaneous bleed in the thigh as well. More serious problems, however, need to be investigated, especially in teenagers: rhabdomyosarcoma of the quadriceps, Ewing's sarcoma, and osteosarcoma should be considered. At a minimum, plain radiographs should be obtained. If sarcoma is suspected, the patient should undergo MRI.

9. **How is a quadriceps contusion initially treated? How is its progress monitored?**
Acutely: rest, ice, a compressive wrap, and elevation are used to reduce bleeding. The three most important parameters to follow are pain, swelling, and the restriction of passive knee flexion. The ability to fully flex the knee is the last function to return to normal and is, therefore, the best indicator for return to sport.

10. **How soon can a player return to sports following a quadriceps contusion?**
Although technically a bruise, this injury has a wide spectrum of severity. Players with mild contusions can return to sports almost immediately, whereas those with severe contusions may be out for more than 6 weeks.

11. **What is the consequence of a premature return to participation following a quadriceps contusion?**
Repeat interstitial hemorrhaging. This can lead to significant exacerbation of the injury with marked delay in subsequent resolution. It is very important to be sure that this injury has completely resolved before returning the athlete to sports, particularly contact sports.

12. **How do meniscal tears present in young patients?**
Meniscal tears in youths are usually associated with significant injuries that result from a memorable event. They produce pain, swelling, and limping. They rarely result from trivial episodes, as can happen in adults. There is often associated injury to the ligaments in youths, particularly the anterior cruciate ligament (ACL) and the medial collateral ligament. The youth with spontaneous or gradual onset of joint line pain in the knee rarely has a torn cartilage unless it is secondary to a congential discoid meniscus.

13. **At what age do meniscal tears begin to occur?**
Tearing of a normal meniscus rarely occurs before 12 years of age. A discoid meniscus is a congenitally abnormal cartilage and can present at almost any age.

14. **How does a discoid meniscus become symptomatic?**
Discoid menisci can be thick and bulbous (i.e., Wrisberg's type), which causes them to snap when the knee performs a range of motions. Discoid menisci can also tear spontaneously in very young children.

15. **What portion of the meniscus has a blood supply that aids in the healing process, either spontaneously or with surgical repair?**
Microangiographic studies have shown that the menisci are not completely avascular structures, as was once thought. Approximately one third of the meniscus closest to the capsule has a blood supply that facilitates healing. Children and adolescents have a high percentage of detachments and longitudinal tears near the capsular margin, both of which are good candidates for repair. With proper selection and technique, repair should be 80–90% successful, with minor deterioration over time.

16. **What is the expected outcome of meniscectomy in youths?**
Initially, meniscectomy should relieve the symptoms of a torn cartilage. A small percentage of patients then begin to develop symptoms between 3 and 5 years later. Seventy-five percent of these patients at 30 years will show degenerative articular changes radiographically, although only 30% will be clinically symptomatic. Presumably, most of these patients will develop debilitating arthritis in their 40s and 50s. The long-term affects of arthroscopic partial meniscectomy are still not known, but they may not be completely favorable. All reasonable efforts should be made to preserve a torn meniscus in a young person.

17. **Name the naturally occurring plicae of the knee.**
- Suprapatellar plica
- Medial patellar plica
- Infrapatellar plica
   See Fig. 37-2.

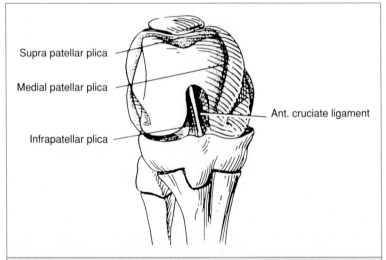

Figure 37-2. Plicae are synovial folds, and three major ones are commonly present in the knee. A suprapatellar plica can partially or completely divide the suprapatellar pouch from the rest of the knee joint. The medial patellar plica is the one that most commonly becomes symptomatic. The infrapatellar plica (i.e., the ligamentum mucosum) lies directly in front of the anterior cruciate ligament. (From Busch MT: Sports medicine. In Morrissy RT [ed]: Lovell and Winter's Pediatric Orthopaedics, 4th ed. Philadelphia, Lippincott-Raven, 1996, p 1306.)

18. **Which plica is most often symptomatic?**
Plicae are normally occurring structures that are remnants from the embryologic development of the knee joint. Initially, three cavities form, and as these coalesce, their fusion is incomplete; the remaining small septae form the plicae. Plicae are rarely symptomatic, with the exception of the medial plica.

19. **Name the two most common ways for a patient with symptomatic medial plica to present.**
- **Acute:** Often, plicae become symptomatic after the patient sustains a direct blow (e.g., from a fall) to the area. It is believed that the plica and overlying synovium become thickened and

then begin to catch or impinge where they previously had not. The youngster may experience persistent pain with attempts to resume activities and occasionally presents with an acutely locked knee. The knee is typically held in flexion, with the youngster refusing to fully extend it, blocking because of pain.

- **Chronic:** Characterized by a gradual onset of pain, this is particularly associated with sports that involve running. Patients who pronate as they walk and run may develop pain symptoms over the anteromedial portion of the knee joint. This usually follows the onset of a new sports season or with a sudden increase in training levels. Participants in track, cross country, soccer, football, and cycling are especially vulnerable.

20. **True or False: The ACL is rarely ruptured in children because the physeal plates are weaker and break first, thereby acting as a safety valve.**
    False. Although the physeal plates of the distal femur and the proximal tibia can act as the "weak link in the chain" and may fracture prior to disruption of the ACL, concurrent injuries may occur. Depending on the rate and mechanism of loading, the ACL can fail first, although this is less common before skeletal maturity and is rare in children under the age of 8. Rupture of the ACL should always be considered in the differential diagnosis of a young person with an acute knee injury and swelling. ACL injuries are sometimes associated with femur fractures, and a Lachman examination should be routinely done in the course of evaluating and treating a femur fracture in youths.

21. **Should an ACL sprain be treated by casting of the knee?**
    As in adults, the ACL has a very limited capacity to heal. The blood supply comes from each end and is often disrupted with the sprain because it is located in the center of the knee joint. Factors within the synovial fluid may impair healing as well. Rigid immobilization has not been shown to improve outcome. Following acute injury, the knee is rested with a brace or knee immobilizer until the swelling and pain begin to subside. Aspiration may be indicated for a very tense and painful hemarthrosis. As the knee recovers from this acute phase, a definitive treatment plan can be formulated and the injury better evaluated. The natural history of an untreated complete ACL sprain in young athletes is very unfavorable, with rates of reinjury approaching 90%.

22. **Can the ACL be safely reconstructed in a skeletally immature person?**
    To best restore the biomechanical properties of the ACL, a graft must be placed in as nearly an anatomic location as possible. Nonanatomic reconstructions (such as iliotibial band tenodesis) almost always stretch out and fail due to their anisometric nature. The ACL is a structure that spans from epiphysis to epiphysis. Most anatomic reconstruction techniques require the placing of drill holes through the proximal tibia and the distal femur. In the skeletally immature individual, these cross the physeal plates and therefore create a risk for a growth plate injury, which could result in either the shortening or the angular deformity of the limb. Most studies of ACL reconstruction in young adolescents suggest that in spite of this, clinically significant growth impairment is uncommon. The graft should not contain a bone block that crosses the physeal plate as that might promote the development of a physeal bar.
    Key growth issues need to be considered in making the best decision about ACL reconstruction in skeletally immature youths. Bone age (ascertained by comparing a radiograph of the patient's left hand to a series of standards in an atlas) is probably the most reliable indicator of growth remaining.

- **Boys (bone age) > 14 years and girls > 12 years:** Less than 5% of the growth of the distal femur and tibia occur in the last year of growth, so, generally, these patients can be treated in almost any conventional manner as the risk of a growth disturbance leading to a clinically significant limb-length inequality or angular deformity is almost nil.

- **Boys (bone age) 12–14 years and girls 10–12 years:** For youths approaching skeletal maturity, there is a risk of clinically significant complications to drilling across the physeal plates and spanning a graft across from metaphysis to metaphysis. Keeping the bone tunnels small and using only soft tissue in the graft, such as autologous hamstring grafts and tibial anterior or posterior allografts, are generally preferred techniques.
- **Boys (bone age) < 12 years and girls < 10 years:** In youths with several years of growth remaining, there are little clinical data, but documented complications are known and suggest that these very immature youths should generally be treated nonoperatively. For those younger patients with ACL deficiency who fail nonoperative care of a repairable meniscus tear, physeal-sparing procedures, such as the Micheli or Anderson procedures, are probably the best choice.

23. **Is surgical intervention necessary for posterior cruciate ligament (PCL) injuries in youths?**
Fortunately, PCL injuries are much less common than ACL injuries in children and adults. They can be associated with bony avulsions from either the femoral or tibial ends. Bony avulsion is an indication for primary repair of a PCL injury in a skeletally immature individual. Midsubstance ruptures are treated expectantly; reconstruction in youths is rarely necessary.

24. **Compared with the other ligaments about the knee, what is unique about the tibial insertion of the medial collateral ligament (MCL)?**
Distally, the MCL inserts into the metaphysis of the proximal tibia. Its femoral origin is from the epiphysis of the femur. The lateral collateral ligament originates from the epiphysis of the femur and inserts into the epiphysis of the fibula. Only the tibial end of the MCL inserts into a metaphysis spanning the physeal plate. The cruciate ligaments arise and insert into epiphyses.

25. **What imaging study should be performed if a severe-grade MCL sprain is suspected in a skeletally immature individual?**
Plain radiographs should always be performed to look for physeal and epiphyseal fractures in skeletally immature individuals with clinical instability at the knee. Physeal fractures are more common than complete MCL sprains in youths. If the fracture is nondisplaced, it may not be apparent on plain radiographs, so a valgus stress radiograph should be obtained if the knee is clinically unstable and the plain radiographs appear normal. This should not be done so forcefully as to further injure the physeal plate. If the diagnosis remains uncertain, MRI may be needed.

26. **What is the most likely diagnosis for a 14-year-old male basketball player who sustains an inversion injury of the ankle and presents with lateral ankle swelling and tenderness?**
Most males are still skeletally immature at 14 years of age, and if the physeal plate of the distal fibula is still open, fracture is a strong possibility. The other likely diagnosis is sprain of the anterior talofibular ligament. In more-severe ankle sprains, the calcaneal fibular ligament can be involved as well.

27. **What physical examination finding best differentiates a physeal fracture of the distal fibula from an ankle sprain?**
Although there may be generalized swelling that is diffusely tender, you should specifically examine for tenderness to percussion over the physeal plate, typically about 15–20 mm proximal to the tip of the fibula. Comparing the tenderness in the area of the anterior talofibular ligament to the pain produced with gentle digital percussion over the physis is often helpful in separating a physeal fracture from an ankle sprain.

KEY POINTS: LOWER-EXTREMITY SPORTS INJURIES

1. Apophyseal injuries around the hip and pelvis are common problems in young athletes; these include apophysitis and apophyseal avulsion fractures. Left untreated, apophysitis in any location can lead to an apophyseal avulsion fracture.

2. Slipped capital femoral epiphysis (SCFE) is the most common adolescent cause of hip pain and must not be overlooked as there are serious consequences of delayed diagnosis due to the potential risks of avascular necrosis of the femoral head and chondrolysis. The complaint in SCFE may be insidious in onset, presenting with pain in the hip, thigh, or knee.

3. Quadriceps contusions should not be viewed as simple bruises, and they can be very disabling injuries. Complications include formation of heterotopic bone, stiffness of adjacent joints, residual muscle weakness, and repeat bleeding.

4. Meniscal injuries can occur in youths, and the long-term outcomes following total meniscectomy are not favorable. As a result, the diagnosis needs to be considered and the possibility of meniscal repair strongly considered in the treatment. The most common reason for a meniscal tear in juveniles is discoid lateral meniscus.

5. The synovial plica of the knee can be a source of pain and locking but must not be blamed for the cause of knee pains in most adolescents. The plica can cause real symptoms but is also a diagnosis of exclusion.

6. Treatment of anterior cruciate ligament injuries in youths involve consideration of multiple factors, basically weighing the risk of reinjury versus growth remaining and the risk of growth-related complications. These influence the decision to treat, as well as the techniques and the graft selection.

28. **What occult congenital foot anomaly is associated with an increased incidence of ankle sprains?**
Talar coalitions are anomalies resulting from failure of segmentation of the hindfoot bones. The two most common are the calcaneonavicular and talocalcaneal (i.e., subtalar) coalitions. Motion of the subtalar joint is particularly important in compensating for inversion or eversion moments produced by walking, running, and suddenly changing direction. By restricting intrinsic hindfoot motion, tarsal coalitions increase inversion and eversion stresses at the ankle joint and are thereby associated with an increased rate of ankle sprains and recurrent ankle injuries.

29. **Consider a young athlete with an inversion injury to an ankle looking much like a sprain. Can there be a fracture present in the physis (such as the distal fibula) in spite of a normal radiograph?**
The most common physeal fracture pattern from an inversion injury of the ankle is a Salter-Harris type I injury. These are often nondisplaced and result in a normal-looking bone (with soft tissue swelling present). The diagnosis of fracture in these cases is based primarily on the physical examination findings. When in doubt, assume and treat for a nondisplaced physeal fracture.

30. **What other fractures are typically associated with inversion injuries of the foot and ankle?**
Fractures at the base of the fifth metatarsal often result from inversion mechanisms. Originally, these were thought to result from an avulsion mechanism based on pull of the peroneus

brevis. Some studies suggest that the culprit is actually the band of the lateral plantar fascia, which inserts on the plantar base of the fifth metatarsal. In runners, the proximal portion of the fifth metatarsal can be an area of stress concentration (and stress fracture) resulting from excessive training. This can subsequently fracture, either from repetitive use or from an inversion injury.

31. **How are fractures at the base of the fifth metatarsal treated?**
Localizing the fracture is important. Transverse fractures through the metaphysis that extend lateral to medial above the articulation with the cuboid are referred to as *Jones fractures*. When associated with a chronic stress reaction, these fractures are very prone to delayed union and nonunion. The most common treatments are nonweightbearing immobilization in a cast for 6–12 weeks and acute internal fixation with a screw, if indicated.

More-proximal fractures often heal with minimum treatment, including compressive wraps and hard-soled shoes; however, delayed unions and refractures can occur, particularly in highly active young athletes such as gymnasts. For these individuals, cast immobilization is warranted until radiographic healing is evident.

32. **What normal structure can be mistaken for a fracture of the base of the fifth metatarsal?**
The apophysis at the base of the fifth metatarsal typically appears in girls of 9–11 years of age and in boys of 11–14 years of age. The small ossified portion can be mistaken for a fracture fragment; however, the apophysis runs parallel to the shaft of the fifth metatarsal, whereas most fractures are perpendicular to the longitudinal axis of the metatarsal. Apophysitis at this location is known as Iselin's disease.

BIBLIOGRAPHY

1. Andrish J: Meniscal injuries in children and adolescents: Diagnosis and management. J Am Acad Orthop Surg 4:231–237, 1996.
2. Boden B, Osbahr D: High-risk stress fractures: Evaluation and treatment. J Am Acad Orthop Surg 8:344–353, 2000.
3. Busch M: Sports medicine. In Morrissy RT (ed): Lovell and Winter's Pediatric Orthopaedics, 5th ed. Philadelphia, Lippincott-Williams & Wilkins, 2001, pp 1273–1318.
4. Kocher MS, Klingele K, Rassman : Meniscal disorders: Normal, discoid, and cysts. Orthop Clin North Am 34:329–340, 2003.
5. Kocher MS, Tucker R: Pediatric athlete hip disorders. Clin Sports Med 25:241–253, 2006.
6. Lo IK, Bell DM, Fowler PJ: Anterior cruciate ligament injuries in the skeletally immature patient. Instr Cours Lect 47:351–359, 1998.
7. Lynch LA, Renstrom PA: Treatment of acute lateral ankle ligament rupture in the athlete. Conservative versus surgical treatment. Sports Med 27(1):61–71, 1999.
8. Metzmaker J, Pappas A: Avulsion fractures of the pelvis. Am J Sports Med 13:349–358, 1985.
9. Moeller JL: Pelvic and hip apophyseal avulsion injuries in young athletes. Curr Sports Med Rep 2(2):110–115, 2003.
10. Quill GE Jr: Fractures of the proximal fifth metatarsal. Orthop Clin North Am 26:353–361, 1995.
11. Ryan JB, Wheeler JH, Hopkinson WJ, et al: Quadriceps contusions: West Point update. Am J Sports Med 19:299–304, 1991.
12. Stanitski C: Anterior cruciate ligament injury in the skeletally immature patient. J Am Acad Orthop Surg 3:146–158, 1995.

LEG-LENGTH DISCREPANCY

Colin F. Moseley, MD, CM, Noelle Cassidy, MB, and Robert M. Bernstein, MD

CHAPTER 38

1. **What is a leg-length discrepancy (LLD)?**

   This is a measurable difference in the overall lengths of the two legs. LLDs can be subdivided into true, apparent, and functional LLDs.

2. **What is anisomelia?**

   This is defined as inequality between paired limbs. It is usually a term used in reference to limbs in which hemiatrophy or hemihypertrophy is apparent.

3. **What is true LLD?**

   Sometimes referred to as the *anatomic discrepancy*, this is the measurable difference in the overall lengths of the two legs from the anterior superior iliac spine (ASIS) to the medial malleolus, with both legs placed in the same anatomic attitude.

4. **What is apparent LLD?**

   This is the measurable difference in the two legs from the umbilicus or xiphisternum to the medial malleolus.

5. **Why might the true and apparent LLDs be different?**

   There are times when these measurements are not equal. This occurs when the overall lengths of the two legs may be the same, but, because of a contracture around the hip, one leg seems short. For example, an abduction contracture of the hip will make the apparent and functional lengths of that leg appear to be short even though there is no true LLD.

6. **What is a functional LLD?**

   This is best determined clinically by placing blocks under the short leg of the patient to level the pelvis while the patient is standing. This discrepancy is what the patient notices in the upright position and takes into account any differences in the pelvis and foot.

7. **Which discrepancy is more important?**

   All are important, but functional discrepancy is what is most important to the patient. In fact, sometimes the tilt of the pelvis and the posture of the trunk and spine are more important than the actual LLD.

8. **How do you assess a patient with LLD?**

   Clinically

   - Level the pelvis by placing blocks under the short leg, with the patient standing.
   - Measure the distance from the ASIS to the medial malleolus (for true LLD).
   - Measure the distance from the umbilicus or xiphisternum to the medial malleolus (for apparent LLD).
   - Observe the patient's walking gait.

Radiographically

- Scanogram
- Teleoroentgenogram
- Orthoroentgenogram
- Computed tomography (CT) scan

9. **What is a teleoroentgenogram?**

This is a single 3-foot radiograph taken of the lower extremities. The advantages of this are that measurements are not affected by patient movement and that entire bones are shown so that malalignments or lesions in the bone will be apparent. The disadvantage is that it distorts the results by magnification at the upper and lower ends of the film; as the child gets bigger, the distortion gets bigger. In addition, the large film size makes handling and storage difficult.

10. **What is an orthoroentgenogram?**

This is also a 3-foot radiograph, but the hip, knee, and ankle are taken in three separate exposures with the beam directly perpendicular to the film over the three joints. This avoids the magnification problems seen with teleoroentgenograms. Again, the large film size makes storage difficult.

11. **What is a scanogram?**

This is currently the most popular way of measuring the lengths of the femur and tibia. It is a series of radiographs, with the hips, knees, and ankles exposed separately to avoid magnification errors, taken with the child lying supine next to a radiographic tape measure. The machine and film are moved to take each set of radiographs. A small, easily stored and handled film is produced. Disadvantages of this method include the possibility that that the child will move between exposures. Malalignments and intraosseous lesions may be missed since the entire extremity is not included on the film. Discrepancies in foot size or pelvic shape are not included if scanogram calculations alone are used.

12. **How can the method of performing a scanogram be modified to eliminate errors arising from hip or knee contractures?**

Perform the scanogram with the leg in the lateral or posteroanterior (PA) position, shooting each bone separately if necessary.

13. **Is radiologic measurement of leg length enough to evaluate the child's growth pattern?**

The leg-length measurements mean nothing by themselves and must be correlated with development. In children under 7 years of age, it suffices to relate the lengths to age, but after the age of 7 years it is best to use skeletal age to account for the variation in maturation among children. Therefore, after the age of 7 years, routinely take left-hand and wrist radiographs to determine bone age as an adjunct to the scanogram.

14. **How are limbs measured on a CT scan?**

A scout film of the leg is taken. The technician places points on the ends of the bones, and the computer measures the distance between the points. There may be less potential for error because of angular deformities and, in the right circumstances, less radiation and less cost than conventional techniques.

15. **What are the causes of LLD?**

See Table 38-1.

TABLE 38-1. CAUSES OF LEG-LENGTH DISCREPANCY (LLD)
Acquired
Traumatic
Femoral or tibial length malunion or overgrowth
Growth due to a growth-plate fracture
Paralytic (reduces the growth rate of a limb)
Polio, cerebral palsy
Vascular
Hemangioma
Klippel-Trénaunay-Weber syndrome
Neoplastic
Wilms' tumor
Radiation treatment
Infectious
Congenital
Hemihypertrophy
Congenital short femur
Proximal femoral focal deficiency
Fibular hemimelia
Hip dislocation
Posteromedial bow of the tibia
Positional
Pelvic obliquity
Hip contracture

16. **At what age is overgrowth of a fractured femur a problem that can result in LLD?**
The problem of growth acceleration is most consistent between 2 and 10 years of age. There seems to be a potential for overgrowth of the fracture limb; thus, the recommendation is to accept fractures that are healing approximately 1–1.5 cm short in order to avoid LLD at skeletal maturity.

17. **Why does overgrowth occur after a fracture?**
This may be related to local hyperemia induced by the fracture and remodeling. As the healing process comes to an end, so does the enhancement of growth, so the overgrowth does not continue more than $1\frac{1}{2}$ years after the fracture.

18. **What is the Galeazzi sign?**
Have the child lie supine with the knees flexed and the feet on the table. If the knees are at different heights, this implies that one leg is shorter than the other. Careful observation can help you discern whether the difference is in the femur or the tibia.

19. **What kinds of problems can LLD cause?**
    - **Inefficient gait:** As the discrepancy gets larger, the gait gets less efficient.
    - **Cosmetic problems:** As children get older, they may not like how they look.
    - **Arthritis:** There is soft evidence that the hip of the longer leg is less covered and may be predisposed to arthritis.
    - **Scoliosis and low-back problems:** There is also soft evidence that living with an LLD can produce spinal deformity and back pain as an adult.

20. **What are the consequences of LLD in a child?**
    Small amounts (0–2 cm) are of little consequence. Larger amounts are more difficult to hide and result in a larger energy expenditure during gait because of the up-and-down motion of the body mass.
    - 1 cm: Probably of no consequence; many people with LLDs in this range do not even know that they have an LLD
    - 1–2 cm: Easily hidden by the child's slightly bending one knee, hiking the pelvis, or walking on tiptoe
    - >2 cm: Produces a noticeable limp

21. **What are the consequences of an LLD in an adult?**
    As the ratio of body mass to muscle strength increases with growth, the ability of the person to compensate for the discrepancy decreases. Thus, a child might be able to hide a 5-cm discrepancy by bending the knee, but a full-grown adult cannot and pistons up and down, utilizing significantly more energy to walk.

22. **Is an LLD ever beneficial?**
    Surprisingly, yes. When the short leg is stiff or weak and a brace is required to stiffen the knee, hip, or ankle, it can be an advantage to be a little short (1–2 cm) so that the limb does not scuff the ground during the swing phase. Also, patients with deformities of the lumbar spine sometimes must stand with the pelvis tilted in order to make their trunks erect, and an LLD can accommodate this need. This example emphasizes the benefit of assessing functional LLD.

23. **Does LLD cause scoliosis?**
    When a patient with LLD is standing with both feet on the ground, there is pelvic obliquity and subsequent functional scoliosis to keep the trunk upright. Little time is spent in this position, however; thus, the effects on the spine are probably minimal. Keep in mind that some diseases that cause LLD can also cause scoliosis (e.g., polio).

24. **Does LLD cause back pain?**
    This is controversial. LLD up to 2.5 cm is unlikely to cause back pain.

25. **Who should manage this condition?**
    Because analysis, prediction, and treatment techniques require special expertise, these patients should be treated by pediatric orthopaedic surgeons with a special interest in this subject.

26. **What are the guidelines for selecting the appropriate treatment?**
    See Table 38-2.

27. **What are the limitations of a shoe lift?**
    Shoe lifts smaller than 2 cm can fit inside a shoe and thus can be moved between different pairs of shoes. Shoe lifts larger than 2 cm must be attached to the sole of the shoe and thus are permanent and may be unsightly. If the lift is larger than 5 cm, it can potentiate ankle instability, and an ankle/foot orthotic (AFO) extension is often indicated.

TABLE 38-2. GUIDELESS FOR THE APPROPRIATE TREATMENT OF LEG-LENGTH DISCREPANCY (LLD)	
LLD at Maturity	**Treatment Options**
<2 cm	No treatment required
2–6 cm	Shoe lift, epiphyseodesis, or femoral shortening to equalize the leg lengths
6–8 cm	Leg lengthening
6–20 cm	Combination of lengthenings, shortening, and epiphyseodesis
>20 cm	Amputation and prosthetic fitting

28. **What means are available to perform an epiphyseodesis?**
   - **Percutaneous:** This method involves the destruction of the growth plate medially and laterally under fluoroscopic guidance by means of a drill. This is now the most popular method used for this procedure, and it is usually performed through small stab incisions on the medial and lateral aspects of the growth plate.
   - **Staples:** Blount introduced the use of three medial and three lateral staples to arrest growth, with the assumed advantage that the procedure is potentially reversible by removal of the staples. Permanent epiphyseodesis occasionally occurred, however, and the staples sometimes backed out and necessitated reoperation. This technique is now of historical interest only.
   - **The Phemister technique:** A rectangular block of bone, two thirds on the metaphyseal side and one third on the epiphyseal side, is removed and replaced in the reverse position. This technique has been abandoned in favor of the percutaneous approach.

29. **What are the limitations of femoral shortening?**
   A femur can be acutely shortened up to approximately 5 cm. Any more than this and the quadriceps may not recover its preoperative strength. The wound also becomes more difficult to close.

30. **What are the contributions of the major physes in the total growth of the lower extremity?**
   - **Proximal femur (i.e., the capital physis):** 15%
   - **Distal femur:** 37%
   - **Proximal tibia:** 28%
   - **Distal tibia:** 20%

31. **How much does the femur grow from its proximal and distal physes?**
   - **Proximal:** 25%
   - **Distal:** 75%

32. **How much does the tibia grow from its proximal and distal physes?**
   - **Proximal:** 60%
   - **Distal:** 40%

33. **What work-up should a patient with hemihypertrophy undergo?**
   Because of the association between Wilms' tumor and hemihypertrophy, a patient with the diagnosis of hemihypertrophy should undergo an abdominal ultrasonogram yearly until the age of 5 years. In order to avoid excessive investigation, understand that this relationship is with hemihypertrophy, not hemiatrophy or congenital short limb.

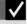

KEY POINTS: LEG-LENGTH DISCREPANCY

1. In a growing child, always plan correction based on the predicted discrepancy at maturity, not the present discrepancy. Failure to observe this rule is the most common source of error.

2. Appreciate that lengthening procedures are difficult and risky. Lengthening is a procedure of last resort and is rarely done for discrepancies anticipated to be less than 6 cm since other good options are available.

34. **How can you predict the ultimate LLD at maturity?**
There are currently four methods available for use:
- The Green-Anderson method
- The Menelaus method
- The Moseley straight-line graph
- The multiplier method

   Both the Green-Anderson method and the Moseley straight-line graph method utilize the information published by Anderson and Green, who compiled information relating the leg lengths of children to chronological and skeletal age. From these graphs, one can determine the growth percentile of the child and the growth remaining in the long leg. Both the Green-Anderson and the Moseley methods utilize exactly the same information, but in different ways.

   The Menelaus method is based on the assumptions that the distal femur grows approximately $\frac{3}{8}$ inch per year and the proximal tibia grows $\frac{1}{4}$ inch per year, that boys stop growing at age 16 and girls at age 14, and that the discrepancy increases by $\frac{1}{8}$ inch per year. Using this method, one can make fairly good predictions for those patients whose skeletal maturity corresponds to their chronological age and who are in their later years of growth.

   Paley has published the multiplier method, and again this is derived from the original Anderson data. The multiplier is the inverse of the percentage of mature leg length achieved and is age- and sex-specific. For congenital deformities, the current LLD is multiplied by this factor to give the predicted LLD at maturity.

35. **What are the advantages of a leg-lengthening procedure?**
There are two distinct advantages to leg lengthening. One is that the procedure is almost always performed on the abnormal (i.e., the short) limb. Parents are much more likely to understand and accept this. The other advantage is that the patient achieves a height that is appropriate for the long, normal leg. Patients and parents recognize that there are social benefits to being tall.

36. **What are the disadvantages of a leg-lengthening procedure?**
Lengthening requires a prolonged treatment time, with the potential for major complications to arise at any stage during the actual lengthening period, during the consolidation period, or following removal of the lengthening device. Numerous hospital clinic visits are necessary during the lengthening process. The patient and family must be committed to the treatment and all that it entails and must comply with instructions regarding the actual lengthening and physical therapy to maintain joint motion. The majority of patients undergoing a lengthening will have some complications and many have major complications.

37. **How is a bone lengthened?**
An appropriate lengthening device is chosen and applied to the bone to be lengthened using pins, wires, or a combination of these. An osteotomy is performed, preferably in metaphyseal bone. The lengthening process occurs in three phases, as follows:
- **Wait period:** 7–10 days to allow the healing process to begin.

- **Lengthening:** Distraction proceeds at 1 mm per day until the target correction is achieved or a problem provides a reason to stop.
- **Consolidation:** The device stays in place for several months until the bone in the lengthening gap becomes strong enough for its removal.

38. **What types of lengthening devices are available?**

There are a number of lengthening devices on the market. All are similar in that (1) they must be fixed to the bone above and below the site to be lengthened, and (2) they utilize one or more threaded rods that are turned gradually to achieve the desired length. The devices differ in complexity and the method of fixation.

- **Simple lengthening devices:** These allow only distraction at the lengthening site. In general, they are half-pin external fixators that are attached to the bone by large threaded pins. The pins stick out through the skin on one aspect of the leg and are attached to the device. Once attached, they do not allow angular or rotational changes of the bone. Examples include the Orthofix device.
- **Complex lengthening devices:** These allow gradual angular and rotational changes, as well as distraction, to lengthen the bone. In general, they are attached to the bone by thin, tensioned wires that are inserted completely through the limb. The wires are attached to rings that surround the limb. The rings are attached to each other by threaded rods and hinges. Using these devices, complex deformities can be corrected at the same time as the bone is lengthened. Examples include the Ilizarov device. The Taylor spatial frame uses a complex computer-controlled system for correcting complex deformities in three planes.
- **Lengthening nails:** These are on the horizon but are not yet in widespread use. They have the very significant advantages that they are entirely internal and can be left in place for a long time, thereby avoiding the complication of fracture through the lengthening gap.

39. **How fast should a limb be lengthened?**

In general, the soft tissues are the rate-limiting factor. Ilizarov suggested that the nerves are the most sensitive to stretch and seem to regenerate at approximately 1 mm/day, so most lengthenings are now performed at this rate. This 1 mm/day can be achieved with a 0.25-mm lengthening approximately every 6 hours. This has also been shown to be the optimal rate for bone regenerate formation but, if bone regeneration appears inadequate by x-ray, it is possible to slow, stop, or even reverse temporarily the lengthening.

40. **How long will an external fixator need to be used?**

The fixator needs to support the bone until it has matured enough to tolerate full weightbearing without external support. The rule of thumb is that the total time is usually about 1 month/cm lengthened. Thus, for a 60-mm lengthening, the fixator would be on 60 days for the lengthening plus an additional 120 days for consolidation. The radiographic appearance of the lengthening site is of prime importance in deciding when to remove the fixator, and the presence of three cortices is often taken as the prerequisite.

41. **When a patient is undergoing a lengthening procedure, why should you always check the blood pressure?**

Acute hypertension can occur. The mechanism is not clear, but shortening the lengthening gap resolves this problem reliably. After the blood pressure has returned to normal, the lengthening can be resumed and the hypertension may not recur.

42. **What can the patient and the parents do to ensure success?**

The child's participation, and therefore the support by parents, is an essential ingredient for success. In particular, in femoral lengthening, it is essential for the patient to participate vigorously in an exercise program to maintain knee motion. Maintaining full knee extension is especially important because a loss of even a few degrees of extension can be a harbinger of knee subluxation. It is a good idea to make a contract with the family at the start to establish that lengthening will not be continued in the face of a flexion contracture of more than 10 degrees.

43. What are some of the most common pitfalls in the treatment of LLD?

- **Making mistakes in arithmetic:** Always be sure to write the measurements on the x-ray film with a soft lead pencil and to check and recheck the measurements and the math on all scanograms prior to making a clinical decision.
- **Focusing too narrowly on the radiologic measurements:** It is essential to assess the functional LLD when deciding upon treatment goals.
- **Correcting the current discrepancy in a growing child:** Be sure to correct the predicted discrepancy at maturity.

44. List some of the recognized complications of leg-lengthening procedures.

- Incomplete corticotomy or osteotomy
- Pin-site irritation
- Pin-site infection
- Joint contractures (e.g., ankle equinus and knee flexion contractures)
- Joint dislocation (e.g., hip or knee)
- Premature consolidation
- Deformity arising in the regenerate (e.g., valgus femur)
- Pin breakage or cut out
- Delayed consolidation of the regenerate, especially associated with cigarette smoking
- Hypertension
- Failure to achieve desired lengthening
- Osteomyelitis
- Fracture or deformity in the regenerate following removal of the fixator device
- Premature spontaneous physeal closure or accelerated physeal growth

BIBLIOGRAPHY

1. Anderson M, Green W, Messner M: Growth and predictions of growth in the lower extremities. J Bone Joint Surg Am 45:1–14, 1963.
2. Anderson M, Messner M, Green W: Distributions of the lengths of normal femur and tibia in children from one to eighteen years of age. J Bone Joint Surg Am 46:1197–1202, 1964.
3. Aronson J: The biology of distraction osteogenesis. In Bianchi Maiocchi A, Aronson J (eds): Operative Principles of Ilizarov. Baltimore, Williams and Wilkins, 1991, pp 42–52.
4. Blount WP, Clarke GR: Control of bone growth by epiphyseal stapling. A preliminary report. J Bone Joint Surg 31:464–478, 1949.
5. Gross RH: Leg length discrepancy: How much is too much? Orthopedics 1:307–310, 1978.
6. Menelaus M: Correction of leg length discrepancy by epiphyseal arrest. J Bone Joint Surg Br 48:336–339, 1966.
7. Moseley C: A straight-line graph for leg-length discrepancies. J Bone Joint Surg Am 59:174–179, 1977.
8. Moseley C: Leg length discrepancy and angular deformity of the lower extremities. In Morrissy RT, Weinstein SL (eds): Lovell & Winter's Pediatric Orthopaedics, 4th ed. Philadelphia, J.B. Lippincott, 1996, pp 849–901.
9. Paley D, Bhave A, et al: Multiplier Method for predicting limb-length discrepancies. J Bone Joint Surg 82-A:1432–1446, 2000.
10. Rang M: Leg length discrepancy. In Wenger DR, Rang M (eds): The Art and Practice of Children's Orthopaedics. New York, Raven Press, 1993, pp 508–533.

CHAPTER 39

LEG ACHES

Richard E. McCarthy, MD

1. **What are leg aches?**

   Leg aches is a term that has been proposed by some to replace the often misunderstood disease entity referred to as *growing pains*. Leg aches refer to generalized pains or discomfort felt in children's legs bilaterally late in the day or at night. They occur in 13% of boys and 18% of girls and have a benign nature and an idiopathic origin. No functional disability or objective signs are associated with leg aches, and they generally resolve spontaneously with the completion of growth. Leg aches may be due to an as yet unknown specific syndrome, and most authors feel that discounting leg aches as growing pains does an injustice to children. It is important that this diagnosis be made by excluding all other possible causes.

2. **What age group is most affected by leg aches?**

   Leg aches generally start at about the age of 4 years, when the discomfort is most pronounced, but they can affect children up to 12 years of age. Pain in the limbs accounts for 7% of pediatrician visits every year.

3. **What are the most common causes of leg aches?**

   The cause is unknown, but the pattern of pain supports the commonly held theory that this is due to fatigue of the muscles in the thighs and calf.

4. **What are the usual patterns of pain?**

   The most common sites of pain are at the front of the thighs, in the calves, and behind the knees. Occasionally, pains are felt in the groin. The pain is generally outside the region of the joints. The pain is typically bilateral; this is important because serious causes of pain in the limbs are usually unilateral. Leg aches usually occur late in the day and in the evening, occasionally awakening a child from sleep. The pain typically is gone in the morning and does not limit the child's activities during the day.

5. **What should be asked of the parents when taking a history of a patient with leg aches?**

   Certainly, the time of day of occurrence and the area of localization of the pain are important. The words used to characterize the pain may reflect a cramping pain of muscle fatigue or the deep, aching pain of bone tumors. The location is important, whether it is bilateral or unilateral or localized to one region of the limb. Whether this is associated with swelling or affects gait or overall health should also be noted. The date of onset of the pain may correspond with initiation of a new sports activity. How long the pain has been present and whether it is a daily pain felt for a few minutes or for hours may shed some light on how serious this problem is. Whether medication helps to relieve the pain may pinpoint the diagnosis; for example, pain secondary to a benign osteoid osteoma typically abates with salicylates. The child's overall constitution needs to be questioned; poor general health and an attitude of malaise may indicate that a hematologic disorder such as leukemia causes the leg aches.

6. **How do I examine a child for leg aches?**

   Examination of the child begins with initial observation. The child who sits in the corner of the examination room playing quietly with toys and then stands to stroll casually or even to run toward the parent may indicate a more benign pattern to the disorder. The movements of the legs or back may be restricted in situations of infection or neurologic disorders. Distracting the child and getting him or her to play with toys or to walk along with the parent will give the examiner an indication of how fluid and natural the gait may be. Range of motion through the hips, knees, and ankles should be checked, as well as examination of the joints to look for swelling, especially along the medial aspect of the parapatellar border.

Starting the examination of the limbs away from the areas of complaint will yield more information, saving a potentially tender area for the last part of the examination. Asking the child to stand on tiptoes and heels and making a game of the examination is especially helpful for a determination of muscle function. Reflexes, including abdominal reflexes, must be checked to rule out any spinal cord abnormalities. The circumference of the thighs and calves may indicate atrophy or hypertrophy of musculature when comparing one side with the other. Measurement of leg lengths may indicate a leg-length inequality such as one might expect with a hemangioma near a growth plate or with atrophy due to a tethered spinal cord. Any restriction in the range of motion, whether it is due to contracture or guarding from pain, may indicate joint disease rather than simple leg aches.

7. **What is the differential diagnosis for leg aches?**
Most unknown causes will fall into the categories of congenital, infectious (i.e., inflammatory), metabolic, tumor, or traumatic (CIMTT). Utilizing the CIMTT mechanism for your approach to unknown causes allows you to consider the differential diagnosis in an orderly fashion. Congenital causes would include disorders such as clubfeet or dislocated hips, which may have produced subtle deformities as yet not diagnosed. Infections, including Brodie's abscesses, may also cause leg aches. Inflammatory disease, including monoarticular juvenile rheumatoid arthritis and other forms of arthritis, should be considered, as should tumors, local or remote. Osteoid osteoma in the upper femur may be hard to diagnose without ancillary studies. Tumors of the spinal cord may produce leg symptoms as well. Other spinal disorders including tethering must be considered. Traumatic causes, including stress fractures, may be subtle; a bone scan may be helpful in making this diagnosis. Specific diseases about the hip must also be considered, such as toxic synovitis, Perthes' disease, and slipped capital femoral epiphyses, which often manifest with a limp or pain in the thigh.

8. **What ancillary studies will help in the initial evaluation of leg aches?**
If there is any question about the motion, function, or tenderness of a specific area, then radiographs must be considered. Knee pain in a child is often referred from the hip. Therefore, when ordering radiographs for knee pain in children, an anteroposterior (AP) pelvis film should be considered as well. When considering a hip disorder, a frog lateral film is also helpful, especially when diagnosing a subtle slipped capital femoral epiphysis. A full-length AP view of the pelvis and both legs can easily be acquired in the smaller child to assess both legs fully. If there is any doubt regarding the diagnosis or if the parents are expecting a radiograph, you should proceed with the study.

Blood studies, including a complete blood cell count with differential and sedimentation rate, may be helpful in certain cases to eliminate the possibility of hematologic disorders such as leukemia or to eliminate suspicion of infectious causes. The use of a bone scan may be necessary when persistence of the symptoms necessitates further examination. Certainly, you would use follow-up repeat examinations and attempts at simple treatment before proceeding to the second line of tests, which includes bone scans, magnetic resonance imaging (MRI), and computed tomography (CT) scans. If you are considering the possibility of a spinal cord origin for the leg aches, then inclusion of the entire spine will put the matter to rest since it is possible that a syringomyelia can cause distal symptoms from its location in the spinal cord.

9. **Do medications help in the treatment of leg aches?**
Some physicians have recommended the use of salicylates or other anti-inflammatories at bedtime to help with treatment of leg aches with an evening or a nocturnal pattern. Others have

utilized stretching exercises in conjunction with the anti-inflammatories and a warm bath prior to bedtime.

KEY POINTS: LEG ACHES

1. History and physical exam are key to understanding the extent of the problem.
2. Occasionally, leg aches are early signs of significant importance.

10. **What are the danger signs to watch for?**
    A persistent pattern of night pain waking the child from sleep, especially with a unilateral location, is worrisome. You might fear the presence of a tumor such as a benign osteoid osteoma. In that case, bone scan results would generally be positive.

11. **What is the expected outcome for the child with simple leg aches?**
    Children outgrow leg aches and grow into normal adults without any restrictions in activities.

12. **What is the most important fact to remember about leg aches?**
    It is critical not to write these off as simply growing pains. A careful history and physical examination may be all that are necessary. Reassurance of the parents and an invitation to return should the pattern of the pain change or persist may be sufficient treatment. For the worrisome child, follow-up visits offer the opportunity for repeat examination and further history-taking. For the child with a limp or functional limitation, additional tests will certainly be necessary to rule out other possible causes. The greatest diagnostic error is to make the diagnosis of growing pains while overlooking a serious underlying condition.

BIBLIOGRAPHY

1. Bowyer SL, Hollister JR: Limb pain in childhood. Pediatr Clin North Am 31:1053–1081, 1984.
2. Peterson H: Growing pains. Pediatr Clin North Am 33:1365–1372, 1986.
3. Staheli LT: Fundamentals of Pediatric Orthopaedics. New York, Raven Press, 1992, pp 2.7, 2.8, 4.1.
4. Wenger DR, Rang M: The Art and Practice of Children's Orthopaedics. New York, Raven Press, 1993, pp 194–198, 223–226.

CHAPTER 40

LIMPING

David E. Westberry, MD, and Jon R. Davids, MD

1. **What is a limp?**
   A limp is defined as an abnormal gait pattern. Limping may be secondary to pain, weakness, or deformity of the musculoskeletal system.

2. **How can a limp be classified?**
   Limping can be classified by the following:
   - A description of the abnormal gait pattern
   - The absence or presence of pain
   - The age of the child at the time of presentation
   - The anatomic region involved

3. **What are the most common abnormal gait patterns associated with limping?**
   - Antalgic gait
   - Trendelenburg gait
   - Stiff-knee gait
   - Equinus gait
   - Steppage gait
   - Short-leg gait

4. **What is an antalgic gait?**
   An antalgic gait is a painful gait. It can be caused by pain in the lower extremity or the back. It is characterized by a decreased duration of the stance phase on the affected limb. To avoid pain, the child will take quick and soft steps (i.e., short stepping) on the involved extremity. If the source of pain is the back (from discitis or osteomyelitis), the child may refuse to walk completely or may walk very slowly to avoid jarring his or her back. The most common causes of an antalgic gait are trauma or infection.

5. **What is a Trendelenburg gait?**
   A Trendelenburg gait (i.e., abductor lurch or compensated gluteus medius lurch) is caused by weakness or inadequate strength of the hip abductor muscles. In this gait pattern, the trunk shifts over the stance phase limb to decrease the load on the ipsilateral hip abductor muscles. This gait is commonly seen in development dysplasia of the hip (DDH), congenital coxa vara, and coxa vara secondary to other conditions such as Perthes' disease or slipped capital femoral epiphysis (SCFE).

6. **What is a stiff-knee gait?**
   A stiff-knee gait is characterized by keeping the knee extended or stiff during the stance phase and is secondary to dysfunction (i.e., weakness or spasticity) of the knee extensors (i.e., the quadriceps).

7. **What is equinus gait?**
   Toe walking, or equinus gait, can be caused by muscle imbalance or poor motor control about the ankle. Bilateral toe walking can be seen in diplegic cerebral palsy, muscular dystrophy, and idiopathic toe walking.

8. **What is a steppage gait?**
A steppage gait is characterized by increased hip and knee flexion during the swing phase to help promote adequate clearance of the foot and ankle. Weakness of the ankle dorsiflexors may be compensated for by a steppage gait.

9. **What does a short-leg gait look like?**
Structural deformity of the musculoskeletal system may result in a limb-length inequality. During the stance phase, an apparent trunk shift over the short limb is seen secondary to increased downward pelvic obliquity in the coronal plane. Circumduction of the long extremity, vaulting of the short extremity, or both, are common compensations. Circumduction of the long side is described as increased hip abduction, upward pelvic obliquity, and increased pelvic rotation on the long side during the swing phase. Vaulting of the short extremity is seen as an early heel rise during the stance phase to assist with clearance of the long side in the swing phase.

10. **What are the essential questions when evaluating a limp?**
   - Is there pain?
   - Is the child sick?
   - Was the onset of the limp sudden or gradual?
   - What type of limp does the child have?
   - Can the source of the pain be localized?
   - Is the limp getting better or worse, or is it staying the same?

11. **What are the most important points in taking the clinical history?**
A thorough history is vitally important in making the diagnosis of the cause of limping. A key differentiating element is whether the limp is associated with *pain*. If pain is present, its location and duration, as well as aggravating and ameliorating factors, should be ascertained. A complete review of systems should be obtained, including any recent systemic illness (with or without fever) or antecedent trauma. Pertinent perinatal history, as well as any previous treatment for the limp, should be included in the medial history. In the absence of pain, the clinical history should establish when the limp began, who first noticed it, and whether it is associated with certain factors such as shoe wear or activities and whether it is consistently or inconsistently present.

12. **What are the most important points in the physical examination?**
The physical examination should be systematic, anatomically based, and comprehensive. The exam should begin with the spine and should work its way down through the pelvis and the lower extremities. The spine should be examined for obvious deformity, noting the sagittal posture of the child as well as palpation for bony tenderness and soft tissue swelling. Each bone should be palpated and each joint put through an active and passive range of motion. Each joint should be examined for point tenderness, swelling, erythema, and warmth. Stress testing should be performed on all ligamentous and tendinous structures. Manual muscle testing for strength and selective control should be performed at all levels. Proximal muscle weakness (usually associated with muscular dystrophies) can be appreciated by asking the child to rise from a seated position on the floor (i.e., the Gower maneuver); use of the hands on the thighs to substitute for weak hip extensors constitutes a positive finding.

13. **How do I use observational gait analysis?**
Observational gait analysis should be performed with the child wearing the least amount of clothing possible. It should be done in a long hallway, and the child should be observed in both the coronal (i.e., walking toward and away from the observer) and sagittal (i.e., walking past the observer in both directions) planes. Global assessment should focus on speed, stability, balance, and symmetry. Observations of the ankle in the sagittal plane should include the following:

- The heel strike at initial contact
- Flat foot in midstance
- Timing of the heel rise (just prior to the opposite swing limb contacting the floor)
- Alignment in the swing phase

The foot-progression angle and hindfoot alignment in stance and swing are the most important observations made of the foot and ankle in the coronal plane. The knee is observed primarily in the sagittal plane. Attention should be directed to its position at the following moments:

- At initial contact (extended)
- During the loading response (a small flexion wave)
- During the swing phase (a large flexion wave)

The hip should be fully flexed at the beginning of the stance phase and fully extended at the end of the stance phase. The pelvis should exhibit minimal dynamic deviations in all planes. The trunk should be stable throughout the gait cycle. The upper extremity should exhibit a reciprocal swinging pattern that is out of phase with the ipsilateral lower extremity. For small children who may be uncooperative or afraid, asking them to walk toward an object or to attempt to pick up a toy or a piece of candy off of the floor may give clues to the source of the limp. Bending at the knee instead of through the lumbar spine may lend evidence toward the spine as the source of pain.

14. **What is the clinical algorithm for the evaluation of a *painful* limp?**

The most common causes of a painful limp in a child include trauma, infection, inflammation, and tumor. The history and physical should focus on the duration of symptoms and the location of the source of pain. Swelling, discoloration, limitation of motion, and point tenderness should be noted. Plain radiographs of the involved extremity may demonstrate the presence of fracture (i.e., acute trauma), periosteal new-bone formation (i.e., subacute fracture, infection, or tumor), radiolucency (i.e., osteomyelitis), or structural deformity (i.e., Perthes' or SCFE). In a limping toddler in whom symptoms cannot be localized, a plain film of the entire lower extremity from hip to feet may be helpful.

Appropriate laboratory studies include the complete blood count, the erythrocyte sedimentation rate, and the C-reactive protein. Evaluation of these studies helps to differentiate between acute infectious etiologies and other noninflammatory causes of limp. Although the presence of other serologic indicators of rheumatologic disease (such as antinuclear antibody, rheumatoid factor, and HLA-B27) may be helpful clinically, the absence of these markers does not rule out the presence of this group of diseases. Further imaging can be obtained with computed tomography (CT) to provide increased bony detail or magnetic resonance imaging (MRI) to provide increased soft tissue detail. Ultrasound of the hip joint can provide evidence for the presence of a hip joint effusion, but it cannot differentiate between transient synovitis and acute septic arthritis. When the location of the cause of a painful limp cannot be determined, which may be the case in infants and younger children, a nuclear medicine scan (usually a three-phase technetium-99m bone scan) is the most effective imaging study.

KEY POINTS: LIMPING

1. The most common causes of limp are trauma, infection, inflammation, and tumor.

2. To accurately diagnose the cause of a limp, a complete history and physical exam, with appropriate laboratory evaluation and medical imaging, are required.

3. The differential diagnosis for limp is age-specific. Common causes of limp in a young child are different from those in the older child and adolescent.

15. **What is the clinical algorithm for the evaluation of a *nonpainful* limp?**

In the absence of pain, the differential diagnosis should focus on structural musculoskeletal (congenital and developmental), neurologic, and metabolic diseases. The key elements of the physical examination include the assessment of limb length and limb girth, as well as the neurologic evaluation. Limb length is best assessed with the patient standing and the examiner palpating the iliac wings. Wooden blocks are placed beneath the short side until the limb lengths are equalized. This method relies on both proprioception and visual assessment and is more accurate than methods that involve measuring from either the umbilicus or the anterosuperior iliac spine to the medial malleolus when the patient is supine.

The neurologic examination should include assessment of muscle strength and selective control (i.e., manual muscle testing), sensation, spasticity, and deep tendon reflexes. Diagnostic laboratory studies are appropriate only when considering muscle and metabolic diseases. Plain radiographs are appropriate when considering structural problems such as hip dysplasia or femoral hypoplasia. Limb lengths may be determined by plain radiography (i.e., orthoroentgenography) or by CT scan. Electrodiagnostic studies (i.e., nerve conduction studies and electromyography), muscle biopsy, and chromosomal analysis are appropriate only after the more common problems have been ruled out.

16. **What are the most common causes of limp in a child of 0–5 years of age?**

An accurate diagnosis of the etiology of limping in this group is often challenging, but it is also the most critical (Table 40-1). Many children in this group are learning to walk and demonstrate an immature gait pattern characterized by a wide base of support and a toe-strike foot pattern. A typical mature gait pattern is established by age 3–7. Irritability, refusal to stand, or not using the extremity are common descriptions of the child's presentation. The history from the child's caretakers may be vague, and the child may not cooperate with the exam. The physician's goal is rule out the more serious causes of limping, including septic arthritis, osteomyelitis, hip dysplasia, fracture, tumor, and nonaccidental trauma. Limited hip motion accompanied by fever, an inability to walk, an elevated sedimentation rate (>40 mm/hr), and an elevated white blood cell (WBC) count (>12,000 cells/cmm) are suggestive of septic arthritis and warrant urgent hip aspiration. Growing pains usually do *not* cause limping. Instead, growing pains are characterized by transient aching in the legs or knees at night that typically are variable, intermittent, and resolve over time.

17. **What are the most common causes of a limp in a child of 5–10 years of age?**

Children in this age group are generally able to give a good clinical history and to cooperate with the physical examination. Although infection is still a common cause of limping in these children, other conditions related to growth (e.g., apophysitis) and increased physical activity (e.g., fractures and sprains) are frequently seen (Table 40-2). This is the most common age group for presentation of Perthes' disease, transient synovitis of the hip, and Duchenne's muscular dystrophy.

18. **What are the most common causes of a limp in a child of 10–15 years of age?**

Limping in this age group is more commonly due to acquired causes related to increased levels of physical activity, also known as overuse injuries, particularly about the hip and knee (Table 40-3). The adolescent growth spurt is often accompanied by apophysitis and the peripatellar pain syndrome. Once the physes have closed, athletic injuries in teenagers become similar to those seen in adults. This is the most common age group for the presentation of slipped capital femoral epiphysis and spondylolysis or spondylolisthesis. Children who develop Perthes' disease at this age have a distinctly worse outcome than those who present in the younger age group.

TABLE 40-1. COMMON CAUSES OF LIMP IN A CHILD OF 0–5 YEARS OF AGE

Ankle/Foot	Knee/Tibia	Hip/Femur	Pelvis/Spine	Other
Clubfoot	Septic arthritis	Hip dysplasia	Discitis	Nonaccidental trauma
Osteomyelitis	Osteomyelitis	Synovitis	Osteomyelitis	Cerebral palsy
Juvenile rheumatoid arthritis	Toddler's fracture (tibial)	Septic arthritis		Acute lymphocytic leukemia
	Discoid lateral meniscus	Osteomyelitis		Congenital limb-length inequality (femoral, tibial, or fibular)
	Congenital patellar dislocation			Acquired limb-length inequality (i.e., Ollier's disease or neurofibromatosis)
	Juvenile rheumatoid arthritis			
	Infantile tibia vara (i.e., Blount disease)			

TABLE 40-2. COMMON CAUSES OF LIMP IN A CHILD OF 5–10 YEARS OF AGE			
Ankle/Foot	**Knee/Tibia**	**Hip/Femur**	**Pelvis/Spine**	**Other**
Calcaneal apophysitis (i.e., Sever's disease)	Tibial tubercle apophysitis (i.e., Osgood-Schlatter disease)	Perthes' disease	Discitis	Muscular dystrophy
Navicular osteochondritis (i.e., Köhler's disease)	Osteochondritis dissecans	Synovitis	Osteomyelitis	Hereditary motor sensory neuropathy (i.e., Charcot-Marie-Tooth disease)
Tarsal coalition	Growing pains	Septic arthritis	Septic arthritis	Friedreich's ataxia
Trauma (i.e., fractures or sprains)	Trauma (i.e., fractures or sprains)	Osteomyelitis	Spondylolysis	
Juvenile rheumatoid arthritis	Tumor (i.e., osteochondroma, unicameral bone cyst, nonossifying fibroma, Ewing's sarcoma, or osteogenic sarcoma)	Tumor (i.e., unicameral bone cyst, nonossifying fibroma, Ewing's sarcoma, or osteogenic sarcoma)		
Osteomyelitis				
Cavus foot				

TABLE 40–3.   COMMON CAUSES OF LIMP IN A CHILD OF 10–15 YEARS OF AGE

Ankle/Foot	Knee/Tibia	Hip/Femur	Pelvis/Spine	Other
Tarsal coalition	Tibial tubercle apophysitis (i.e., Osgood-Schlatter disease)	Slipped capital femoral epiphysis	Pelvic apophyseal avulsions or apophysis	Hereditary motor sensory neuropathy (i.e., Charcot-Marie-Tooth disease)
Accessory navicular calcaneal apophysitis (i.e., Sever's disease)	Patellar apophysitis (i.e., Sinding-Larsen)	Perthes' disease	Osteitis pubis	
5th metatarsal apophysitis	Peripatellar pain syndrome	Hip dysplasia (i.e., subluxation)	Spondylolysis	
Stress fracture (calcaneus or metatarsals)	Patellare dislocation (acute or recurrent)	Tumor (i.e., Ewing's sarcoma or osteosarcoma)	Spondylolisthesis	
Trauma (fractures or sprains)	Ligament injuries		Lumbar (i.e., Scheuermann's disease)	
	Osteochondritis dissecans		Diastematomyelia	
	Meniscal injuries		Tethered cord	
	Tumor (i.e., osteochondroma, Ewing's sarcoma, or osteosarcoma)			

BIBLIOGRAPHY

1. Bucholz RW, Lippert FG, Wenger DR, Ezaki M: Orthopaedic Decision Making. St. Louis, Mosby, 1984, pp 214–220.

2. Flynn JM, Skaggs DL: Staying Out of Trouble in Pediatric Orthopaedics. Philadelphia, Lippincott Williams & Wilkins, 2005, pp 144–151.

3. Flynn JM, Widmann RF: The limping child: Evaluation and diagnosis. J Am Acad Orthop Surg 9:89–98, 2001.

4. Herring JA: Tachdjian's Pediatric Orthopaedics, 3rd ed. Philadelphia, WB Saunders, 2002, pp 83–94.

5. Lloyd-Roberts GC, Fixsen JA: Orthopaedics in Infancy and Childhood, 2nd ed. London, Butterworth-Heinemann, 1990, pp 215–216.

6. Phillips WA: The child with a limp. Orthop Clin North Am 18:489–501, 1987.

7. Scoles PV: Pediatric Orthopedics in Clinical Practice, 2nd ed. Chicago, Year Book Medical Publishers, 1988, pp 1–22.

8. Staheli LT: Fundamentals of Pediatric Orthopaedics, 3rd ed. Philadelphia, Lippincott Williams & Wilkins, 1998, pp 40–41.

9. Sutherland DH: Gait Disorders in Childhood and Adolescence. Baltimore, Williams & Wilkins, 1984, pp 51–64.

10. Tolo VT, Wood B: Pediatric Orthopaedics in Primary Care. Baltimore, Williams & Wilkins, 1993, pp 278–283.

11. Wenger DR, Rang M: The Art and Practice of Children's Orthopaedics. New York, Raven Press, 1993, pp 50–76.

CHAPTER 41

INTOEING AND OUT-TOEING

Lynn T. Staheli, MD

1. **What is intoeing?**

   Intoeing is a medial rotation of the foot in the transverse plane relative to the direction in which the child is walking. Sometimes when families describe their child's problem as a turning in of the feet, this may describe either intoeing or flatfoot. Ask for more information to make this distinction.

2. **How common is intoeing?**

   Intoeing is very common; torsion problems account for the greatest number of referrals of children to orthopaedists.

3. **Is intoeing abnormal?**

   Usually not. We define abnormal conditions as those that fall beyond 2 standard deviations (SDs) from the mean. Many normal children who intoe fall within the normal range and may be considered to have a developmental variation—that is, a variation of normal that resolves spontaneously. If the rotational deformity is severe and falls outside this 2-SD range, we describe the condition as a torsional deformity.

4. **What is the natural history of intoeing?**

   The lower limb shows a triphasic sequence of rotational development, as follows:
   - **Embryonic phase:** Initially, the limb bud is formed with the great toe in a preaxial position—that is, with the great toe pointing laterally. Over the next few weeks of embryonic development, the limb rotates medially to bring the great toe to the midline.
   - **Fetal phase:** The second phase includes the remainder of intrauterine life and early infancy. During this intrauterine period, the lower limbs are positioned in lateral rotation in the uterus. This results in a lateral rotation contracture of the hips. This lateral rotational contracture resolves during early infancy.
   - **Childhood phase:** The third phase occurs during infancy and childhood. Both the tibia and the femur gradually rotate laterally with growth.

5. **What is the background of the conditions that cause intoeing?**

   There are several known causes of rotational deformities.
   - **Developmental variations:** The reason for the wide range of normal is unclear. We are not aware of any functional reasons to account for this development sequence. Normal variability accounts for the majority of rotational problems.
   - **Genetic causes:** In other children, the pattern of limb development appears to be genetic. Medial femoral torsion is often seen in both a girl and her mother. Medial tibial torsion has been described to run in certain families. It is likely that we inherit the shape of the lower limbs, just as we do any other physical characteristic. Examining the parents of children with rotational problems often uncovers a more subtle rotational deformity in the parent similar to that of the child.
   - **Intrauterine position:** Intrauterine position is the likely cause of lateral rotational contracture of the hip, metatarsus adductus, and possibly medial tibial torsion.

6. **What conditions cause intoeing?**

The clinical conditions include medial femoral torsion, medial tibial torsion, and forefoot adductus. Often, deformities are multiple. For example, in the infant, forefoot adduction (i.e., metatarsus adductus) and medial tibial torsion often exist together, each contributing to the degree of intoeing.

7. **What is the rotational profile?**

The conditions that cause intoeing can be differentiated by measuring the child's rotational profile and comparing these values with published normal values. This profile is determined by physical examination. The values may be measured but, for practical reasons, are usually estimated and are expressed in degrees. These values document the level and severity of the problem. The rotational profile includes several measurements:

- **Foot progression angle (FPA):** This is the number of degrees the foot turns in or out relative to the direction of walking. Intoeing values have a minus sign preceding the number of degrees. Usually, mild intoeing is 0 to 10 degrees, moderate is 10 to 20 degrees, and severe is more than 30 degrees of intoeing. Most children and adults will walk in an out-toeing with an FPA between 0 and 30 degrees. When estimating the FPA, focus on one foot at a time. Because the FPA will often change with each step in the infant or young child, make your estimates based on an average number of steps.
- **Arc of hip rotation:** This measures the arc of motion with the child prone. Flex the knees to a right angle and rotate both thighs concurrently. Let the limbs fall to the level of maximum rotation without force. If necessary, rotate both limbs concurrently to the level of the pelvis. Measure both medial rotation (MR) and lateral rotation (LR). When measuring LR, it is necessary for the patient's legs to be crossed. Measure the maximum rotation as the vertical-tibial angle. The normal values change with age. The arc of hip rotation during early infancy is primarily lateral due to contracture secondary to the intrauterine position. In late infancy and early childhood, the arc shows similar values for MR and LR. Later in childhood and in the teen years, LR exceeds MR as the femur rotates laterally, which is associated with declining degrees of femoral anteversion. During childhood, the upper range of MR is about 70 degrees for girls and 60 degrees for boys. Girls tend to intoe slightly more than boys. Normally, the total arc of motion is about 90 degrees, but this will be greater in individuals with ligamentous laxity and less in tight-jointed individuals. Beware of asymmetric hip rotation. This is often a sign of hip disease and is the basis of the hip rotation test (HRT) used for screening for hip disease. Asymmetric hip rotation is an indication for radiography of the pelvis.
- **Thigh-foot angle (TFA):** This is a measure of tibial rotation. With the foot in a quiet resting position, estimate this angle by comparing the axis of the foot with that of the thigh. Precede the number of degrees with a minus sign if the axis of the foot is turned in (i.e., medial) compared with the axis of the thigh. The TFA rotates laterally with increasing age. A minus value for TFA is often seen in infants. A minus value during childhood or the teen years that falls outside the normal range is referred to as medial tibial torsion (MTT). The upper range of normal is plus 30 degrees. Values beyond that level are abnormal and are described as lateral tibial torsion (LTT).
- **Foot:** The shape of the sole of the foot is easily assessed with the patient prone. Normally, the lateral border is straight. A convex lateral border is indicative of forefoot adductus (right foot in Fig. 41-1).

8. **What are the pitfalls of diagnosis?**

To avoid overlooking underlying disease when assessing a child with a rotational problem, first order a screening examination to make certain that the rest of the musculoskeletal system is normal. Assess hip abduction and symmetry to rule out hip dysplasia. Be aware that children with mild diplegia or hemiplegia (i.e., cerebral palsy) may present with a rotational problem. Out-toeing in the older child or teenager may be a sign of slipped capital femoral epiphysis.

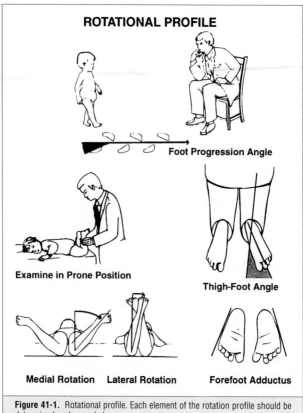

Figure 41-1. Rotational profile. Each element of the rotation profile should be determined and recorded.

9. **Is age at presentation useful in diagnosis?**
   Yes. In early infancy, inward rotation of the feet is usually due to metatarsus adductus. In the toddler, intoeing is most likely due to MTT. Intoeing in early childhood (especially in girls) is most likely due to medial femoral torsion.

10. **Does intoeing require treatment?**
    Not usually. The vast majority of cases will resolve spontaneously over time. The conditions that are most likely to require treatment are rigid forefoot adductus (i.e., metatarsus varus) and severe intoeing that persists into late childhood or the teen years.

11. **Are shoe modifications, braces, or night splints useful?**
    No, with one exception: in metatarsus varus. In the past, intoeing children were prescribed all sorts of devices: twister cables, night splints, shoe wedges and inserts, and so forth. Every study has shown these devices to be ineffective; the improvement is due to natural history, not treatment. Not only are the devices ineffective and usually unnecessary, but they probably also harm the child and are expensive for the family.

12. **Does intoeing ever persist and cause disability?**
    Yes. Like everything else in medicine, exceptions do occur. Rarely, metatarsus varus, MTT, and femoral torsion may persist. The frequency of persistent disease severe enough to produce

symptoms is less than 1%. I believe that these severe persistent deformities are often genetically based and are different from the usual developmental variations. The disability is usually functional and cosmetic.

13. **Does a rotational deformity at one level cause problems in other joints or in the spine?**
No. This cascading of problems is frequently described to justify various treatments but is unfounded.

14. **Is surgical correction of intoeing ever necessary?**
Rarely. Operative rotational osteotomy of the femur or tibia is indicated only for a severe disabling deformity that persists beyond the age of 10 years.

15. **How can I convince the family that observation is best?**
   - Take the family's concerns seriously. This is a real concern to them. See what is bothering the family. For example, if the family members are concerned about how much the child intoes while running, watch the child run.
   - Make an accurate diagnosis by performing a screening examination and the rotational profile. Thoroughness will instill confidence. Knowing the cause of the rotational problem makes possible a more accurate prediction of the natural history.
   - Provide reassurance. Explain the natural history and the reason why letting the condition resolve without interference is best for the child.
   - Offer to follow the progress if the family wishes.

16. **How long do rotational problems take to resolve?**
Resolution is often slow and usually occurs over months or sometimes several years. When told that the condition will resolve on its own, many parents expect this to take only a few weeks or a few months. Orthopaedic time is slow!

17. **When should I refer the child to the orthopaedist?**
   - **For additional reassurance:** The most common indication will be a family who requires additional reassurance. Make certain that you inform the orthopaedist of the reason for the referral—to reassure the family, and not necessarily for treatment.
   - **For uncertain diagnosis:** If the findings are not clear or if an abnormality is found on the screening examination that poses a problem, referral is indicated.
   - **For an older infant or child with stiff forefoot adductus:** The child may be a candidate for cast or brace treatment.
   - **For an older child or adolescent with a disability due to a rotational problem:** If the problem appears to be permanent and disabling, operative correction may be necessary.

18. **If the family insists that something be done, what should I do?**
Prescribe a healthy lifestyle for the child: exercise through play activities, limited television watching, and healthy diet. Avoid mechanical devices since these can be harmful in addition to being ineffective.

19. **Do sprinters intoe?**
In our study of high school sprinters, we found that sprinters have a smaller TFA than control subjects and tend to intoe more often than nonsprinters while running. This suggests that mild MR of the tibia enhances running. We concluded that slight MR allows the toe flexors to be more effective in enhancing push-off.

FOREFOOT ADDUCTUS

20. **What is forefoot adduction?**
Forefoot adductus is a transverse plane deformity in which the forefoot is medially angulated relative to the hindfoot. Forefoot adductus may be due to metatarsus adductus or metatarsus varus, or it may be part of the skewfoot deformity.

21. **What is metatarsus adductus?**
Metatarsus adductus is a common flexible form of forefoot adduction secondary to intrauterine positioning. Like other positional deformities, it improves spontaneously and resolves in the first months or year of life. Treatment is usually unnecessary.

22. **What is metatarsus varus?**
Metatarsus varus is an uncommon form of forefoot adduction that is stiff and is more persistent than the common form. In some cases, the first cuneiform is triangular in shape. Persisting deformity produces little disability. It is not a cause of bunions. Since the disability is only cosmetic, correction with serial corrective casts or bracing may be appropriate. Operative correction should be avoided because the risk of complications exceeds the benefits.

23. **What are skewfeet?**
Skewfeet (also called *Z feet* and *serpentine feet*) are a rare, complex deformity including forefoot adduction, midfoot abduction, and heel valgus. This deformity is often present in loose-jointed children, is sometimes familial, is often bilateral, but is often asymmetric in severity. The natural history is poorly understood, and the potential for disability in adult life is uncertain. Nonoperative treatment is not effective. Delay operation correction until mid-childhood, and correct the deformity by lengthening the calcaneus and the first cuneiform.

24. **How should flexible forefoot adductus in the infant be managed?**
First examine the hips to rule out hip dysplasia. Note the degree of flexibility of the foot. The more flexible the foot, the more rapid the resolution. Some physicians ask the parents to massage or stretch the foot. I do not recommend this because it is unlikely to make any difference, and, if the condition persists, the parent will feel responsible for the failure of treatment. The severity can be documented by clinical description, tracing the shape of the foot on paper, recording the shape of the foot with a copy machine or photography. Radiographs are not appropriate. See the infant again in 3–4 months. Most will improve. Stiff adductus or a failure of improvement are indications for treatment. Most primary care physicians will elect to refer infants requiring treatment to an orthopaedist.

Braces or casts that extend above the knee are most effective. The knee is flexed to 90 degrees, and the foot is laterally rotated to the position of maximum comfort. This stabilizes the hindfoot. The forefoot is then abducted and held in either the cast or a long-leg brace. Short-leg braces or casts are much less effective because the rotation of the hindfoot is poorly controlled.

TIBIAL TORSION

25. **What is tibial torsion?**
Tibial torsion is a deformity in which the horizontal plane of the tibia is rotated medially or laterally beyond the normal range (plus or minus 2 SD). The deformity may be medial (i.e., internal) or lateral (i.e., external). MTT is common in the toddler. LTT is most common in late childhood or adolescence. In contrast to femoral torsion, tibial torsion is often asymmetric and

may be unilateral. Since the human tibia tends to rotate to the right, unilateral MTT is more common on the left, and LTT is more common on the right.

26. **Should tibial torsion be treated with a night splint?**
This is controversial. The evidence indicates that resolution occurs with or without treatment. Splints are a hassle for the family and the child. If you use splints, restrict their use to nighttime only. Daytime devices are clearly much more harmful because they may limit play and alter the child's self-image. I do not recommend treatment of tibial torsion during infancy or early childhood.

27. **When is surgical correction necessary?**
Operative correction of tibial torsion is rarely necessary. MTT continues to improve until growth is complete. LTT increases with growth, is more serious, and is more likely to require operative correction than MTT. The severity of deformity that requires correction is influenced by the rotational status of the femur since femoral rotation can aggravate or compensate for tibial torsion. Generally, if the TFA is more medial than minus 10 degrees or more lateral than plus 40 degrees, operative correction may be considered.

28. **How is tibial torsion corrected surgically?**
The tibia is divided transversely and is rotated to correct the deformity. The osteotomy is best performed in the tibia at about 2 cm above the distal growth plate. The osteotomy is fixed with crossed smooth pins that are left protruding through the skin for ease in removal. If rotation of more than 25 degrees is required, the fibula may also require division. A long-leg cast is necessary to supplement the cross-pin fixation. The leg is immobilized for 7–8 weeks. Both tibias can be corrected at the same time, but the child will require a wheelchair for mobility while the osteotomies heal. Although correction can also be achieved with proximal tibial osteotomy, upper tibial osteotomy is more likely to be complicated by compartment syndrome or peroneal nerve palsy.

FEMORAL TORSION

29. **What is femoral torsion?**
Femoral torsion is an abnormal twisting (i.e., rotation in the transverse plane) of the femur. This femoral twisting is defined as the angular difference between the axis of the upper femur and that of the knee. Since the hip is a ball-and-socket joint that allows about 90 degrees of rotation, the axis of the upper femur rather than the joint serves as the proximal point of reference. Normally, the upper femur is anteverted—that is, the head and neck are angled forward relative to the rest of the femur. Increased anteversion allows increased medial hip rotation equivalent to a medial rotational deformity. The upper femur may be retroverted or angled posteriorly. Retroversion is uncommon and results in increased LR of the hip. An abnormal increase in anteversion or retroversion is sometimes called antetorsion and retrotorsion. For consistency, we prefer the terms medial femoral torsion (MFT) and lateral femoral torsion (LFT).

30. **What is the natural history of anteversion?**
At birth, femoral anteversion averages 40 degrees. Anteversion spontaneously decreases with growth and averages 10 degrees for adult men and 15 degrees for adult women.

31. **What are the clinical features of MFT?**
MFT usually first becomes clinically noticeable in early childhood. We believe that MFT is not seen in infancy because it is masked by the LR contracture of the hip. As this contracture resolves, abnormalities in the shape of the femur become apparent and the clinical features of MFT may develop.

MFT is more common in girls and may be familial. It is not uncommon for the mother to describe having the same problem as her child. Examination of the parents often shows a milder degree of MFT. The child with MFT intoes and stands with the patella pointing medially, which is sometimes described as the cross-eyed or squinting patella. Running is awkward and is described as an eggbeater running style. The child sits with the legs medially rotated, described as the reverse tailor or M position. MR of the hip is increased, and LR is decreased. Usually, we consider MFT to be mild if medial hip rotation is 70–80 degrees, moderate if between 80 and 90 degrees, and severe if more than 90 degrees.

32. **Are radiographs or other imaging studies necessary?**
Usually not. Although the degree of femoral anteversion can be measured with special imaging studies, imaging is not necessary unless hip rotation is asymmetric or operative correction is planned.

33. **What happens without treatment?**
MFT usually peaks in severity between the ages of 4 and 6 years and then improves. After that, the condition becomes muted. In less than 1% of cases, the condition is severe, and disability persists into late childhood or adolescence. The child continues to intoe, running is awkward, and the altered function and appearance pose a problem. For these rare cases, operative correction may be appropriate.

34. **Does the use of twister cables or night splints change the natural history of MFT?**
No. Such treatment simply adds another disability for the child and should be avoided.

35. **Does MFT cause osteoarthritis of the hip or functional problems in adult life?**
No. In the past, MFT was thought to cause arthritis and severe functional problems in adult life. We studied the relationship between measured anteversion in adults with osteoarthritis and control subjects and found no relationship. We also found no relationship between anteversion and physical performance in adults. Operative correction of MFT should not be considered prophylactic.

36. **How should I manage femoral torsion?**
Manage the family's concerns, as described previously. Emphasize the natural history of spontaneous resolution. Encourage the family and child not to focus on the problem. Discourage the family from telling the child, "Turn your feet out," or "Don't sit that way." Do not allow them to insist that the child take ballet lessons. Encourage the family to explain the reasons for this method of management to other family members or the preschool staff. Offer to discuss the problems with other concerned adults. If the family insists on doing something, encourage a healthy lifestyle for the child, as discussed previously. If additional reassurance is necessary, it may be time to get a second opinion from an orthopaedist who deals with such problems frequently.

37. **Are orthotics useful in the management of MTF?**
No. Changing the position of the foot will not affect the bony configuration of the femur. In addition, MFT does not lead to foot deformities, and foot problems do not cause MFT.

38. **How is MFT corrected surgically?**
MFT may be corrected operatively if the deformity is severe (i.e., an MR of 90 degrees or an LR of 0 degrees) and if the child has a significant cosmetic and functional disability and is older than 10 years. The correction is achieved with a rotational femoral osteotomy. This may be

performed at any level, but we have found that correction at the proximal femoral level is best. The femur is divided transversely and the distal fragment rotated 45 degrees laterally. Whether a cast is necessary depends on the rigidity of the internal fixation. Operative correction is effective and permanent, usually corrects the problem, and improves function but is not without risks; it should be undertaken only for a severe deformity.

OUT-TOEING

39. What is out-toeing?
The feet are normally turned out in relation to the direction of walking. We naturally out-toe. The normal range throughout most of life is from neutral position to about 30 degrees of out-toeing.

40. What are the causes of out-toeing?
Physiologic lateral rotation contracture of infancy. Most infant feet turn out when first supported in the upright position. This pattern resolves during the first year. We often see infants because one foot turns out. This is usually due to the combination of bilateral physiologic LR contracture of infancy and unilateral MTT on the opposite side. It is usually the right foot that is turned out since unilateral MTT is more common on the left side. No treatment is required.

LTT can be a major problem. Since the tibia normally rotates laterally with growth, LTT tends to become worse. Sometimes it becomes severe enough to require correction with a tibial osteotomy. LTT has been found to be associated with osteochondritis dissecans and Osgood-Schlatter disease.

LFT, or retrotorsion, is very rarely severe enough to require operative correction. It may be a risk factor in developing a slipped capital femoral epiphysis. Some evidence suggests that it may increase the risk of osteoarthritis of the hip in later adult life.

Lateral torsion is more serious than medial torsion. We have traditionally focused most on intoeing. Out-toeing is being recognized as the more serious problem as it worsens with growth and is associated with significant problems.

KEY POINTS: INTOEING AND OUT-TOEING

1. With growth, the lower limb normally externally rotates.

2. Intoeing spontaneously improves, whereas out-toeing may become more severe.

3. Out-toeing has the potential of causing many more problems than intoeing.

4. Nonoperative measures do not correct femoral or tibial torsion.

5. Avoid treating the child to satisfy the parents. Unnecessary treatment is harmful for children.

TORSIONAL MALALIGNMENT

41. What is the torsional malalignment syndrome (TMS)?
The combination of MFT and LTT is the most common form. The FPA is normal, but the knee is rotated medially during walking or running. A less common form is the reverse: LFT and MTT.

42. **What are the clinical features of TMS?**

TMS is usually seen in teenaged patients who complain of knee pain. The pain is patellofemoral in origin, with symptoms of chondromalacia patellae, sometimes patellar subluxation, or, rarely, dislocation. Because the knee is rotated medially, the quadriceps tends to displace the patella laterally, causing or aggravating patellofemoral instability.

43. **How should TMS be managed?**

First, apply the routine treatment for chondromalacia—that is, activity modification or restriction, nonsteroidal analgesics, and so forth. Avoid lateral releases. In rare situations, correction with a double osteotomy may be required to correct the underlying bony deformity.

44. **Can TMS be prevented?**

Not at present. We are unable to predict which children are likely to develop TMS. Nonoperative management does not change the torsion of the femur or tibia, and prophylactic single-level osteotomy would likely cause a great number of complications. Possibly in the future, prospective natural history studies will make it possible to predict which children are at risk, and we will be able to selectively correct single-level torsional deformities before compensatory deformity develops.

BIBLIOGRAPHY

1. Lincoln TL, Suen PW: Common rotational variations in children. J Am Acad Orthop Surg 11:312–320, 2003.
2. Staheli LT, Corbett M, Wyss C, King H: Lower-extremity rotational problems in children. J Bone Joint Surg 67A:39–47, 1985.

CHAPTER 42

BOWLEGS AND KNOCK KNEES

Peter M. Stevens, MD

1. **What should be asked in the history of a child with bowlegs or knock knees?**
   The age at presentation and the observed trend (worsening versus improving) are critically important. Up until the age of 2, there is a prevalence of physiologic bowlegs. Between the ages of 3 and 6 years, knock knees are exceedingly common. The onset or persistence of angular deformities after these respective ages should be viewed with suspicion. Likewise, asymmetric deformities and those associated with functional impairment or pain should be investigated and documented radiographically. A history of trauma, infection, or tumor may account for local or regional growth disturbance, causing clinical deformity.

   The family history is relevant and may underscore the parents' concerns. Persistent familial angular deformities, especially in family members affiliated with short stature, should raise concerns about metabolic disorders or inheritable skeletal dysplasias. On the other hand, spontaneous resolution of deformities in older siblings or parents may prove to be reassuring. The pre- and perinatal histories, along with information about growth and development milestones, are also relevant. Early walking may be associated with bowlegs; late walking may imply neuromuscular disease.

2. **What are the physical findings?**
   With **bowlegs**, when a person stands erect with his or her feet together and ankles touching, the knees should touch as well. Any separation between the knees is indicative of bowlegs; the greater the distance, the more serious the implications. Although you can make a qualitative assessment of infants, this deformity is not typically noted before the child can stand. In these young children, physiologic ligamentous laxity will accentuate the bow. Documented by tape measure (or finger breadths) as the intercondylar distance, this is a very reproducible measurement that even the parents can monitor. Concomitant torsion deformities often include outward torsion of the femora and inward torsion of the tibiae, each of which contributes to the bowed appearance. The child usually has an intoeing gait pattern and may be prone to tripping. You may observe some lateral thrust of the knee during gait due to physiologic ligamentous laxity. The findings are typically symmetrical, and the limb lengths are equal. Progressive, asymmetric, or unilateral bowing or associated limb-length discrepancy should raise suspicion regarding underlying disease and should prompt further investigation, starting with radiographs.

   With **knock knees**, the distance measured between the ankles when the child is standing erect with knees touching reflects the presence and severity of knock knees. Once again, ligamentous laxity, particularly in younger children, will accentuate the deformity. The intermalleolar distance may be readily measured and recorded by the parents, serving as an indicator of severity and progression. There is often coexisting outward torsion of the femur or tibia. In adolescence, the combination of inward femoral torsion and outward tibial torsion, known as *miserable malalignment,* may produce the appearance of knock knees. This is best documented in the prone position, recording the torsional profile. In more severe cases, you may note lateral tilt and even instability of the patella. The gait pattern is marked by circumduction, which is more pronounced with running. When knock knee is unilateral or associated with limb-length inequality, there may be underlying disease and progressive deformity. Idiopathic genu valgum developing or persisting in a teenager is typically bilateral and is unlikely to resolve spontaneously.

3. **What imaging studies are appropriate?**

A standing, full-length anteroposterior (AP) radiograph of the lower extremities, with both knees extended and the patellae pointing straight forward, will provide useful information pertaining to the major joints and their respective epiphyses. The tilt of the pelvis and the comparative length of the long bones are readily ascertained; note the contour of the shaft as well as the quality of the trabecular bone and the growth plates. By drawing a plumb line from the center of each femoral head to the center of the ankle, you can readily see where the center of gravity passes relative to the knee. By adolescence, this line, which is called the *mechanical axis*, should bisect the knee (Fig. 42-1). The angle subtended by the articular surfaces of the tibia and femur and their respective shafts should also be measured.

In a symptomatic patient with knock knees, a patellar sunrise view, taken with the knees flexed 30 degrees, may reflect the lateral patellar tilt of subluxation.

For persistent or increasing clinical deformities, follow-up radiographs are indicated annually (or semiannually) to document progression and to plan intervention. In adolescents, the status of the growth plates should be noted, particularly if hemiepiphysiodesis is being contemplated. It may be helpful to obtain an AP radiograph of the hand to assess skeletal maturity. Other imaging studies such as scanography, computed tomography (CT), or magnetic resonance imaging (MRI) are seldom beneficial.

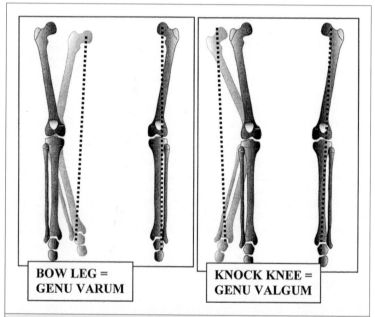

BOW LEG = GENU VARUM

KNOCK KNEE = GENU VALGUM

Figure 42-1. Note the mechanical axis *(dotted line)* in genu varum and genu valgum. Normally, on a standing radiograph, a line drawn from the center of the femoral head to the center of the ankle should bisect the knee. With normal alignment, the knee and physes are protected, able to resist intermittent compression due to gravity and activities while shielded from shear stress. Likewise, the collateral ligaments are protected and are able to stabilize the knee and the patella.

4. **Are laboratory studies useful?**

In rare cases when metabolic disturbances are suspected to be the cause of the deformity, it is helpful to assess serum and urinary calcium and phosphate, along with alkaline phosphatase and, occasionally, thyroid function tests. Genetic anomalies may also be documented by chromosomal analysis in selected patients.

5. **Do these conditions require treatment? By whom?**
Primary care providers or trained health care professionals may safely triage and manage most patients, referring only those with suspicious or recalcitrant deformity. In the overwhelming majority of children with bowlegs presenting before the age of 2 and those with knock knees presenting before age 6, the condition will resolve spontaneously. The natural history of each condition is typically benign because the deformities are self-correcting. Therefore, the current philosophy is that corrective shoes and bracing are superfluous and represent an unnecessary expense. Despite parent education and reassurance, it is still wise to see the children annually until your prediction is fulfilled and their legs are straight.

The minority of children who do not follow the expected course or those with unilateral deformity, limb-length inequality, or pain should be referred for evaluation by an orthopaedist. His or her role is to determine the cause and to intervene judiciously. The goal of intervention is to achieve and maintain straight legs of equal length, alleviating (or averting) pain and instability. The historic approach of applying braces has yielded to an all-or-nothing philosophy; physiologic deformities are best observed, whereas pathologic problems should be treated surgically.

6. **What are the controversies with bracing?**
Parental anxiety, often compounded by pressure from grandparents, may produce an atmosphere of "don't just stand there, do something!" Often a parent or relative wore braces or corrective shoes and obtained a good result. It may prove difficult to convince them that the satisfactory outcome was despite, rather than due to, the treatment. Having excluded pathologic bowing or knock knee, the managing physician must educate the concerned parents regarding the benign natural history of these deformities.

I find it helpful to date and label a diagram of the legs, comparing sequential measurements on a semiannual or annual basis. For the extreme skeptics, I am apt to show them before and after radiographs of another child who outgrew the problem without treatment. I further explain that bracing requires three-point fixation with the knee locked in extension—a very unphysiologic situation. Pointing out the ligamentous laxity at the knee, I explain that bracing may exacerbate ligamentous stretch without producing documented beneficial effect on the growth plates. The cost of unnecessary bracing is also an important consideration.

A lingering controversy is the potential benefit of bracing children with bowlegs due to type I (i.e., mild) Blount disease. This is a pathologic condition involving the posteromedial growth plate of the proximal tibia. Given the difficulties of radiographic analysis, including interobserver error, many of these children may actually have physiologic bowing and be destined for spontaneous resolution.

Adolescent idiopathic knock knees behave differently; these patients frequently have anterior knee pain and functional limitations. One controversy pertains to the type and severity of symptoms deemed worthy of intervention. Recognizing that conservative management, such as exercises, physical therapy, and bracing, are of no lasting benefit, one is left with the options of limiting sports and activities versus surgical intervention.

Most patients are unwilling to accept the deformity and adopt a sedentary lifestyle, hoping to reduce symptoms and avoid arthritis. Furthermore, activities of daily living such as kneeling, squatting, sitting, and descending stairs may produce pain. These patients are apt to seek out more aggressive treatment.

7. **What about hemiepiphysiodesis?**
Another controversy pertains to the preferred timing and technique of hemiepiphysiodesis to change the angle of growth, thereby straightening the limb (Fig. 42-2). The traditional method of surgical ablation of the physis, be it by open or percutaneous technique, produces permanent

closure. Therefore, timing must be perfect to avoid overcorrection. Unfortunately, estimation of skeletal maturity is imprecise (±1 year), so you must follow these patients closely and be prepared to arrest the opposite side of the growth plates to preserve a neutral mechanical axis. If this opportunity is missed, the patient may overcorrect and have to undergo corrective osteotomy.

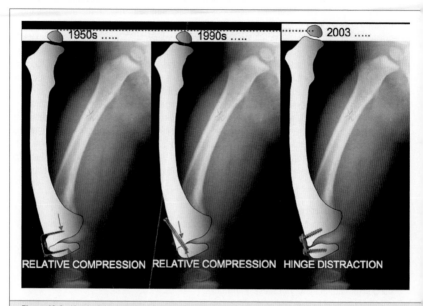

RELATIVE COMPRESSION   RELATIVE COMPRESSION   HINGE DISTRACTION

Figure 42-2. Hemiepiphysiodesis. Extraperiosteal application of a two-hole plate and screws provides a simple solution to the problems posed with staples or transphyseal screws. Rather than confronting the physis, the plate acts as a tension band, allowing continued growth to correct the angular deformity around a focal hinge point. This technique may be used in patients of any age.

KEY POINTS: BOWLEGS AND KNOCK KNEES

1. Growing children may go through phases during which *physiologic deformities* (bowlegs up to the age of 2 years and knock knees until the age of 6 years) are commonly encountered.

2. Intoeing often accompanies bowing, whereas out-toeing may accompany knock knees.

3. The characteristic features of *physiologic deformities* are that they tend to be symmetric and painless, and they improve with observation alone; no intervention is warranted. Corrective shoes and "Forrest Gump" braces are of no proven benefit; these are self-limiting conditions. The key is parent education and as-needed follow-up.

4. In contradistinction, *pathologic deformities* may be unilateral (or bilateral), causing gait disturbance and pain.

5. Pathologic deformities typically do not respond to brace treatment because braces are supportive rather than corrective. These deformities progress with growth.

6. Before resorting to corrective osteotomy, guided growth, redirecting one or more physes, may be the most appropriate treatment.

8. **What about the need for osteotomy?**

Osteotomy of the tibia and fibula, the femur, or all, is the classic approach for deformity correction (after all, *orthopaedic* literally means *straight child*). Compared to guided growth, this is a maximally invasive technique that involves cutting and stabilizing bones; this usually requires the application of pins or plates plus casts and restricted weight-bearing for several weeks while the bones are healing. Preoperative planning should be employed to preserve or restore equal limb lengths and a horizontal knee while neutralizing the mechanical axis. Osteotomies of the proximal tibia have earned a reputation for frequent complications, most notably compartment syndrome and peroneal nerve injury. Although some consider osteotomies to be definitive, further growth may still produce recurrent deformities. Therefore, these patients need to be followed until maturity.

9. **What is guided growth?**

Instrumented hemiepiphysiodesis for angular correction was first popularized by Blount in the 1950s. Employing reinforced staples, he was able to address genu valgum and genu varum by placing 2 or 3 staples at the apex of the deformity. This technique was traditionally reserved for adolescents because of concerns about premature physeal closure. With the advent of fluoroscopy, the technique was refined and the indications extended to younger children with a variety of physeal pathologies (Fig. 42-3). However, on occasion, staple migration or breakage

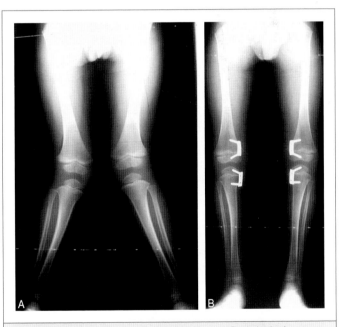

Figure 42-3. Guided growth offers an attractive alternative. By placing hardware (previously, staples; now, a two-hole plate and screws) around a physis, you may induce an angular change with continued growth. Provided that the periosteum is carefully spared, this method is a reversible means of manipulating the physis for deformity correction. Therefore, timing is not so critical; even young children with pathologic angular deformities may be successfully managed with a hinge plate, thus avoiding the need for angular correction. The plate or plates are removed when the legs are straight; further growth is monitored. *A,* Radiograph of a 6-year-old child with skeletal dysplasia. *B,* Radiograph of the same patient 12 month after application of guided growth.

may thwart correction or require unanticipated revision surgery. Enthusiasm for this method has waxed and waned accordingly.

Metazeau proposed the insertion of transphyseal screws in the medial femur or tibia to correct valgus and lateral screws to correct varus. This technique has gained limited popularity, partly due to concerns about potential damage to the physis. There are no documented cases of continued growth following screw removal. The technique may not be reversible, and, therefore, applications may be limited to adolescents with a finite (although sometimes unpredictable) amount of growth remaining.

10. **What is the prognosis?**
The prognosis is determined by the stability of the knee (including the patella), the orientation of the joint surface (parallel to the ground), and the location of the mechanical axis at maturity (females, age 14; males, age 16). With these attributes and a good range of motion and muscle strength, the knees should function well for decades.

- **Bowlegs:** If the mechanical axis falls in the medial compartment or medial to the knee, regardless of the cause, eccentric and pathologic compression of the medial meniscus and articular cartilage will accelerate the degenerative process, leading to secondary arthritis. In advanced cases, the lateral ligaments yield to excessive tensile forces, exacerbating this process. Once the medial articular cartilage has worn away, bone erosion ensues.
- **Knock knees:** With significant knock-knee deformities, the mechanical axis may produce pathologic compression of the lateral compartment, combined with tensile stresses on the medial ligaments and shear forces on the patella. The net result is patellar tilt and, in some instances, instability, along with accelerated water and degenerative arthritis involving the patellofemoral joint and the lateral compartment of the knee.

BIBLIOGRAPHY

1. Brooks W, Gross R: Genu varum in children: Diagnosis and treatment. J Am Acad Orthop Surg 3:326–335, 1985.
2. Heath DH, Stahell L: Normal limits of knee angle in children: Genu varum and genu valgum. J Pediatr Orthop 13:259–262, 1993.
3. Kling T, Hensinger R: Angular and torsional deformities of the lower extremities in children. Clin Orthop 176:136–147, 1983.
4. Mielke C, Stevens P: Hemiepiphyseal stabling for knee deformities in children younger than ten. J Pediatr Orthop 16:423–429, 1996.
5. Nouth F, Kuo LA: Percutaneous epiphysiodesis using transphyseal screws (PETS): Prospective case study and review. J Pediatr Orthop 24:721–725, 2004.
6. Salenius P, Vankka E: The development of the tibiofemoral angle in children. J Bone Joint Surg 57:259–261, 1975.
7. Shopfner CE, Colin CG: Genu varus and valgus in children. Radiology 92:723–732, 1969.
8. Stevens P, Holmstrom M: Genu valgum. Pediatric emedicine.com, 2002.
9. Zuege R, Kempken TG, Blount WP: Epiphyseal stapling for angular deformity at the knee. J Bone Joint Surg 61:320–329, 1979.

VII. FOOT AND ANKLE PROBLEMS

CHAPTER 43

FOOT PAIN

Matthew B. Dobbs, MD

1. **How do children present with foot pain?**
   Infants will withdraw the limb when the foot is touched or manipulated. Toddlers may limp or refuse to bear weight. Older children demonstrate an antalgic limp and may be able to isolate the pain to a specific site.

2. **What are the physical findings?**
   Most causes of foot pain are unilateral. This permits comparison between the two feet. The involved foot may be swollen, warm, red, or locally tender. Both acute and chronic problems may demonstrate limited motion, particularly in the subtalar joint. The normal callus distribution between the hindfoot and forefoot may be changed if there is a chronic problem leading to an abnormal weight-bearing position for the foot.

3. **What is the differential diagnosis for foot pain in infants, children, and adolescents?**
   See Table 43-1.

TABLE 43-1.	DIFFERENTIAL DIAGNOSIS FOR FOOT PAIN ACCORDING TO AGE	
<4 years	**4–10 years**	**>10 years**
Toddler's fracture (tibia or foot)	Fracture	Stress fracture
Osteomyelitis, septic arthritis	Osteomyelitis, septic arthritis	Osteomyelitis, septic arthritis
Juvenile rheumatoid arthritis	Osteochondritis dissecans	Osteochondritis dissecans
Foreign body in the foot	Sever's apophysitis	Juvenile rheumatoid arthritis
Benign or malignant tumor	Accessory tarsal navicular	Accessory tarsal navicular
Flatfeet	Foreign body in the foot	Tarsal coalition
Growing pains	Benign or malignant tumor	Benign or malignant tumor
	Flatfeet	Flatfeet
	Growing pains	Growing pains
	Osteochondrosis	Osteochondrosis

4. **Why is taking a good history important?**
   The history often provides clues to obtaining an accurate diagnosis. The pattern, onset, and duration of pain often suggest the origin. Acute onset of pain over a few days makes one suspicious for trauma, infection, or malignancy, whereas gradual worsening over months suggests mechanical or inflammatory symptoms. It is also important to note the timing of pain. Morning pain and pain after inactivity are more characteristic of an inflammatory process. Pain after activity may suggest a stress fracture or an osteochondral lesion. Night pain that wakes a

child from sleep may represent growing pains but also raises the concern for a tumorous process. A past medical history focusing on recent trauma or exposure to infectious diseases can be very helpful. Recent infections may render the child susceptible to opportunistic bone and joint infections. The review of systems should explore whether there is a history of recent fever or weight loss, suggestive of infection or malignancy.

5. What is essential in the physical examination of a child with foot pain?
The child should be dressed in such a way that the examiner can see and examine the entire lower extremities. You should first watch the gait of the child to observe limp and symmetry of gait. Next, with the child on the examining table, you should inspect for asymmetry, erythema, deformity, swelling, and rashes. Puncture wounds or foreign bodies should be sought on the plantar aspect of the foot in ambulators. Palpation of the lower extremity to locate the point of maximum tenderness is often the most revealing part of the physical examination. Knowing the exact location of the pain often significantly limits the differential diagnosis. It is important to examine every joint of the lower extremity, especially in those cases in which it is difficult to localize the pain.

6. What imaging studies should be obtained?
Anteroposterior and lateral radiographs that visualize the joint above and below the joint of maximum tenderness are warranted. If the history and physical examination fail to localize the site of pain, then a triphasic technetium-99m bone scan is an option.

7. When are laboratory tests indicated?
Laboratory testing is indicated in any child who presents with an acute nontraumatic limp and signs of fever or malaise. Appropriate tests include a complete blood cell count with differential, erythrocyte sedimentation rate (ESR), a C-reactive protein, rheumatologic factor, and antinuclear antibody levels.

8. What are growing pains?
Growing pains are common in childhood and may affect up to 20% of all children at some time. This is a diagnosis of exclusion and is typically seen in children from 2–12 years of age who have benign pain in the calf, foot, knee, or thigh that is precipitated by exercise and routine physical activities. These pains usually occur in the afternoon, the evening, or the middle of the night but are never present in the morning. They often are relieved with massage or analgesics. The physical examination is unremarkable, and the laboratory studies are always normal. In most children, the problem spontaneously resolves by the age of 8 years. There are children who have exaggerated but benign pains that are similar to growing pains. These pains are often more frequent, more intense, can be present at any time of the day, and are increased by physical activity. These children often have hypermobile joints on exam. This ligamentous laxity in the feet can result in pes planus with pronation and pain in the medial side of the arch. The use of custom shoe inserts or orthotics placed inside inexpensive sneakers leads to symptomatic relief in nearly all cases. The inserts can be discontinued at any age, and a clinical trial can be performed to determine the need for their continued use.

9. What is a flexible flatfoot with a shortened tendo Achillis?
There is a small group of patients with a flexible flatfoot who gradually develop a shortened Achilles tendon, which limits hindfoot dorsiflexion. The heel becomes locked in valgus and equinus by the shortened heelcord. Pedal dorsiflexion during the stance phase of gait is transferred forward to the midfoot, leading to a flattened medial longitudinal arch and a painful callus beneath the talar head. Associated forefoot pronation creates a painful rigid flatfoot. Weight-bearing radiographs of this type of flatfoot show plantar sag in the midfoot. When a heelcord-stretching program is unsuccessful, there is the occasional need for a calcaneal neck lengthening osteotomy and Achilles tendon lengthening, both to relieve the hindfoot equinus and to lengthen the lateral column of the foot.

10. **What are the most common sports-related heel injuries?**
These include Achilles tendinitis, retrocalcaneal and Achilles bursitis, plantar fasciitis, calcaneal bursitis, calcaneal apophysitis, and calcaneal stress fracture. The specific diagnosis is made according to the anatomic location of pain, which may be accompanied by local swelling.

11. **What is Severs disease?**
Severs disease, or calcaneal apophysitis, is one of the most common overuse syndromes seen in growing children. It most commonly occurs in the age range of 6–12 years and is thought to be due to repeated microtrauma. Affected children present with activity-related pain over the posterior aspect of the calcaneus. Physical examination reveals tenderness to compression over the calcaneal apophysis. If the patient has bilateral symptoms, radiographs are often not necessary. In unilateral cases, however, radiographs of both feet should be obtained to rule out other causes of heel pain, including stress fractures, infection, and neoplastic lesions. Sever's disease is a self-limiting condition. Treatment includes activity limitation, casting, or both.

12. **What other conditions can cause heel pain?**
Soft tissue and osseous infections (e.g., a nail puncture wound) can occur. Bone tumors are uncommon, and malignant tumors are especially rare. Benign osteoblastoma, osteoid osteoma, and calcaneal cysts can occur. Ewing's sarcoma involving either the calcaneus or the talus is the most common hindfoot osseous malignancy. A tarsal tunnel syndrome can develop from a bone prominence (i.e., talocalcaneal coalition) or from mechanical stress to the posterior tibial nerve in the tarsal tunnel.

13. **What types of problems limit subtalar motion?**
These include congenital conditions (e.g., tarsal coalition); trauma, especially occult calcaneal fractures; and acquired inflammatory conditions including pauciarticular juvenile rheumatoid arthritis, inflammatory bowel disease, spondyloarthropathies, and juvenile-onset ankylosing spondylitis. These conditions can present with insidious onset of pain, swelling, and restricted inversion and eversion in the subtalar joint.

14. **What is tarsal coalition?**
A tarsal coalition refers to the union of two or more tarsal bones by fibrous, cartilaginous, or bone tissue. The most common sites of coalition are between the calcaneus and the navicular and between the talus and calcaneus. They occur in approximately 1% of the population, with a 2:1 male-to-female distribution. Symptoms most commonly develop when the coalition begins to ossify, with the calcaneonavicular coalition presenting between 8 and 12 years and the talocalcaneal coalition presenting between 12 and 16 years. Pain is the initial complaint and is usually insidious in onset. The pain in the talocalcaneal coalition can be poorly localized in the hindfoot, whereas calcaneonavicular coalition usually causes pain laterally in the area of the coalition. Subtalar motion is restricted to absent. The hindfoot is usually in valgus and the forefoot in abduction; the peronei may be contracted. Calcaneonavicular coalitions can be visualized on an internal oblique radiograph of the foot (Fig. 43-1), whereas coronal plane computed tomography (CT) scans are necessary to document the talocalcaneal coalition, which is most commonly located in the area of the sustentaculum tali. Symptomatic coalitions are best managed by excision of the bar. Triple arthrodesis is reserved for major coalitions involving more than one joint or for symptomatic degenerative arthritis.

15. **What condition can cause pain in the midfoot?**
Köhler disease is an osteochondrosis that affects the tarsal navicular. It is a self-limited condition characterized by pain or swelling in the area of the tarsal navicular in association with characteristic radiographic findings. It occurs in the age range of 4–7 years, with 80% of cases occurring in boys. The cause is unknown, but it is thought to be related to repetitive trauma. Physical findings include soft tissue swelling, erythema, and tenderness to palpation over the

tarsal navicular. Active and passive range of motion are normal. Radiographic findings include flattening and patchy ossification of the navicular bone, with preservation of its joint surfaces. Treatment of the condition is designed to relieve symptoms and not to hasten the reparative process. This can be usually be accomplished with cast immobilization and rest until the patient is asymptomatic, which is usually in 3–4 weeks. Without treatment, most patients have intermittent symptoms for 1–3 years that are activity related and are relieved by rest. Radiographic improvement is noted over the following year, and no long-term disabilities have been reported in patients despite lack of treatment (Fig. 43-2).

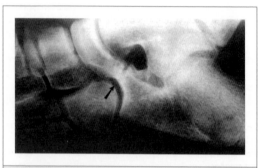

Figure 43-1. Tarsal coalition. The 45 degree oblique radiograph illustrates the calcaneonavicular bar.

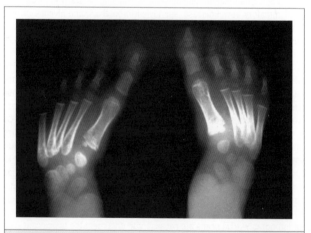

Figure 43-2. Köhler's disease. The avascular necrosis demonstrates bone resorption and sclerosis but retains its articular relationships.

16. **What is an accessory navicular bone?**
    An accessory navicular bone is another unique midfoot problem and occurs in 10% of patients older than the age of 5 years, with symptoms more commonly developing in girls. Pain and tenderness are localized to the prominent medial accessory navicular. An external oblique radiograph may be needed to visualize this accessory ossification center. Technetium bone scanning may show local increased uptake. Conservative management includes short-term use

of a walking cast or foot orthotic. Occasionally, this condition requires surgical resection because of the bursitis that develops between the navicular and its accessory bone.

17. **What are causes of pain in the forefoot?**

Freiberg infraction is a type of osteochondrosis characterized by aseptic necrosis of the metatarsal head, the second metatarsal being most often affected. This is most commonly encountered in the 13–18 year age group and has a predilection for female athletes. Clinically, patients present with pain and tenderness around the second metatarsophalangeal joint. This clinical finding should lead to radiographic evaluation. Radiographically, the second metatarsal head may have a flattened, enlarged appearance, with areas of increased sclerosis and fragmentation. The affected metatarsophalangeal joint may be narrowed, and secondary degenerative changes may be present in long-standing disease. The natural history is variable. Many cases are self-limited, with revascularization of the metatarsal head. Some cases, however, result in significant deformity and secondary degenerative changes at the metatarsophalangeal joint. Initial treatment includes decreasing activities and using metatarsal pads inserted in the shoe. In more acute cases, casting may be beneficial. Surgery is reserved for chronic problems.

18. **What are stress fractures?**

Stress fractures in the young athlete generally involve the diaphysis of the metatarsals. Initially, the pain is present with activity, but later it becomes constant with all weight-bearing. Physical examination will demonstrate well-localized pain. Swelling may not be a prominent finding. Repetitive running activities are more likely to lead to a metatarsal fracture, whereas basketball is associated with fractures of the hindfoot. This is particularly true in the older child with a less-flexible foot and greater bone rigidity. Nondisplaced fractures can be treated with rest and decreased activity for 6 weeks. More symptomatic stress fractures may require cast immobilization.

19. **What are unique problems causing ankle pain?**

Osteochondritis dissecans of the talus occurs in adolescent athletes and is more frequently found in males. A deeply aching sensation that is poorly localized may be the presenting complaint. This can be clinically distinguished from a chronic ankle sprain by the absence of tenderness over the anterior talofibular ligament. Swelling, bruising, and a limited range of motion of the ankle may be noted. A bone scan may be diagnostic if routine radiographs fail to demonstrate the lesion. Arthroscopic management may be required.

Dysplasia epiphysealis hemimelica is an uncommon skeletal lesion that describes isolated overgrowth of either the medial distal tibia or the talus. Children present within the first few years of life with an asymmetric swelling of the joint with associated limited range of motion or pain. Radiographs demonstrate an irregular enlargement of the involved growth center. Treatment depends on the symptoms and the degree of deformity, and the process completes its course at skeletal maturity. Attempts at surgical excision of the immature mass may lead to regrowth of the lesion and may also remove normal articular cartilage from the joint surface.

20. **What are other unusual causes of foot pain?**

Reflex sympathetic dystrophy can result from minor trauma and is associated with localized skin blanching or venous discoloration, increased or decreased skin temperature, and exquisite local tenderness and pain out of proportion to the original injury. Alternating contrast baths and the use of medication may be required in addition to immobilization in a weight-bearing cast.

A crushing type of pedal injury may result in a compartment syndrome. Pain on passive dorsiflexion of the foot and evidence of decreased circulation are important clues. Increasing pain in the foot with complaints of numbness or tingling in the toes is worrisome. The presence of pulses should not preclude this diagnosis, which can be confirmed by increased compartment pressure measurements. Prompt fasciotomy will be required to avoid amputation.

KEY POINTS: FOOT PAIN

1. Taking a good history is the key to obtaining an accurate diagnosis.

2. It is important to differentiate between flexible and rigid flat feet.

3. Tarsal coalition is an important cause of a rigid flatfoot in children and adolescents.

21. **What types of tumors can occur in children?**

There are a variety of benign bone tumors in the pediatric population. Osteoid osteoma is most common in the first decade, and the foot and tarsal bones are a common site. The radiographs demonstrate a radiolucent nidus generally surrounded by dense reactive bone. An osteoid osteoma generally presents with pain, classically greater at night, and is relieved by salicylates. The tumor can be managed by surgical resection, or the pain can be controlled with nonsteroidal anti-inflammatory medication. Osteoblastoma of the hindfoot and enchondroma of the metatarsals or proximal phalanges are also found. The calcaneus is the most common pedal site of a unicameral bone cyst. An aneurysmal bone cyst is an expansile cystic lesion that presents in the first 2 decades of life with swelling and pain and is generally localized in the metaphysis of the phalanges or the calcaneus.

Leukemia and Ewing's sarcoma are the two most frequent causes of malignant bone lesions. Synovial sarcoma is the most common malignant neoplasm of soft tissue. Its average age of presentation is 13 years, and it generally occurs in the soft tissues of the midfoot and hindfoot.

This is a slow-growing lesion that presents as a painless enlarging mass in close proximity to a joint. Radiographic analysis reveals a soft tissue mass arising in proximity to a joint or tendon sheath, which may have some calcification. A magnetic resonance imaging (MRI) scan shows an oval tumor with the same density as muscle.

BIBLIOGRAPHY

1. Angermann P, Jensen P: Osteochondritis dissecans of the talus: Long term results of surgical treatment. Foot Ankle 10:161–163, 1989.

2. Flynn JM, Widmann RF: The limping child: Evaluation and diagnosis. J Am Acad Orthop Surg 9:89–98, 2001.

3. Gould N, Moreland M, Alvarez R, et al: Development of the child's arch. Foot Ankle 9:241–245, 1989.

4. Harris RI, Beath T: Hypermobile flat-foot with short tendo-Achillis. J Bone Joint Surg Am 30:116–138, 1948.

5. Ippolito PT, Pollini R, Falez R: Köhler's disease of the tarsal navicular: Long-term follow-up of 12 cases. J Pediatr Orthop 4:416–417, 1984.

6. Jacob RF, McCarthy RE, Elser JM: Pseudomonas osteochondritis complicating puncture wounds of the foot in children: A 10 year evaluation. J Infect Dis 106:657–661, 1989.

7. Kirby EJ, Shereff MJ, Lewis MM: Soft tissue tumors and tumor-like lesions of the foot: An analysis of eighty-three cases. J Bone Joint Surg 71A:621–626, 1989.

8. Mosca VS: Flexible flatfoot and skewfoot. J Bone Joint Surg 77A:1937–1945, 1995.

9. Murari TM, Callaghan JJ, Berrey BH Jr, Sweet DE: Primary benign and malignant osseous neoplasms of the foot. Foot Ankle 10:68–80, 1989.

10. Olney BW, Asher MA: Excision of symptomatic coalition of the middle facet of the talocalcaneal joint. J Bone Joint Surg Am 69:539–544, 1987.

11. Scott RJ: Acute osteomyelitis in children: A review of 116 cases. J Pediatr Orthop 10:649–652, 1990.

12. Staheli LT, Chew DE, Corbett M: The longitudinal arch: A survey of eight hundred and eighty-two feet in normal children and adults. J Bone Joint Surg 69A:426–428, 1987.

13. Sullivan VA: Pediatric flatfoot: Evaluation and management. J Am Acad Orthop Surg 7:44–53, 1999.

BUNIONS

Matthew B. Dobbs, MD

CHAPTER 44

1. **What is a bunion?**

   A bunion is an abnormal prominence on the medial side of the first metatarsal head, with its accompanying bursa. A juvenile bunion or hallux valgus deformity has its onset in the preteen or teenage years, when the growth plates of first metatarsal and proximal phalanx are still open. By definition, a bunion deformity is greater than 14 degrees of lateral deviation of the hallux on the first metatarsal with an increased first-cuneiform–first-metatarsal angle, metatarsus primus varus, hallux valgus, and malrotation of the great toe.

2. **How is the deformity documented?**

   Standing anteroposterior and lateral radiographs of the foot are necessary to evaluate juvenile hallux valgus. The most notable and commonly recorded measurements are (1) the first-second intermetatarsal angle, (2) the first metatarsal-proximal phalanx angle, as well as (3) distal metatarsal articular angle (DMAA), (4) metatarsophalangeal (MTP) joint congruity, and (5) the relative lengths of the metatarsals (Fig. 44-1).

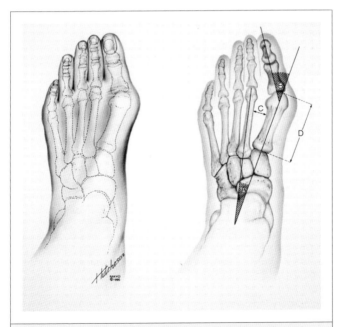

Figure 44-1. *Left,* Bunion deformity with underlying bone. *Right,* Radiographic bunion deformity measurements. *A,* First-second metatarsal angle. *B,* First metatarsal-proximal phalanx angle. *C,* First-second intermetatarsal distance. *D,* Length of the first metatarsal.

3. **What is the incidence of adolescent bunions?**
    The incidence is unknown. They are much more common in girls than in boys, with girls accounting for over 80% of operative cases.

4. **What is the cause of bunions?**
    Although the cause is unknown, there is a strong genetic component with case reports suggesting X-linked–dominant, autosomal-dominant, and polygenic transmission. In the typical patient, there is no congenital abnormality or underlying neurologic deficit. Bunions are commonly found in patients with neuromuscular disease (e.g., cerebral palsy), connective tissue disorders (e.g., Ehlers-Danlos syndrome), or relative shortening of the second metatarsal (e.g., multiple hereditary osteochondromatosis). Juvenile hallux valgus does not appear to be related to the use of constrictive shoewear.

5. **What complaints accompany bunions?**
    Most adolescents with hallux valgus are asymptomatic. Complaints are usually centered around the appearance or pain. Pain is typically a problem with shoewear and is located in the prominent bursa over the medial side of the head of the first metatarsal. The bursal irritation is caused by pressure from the shoe on the first metatarsal head. There may also be pain associated with the overlapping of the second toe on the distal end of the hallux. Intra-articular pain is rare in juvenile hallux valgus. Cosmetic concerns are frequently important to adolescents. A teenager's desire to wear footwear similar to that of peers is great. As females get older, the increasing desire to wear higher heels and stylish shoes increases shoe-fitting difficulties. Parental concern about cosmesis and future function impairment is common and is difficult to separate from more objective concerns. Function impairment associated with bunions is extremely rare in adolescents.

6. **What is the natural history?**
    The natural history of juvenile hallux valgus is not known. Most experts concur that congruous joints with juvenile hallux valgus are stable and are less likely to progress than those with subluxation.

7. **What are the options for management?**
    The goal of treatment is to relieve pain and not to address strictly cosmetic concerns. Depending on the circumstances, this may be accomplished through either nonoperative or operative modalities. Most patients with juvenile hallux valgus can be managed with conservative measures.

8. **What are the choices for nonoperative treatment?**
    The goal of conservative management is to relieve symptoms without actually correcting the deformity. This is best accomplished by the use of shoes with an adequate toe box and a low heel. A running shoe is the most acceptable shoe that meets these requirements for this age group. Finding dress shoes that meet these requirements can be difficult. Mechanically stretching the forefoot width of the shoe with a bunion stretcher can effectively reduce external pressure. Use of a variety of splints to hold the great toe in a more neutral position has not been found to have a lasting corrective effect.

9. **When is surgery indicated?**
    Surgery is indicated only when prolonged attempts at conservative management have failed to relieve the pain over the first metatarsal head. The age of the patient at the time of surgery is also a consideration since open physes are thought to contribute to an increased incidence of recurrent deformity in the juvenile patient. Poor results with high complication rates have been reported in up to 60% of cases.

10. **What types of operations are available for treatment of bunion deformity?**
More than 130 operations have been described for the treatment of bunions. These can be divided into several major groups: simple bunionectomy (i.e., surgical excision of the prominent exostosis), soft tissue procedures such as tenotomies, lateral capsular release or medial capsular tightening to align the MTP joint, osteotomies to change bone alignment, arthroplasty (both bone resection and replacement with artificial substances), and arthrodesis.

11. **Why are there so many operations?**
This suggests that a universally satisfactory operation is not available and that different manifestations of the problem require different operations. It is well known that the risks of a poor outcome and complications are higher in adolescent patients.

12. **What is the goal of surgical correction of a bunion deformity?**
The goal is to correct the deformity at the site of deformity in order to relieve pain and functional disability while maintaining a flexible first MTP joint.

13. **How do you choose which operation is best for a given patient?**
The most important consideration when choosing which bunion operation to perform is whether the MTP joint is subluxed. Surgical treatment for a juvenile hallux valgus deformity with a subluxated MTP joint must include a distal soft tissue realignment. A medial cuneiform or base of the first metatarsal osteotomy should be combined with the soft tissue realignment if the subluxation is combined with a first-second intermetatarsal angle greater than 8 degrees. The treatment of a juvenile hallux valgus deformity with a congruous MTP joint involves osteotomies to correct the bone deformities and to realign both the joint and the first ray. Typically, a distal metatarsal osteotomy is used to correct the DMAA, whereas a proximal first metatarsal osteotomy or a medial cuneiform osteotomy is used to correct the first-second intermetatarsal angle (Fig. 44-2).

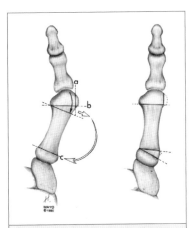

Figure 44-2. *Left,* First metatarsal double osteotomy. *a,* Excision of metatarsal head prominence. *b,* Closing wedge osteotomy (excision of medially based wedge). *c,* Transverse osteotomy in proximal metatarsal. *Right,* Distal osteotomy closed. The wedge of bone removed from the distal closing metatarsal osteotomy is inserted into the proximal metatarsal and becomes an opening wedge osteotomy, which makes the first ray parallel to the second ray. The metatarsalphalangeal (MTP) joint relationships (DMAA) are unchanged. Mathematically, there is no shortening of the first metatarsal since the wedge removed distally is placed proximally. The first-second intermetatarsal angle, the first metatarsophalangeal angle, and the first-second intermetatarsal distance are all decreased.

14. **What are the disadvantages of corrective osteotomies?**
They are major procedures that require 2–3 days of hospitalization, and, if done bilaterally concurrently, require nonweightbearing for 2–4 weeks. Patients who have an osteotomy of any type usually note loss of plantar flexion in the metatarsalphalangeal (MTP) joint. There is usually no loss of dorsiflexion or of plantar flexion strength, and running and jumping abilities are not altered. The loss of plantar flexion has little if any accompanying functional impairment (the only one being the inability to flex the toe down, e.g., over a starting platform for competitive swim races).

15. **Why are surgical results less good in adolescents than in adults?**
Postoperative complications are frequent after surgical correction of juvenile hallux valgus and include recurrence as a result of further epiphyseal growth, overcorrection to hallux varus, avascular necrosis of the metatarsal head, metatarsalgia, joint stiffness, and growth arrest secondary to injury of the growth plates at the proximal ends of the first metatarsal and proximal phalanx.

KEY POINTS: BUNIONS

1. Standing anteroposterior and lateral radiographs of the foot are necessary to evaluate juvenile bunions (i.e., hallux valgus).

2. Although the cause is unknown, there is a strong genetic component with case reports suggesting X-linked dominant, autosomal-dominant, and polygenic transmission.

3. Most adolescents with hallux valgus are asymptomatic. Complaints are usually centered around the appearance or pain.

4. The natural history of juvenile hallux valgus is not known. Most experts concur that congruous joints with juvenile hallux valgus are stable and are less likely to progress than those with subluxation.

5. The most important consideration when choosing which bunion operation to perform is whether the metatarsophalangeal (MTP) joint is subluxed. Surgical treatment for a juvenile hallux valgus deformity with a subluxated MTP joint must include a distal soft tissue realignment.

16. **Which procedures do not work well in adolescents, and why?**
Simple bunionectomy (i.e., removal of the medial side of the head of the first metatarsal) is associated with poor results primarily because of increasing deformity as the patient grows. Resection arthroplasty and fusion of the joint reduce function, which is usually unacceptable in young patients who desire to be active.

17. **What are the disadvantages of resection arthroplasty?**
Procedures that remove the proximal end of the first phalanx to straighten the toe make it floppy and weak. Walking on tiptoes without shoes is difficult, and the remaining proximal end of the phalanx may eventually rub against the head of the first metatarsal, causing degenerative changes.

18. **What is the difficulty with fusion of the MP joint?**
Fusion of the joint determines permanently the angle of alignment between the proximal phalanx and the first metatarsal. The height of the heel of the shoe must always be the same thereafter to accommodate this angle. For a male, an angle of a few degrees of dorsiflexion is comparable with normal shoewear. The female would be limited in the choice of shoe heel height, which is often more problematic.

BIBLIOGRAPHY

1. Aronson J, Nguyen LL, Aronson EA: Early results of the modified Peterson bunion procedure for adolescent hallux valgus. J Pediatr Orthop 21:65–69, 2001.

2. Beadling L: Juvenile hallux valgus: Adapt surgery to address DMAA. In Orthop Today, October 1995, p 26.

3. Bordelon RL: Evaluation and operative procedures for hallux valgus deformity. Orthopedics 10:38–44, 1987.

4. Geissele AE, Stanton RP: Surgical treatment of adolescent hallux valgus. J Pediatr Orthop 10:641–648, 1990.

5. Helal B: Surgery for adolescent hallux valgus. Clin Orthop 157:50–63, 1981.

6. Luba R, Rosman M: Bunions in children: Treatment with a modified Mitchell osteotomy. J Pediatr Orthop 4:44–47, 1984.

7. Mann RA: Etiology and treatment of hallux valgus; bunion surgery: Decision making. Orthopedics 13:951–957, 1990.

8. Peterson HA, Newman SR: Adolescent bunion deformity treated with double osteotomy and longitudinal pin fixation of the first ray. J Pediatr Orthop 13:80–84, 1993.

9. Vittetoe D, Saltzman C, Krieg J, et al: Validity and reliability of the first distal metatarsal articular angle. Foot Ankle Int 15:541–547, 1994.

10. Zimmer TJ, Johnson KA, Klassen RA: Treatment of hallux valgus in adolescents by the Chevron osteotomy. Foot Ankle 9:190–193, 1989.

CHAPTER 45

TOE DEFORMITIES

David A. Spiegel, MD, and Peter L. Meehan, MD

CURLY TOES

1. What is a curly toe?

A curly toe is a common deformity in which the proximal interphalangeal (PIP) joint of the toe is flexed and medially deviated, associated with lateral rotation at the distal interphalangeal (DIP) joint (i.e., the nail faces laterally; Fig. 45-1). The curly toe underlaps the adjacent toe. These deformities are often familial and bilateral, and the underlying cause is congenital tightness of the toe flexors. The third and fourth toes are most commonly involved.

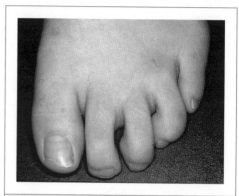

Figure 45-1. Curly toes involving the second, third, and fourth toes.

2. What is the natural history of the curly toe?

Most patients will be asymptomatic, and approximately 25% will resolve spontaneously.

3. Do curly toes require treatment?

It is uncommon for pain or problems with shoe wear to develop, so treatment is rarely needed. Surgery should be delayed until the child is 5–6 years of age.

4. What treatment options are available for curly toes?

Taping of the toes in the corrected position will result in temporary resolution; however, the deformity recurs when the tape is removed. Two treatment options can be considered for children with persistent deformity and associated pain or loss of function. Release of the long toe flexor (with or without the short toe flexor) has been effective. Some authors have recommended the Girdlestone-Taylor procedure, in which the flexors are transferred to the extensors. One study found equivalent results with these two procedures.

OVERRIDING FIFTH TOE

5. What is an overriding fifth toe?

This is a familial deformity in which the fifth toe is dorsiflexed and adducted and overrides the fourth toe (Fig. 45-2). There is also external rotation, and the toenail faces laterally. The problem is usually bilateral. In contrast to a curly toe, which is flexible and underlies the adjacent toe, the overriding, or varus, fifth toe is a rigid deformity.

6. **What is the natural history of the overriding fifth toe?**
   Approximately 50% of patients will develop symptoms—usually pain and callus formation from irritation against the shoe.

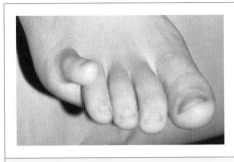

Figure 45-2. Overriding fifth toe.

7. **What treatment options are available for the overriding fifth toe?**
   Treatment is indicated for persistent symptoms despite shoe modifications. Conservative options such as stretching, taping, or splinting are ineffective. Surgical treatment involves release of the contracted metatarsophalangeal joint capsule, lengthening of the extensor tendon, and pinning the toe in the corrected position. A dorsal incision is generally avoided as contracture of the scar can lead to recurrent deformity. In addition to this soft tissue release, some authors also remove the proximal phalanx and create a syndactyly between the fourth and fifth toes. Complications of proximal phalangectomy may include pain over the fifth metatarsal (up to 25% of cases), hammer toe deformity (up to one third of cases), and a bunionette deformity.

SUBUNGUAL EXOSTOSIS

8. **What is a subungual exostosis?**
   Subungual exostosis is a benign growth of bone and cartilage that arises on the dorsal and medial surface of the distal phalanx of the toe, usually under the nail (Fig. 45-3). The great toe is most commonly involved, and the growth is felt to be due to repetitive trauma. Patients usually present in the second or third decade. The clinical and plain radiographic findings are diagnostic.

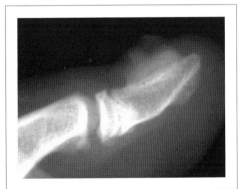

Figure 45-3. Subungual exostosis on the dorsum of the terminal phalanx of the great toe.

9. **What are the symptoms of subungual exostosis?**
   The enlarging mass can cause pain. Problems associated with larger masses include deformity of the nail and sometimes ulceration, with or without secondary infection.

10. **What is the treatment of subungual exostosis?**
    Surgical excision is required, and the nail must be removed to accomplish this. Recurrence may be observed in approximately 15% of patients.

FREIBERG'S INFRACTION

11. **What is Freiberg's infraction?**
    Freiberg's infraction is a disease of unknown etiology in which there is avascular necrosis of one or more metatarsal heads. The second metatarsal head is most commonly affected, and rarely this can involve the third or fourth metatarsal head. The etiology is unknown but may result from repetitive stress, and in most cases the affected metatarsal is the longest in the foot. Adolescent females are most commonly affected.

12. **What are the clinical and radiographic features?**
    Most patients present with pain in the plantar aspect of the infected metatarsal head, and physical findings may include tenderness and swelling in this region as well as stiffness of the metatarsophalangeal (MTP) joint. Radiographically, there is irregularity of the metatarsal head with enlargement, flattening, and sclerosis. Narrowing of the joint space may be observed later in the disease process.

13. **What is the management of Freiberg's infarction?**
    Many patients respond to symptomatic measures such as activity modification, nonsteroidal anti-inflammatory drugs, and shoe modifications to relieve the weight-bearing stresses over the affected metatarsal head. Those with a greater degree of symptoms may be treated, initially by a short-leg walking cast for several weeks and then by shoe modifications.

14. **What options can be considered if a nonoperative treatment fails to relieve the symptoms?**
    Several operative approaches have been reported, but the existing literature is unable to support one method over the others. Options include joint exploration and removal of loose bodies, curettage of the metatarsal head and placement of a cancellous bone graph, dorsiflexion osteotomy of the metatarsal head to reduce stresses, shortening osteotomy of the metatarsal head, excision of the metatarsal head, debridement and interposition with a tendon of the extensor digitorum longus, and, finally, the use of a titanium hemi-implant.

HAMMERTOES

15. **What is a hammertoe?**
    The hammertoe involves a flexion deformity at the PIP joint, usually with a hyperextension deformity at the MTP joint. There may be flexion at the DIP joint as well. The second toe is most commonly affected, and this metatarsal may be longer than normal. Over time, irritation from the shoe may result in a painful callous over the PIP joint dorsally. If a DIP joint is flexed, then irritation and discomfort may occur over the toenail, which is in a weight-bearing position.

16. **What treatment options are available?**
    Nonoperative treatment is ineffective. Patients with flexible deformities may be treated by release of the flexor tendon. An alternative is to transfer the flexors to the extensors. In older patients with rigid deformities, options include fusion of the PIP joint and resection (partial or complete) of the proximal phalanx.

CLAW TOES

17. **What are claw toes?**
    In a claw toe, there is extension at the MTP joint, flexion at the PIP joint, and flexion at the DIP joint (Fig. 45-4). The deformities may be flexible or rigid, and often all of the toes are involved unilaterally or bilaterally. Irritation may occur from the shoes rubbing against the dorsal surface

of the PIP or DIP joint. With dorsiflexion at the MTP joint, there may be excessive pressure over the plantar surface of the metatarsal heads, resulting in callous formation.

18. **What is the etiology of claw toes?**
In many cases, claw toes are associated with an underlying neurologic diagnosis such as Charcot-Marie-Tooth disease (Fig. 45-5). Especially when unilateral, occult spinal dysraphism must be ruled out. A posteroanterior (PA) radiograph of the spine is suggested to rule out any overt signs of spinal dysraphism such as a widening of the interpedicular distance. Magnetic resonance imaging (MRI) of the neural axis is often recommended, and neurologic consultation should be considered. Claw toes are often associated with cavus feet.

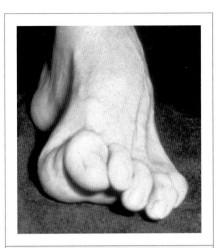

Figure 45-4. Cavus foot and claw toes.

19. **What treatment options are available?**
Nonoperative treatment measures are ineffective. Operative treatment is required for patients with persistent symptoms— usually pain over the dorsum of the PIP joint. For patients with flexible deformities associated with a cavus foot, correction of the cavus may be associated with spontaneous improvement of the claw toes. For patients with long-standing rigid deformities, surgical treatment involves releasing the contracted dorsal capsule of the MP joint, fusing the PIP joints, transferring the long toe extensor to the metatarsal neck, and finally suturing the distal portion of the long toe extensor to the short toe extensor. This may be performed at the same time as correction of the cavus foot, or it may be staged.

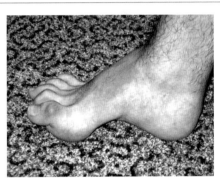

Figure 45-5. Foot of a patient with Charcot-Marie-Tooth disease.

POLYDACTYLY

20. **What is polydactyly?**
Polydactyly represents duplication of a toe and is the most common congenital toe deformity. The fifth is toe is duplicated most often (called *postaxial polydactyly*), and the deformity is bilateral in 50% of patients. Polydactyly may be seen in association with certain syndromes, including Ellis-van Creveld syndrome, longitudinal deficiency of the tibia, and Down syndrome. Polydactyly of the hand is present in approximately one third of those with polydactyly of the foot. The extra digit may be rudimentary or well formed.

21. **What are the clinical consequences of polydactyly?**
    In addition to cosmetic concerns, difficulties with shoe wear are common when there is also duplications of the metatarsal head. (It widens the foot.)

22. **What is the recommended treatment for patients electing to have surgery?**
    Surgical excision of the duplicated digit and the associated metatarsal can improve the cosmetic appearance of the foot and enable the patient to wear regular shoes. The procedure is generally performed between 9 and 12 months of age. Radiographs are required to define the bony anatomy. Most of the time it is best to remove the outer digit. However, in some cases, an inner digit must be removed for the best functional and cosmetic result. Muscle and soft tissue balancing may also be required.

HALLUX VARUS

23. **What is hallux varus?**
    Hallux varus is a congenital or acquired deformity in which there is medial deviation of the great toe at the MTP joint (Fig. 45-6). This deformity may be seen in isolation (in soft tissue contracture) or following bunion surgery (from excessive resection of the metatarsal head medially). Hallux varus may be associated with other malformations of the foot such as complete or partial duplication of the great toe or with generalized skeletal dysplasias such as diastrophic dysplasia.

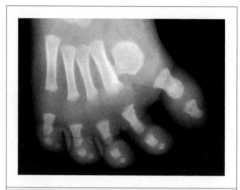

Figure 45-6. Plain radiograph of hallux varus.

24. **What symptoms are associated with hallux varus?**
    Patients will have difficulty in wearing standard shoes in addition to cosmetic concerns.

25. **What treatment options are available?**
    In milder cases in which the deformity is flexible and is not associated with either an osseous abnormality or a syndrome, the deformity may improve spontaneously with time. If the deformity is rigid, surgical treatment is required. Surgical treatment addresses the underlying pathoanatomy and often requires release of medial soft tissue contracture, including the MTP joint, and syndactylization of the great toe to the second toe is often recommended. Depending on the local anatomy, resection of accessory ossicles or a bony osteotomy may be required. Additional procedures reported include reefing of the lateral MTP joint capsule, as well as extensor hallucis brevis rerouting. Fusion of the first MTP joint is reserved for salvage. When hallux varus complicates bunion surgery, bone grafting of the medial side of the first metatarsal head may be effective.

SYNDACTYLY

26. **What is syndactyly?**
    Syndactyly represents congenital webbing of the toes and may be incomplete or complete (extending to the tip of the toes). Whereas a simple syndactyly involves just the skin, in a

complex syndactyly there is also a failure of separation of the phalanges. In some cases, the toenails are confluent.

27. **What are the clinical consequences of syndactyly?**
Simple syndactyly does not typically lead to any functional problems, and thus the only issue is cosmesis. In complex syndactyly, there may be a tethering of longitudinal growth that results in a flexion deformity of the toes, which may result in pain and difficulties with shoe wear.

28. **What treatment options are available for syndactyly?**
For simple syndactyly, no treatment is required. Surgical release of the syndactyly necessarily involves skin grafting, so the scarring created by the surgery may be more of a cosmetic concern than the syndactyly. Scar contracture may also result in progressive deformity and the need for additional procedures. For cases of complex syndactyly in which the deformity results in pain or difficulty wearing shoes, surgical separation should be considered.

INGROWN TOENAILS

29. **What causes an ingrown toenail?**
An ingrown toenail is caused by encroachment of the soft tissues under the toenail, and this most commonly occurs in the great toe on either the medial or lateral side. In some cases, a U-shaped malformation of the nail may predispose to this problem. Mechanical irritation of the soft tissue adjacent to the nail creates inflammation and, often, a secondary infection.

KEY POINTS: TOE DEFORMITIES

1. The etiology of toe deformities is variable, and treatment is required in a subset of patients with symptoms or functional problems.

2. An underlying neuromuscular problem should be suspected in a patient with claw toes.

3. Subungual exostosis is a benign osteocartilaginous growth that elevates or erodes the nail and requires surgical excision.

4. Freiberg's infraction describes avascular necrosis of a metatarsal head, which frequently results in pain and occasionally requires surgical treatment if activity modification and orthoses fail to relieve the symptoms.

5. Syndactyly (i.e., webbing of the toes) may be simple (skin only) or complex (with bony fusion of the two toes), the latter often requiring surgical separation.

6. An ingrown toenail requires surgical treatment for recurrent or recalcitrant infection, and the most common procedure is partial removal of the nail, with or without ablation of the germinal matrix.

30. **What are the contributing preventable causes?**
If the nail is trimmed improperly, the corner can grow into or under the nail fold. A toenail should always be trimmed straight across; if the corners are rounded, the nail may grow into the medial or lateral soft tissues. Repetitive trauma to the toenail resulting from shoes that are too short or too narrow may also contribute.

31. **What is the recommended treatment for cases in which there is no active infection?**

If the problem is mechanical irritation, placement of gauze under the leading edge of the nail with daily warm-water soaks, followed by application of an antibiotic ointment, is effective. Treatment is continued until the margin of the nail grows out beyond the end of the soft tissue. Shoe modification and activity restrictions should also be considered to alleviate any coexisting mechanical trauma.

32. **What is the recommended treatment for active cellulitis?**

In addition to the local measures described above, an oral antistaphylococcic antibiotic should be prescribed.

33. **What are the indications for removal of the nail?**

Nail avulsion is indicated in order to control infection or if the nail is U-shaped and there have been problems with recurrence or persistent infection. In these cases, either the medial or lateral margin of the nail should be excised and the corresponding portion of the germinal matrix should be ablated (with excision or phenol) to prevent recurrence. There is an increased risk of postoperative infection when phenol is used. Other techniques described include a wedge excision of the nail fold (in addition to removal of the germinal matrix) in order to reduce the convexity of the nail fold. Partial matricectomy followed by a lateral fold advancement flap has also been used with success. Complications of these procedures include recurrence, formation of a nail spicule, and the need for reoperation.

BIBLIOGRAPHY

1. Coughlin MJ: Lesser toe abnormalities. Instr Course Lect 52:421–444, 2003.
2. Hamer AJ, Stanley D, Smith TW: Surgery for curly toe deformity: A double-blind, randomized, prospective trial. J Bone Joint Surg 75B:662–663, 1993.
3. Islam S, Lin EM, Drongowski R, et al: The effect of phenol on ingrown toenail excision in children. J Pediatr Surg 40(1):290–292, 2005.
4. Janecki CJ, Wilde AH: Results of phalangectomy of the fifth toe for hammertoe: The Ruiz-Mora procedure. J Bone Joint Surg 58A:1005–1007, 1976.
5. Letts M, Davidson D, Nizalike J: Subungual exostosis: Diagnosis and treatment in children. J Trauma 44:346–349, 1998.
6. Miller-Breslow A, Dorfman HD: Dupuytren's (subungual) exostosis. Am J Surg Pathol 12:368–378, 1988.
7. Operation: An over-riding fifth toe. J Bone Joint Surg 50B:78–81, 1968.
8. Ross ERS, Menelaus MB: Open flexor tenotomy for hammertoes and curly toes in childhood. J Bone Joint Surg 66B:770–771, 1984.
9. Rounding C, Bloomfield S: Surgical treatments for ingrown toenails. Cochrane Database Syst Rev 18(2):CD001541, 2005.
10. Vanore JV, Christensen JC, Kravitz SR, et al: Diagnosis and treatment of first metatarsal phalangeal joint disorders. Section 3: Hallux varus. J Foot Ankle Surg 42:137–142, 2003.
11. Venn-Watson EA: Problems in polydactyly of the foot. Orthop Clin North Am 7:909–927, 1976.

CHAPTER 46

NAIL PUNCTURE

David A. Spiegel, MD

1. **What questions should be asked during the initial history?**
   It is important to identify the penetrating object and to assess the likelihood of a retained foreign body, as well as where the injury occurred, whether or not shoes were worn (and what type of shoes), the time between injury and presentation, and when the patient last had a tetanus booster.

2. **What is the most likely cause of a puncture into the foot?**
   Nail injuries are most common. Foreign bodies may include glass, rubber, sewing needles, tacks, toothpicks, and wood.

3. **What is the role of imaging in the evaluation of puncture wounds to the foot?**
   Plain radiographs should be obtained if a foreign body is suspected, recognizing that plastic, aluminum, and wood can be radiolucent. Additional imaging studies such as ultrasound, computed tomography (CT), or magnetic resonance imaging (MRI) may be considered when plain films are normal. Some authors recommend a bone scan or an MRI to rule out osteomyelitis.

4. **What is the initial management of this injury?**
   Patients should receive a tetanus booster if appropriate. Most patients may be managed by a limited irrigation (using a needle) under local anesthesia. It may be helpful to saucerize the wound first by excising the cornified epithelium at the edges and then removing any debris just below the surface. One recent study found that, with surface cleansing alone, 8% of patients developed an infection and 3% had a retained foreign body. Puncture wounds of greater severity with obvious contamination should be treated by irrigation and debridement in the operating room.

5. **Is there a role for prophylactic antibiotics?**
   There is insufficient evidence to support routine prophylactic antibiotics acutely.

6. **What should be done if a retained foreign body is suspected at the time of the initial presentation?**
   The patient should be treated with a formal wound exploration in the operating room, and cultures should be obtained. The location of the injury dictates how extensive the exploration should be. If the object penetrates the region adjacent to a joint, the joint should be explored and irrigated.

7. **What is the usual outcome?**
   Most patients will do well with the steps outlined previously. Cellulitis will develop in approximately 8–15% of patients, usually within several days of the initial injury. Osteomyelitis will be seen in 0.6–1.8% of patients, and the symptoms usually occur 7–10 days after the injury.

8. **What instructions should be given to the family?**
   The symptoms should improve after the first couple of days as the inflammation subsides. If the pain persists or increases or if swelling, redness, or drainage occur, the patient should return for a follow-up evaluation.

KEY POINTS: NAIL PUNCTURE

1. Most puncture wounds to the foot can be treated effectively by limited irrigation in the emergency department.

2. Prophylactic antibiotics remain controversial.

3. If a foreign body is present or suspected, a formal exploration in the operating room should be performed.

4. Cellulitis (8–15%, presenting within several days) and osteomyelitis (up to 2%, presenting after 7–10 days) are rare and require irrigation and debridement in the operating room.

5. Soft tissue infection is most commonly caused by staphylococci, whereas septic arthritis or osteomyelitis is often due to *Pseudomonas* species, especially if the patient is wearing sneakers at the time of injury.

9. **What should be done if a patient returns with evidence of cellulitis?**
Local wound care and antibiotics are not likely to cure the infection. The wound should be explored surgically, and cultures should be obtained. Aspirates placed in blood culture bottles may have a higher yield than routine cultures. Any foreign body should be identified and removed, and if the track extends near a joint, then a joint exploration should be performed. If the track extends near any osseous structure and osteomyelitis is suspected, then the bone should be curetted and cultures taken. A large needle can be used to aspirate the bone, and the aspirate should be placed in blood culture bottles to increase the yield over standard cultures.

10. **What are the most likely organisms involved in cellulitis or osteomyelitis?**
The most common organism leading to soft tissue infection is staphylococcus. *Pseudomonas* should always be suspected in cases of septic arthritis or osteomyelitis, particularly if the patient was wearing sneakers at the time of injury. This organism often proliferates in the foam rubber of the sole of sneakers but also can be found in work boots or in any warm and moist environment. Less commonly, gram-negative bacteria and atypical acid-fast organisms can result in infection, especially in the compromised host.

11. **How long should antibiotics be continued?**
A thorough debridement is the most important step in achieving resolution of the infection. Empiric broad-spectrum coverage is started and later modified based on the cultures and sensitivities. For a soft tissue infection alone, 7–10 days is a reasonable course. For cases with established osteomyelitis, a longer duration of therapy may be indicated; 7 days to 6 weeks have been recommended, depending upon the underlying organism, the host defense, and the response to treatment. The clinical response is monitored closely as the laboratory studies are typically not helpful in establishing the diagnosis or in monitoring the response to treatment.

BIBLIOGRAPHY

1. Eidelmann , Bialik V, Miller Y, et al: Plantar puncture wounds in children: Analysis of 80 hospitalized patients and late sequelae. Isr Med Assoc J 5(4):268–271, 2003.

2. Fitzgerald RH, Cowan JDE: Puncture wounds of the foot. Orthop Clin North Am 6:965–972, 1975.

3. Jacobs RF, McCarthy RE, Elser JM: Pseudomonas osteochondritis complicating puncture wounds of the foot in children: A ten-year evaluation. J Infect Dis 160:657–661, 1989.

4. Jarvis JG, Skipper J: Pseudomonas osteochondritis complicating puncture wounds in children. J Pediatr Orthop 14:755–759, 1994.

CHAPTER 47

METATARSUS ADDUCTUS

Frederick R. Dietz, MD

1. What is metatarsus adductus?

Metatarsus adductus is a congenital foot deformity characterized by adduction (i.e., turning inward) of the forefoot with respect to the hind foot (Fig. 47-1). The curvature occurs in the midfoot at the tarsometatarsal joints. The lateral border of the foot has a convex contour with prominence of the base of the fifth metatarsus. There is no abnormality of the hindfoot—the static position and range of motion of the ankle and subtalar joints are normal.

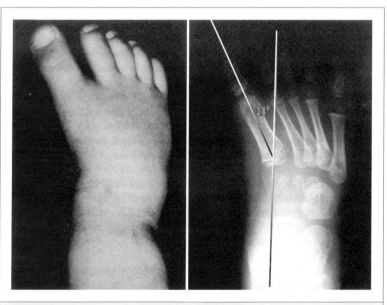

Figure 47-1. Metatarsus adductus. The clinical and radiographic findings document that the adduction occurs at the metatarsocuneiform joints.

2. How common is metatarsus adductus?

It occurs in approximately 1 in 1000 births. Metatarsus adductus occurs with equal frequency in boys and girls and is bilateral 50–80% of the time.

3. What causes metatarsus adductus?

Metatarsus adductus is a late-pregnancy molding deformity (as is calcaneal valgus foot deformity). It occurs more often when fetal crowding at the end of pregnancy is more common, as in first pregnancies, twin pregnancies, and oligohydramnios.

4. **What is the natural history of metatarsus adductus?**
   In the first year of life, 90% of cases will resolve spontaneously or with stretching exercises. An additional 5% of cases will resolve during the early walking period (i.e., 1–4 years of age). If not treated, 4–5% will persist. Long-term follow-up studies have shown that residual metatarsus adductus causes no problems. Arthritis does not develop, foot function is normal (in fact, a disproportionate number of world class sprinters have metatarsus adductus), and shoe fitting is generally not a problem. Feet that are stiffer (i.e., cannot be passively abducted to a neutral alignment) in infancy are less likely to correct spontaneously.

5. **Should metatarsus adductus be treated? If so, how?**
   Given the benign natural history of this deformity, treatment is not necessary. Nonetheless, some families are distressed by the appearance of the foot, and effective, nonrisky treatment is available. Treatment initially consists of teaching parents appropriate stretching exercises performed after diaper changes or several times a day. The parents are taught to hold the heel in a neutral position and to manually abduct the forefoot using a thumb placed over the lateral cuboid as the fulcrum for correction. The exaggerated forefoot abduction position should be maintained for a few seconds, and the stretching should be repeated 10 times at each session. It is critical that parents be taught the correct stretching technique. If stretching is done by abducting the forefoot without blocking the calcaneal-cuboid area, heel valgus may result without correction of the adductus, resulting in a skewfoot. Skewfoot often becomes painful and is difficult to treat, and most cases are caused by inappropriate manipulation of metatarsus adductus. Inappropriate stretching is the only mistake one can make in treating metatarsus adductus.
   If the deformity is still cosmetically distressing to the family when the patient is about 5 months of age, I place two or three sets of casts at 2-week intervals. The foot is manipulated as described above, and then an above-the-knee cast is placed, with the knee bent 90 degrees and the plaster molded with abduction of the forefoot, with the calcaneal-cuboid area as the counter fulcrum. This will resolve the deformity in almost all cases. If the deformity is very severe, stiff, or recurrent, bracing after correction for a period of months may help ensure maintenance of the correction. Casting at 5 months of age means that I cast some feet that would resolve. However, I have had little success in casting feet at crawling and walking ages.

KEY POINTS: METATARSUS ADDUCTUS

1. Metatarsus adductus is a late-pregnancy molding deformity and resolves spontaneously in most cases.

2. Stretching exercises must be done properly, using the calcaneal-cuboid joint as the fulcrum for abducting the forefoot.

3. Manipulation and casting is effective for cosmetically unacceptable deformities.

4. Even if metatarsus adductus persists and is uncorrected, the feet will function normally without pain or arthritis and almost always without problems with shoes.

6. **How does the condition differ from talipes equinovarus and skewfoot?**
   A rigid clubfoot has a hindfoot that is fixed in equinus, inversion, and cavus, as well as adductus of the midfoot.
   Skewfoot is more difficult to distinguish on infant examination. Its medial skin crease is located at the more distal naviculocuneiform joint. The heel in the skewfoot is in valgus, and this condition rarely has an associated contracture of the abductor hallucis muscle. This

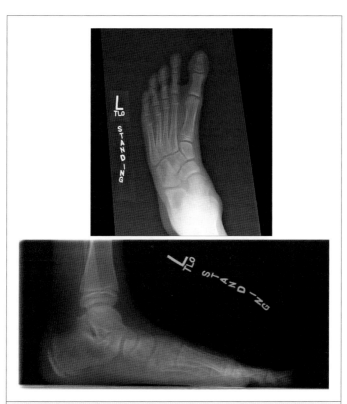

Figure 47-2. Serpentine foot. The anteroposterior (AP) radiograph demonstrates hindfoot valgus, lateral subluxation of the navicular bone, and adduction of the forefoot localized to the cuneonavicular joint.

complex foot deformity combines heel valgus with a lateral subluxation of the talonavicular joint (midfoot) and adduction of the forefoot, which explains its common nickname of *Z foot* (Fig. 47-2). The differentiation of metatarsus adductus from skewfoot is important because serial casting of the skewfoot is inappropriate and could lead to the development of a significant iatrogenic flatfoot as the congenital midfoot lateral subluxation becomes exaggerated. In my experience, idiopathic skewfoot is much less common than skewfoot created by inappropriate stretching of metatarsus adductus.

BIBLIOGRAPHY

1. Berg EE: A reappraisal of metatarsus adductus and skewfoot. J Bone Joint Surg Am 68:1185–1196, 1986.

2. Farsetti P, Weinstein SL, Ponseti IV: The long-term functional and radiographic outcomes of untreated and non-operatively treated metatarsus adductus. J Bone Joint Surg Am 76:257–265, 1994.

3. Ghali NN, Abberton MJ, Silk FF: The management of metatarsus adductus et supinatus. J Bone Joint Surg Br 66:376–380, 1984.

4. Mosca VS: Flexible flatfoot and skewfoot. J Bone Joint Surg Am 77:1937–1945, 1995.

5. Peterson HA: Skewfoot (forefoot adduction and heel valgus). J Pediatr Orthop 6:24–30, 1986.

6. Ponseti IV, Becker JR: Congenital metatarsus adductus: The results of treatment. J Bone Joint Surg 48A:702–711, 1966.

CHAPTER 48

IDIOPATHIC CLUBFOOT

Frederick R. Dietz, MD

1. **What is idiopathic clubfoot?**
   A congenitally deformed foot that points downward and is turned inward. If the baby could walk, it would look as though the baby were walking on the top of the foot. The four components of a clubfoot are ankle equinus (i.e., the whole foot points down), heel varus (i.e., the back of the foot is turned inward), midfoot adductus (i.e., the foot is curved inward in the middle of the foot), and midfoot cavus (i.e., there is an abnormally high arch). The key feature of a clubfoot is that the deformities are rigid. That is, the foot cannot be passively brought to a normal-looking foot position. The foot deformities seen in idiopathic clubfoot can be seen in various combinations in babies with myelomeningocele, arthrogryposis, and various syndromes. These are called *syndromic clubfeet* or *neurogenic clubfeet* and are not the same entity as idiopathic clubfoot, which occurs in otherwise normal babies.

2. **How common is clubfoot?**
   The overall incidence of clubfoot in the Caucasian population is a little more than 1 per 1000 births. Much higher incidence is reported in Polynesians, and a lower incidence is reported in Asian populations.

3. **Is clubfoot more common in boys or girls? Are both feet deformed?**
   Boys are affected twice as often as girls, and 50% of cases are bilateral.

4. **When a child is born with a clubfoot, what are the chances that a subsequent baby will have a clubfoot?**
   Overall, the risk of a second child having a clubfoot is 2–4%. In some families, clubfoot shows up more often than this, and in other families it occurs only once. In general, families with more members with clubfoot have a higher likelihood of subsequent children with clubfoot than do families with fewer affected members.

5. **What are the causes of clubfoot?**
   The cause of clubfoot is unknown. There may be more than one cause. Analysis of the inheritance of clubfoot suggests that a significant proportion (70%) have a genetically inherited predisposition.

6. **What are the etiology theories?**
   Regardless of genetic predisposition, researchers have postulated many theories for causing clubfoot, including fetal development arrest, a germ plasm defect, retracting fibrosis, and myogenic and neurogenic theories. There is *no* evidence that intrauterine molding causes clubfoot.

7. **Can clubfoot be diagnosed prenatally?**
   Yes. Ultrasound can make the diagnosis of clubfoot in most fetuses between 14 and 24 weeks. Ultrasound may overdiagnose clubfoot (especially in unilateral clubfoot), and ultrasound has difficulty distinguishing between idiopathic clubfoot and neurogenic or syndromic clubfoot (especially in bilateral cases).

8. **Are all clubfeet the same?**
   No, there are various degrees of severity. Some feet can be corrected by two or three casts. Others require four to six casts. There is a small group of difficult feet that tend to slip out of their casts and may require eight to twelve casts or surgical correction.

9. **How do you classify the severity of a clubfoot?**
   There is no scheme to determine how difficult a foot will be to correct at birth. Several rating schemes (including Pirani and Demiglio) can be used to track the progression of treatment, but none has been shown to be predictive.

10. **When should treatment begin?**
    Within the first week or two after birth. Clubfoot treatment is not an emergency, but treatment is more effective and rapid if initial treatment is not delayed by more than 2–4 weeks. Most feet in babies of less than 9 months of age can be corrected by manipulation and casting by the Ponseti technique.

11. **How does one treat a clubfoot?**
    The standard of care in the United States and much of the rest of the world is the Ponseti technique. This technique was developed by Dr. Ignacio Ponseti in the early 1950s. It has been shown to give more rapid and constant correction than any other technique of manipulation and casting. Other techniques, such as the Kite method, were more commonly used until the last decade and resulted in many uncorrected clubfeet requiring surgical reconstruction by lengthening tendons and releasing joint capsules.

12. **How is the Ponseti technique performed?**
    The cavus is reduced by supination of the forefoot until the forefoot is in normal alignment with the hindfoot. Then, the lateral head of the talus is used as the fulcrum while the foot is abducted. This reduces the adduction of the midfoot and the varus of the hindfoot. In 10% of clubfeet, the foot will dorsiflex and fully correct with this maneuver alone. In 90% of feet, the deformity will be corrected except that the foot will not fully dorsiflex. A percutaneous tenotomy of the Achilles tendon is then performed to speed correction and to avoid creation of a rocker-bottom foot.

13. **How often is the cast changed?**
    Casts are changed every 5–7 days. Cast changes more often than every 5 days do not allow sufficient time for the tissues of the foot to remodel.

14. **What happens to the Achilles tendon after it is cut?**
    The tendon regrows within 2–3 weeks. Weakness is never a problem after tenotomy.

15. **After the feet are corrected, can the deformity recur?**
    Most deformities will recur if appropriate bracing is not done after the initial correction. The deformity will recur in over 90% of feet that are not braced and in only 5% of feet that are braced.

16. **What is appropriate bracing?**
    An abduction foot orthosis (often called a *Denis-Browne splint*) is used 23 hours per day for the first 2–3 months after correction and then is used during naps and nighttimes.

17. **How long is bracing necessary?**
    Most children will wear the brace until they are 3–4 years old. Then many children will refuse to wear the brace. This is usually enough time to avoid recurrent deformity. Some children will wear the brace until 5 years of age. Recurrence in this group is rare.

18. **How successful are manipulation and casting with or without percutaneous tenotomy?**
Most experienced practitioners of the Ponseti technique will be able to correct over 90% of clubfeet without major operations.

19. **What are the results of the Ponseti technique?**
The longest follow-up study (an average age of 35 year after treatment) has shown that clubfeet treated by this technique do as well as nonclubfeet with respect to function and pain. The feet are always stiffer and slightly smaller than normal feet, but they function normally.

20. **What if the deformity recurs in spite of bracing or if the family does not use the brace?**
In infancy, the same manipulation and casting can regain the correction. Usually two or three casts are necessary. If the deformity begins to recur in children older than $2\frac{1}{2}$ years of age, an anterior tibial tendon transfer to the third cuneiform is performed. Sometimes a lengthening of the Achilles tendon is required at the same time if there is not sufficient dorsiflexion.

KEY POINTS: IDIOPATHIC CLUBFOOT

1. Clubfoot is a rigid deformity at birth.

2. The etiology is unknown.

3. Treatment with manipulation and casting should be started soon after birth.

4. Successful treatment by the Ponseti technique results in functionally normal feet in most cases.

21. **How do you know when an anterior tibial tendon transfer is necessary? What are the results of this surgery?**
If the child is older than 2½ years of age and begins walking on the toes and the outside of the foot, the tendon transfer is appropriate. A transfer of the anterior tibial tendon does not cause additional stiffness or weakness of the foot, and the results at least 35 years later are as good as for patients who did not require a tendon transfer.

22. **What do you do if you cannot correct the foot with manipulation and casting initially or after a recurrence and the foot is too stiff for a tendon transfer?**
In these uncommon feet, the plantar fascia and tight intrinsic muscles are divided, a Z-plasty is performed of the tendo Achillis and tibialis posterior, and the tight capsules are divided so that the navicular can be reduced onto the head of the talus, the cuboid can be reduced onto the end of the calcaneus, and the whole foot can be brought out of equinus. The lengthened tendons are then sutured with the foot held in a plantigrade position.

23. **What are the results of the major surgical release of joint capsules and tendon lengthening?**
There are very few long-term studies of clubfeet undergoing major surgical release. The best study suggests that these feet become painful and weak in early adulthood in most patients and do not function nearly as well as those treated by manipulation and casting and tendon transfer (if needed).

24. **What information is important to communicate to the family up front?**
It is especially important to tell the family that there will be calf atrophy, that the calf atrophy was already present at birth, and that the clubfoot will be on average one-half shoe size smaller than

the normal foot. Although most feet will function normally, they will be stiffer than a normal foot. The correction of the foot by the practitioner is usually straightforward and is accomplished in the first 2 months of life. It is then the family's responsibility to avoid recurrence by using the brace as directed. Approximately 5% of feet that are successfully braced will recur, whereas 90% of feet that are not braced will recur.

25. **What are the controversies?**
   - How old can the child be when the Achilles tendon is lengthened percutaneously, versus a Z-lengthening, without compromising strength?
   - How best to recognize and treat the "atypical" or "complex" clubfoot. These feet have a deep transverse crease in the sole and are in severe equinus at the ankle with a deep posterior crease. Over-abduction causes a mid foot breach and the equinus causes cast slippage at the third or fourth cast. Recognition and codified treatment of this subgroup is necessary.
   - How much dorsiflexion is satisfactory in a recurrent deformity? Specifically, when should a posterior release of the ankle joint be performed in addition to a lengthening of the Achilles tendon to gain more dorsiflexion?

BIBLIOGRAPHY

1. Carroll NC: Surgical treatment for talipes equino-varus. Op Tech Orthop 3(2):115, 1993.
2. Cooper DM, Dietz FR: Treatment of idiopathic clubfoot. A thirty-year follow-up note. J Bone Joint Surg Am 77:1477–1489, 1995.
3. Crawford AH, Marxen JL, Osterfeld DL: The Cincinnati incision: A comprehensive approach for surgical procedures of the foot and ankle in childhood. J Bone Joint Surg 64A:1355–1358, 1982.
4. Dietz F: The genetics of idiopathic clubfoot. Clin Orthop 401:39–48, 2002.
5. Evans D: Relapsed clubfoot. J Bone Joint Surg 43B:722, 1961.
6. Flynn JM, Donohoe M, Mackenzie WG: An independent assessment of two clubfoot-classification systems. J Pediatr Orthop 18:323–327, 1998.
7. Herzenberg JE, Carroll NC, Christofersen MR, et al: Clubfoot analysis with three-dimensional computer modeling. J Pediatr Orthop 8:257–263, 1988.
8. Kite J: Principles involved in the treatment of congenital clubfoot. J Bone Joint Surg 21:595–606, 1939.
9. Kuo KN, Hennigan SP, Hastings ME: Anterior tibial tendon transfer in residual dynamic clubfoot deformity. J Pediatr Orthop 21:35–41, 2001.
10. Laaveg SJ, Ponseti IV: Long-term results of treatment of congenital clubfoot. J Bone Joint Surg 62A:23–31, 1980.
11. Levin MN, Kuio KN, Harris GF, Matesi DV: Posteromedial release for idiopathic talipes equinovarus. A long-term follow-up study. Clin Orthop 242:265–268, 1989.
12. Lourenco AF, Dias LS, Zoellick DM, Sodre H: Treatment of residual adduction deformity in clubfoot: The double osteotomy. J Pediatr Orthop 21:713–718, 2001.
13. McKay DW: New concepts of and approach to clubfoot treatment. Section 1: Principles and morbid anatomy. J Pediatr Orthop 2:347–356, 1982.
14. McKay DW: New concept of and approach to treatment. Section 2: Correction of clubfoot. J Pediatr Orthop 3:10–21, 1983.
15. Ponseti IV: Current concepts review treatment of congenital club foot. J Bone Joint Surg 74A:448–453, 1992.

CHAPTER 49

FLATFOOT

Vincent S. Mosca, MD

1. **What is a flatfoot?**
   Flatfoot describes a foot shape in which the medial longitudinal arch is depressed toward the ground. There is a sagging of the midfoot, valgus alignment of the hindfoot, abduction of the forefoot on the hindfoot, and an outward rotation of the foot in relation to the leg. There are no universally accepted clinical or radiographic criteria for differentiating a foot with a low normal arch from a flatfoot.

2. **How common are flatfeet?**
   It is hard to say with certainty because a strict definition does not exist. Nevertheless, based on footprint and radiographic studies, flatfeet are present in most children and in more than 20% of adults.

3. **Are there different types of flatfeet?**
   There are three types of flatfoot in normal, healthy individuals: (1) hypermobile or flexible flatfoot, (2) flexible flatfoot with a short Achilles tendon, and (3) rigid flatfoot. The flatfoot shape can also be seen in individuals with underlying neuromuscular disorders.

4. **Why is it important to classify flatfoot into different types?**
   To help with prognosis. The flexible or hypermobile flatfoot accounts for almost all flatfeet in children and approximately two thirds of flatfeet in adults. It is of little or no clinical concern as a cause of disability. The flexible flatfoot with a short Achilles tendon is rarely seen in children and accounts for about 25% of flatfeet in adults. It has the potential for causing pain and disability. The third and least-frequent type of flatfoot is the rigid type. It is seen most commonly in feet with tarsal coalitions. Pain and disability are evident in about one quarter of affected individuals.

5. **How do you differentiate the types of flatfoot on clinical examination?**
   A flexible flatfoot has good mobility of the subtalar joint. The foot has the characteristic flat appearance when the individual stands erect. The flexibility is characterized by inversion of the hindfoot to neutral (or even varus) and elevation of the medial longitudinal arch when the heel is elevated off the ground during toe-standing. The arch is also evident when the foot is dangling in the air, as when the individual is seated on an examining table with the foot off the ground.

   The common benign flexible flatfoot has normal excursion of the ankle joint and Achilles tendon (triceps surae musculotendinous complex). To assess this accurately, the subtalar joint is inverted to the neutral position and the ankle is dorsiflexed while the knee is held in flexion. The knee is then extended while maintaining inversion of the subtalar joint and attempting to maintain dorsiflexion of the ankle. The ankle should maintain at least 10 degrees of dorsiflexion above neutral when the knee is extended. A flexible flatfoot with less than 10 degrees of dorsiflexion, due to contracture of the Achilles tendon, is more likely to cause pain and disability than one with more excursion.

   A rigid flatfoot has a stiff subtalar joint that does not change shape during toe standing. The heel will of course elevate, but the sagging of the midfoot and the valgus alignment of the hindfoot will still be evident.

6. **What causes a flexible flatfoot?**
The shapes of the bones and the laxity of the ligaments of the foot determine the height of the longitudinal arch. Muscles are important for balance and function but not for structure. Flexible flatfeet often run in families and are more common in certain ethnic and racial groups. Therefore, one must conclude that a flexible flatfoot is genetically determined.

7. **What is the natural history of arch development in the child?**
There is spontaneous elevation of the longitudinal arch of the foot in most children during the first decade of life. Clinical footprint and radiographic studies confirm this finding.

8. **Can shoes, braces, and orthoses affect the natural history of arch development?**
No. Only two prospective controlled studies have been performed to answer this question, and both found no beneficial effect of shoes or orthoses in the development of the longitudinal arch.

9. **What causes a rigid flatfoot?**
The most common cause of a rigid flatfoot is a tarsal coalition, an autosomal-dominant condition that affects 1–2% of the population. It is due to failure of differentiation and segmentation of the primary mesenchyme that forms the tarsal bones. The most common sites for a coalition are between the calcaneus and navicular and between the talus and calcaneus. The coalitions undergo metaplasia from fibrous (syndesmosis) to cartilaginous (synchondrosis) to osseous (synostosis) unions during childhood and adolescence.

Other causes of a rigid flatfoot include congenital vertical talus, juvenile rheumatoid arthritis, septic arthritis, and traumatic arthritis following intra-articular fracture of the subtalar joint.

10. **What is the most likely cause of progressive flattening of the longitudinal arch in a child?**
A tarsal coalition produces a progressive flattening of the longitudinal arch in childhood. A flexible flatfoot, with or without a short Achilles tendon, is almost always present from birth and shows a progressive elevation or no change in arch height during the growth of the child.

11. **Should radiographs be obtained when evaluating the flatfoot?**
Radiographs are not indicated when evaluating the asymptomatic flatfoot in a child who presents because of parental concern about the shape of the foot. Physical examination is all that is required. Radiographs may be indicated for the child with a flexible flatfoot or a flexible flatfoot with a short Achilles tendon who has foot pain, particularly if the symptoms are severe or are unrelated to activities and if other signs or symptoms are present.

Weightbearing anteroposterior, lateral, oblique, and axial Harris-view radiographs should be obtained for the adolescent with a painful rigid flatfoot. A calcaneonavicular coalition is best seen on the 45-degree oblique radiograph. The axial Harris view may show a talocalcaneal coalition, but the definitive imaging study for demonstration of a coalition at this site is the computed tomography (CT) scan.

12. **Is it true that flexible flatfeet never hurt?**
No. Many individuals with flexible flatfeet have generalized laxity of their ligaments. Children will sometimes report activity-related pain and fatigue as well as nocturnal aching pain in their feet, ankles, and legs. It is thought that these symptoms represent an overuse syndrome caused by muscles overworking to compensate for the excessively lax ligaments. In these situations, use of over-the-counter or, less commonly, molded foot orthoses may diminish or eliminate symptoms.

13. **Are there other benefits from the use of orthoses?**
Yes. Orthoses may change the pattern of wear and increase the useful life of shoes.

14. **How does pain manifest in the flexible flatfoot with a short Achilles tendon?**
There is pain, redness, and callus formation in the arch area under the plantar-flexed head of the talus. This is a specific site of pain and tenderness that differentiates it from the activity-related, generalized aching occasionally seen in the isolated flexible flatfoot.

15. **What can be done for pain and disability in the patient with flexible flatfoot with a short Achilles tendon?**
Foot orthoses may exacerbate symptoms in this condition and are not recommended. Pressure is already being concentrated under the head of the talus because the tight Achilles tendon is forcing it to the ground. An arch support will increase the pressure in this area and cause more pain. Stretching the Achilles tendon may be beneficial. A block is placed under the first and second metatarsal heads to invert the subtalar joint. The knee is extended. The child leans into a wall, keeping the heel on the ground. Aching is experienced in the popliteal fossa and proximal calf during effective stretching.

KEY POINTS: FLATFOOT

1. Flexible flatfoot is a normal foot shape that is present in most children and in a high percentage of adults.

2. The longitudinal arch elevates in most children through normal growth and development.

3. The arch cannot be created by means of special shoes, orthotics, braces, or exercises.

4. Flexible flatfoot rarely causes pain or other disability in children and adults.

5. A contracted, or tight, Achilles tendon can cause pain and disability in an otherwise normal flexible flatfoot. This rarely develops before adolescence.

6. Surgery for flatfoot is rarely indicated.

16. **What are the operative management principles for the two types of flexible flatfoot?**
Surgery is rarely, if ever, indicated for the flexible flatfoot.
Surgery is indicated for a flexible flatfoot with a short Achilles tendon when prolonged attempts at nonoperative treatment have failed to relieve the pain and callosities under the head of the plantar-flexed talus. Surgery may be as simple as an Achilles tendon lengthening if the flatfoot deformity is very mild. With more severe deformity, Achilles tendon lengthening should be accompanied by one or more osteotomies that preserve joint motion while correcting deformity. Arthrodesis, even of the small joints of the foot, should be avoided in the child. The technique of placing synthetic implants in the sinus tarsi region of the subtalar joint has been popular among podiatrists but has not been embraced by most pediatric orthopaedic surgeons because of the risks of infection and foreign body reaction. The long-term effects and consequences of these implants are unknown.

17. **What are the treatment principles for the rigid flatfoot?**
A tarsal coalition may become painful as it changes from a cartilaginous to a bony union. This generally occurs between 8 and 12 years of age for calcaneonavicular coalitions and between 12 and 16 years of age for talocalcaneal coalitions. Only symptomatic coalitions should be treated because approximately 75% of coalitions do not cause pain or disability. A radiographically confirmed painful tarsal coalition is treated with a below-the-knee walking cast for 4–6 weeks. The pain should be relieved immediately, thereby confirming that the coalition is the cause of the

pain and not just an incidental finding. A cushion-type, non-arched (flat) over-the-counter shoe insert is recommended following removal of the cast. There is a 30–68% chance that the child will remain free of pain after removal of the cast and will return to regular activities. Surgery is indicated if symptoms recur. Resection of the coalition with interposition of fat, muscle, or tendon is the procedure of choice in most cases. The long-term results of this procedure for calcaneonavicular coalition are very good. The long-term results for talocalcaneal coalitions have not been reported but, based on short-term results, are probably less favorable.

Osteotomy can be used for the correction of severe deformity. Triple arthrodesis should be considered for the foot with established and documented severe painful degenerative osteoarthritis of the subtalar joint complex. It should, therefore, rarely be used in children.

BIBLIOGRAPHY

1. Harris RI, Beath T: Hypermobile flat-foot with short tendo Achilles. J Bone Joint Surg Am 30:116–138, 1948.
2. Mosca VS: Calcaneal lengthening for valgus deformity of the hindfoot: Results in children who had severe, symptomatic flatfoot and skewfoot. J Bone Joint Surg Am 77:500–512, 1995.
3. Mosca VS: Flexible flatfoot and skewfoot: An instructional course lecture of the American Academy of Orthopaedic Surgeons. J Bone Joint Surg Am 77:1937–1945, 1995.
4. Staheli LT, Chew DE, Corbett M: The longitudinal arch: A survey of eight-hundred and eighty-two feet in normal children and adults. J Bone Joint Surg Am 69A:426–428, 1987.
5. Vanderwilde R, Staheli LT, Chew DE, Malagon V: Measurements on radiographs of the foot in normal infants and children. J Bone Joint Surg Am 70:407–415, 1988.
6. Wenger DR, Mauldin D, Speck G, et al: Corrective shoes and inserts as treatment for flexible flatfoot in infants and children. J Bone Joint Surg Am 71:800–810, 1989.

CHAPTER 50

CAVUS FOOT

Vincent S. Mosca, MD

1. **What is a cavus foot?**
   Cavus refers to a fixed equinus (i.e., plantar flexion) deformity of the forefoot in relation to the hindfoot, resulting in an abnormally high arch. The high arch may be along the medial border of the foot or across the entire midfoot. The heel may be in neutral, varus, valgus, calcaneus (i.e., dorsiflexed), or equinus position. There may be an accompanying clawing of the toes.

2. **What causes cavus deformity?**
   Cavus is a manifestation of a neuromuscular disease with muscle imbalance unless proven otherwise. Various patterns of muscle imbalance due to weakness or spasticity cause the various types or patterns of cavus deformity.

3. **What are some specific diagnostic causes of bilateral cavus foot deformity?**
   - Charcot-Marie-Tooth (CMT) disease
   - Dejerine-Sottas interstitial hypertrophic neuritis
   - Polyneuritis
   - Friedreich's ataxia
   - Roussy-Lévy syndrome
   - Spinal muscular atrophy
   - Myelomeningocele
   - Syringomyelia
   - Spinal cord tumor
   - Diastematomyelia
   - Spinal dysraphism tethered cord
   - Muscular dystrophy
   - Cerebral palsy diplegia or tetraplegia (although usually this causes planus deformities)
   - Familial (consider CMT disease)
   - Idiopathic (diagnosis of exclusion; very rare)

4. **What are some specific diagnostic causes of unilateral cavus foot deformity?**
   Traumatic injury of a peripheral nerve or spinal nerve root, poliomyelitis, syringomyelia, lipomeningocele, a spinal cord tumor, diastematomyelia, spinal dysraphism tethered cord, tendon laceration, an overlengthened Achilles tendon, cerebral palsy hemiplegia, old treated or untreated clubfoot, a compartment syndrome of the leg, a severe burn of the leg, or a crush injury of the leg.

5. **What are typical presenting complaints?**
   Patients typically complain of difficulty with shoe fitting, with pressure and pain over the dorsum of the midfoot; pain and callosities under the metatarsal heads and lateral to the base of the fifth metatarsal; clawing of the toes, with pain and callosities over the interphalangeal joints; inversion instability with frequent falling; and a feeling that ankles are "giving out." There is often a history of repeated ankle sprains.

6. **Why should you take a family history?**

CMT disease is an autosomal-dominant disorder and is a common cause of cavus foot deformity. You should also examine the feet of parents and other family members if possible.

7. **What are you looking for on examination?**

The height of the longitudinal arch is only one of the features to be assessed. First, examine the foot with the child standing. Note the varus, neutral, or valgus alignment of the heel. Severe cavus may give the impression of ankle equinus when in fact the equinus is entirely in the forefoot. Therefore, with the child seated, obscure the forefoot from view with your hand and assess dorsiflexion and plantar flexion of the ankle. Then attempt dorsiflexion of the forefoot onto the hindfoot and note, by palpation, the tightness of the plantar fascia. Manually inverting and everting the hindfoot with the ankle in neutral alignment can assess flexibility of the subtalar joint.

The Coleman block test can also be used to assess flexibility of the subtalar joint; it has the advantage of permitting the assessment with the foot in a weightbearing position. Rigid plantar flexion of the first metatarsal and pronation of the forefoot precede rigid inversion deformity of the subtalar joint of the hindfoot. The block test is performed by placing a block under the lateral border of the foot. By thus allowing the forefoot to pronate, a flexible subtalar joint will correct to neutral position and a rigid one will not. This information gives an indication of chronicity and is important for operative planning. Carefully note the areas of excessive callusing on the plantar aspect of the foot. Also note calluses on the dorsum of the interphalangeal joints of the toes. Perform a careful motor, sensory, and reflex examination of the foot and leg. Include tests for position and vibratory sensation.

Examine the spine. Look for scoliosis, kyphoscoliosis, lateral translation of the shoulders with an oblique take-off of the spine from the pelvis, diminished flexibility, and paraspinal muscle rigidity. Note any midline defects, abnormal hairy patches, or dimpling. Check the abdominal reflex. Inquire about urinary incontinence and anal sphincter control.

Examine the upper extremities for neurologic abnormalities (specifically, wasting and weakness of the interosseous muscles of the hand, as seen in CMT).

8. **What radiographs should be obtained?**

Standing anteroposterior and lateral radiographs of the spine are more important in the initial evaluation of the child with a cavus foot than are radiographs of the foot. Look for widening of the interpedicular distance, congenital malformations, atypical-pattern scoliosis (left thoracic), pelvic obliquity with lateral translation of the shoulders over the pelvis, and an opaque central bone spike (as may be seen with diastematomyelia).

Foot radiographs should include standing anteroposterior (AP) and lateral views. As a simple rule of thumb, a straight line normally passes through the axes of the talus and the first metatarsal on the AP and lateral images. A cavus foot is characterized by varus angulation of the axis of the first metatarsal in relation to the axis of the talus on the AP view and plantar angulation of the axis of the first metatarsal in relation to the axis of the talus on the lateral view. The treating orthopaedic surgeon may obtain more detailed and specialized radiographs.

9. **What other studies should be performed?**

Unless there is a known cause of the cavus foot such as poliomyelitis or myelomeningocele, an electromyogram and nerve condition velocity (EMG/NCV) study is indicated. A positive DNA blood test for CMT disease might obviate the need for the EMG/NCV study, but the test is very expensive and identifies only type I (accounting for 70% of cases). The DNA blood test for most of the other types is even more expensive. Creatinine phosphokinase and aldolase blood levels can be obtained. Magnetic resonance imaging of the spine and brain can also be appropriate in certain circumstances. You may choose to obtain a consultation with a pediatric neurologist at this point.

10. **How is the cavus foot deformity treated?**
Once the deformity has been identified, the underlying cause needs to be ascertained. If the underlying cause is untreatable, such as CMT disease, the child should be referred to an orthopaedic surgeon for foot surgery. If the underlying condition is treatable, such as a spinal cord tumor, treatment of that condition should precede treatment of the foot deformity.

11. **What is the role of nonoperative management of the cavus foot?**
There is little role for nonoperative management of the cavus foot deformity because most are progressive and are of advanced severity at the time of diagnosis. The worse the deformity, the more complex the operative reconstruction. Arch supports and shoe modifications might be appropriate in the earliest stages of a developing cavus foot deformity, but this decision should be made by the orthopaedic surgeon, who will know when to proceed with surgery.

12. **What are some relative indications for operative intervention?**
Painful calluses under the metatarsal heads and over the claw toes, difficulty with fitting shoes, abnormal and excessive shoe wear, and painful ankle instability are some indications that surgery should be performed.

KEY POINTS: CAVUS FOOT

1. The cavus foot deformity is a manifestation of a neuromuscular disorder with muscle imbalance until proven otherwise.

2. Diagnosis and treatment (if possible) of the underlying neuromuscular disorder must precede treatment of the cavus foot deformity.

3. There is little role for nonoperative management for the cavus deformity because most are progressive and of an advanced degree of severity at the time of presentation. Delay increases the complexity and difficulty of reconstruction.

4. Reconstruction involves concurrent correction of deformities and balancing of muscle forces.

5. Deformity correction starts with soft tissue releases and proceeds to osteotomies, reserving arthrodeses for salvage procedures in cases of recurrence or extreme deformities.

6. Tendon transfers are based on existing and anticipated patterns of muscle imbalance.

13. **What are the principles of operative management?**
There are two principles: the first is to correct the deformity, and the second is to balance muscle forces so as to maintain deformity correction and to prevent recurrences. These two components of the operative management are carried out concurrently in either one or two closely timed operative sessions.

Correction of the deformities involves release of soft tissue contractures and realignment osteotomies. The contracted plantar fascia is always released. The abductor hallucis is released from the calcaneus. Capsulotomy of the talonavicular joint with release of the spring ligament and the long and short plantar ligaments is carried out if the subtalar joint does not evert to neutral position. The joints should be aligned following these soft tissue releases. The foot is then evaluated for residual bony deformity, which is corrected using one or more osteotomies. These may be performed in the medial cuneiform, the base of the first metatarsal, the cuboid, and the calcaneus. The techniques for correction of deformities are based on the shape and on the rigidity or flexibility of the foot, not on the muscle imbalance.

The choices for tendon transfers relate directly to the specific pattern of muscle imbalance in the child's foot. Consideration must be given to the present and expected future pattern and the severity of muscle weakness.

14. **What about arthrodesis?**

The final principle of management is that arthrodesis should be reserved as a salvage procedure for severe degenerative osteoarthrosis and should not be used as a primary reconstructive technique. Arthrodesis causes stress shifting and premature degenerative osteoarthrosis in adjacent unfused joints such as the ankle.

BIBLIOGRAPHY

1. Mosca VS: The foot. In Morrissy RT, Weinstein SL (eds): Lovell and Winter's Pediatric Orthopedics, 5th ed. Philadelphia, Lippincott Williams & Wilkins, 2001, pp 1151–1215.
2. Mosca VS: Editorial: The cavus foot. J Pediatr Orthop 21:423–424, 2001.
3. Tachdjian MO: Pes cavus. In Clinical Pediatric Orthopedics: The Art of Diagnosis and Principles of Management. Stamford, CT, Appleton and Lange, 1997, pp 48–55.
4. Thometz JG, Gould JS: Cavus deformity. In Drennan JC (ed): The Child's Foot and Ankle. New York, Raven Press, 1992, pp 343–354.

CHAPTER 51

TOE WALKING

Jose Fernando De la Garza, MD

1. **Is there another name for idiopathic toe walking?**
   This entity was first described by Hall, Salter, and Bhalla in 1967 by the name *congenital short tendon calcaneus,* also known as *habitual toe walking* or *tiptoe walking.*

2. **Before what age in normal gait development is toe walking considered a normal condition?**
   Toddlers may walk with the foot in equinus when beginning independent walking. At the age of 2 years, children develop walking patterns similar to those of adults, and by the age of 3 years a mature gait pattern is established. This means that the heel-strike gait should occur by age 3 years.

3. **What is the main reason for consultation?**
   Persistent bilateral toe walking after age 3 years in a developmentally normal child who can usually stand flat-footed when not walking.

4. **How often does this condition have a positive family history?**
   Kallen's series found that 71% of the patients had a positive family history.

5. **What are common causes of an equinus gait?**
   See Table 51-1.

TABLE 51–1. COMMON CAUSES OF AN EQUINUS GAIT	
Category	**Diagnosis**
Congenital	Clubfoot
Idiopathic	Gastrocnemius contracture
	Accessory soleus muscle
	Generalized triceps contracture
Neurologic	Cerebral palsy
	Poliomyelitis
Myogenic	Muscular dystrophy
Functional	Hysterical toe walking

6. **What are the main conditions in the differential diagnosis?**
   - Cerebral palsy (CP), particularly in a mildly diplegic child
   - Muscular dystrophy
   - Tethered cord syndrome
   - Spinal cord tumor

- Spinal dysraphism
- Diastematomyelia
- Acute myopathies
- Idiopathic toe walking (ITW) (a diagnosis of exclusion)

7. **What are the differences between CP and toe walking?**
See Table 51-2.

TABLE 51-2. DIFFERENCES BETWEEN CEREBRAL PALSY AND TOE WALKING		
	Cerebral Palsy	Idiopathic Toe Walking
Spasticity	Usually present at ankle, knee, or hips	Negative
Gait	Permanent equinus	Occasional equinus
Standing	Equinus	Flat-foot standing
Neonatal history	Can be positive for preterm delivery or neonatal asphyxia	Negative

8. **What are the most important aspects of the history?**
- Prenatal history
- Perinatal data, including gestational age at birth and Apgar scores
- Presence of delayed neuromotor skills
- Family history

9. **If, by definition, idiopathic toe walkers do not have a central problem, where is the problem?**
In the Achilles tendon, which is short due to shortening of the soleus or gastrocnemius muscles.

10. **Are there any other diagnostic modalities that help in the differential diagnosis between ITW and mild CP?**
- Dynamic electromyography (EMG)
- Computerized gait analysis

11. **What are the main findings in the dynamic EMG and the computerized gait analysis?**
The data demonstrate lack of heel strike in association with knee flexion at the end of the swing phase in patients with cerebral palsy.

12. **Can EMG differentiate mild diplegic CP and ITW?**
In a study based on an obligatory coactivation during voluntary contraction of the quadriceps or gastrocnemius, the result suggested that EMG testing of resisted knee extension and quad set to identify gastrocnemius coactivation can help differentiate patients with mild CP from those with ITW.

13. **How many degrees of ankle dorsiflexion are needed for a normal gait (i.e., heel-toe walking)?**
One hundred eight or more.

KEY POINTS: TOE WALKING

1. Toe walking is normal in toddlers up to about 3 years of age.

2. Prenatal, perinatal, and developmental history are important in the assessment of toe walking.

3. Surgery for toe walking is indicated if nonoperative methods have failed and if the child is experiencing functional problems due to the toe walking.

14. **What are the treatment strategies for toe walking?**
    1. Strengthening exercises
    2. Serial stretching casts every 2 weeks for 6–10 weeks
    3. Night braces after the stretching cast to maintain the dorsiflexion
    4. Ankle-foot orthotics
    5. Heelcord lengthening

15. **Is there a place for the botulinum toxin in the treatment of the ITW?**
    The botulinum toxin helps to maintain post-treatment improvement and normalizes the ankle EMG pattern during gait.

16. **What is the best way to maintain the dorsiflexion after the stretching exercises or the stretching cast?**
    Place the foot in an ankle-foot orthosis (AFO) in an attempt to break the toe-walking pattern.

17. **When is surgery indicated for ITW?**
    Surgery is reserved for patients in whom physical therapy (i.e., stretching exercises), casts, and orthotics have not been successful. Achilles tendon lengthening is the usual procedure performed to obtain the necessary dorsiflexion for the heel-toe gait pattern.

18. **What is the main complication of surgical treatment?**
    Overlengthening of the Achilles tendon, producing a calcaneus gait, which is worse than the equinus gait.

19. **What would be a simple and fast treatment in a 2-year-old child with ITW?**
    Percutaneous lengthening of the Achilles tendon, followed by a below-knee cast for 4 weeks.

CONTROVERSIES

20. **Is ITW a diagnosis of exclusion, or is it really an unknown central nervous system deficit?**
    EMG studies were conducted in which children with ITW behaved similarly to patients with CP and equinus deformities and differently from the toe-walking control group. Other reports exist in which muscle biopsy specimens in operated patients showed features suggesting a neuropathic process, including predominance of type I muscle fibers and atrophic angulated fibers, thus suggesting a possible neurogenic basis for the condition.

21. **Is there a neurodevelopmental problem associated in a child with ITW?**
    In studies such as Futagi and Suzuki, there were problems with hyperkinesis and clumsiness in 35% of ITW cases.

BIBLIOGRAPHY

1. Brunt D, Woo R, Kim HD, et al: Effect of botulinum toxin type A on gait of children who are idiopathic toe-walkers. J Surg Orthop Adv 13(3):149–155, 2004.

2. Eastwood DM, Broughton NS, Dickens DRV, Menelaus MB: Idiopathic toe-walking: Does treatment alter the natural history? J Bone Joint Surg 78B(Suppl I):77, 1996.

3. Futagi Y, Toribe Y, Ueda H, Suzuki Y: Neurodevelopmental outcome of children with idiopathic toe-walking. No To Hattatsu 33:511–516, 2001.

4. Griffin PP, Wheelhouse WW, Shiavi R, Bass W: Habitual toe walkers: A clinical and electromyographic gait analysis. J Bone Joint Surg 59A:97–101, 1977.

5. Hall JE, Salter RB, Bhalla SK: Congenital short tendo calcaneus. J Bone Joint Surg 49B:695–697, 1967.

6. Kalen V, Adler N, Bleck E: Electromyography of idiopathic toe walking. J Pediatr Orthop 6:31–33, 1986.

7. Kogan M, Smith J: Simplified approach to idiopathic toe-walking. J. Pediatr Orthop 6:790–791, 2001.

8. Morrissy R, Weinstein S: Lovell and Winter's Pediatric Orthopaedics, vol. 2. Philadelphia, J.B. Lippincott, 1996.

9. Policy JF, Torburn L, Rinsky LA, Rose J: Electromyographic test to differentiate mild diplegic cerebral palsy and idiopathic tow-walking. J Pediatr Orthop 6:748–749, 2001.

10. Staheli L: Fundamentals of Pediatric Orthopedics. New York, Raven Press, 1992.

11. Wenger DR, Rang M: The Art and Practice of Children's Orthopaedics. New York, Raven Press, 1993.

VIII. KNEE AND TIBIA PROBLEMS

KNEE PAIN

Carl L. Stanitski, MD

CHAPTER 52

1. **What is the most common type of knee pain?**
   Nonspecific anterior knee pain seen in adolescents is most common. It is often erroneously referred to as *chondromalacia.*

2. **Why is the term *chondromalacia* a misnomer for this condition?**
   The articular surfaces of the patella, femur, and tibia are pristine, and the pain source is not the chondral zone. The condition should be considered idiopathic, and diagnostic efforts should be made to establish a specific diagnosis. *Chondromalacia* should be eliminated as a diagnostic term for this nonspecific complaint.

3. **What is the most common mistake made in the diagnosis of chronic knee pain?**
   Failure to evaluate the hip as a source of pain. Referred pain from the hip can masquerade as knee pain in such conditions as Perthes' disease and stable slipped capital femoral epiphysis.

4. **What is the most helpful technique to evaluate knee pain?**
   Clinical assessment by history and physical examination, including examination of the hip and contralateral knee, has high specificity and sensitivity for diagnosis.

5. **What should routine radiographic views of the knee include?**
   When possible, weight-bearing anteroposterior (AP), lateral, skyline (patellar profile), and tunnel (notch) views. Comparison views of the opposite knee are not routinely done.

6. **When should comparison views of the opposite normal knee be taken?**
   To assess physeal status following an acute injury or for follow-up of a previous physeal injury. They can also used to compare congenital anomaly status (e.g., bipartite patella or discoid meniscus).

7. **When should a bone scan be ordered to help assess knee pain?**
   Bone scintigraphy is helpful when a stress fracture is suspected. The study is also used in cases of reflex sympathetic dystrophy, but in this condition, bone scan results are highly dependent on the stage of the disorder. Quantitative bone scans may be helpful to predict healing potential in cases of juvenile osteochondritis dissecans.

8. **When should a magnetic resonance imaging (MRI) scan be ordered?**
   MRI is a powerful tool in knee disorder diagnosis. Unfortunately, it is commonly misused. The test should be done only after a thorough clinical examination and a standard radiograph review are unable to provide a specific diagnosis. The MRI examination should be ordered by an individual with the expertise to correlate the pertinent clinical findings with the imaging study and who can provide the appropriate definitive treatment for the specific diagnosis. Knee MRI should not be looked upon as a screening examination. Continued progress is being made with MRI technology, but a significant percentage of false-positive and false-negative readings do occur, especially regarding the meniscus in children and adolescents. Clinical correlation, as with results of all studies, is mandatory.

9. **What are pertinent points to be evaluated during history-taking?**
   - Pain characteristics (i.e., onset, duration, change with activity or rest, and night pain)
   - Trauma (macro vs. micro and recent vs. remote)
   - Effect of previous treatments
   - Swelling
   - Giving way
   - Locking
   - Growth velocity

10. **Physical examination should include what assessments?**
   The patient must be appropriately garbed (preferably in shorts) for an accurate examination to be done. The examination should include analysis of general maturity, gait, lower-extremity weight-bearing alignment, muscle definition, leg lengths (by block test), generalized joint laxity, range of motion (active and passive), swelling (extra- and intra-articular), focal tenderness (in the physes, patella, joint lines, tibial tubercle, or collateral ligaments), patellar tracking, and stability (anteroposterior, rotatory, and varus and valgus).

11. **What repetitive stress (overuse) problems can manifest as knee pain?**
   - Osgood-Schlatter disease
   - Stress fractures
   - Minor patellar maltracking
   - Sinding-Larsen-Johansson disease
   - Jumper's knee (i.e., patellar tendinitis)
   - Pathologic plica

12. **What intra-articular conditions should be considered in the differential diagnosis?**
   - Osteochondritis dissecans
   - Pathologic plica
   - Meniscal cyst
   - Discoid meniscus
   - Meniscal tears
   - Cruciate ligament injury

13. **What inflammatory causes should be considered in the assessment?**
   - Juvenile rheumatoid arthritis
   - Pigmented villonodular synovitis
   - Osteomyelitis
   - Hemophilia
   - Septic arthritis
   - Lyme arthritis

14. **Are tumors a likely source of knee pain?**
   Benign and malignant tumors are very uncommon causes of knee pain. Benign lesions that may be symptomatic include osteochondroma, nonossifying fibroma with stress fracture, osteoid osteoma, and chondroblastoma. Malignant tumors, although rare, can cause knee symptoms, especially in adolescence. These include osteosarcoma and Ewing's sarcoma. In very young children, metastases from a neuroblastoma can also cause pain.

15. **What are common presenting complaints in patients with Osgood-Schlatter disease?**
   The condition usually is seen in active young adolescent patients undergoing a period of rapid growth. Activity-related pain is present at the tibial tubercle, with complaints of "good days and

bad days" pain cycles. Pain is particularly aggravated with kneeling, squatting, or jumping. Parents are often concerned about a tumor because of the tubercle's prominence.

16. **Are radiographs needed for patients with suspected Osgood-Schlatter disease?**
Even though the diagnosis usually appears straightforward, radiographs confirm the diagnosis (tubercle enlargement and fragmentation) and may show uncommon, unsuspected additional sources of pain such as tumors or infections.

17. **What treatment is recommended for Osgood-Schlatter disease?**
Patient and parental reassurance about the benign nature of the condition is paramount. They also should be counseled about the cyclic nature of the symptoms and the 12–18 months required for resolution (i.e., the approach of skeletal maturity). Symptomatic treatment with ice massage, knee padding, anti-inflammatory medication, hamstring and quadriceps flexibility exercises, and activity modification (not elimination) leads to satisfactory resolution in most cases. Steroid injections into the tubercle are to be condemned. If a separate ossicle persists, surgical excision may be required.

18. **What is the difference between Sinding-Larsen-Johansson disease and "jumper's knee"?**
The former is a sequela of traction on the immature distal patellar pole by the patellar tendon. It is analogous to Osgood-Schlatter disease and is seen in the preteen age group. The treatment is similar. The latter, seen in adolescents, is an inflammation of the proximal patellar tendon brought about by repetitive stress from jumping. The condition may progress to produce intratendinous degeneration and necrosis.

19. **What other evaluations should be considered in a patient with suspected juvenile rheumatoid arthritis?**
In addition to clinical examination and laboratory parameters (e.g., sedimentation rate and rheumatoid factor) and synovial fluid analysis, slit-lamp examination should be included in the assessment of these patients because children with pauciarticular or monoarticular arthritis are at increased risk of developing iridocyclitis.

20. **What is the cause of a "snapping knee" in a 6- to 10-year-old?**
A discoid meniscus commonly presents with complaints of snapping at the knee. The condition may be asymptomatic (other than the auditory nuisance). Pain and mechanical symptoms result if a tear is present in the abnormally shaped meniscus or if the meniscus is unstable because of congenital absence of the posterior meniscotibial ligament.

KEY POINTS: KNEE PAIN

1. *Chondromalacia* should be eliminated as a diagnostic term for nonspecific anterior knee pain.

2. Knee pain equals hip pain until proven otherwise. Clinical examination of the hip must be included in a knee examination.

3. Magnetic resonance imaging (MRI) should only be ordered for very specific indications. It should not be used as a screening test.

4. Sympathetic dystrophy (i.e., nonspecific regional pain syndrome) does occur in children and adolescents, especially in the lower extremity. It must be considered in anyone with chronic pain complaints out of proportion to the inciting event.

5. Pathologic plicae occur rarely and are clinically diagnosed by focal tenderness, palpable snapping, and reproduction of pain in an arc of 30–70 degrees of flexion.

21. **What is the treatment of a symptomatic discoid meniscus?**
Treatment is dependent on the meniscal morphology and stability. If the meniscus is stable and without a tear, reconfiguration of the meniscus by surgical sculpting, usually by arthroscopic techniques, results in a more normal meniscus shape and size. If a tear is present, either repair or excision (arthroscopically) is done, depending on the tear's characteristics. A tear is commonly horizontal and often is associated with a meniscal cyst, which should be decompressed as part of treatment of the meniscal lesion. If the meniscus is unstable, surgical stabilization is done. All efforts are directed at preserving as much of a meniscus as possible so that its weight-bearing function can continue and prevent premature onset of degenerative joint disease.

22. **How do I know that I am dealing with a bipartite patella and not a fracture?**
Bipartite patellae are common incidental radiographic findings and should not be confused with an acute injury. Radiographic characteristics of a bipartite patella (in contrast to an acute fracture) include regular, smooth fragment margins; no evidence of soft tissue swelling; and an enlarged total size of the patella (main plus accessory fragment). Clinically, there is no pain or tenderness at the site. One caveat: an acute separation following direct trauma can occur at the junction of the fragment and the main patellar body. In this case, clinical signs of acute injury are present and immobilization is undertaken. If there is no clinical evidence of injury, the condition is considered a radiologic curiosity with no intervention required other than informing the patient and family of the condition's presence to avoid future confusion.

23. **What is the prognosis for osteochondritis dissecans?**
The primary prognostic factors are patient age and skeletal maturity. The less mature the patient is, the better the prognosis, with the best results seen in the juvenile form (i.e., before adolescence), in which full recovery is the usual outcome. In the adolescent type (i.e., partial skeletal maturity), outcome is unpredictable. With the adult type (i.e., skeletal maturity), a guarded prognosis is the rule.

24. **What are common presenting symptoms in a patient with osteochondritis dissecans?**
Mechanical-type pain (increasing with activity and diminishing with rest) and intermittent effusion are the most frequent complaints. Locking or catching due to fragment instability are uncommon findings.

25. **What is a knee plica, and how does it cause symptoms?**
The knee has normal synovial folds that are residual embryonic remnants from when the knee cavity was a septated structure. These folds (i.e., plicae) are common findings and are considered variants of normal anatomy. Occasionally, pathologic conditions occur within the plica when the synovium is inflamed owing to acute, direct, or repetitive microtrauma. The inflamed plica becomes enlarged and is trapped between the patella and the femoral condyle. This impingement sets up further inflammatory changes and plica fibrosis. The thickened plica may cause secondary abrasive injury to the underlying articular surfaces.

26. **How can I diagnose a pathologic plica?**
The diagnosis is made on clinical grounds. The patient complains of snapping and catching when the knee is in a specific position of flexion. The pain and snapping are reproduced by direct palpation over the plica (usually medial) when the knee is taken through a flexion arc, usually from 30 degrees to 70 degrees. Standard radiographs show normal findings.

27. **What is the treatment for adolescent anterior knee pain?**
If possible, a specific diagnosis is made, such as Osgood-Schlatter disease. If objective review does not provide a specific diagnosis, the patient and family should be reassured of the nonfatal nature of the condition. A multitude of nonspecific treatments (including taping, braces,

exercises, and physical therapy modalities) have made claims of efficacy, but objective evidence is lacking. The pain commonly abates spontaneously following the adolescent growth spurt.

28. **How common is reflex sympathetic dystrophy (i.e., chronic regional pain syndrome) in this age group?**

This diagnosis is made with increasing frequency as awareness of the condition in this age group becomes more widespread. Unfortunately, it is still commonly missed, with resultant delay in diagnosis and treatment. The diagnosis must be suspected in any patient whose complaints of pain and disability are out of proportion to the precipitating event or injury. Hypersensitivity to the slightest touch is a common finding. The skin vasomotor changes are of late onset, and their absence should not invalidate the diagnosis. Familial and school problems are common associated findings in this poorly understood condition.

29. **What is the prognosis for reflex sympathetic dystrophy in children?**

The prognosis is usually quite good in children, in contrast to adults. Most childhood disease is seen in the lower extremity. Hallmarks of treatment include physical therapy focused on progressive function, anti-inflammatory medication, and counseling.

30. **What is the role of surgery in treating adolescent anterior knee pain?**

Surgery has a very limited role. Indications for surgery are based on specific objective findings. Pain alone is not an indication for surgery.

BIBLIOGRAPHY

1. Bourne MH, Bianco AJ Jr: Bipartite patella in the adolescent: Results of surgical excision. J Pediatr Orthop 10:69–73, 1990.
2. Dietz FR, Mathews KD, Montgomery WJ: Reflex sympathetic dystrophy in children. Clin Orthop 258:225–231, 1990.
3. Hefti F, Beguiristain J, Krauspe R, et al: Osteochondritis dissecans: A multicenter study of the European Pediatric Orthopaedic Society. J Pediatr Orthop Br 8:231–245, 1999.
4. Johnson BL, Eastwood DM, Witherow PJ: Symptomatic synovial plicae of the knee. J Bone Joint Surg Am 75:1485–1496, 1993.
5. Krause BL, Williams JP, Catterall A: Natural history of Osgood-Schlatter disease. J Pediatr Orthop 10:65–68, 1990.
6. Nimon G, Muray D, Sandow M, Goodfellow J: Natural history of anterior knee pain: A 14–20 year follow up of non-operative management. J Pediatr Orthop 18:118–122, 1998.
7. Paletta G, Bednarz P, Stanitski C, et al: The prognostic value of quantitative bone scan in knee osteochondritis dissecans: A preliminary experience. Am J Sports Med 26:36–39, 1998.
8. Raber DA, Freidrich NF, Hefti F: Discoid lateral meniscus in children: Long-term follow-up after total meniscectomy. J Bone Joint Surg Am 80:1579–1586, 1998.
9. Stanitski CL: Anterior knee pain syndromes in the adolescent. J Bone Joint Surg Am 75:1407–1416, 1995.
10. Stanitski CL: Correlation of arthroscopic and clinical examinations with magnetic resonance imaging findings of injured knees in children and adolescents. Am J Sports Med 26:1–5, 1998.

CHAPTER 53

PATELLOFEMORAL DISORDERS

Robert E. Eilert, MD

1. **What is the most common physical finding associated with anterior knee pain in adolescents?**

   Hamstring contracture is frequently associated with an episode of rapid growth. Resolution of this contracture reliably resolves the symptoms of anterior knee pain. The course of stretching exercises necessary to lengthen the hamstring and increase the range of straight leg-raising takes about 6 weeks to complete. The exact mechanism by which stretching of the hamstring contracture relieves anterior knee pain is not proven but seems biomechanically related to a decrease in the patellofemoral reaction force by means of reducing the relative knee flexion at heel strike. Hamstring contracture produces chopped strides clinically, which are especially noted when the patient runs.

2. **What is the usual treatment for patellar pain?**

   Most patellar pain decreases with nonoperative treatment. In adolescents, patellar pain tends to be associated with tightness or contractures. The lateral retinaculum, the hamstrings, the iliotibial band, the quadriceps muscle, the hip rotator muscles, and the triceps surae muscle may be tight or shortened. During physical examination, these structures should be systematically evaluated. Stretching is a major component of therapy for affected individuals. Rest in cases of overuse, strengthening of weak muscles such as the vastus medialis obliquus, and biofeedback to coordinate muscle action are other features of a physical therapy protocol to treat patellar pain.

3. **Can vastus medialis obliquus (VMO) deficiency be corrected with exercise?**

   VMO deficiency can be congenital or associated with injury or inflammation about the knee. In the case of injury or inflammation, the VMO deficiency may be corrected with rest, anti-inflammatories, and an exercise program to strengthen whatever muscle is present and to help rebalance the patella. There is some evidence that patellar subluxation occurs when there is an asymmetric firing of the VMO and the vastus lateralis. This tendency for firing out of sequence—that is, the vastus lateralis firing before the VMO in terminal extension—can be corrected by exercise training, with or without biofeedback.

4. **By what mechanism does lateral release relieve knee pain?**

   Theoretically, lateral release improves anterior knee pain by altering the alignment of the patella. Another theory is that the release divides nerve fibers in the lateral retinaculum and capsule that are the source of the pain. A third theory is that it changes the pressure relationships under the patella, therefore altering the pain symptoms.

   These theories must be correlated with the clinically apparent relief of symptoms following the operative procedure in selected patients. Operative candidates are patients who show decreased medial mobility (as evidenced by the inability to separate the lateral border of the patella from the lateral condyle of the femur) and in whom a vigorous program to strengthen the vastus medialis obliquus and to stretch contractures around the knee does not resolve knee pain.

5. **In acute dislocation of the patella in a child, what is the appropriate treatment?**

   A reasonable argument can be made for removal of osteochondral fragments, which may be detached either at the time of dislocation or during relocation of the patella. Good results have been reported for reconstruction of the medial patellofemoral ligament combined with lateral release if acute reconstruction is chosen.

The outcome of nonoperative treatment in children and adolescents is similar to that obtained with acute surgery, and nonoperative treatment carries far less risk of possible complications such as hemarthrosis, nerve damage, and scarring.

Nonoperative treatment consists of a short period of joint rest followed by a vigorous rehabilitative effort. Using a knee immobilizer or splint during the period for joint rest for 1–2 weeks allows early movement of the joint and isometric exercises while the initial swelling and pain resolve. As soon as the patient begins to tolerate isometric exercise, this can be supplemented by weight resistance in a short arc mode as well as electrical stimulation to the VMO, which was inhibited by the joint swelling and by the stretching associated with lateral dislocation of the patella.

6. **What is the natural history of patellar dislocation?**
Patellar dislocation is usually associated with patellar malalignment, which predisposes the dislocation. Therefore, patellar dislocation has a strong tendency to be recurrent. The greater the severity of the malalignment, the greater is the tendency for the dislocation to recur. Considering age at time of the first dislocation as a factor, the younger the person is, the more likely it is that the dislocation will recur. The frequency of dislocation tends to decrease over time, but each dislocation can produce chondral damage. Degenerative arthritis is a common long-term sequela, with or without surgery to stabilize the patella.

7. **When do you perform a distal versus proximal reconstruction for a dislocation patella?**
The most common reconstruction performed for recurrent dislocation of the patella is a proximal one, which involves lateral retinacular release and some type of medial tightening operation, whether it is plication of the medial capsule or a more sturdy medial vector reconstruction such as use of the semimembranous tendon routed through the patella (using the method of Putti and Dewar).

Distal reconstruction is reserved for those patients in whom the tibial apophysis has closed and there is an increased Q angle. The tibial apophysis is shifted medially while its anterior position is preserved to reduce the Q angle and valgus shift at the patella. The Goldthwait procedure, performed with partial medial routing of the patellar ligament, has been condemned as producing many complications in skeletally immature patients.

8. **Why is surgery more effective for patellar instability than for patellar pain?**
In cases of patellar subluxation or dislocation, the anatomic abnormalities, which contribute to the instability or are produced by dislocation, can be defined with accuracy. Surgical correction can be tailored to address the malalignment with a high degree of success. The cause of patellar pain is often difficult to define in the absence of instability and may not correlate with any specific anatomic abnormality. Indeed, no consensus exists as to the exact cause of many cases of patellar pain. As in other areas of orthopaedic surgery, when a surgical procedure is not designed to address a specific anatomic abnormality, the outcome is less successful.

9. **What common conditions produce referred pain to the knee in children?**
You should always be suspicious of more-proximal lesions that can refer pain to the knee. The obturator nerve, which innervates both the hip and the knee joint, can cause confusing pain patterns that are commonly perceived on the medial side of the knee. Perthes' disease in the younger child or slipped capital femoral epiphysis in the adolescent may present as knee pain. Other diseases such as osteoid osteoma, which often occurs in the region of the lesser trochanter, likewise can be referred distally, so any child with knee pain should have a

careful hip examination. Because of suspicion of a proximal lesion, radiographs should include the entire femur in any case in which symptoms are not resolving with knee treatment. The cardinal sign of an abnormal hip examination finding is decreased internal rotation as detected by the log roll test, which is performed by rolling the lower extremity medially and laterally with the hip in extension.

10. **How do you differentiate patellar subluxation from a torn meniscus?**
The differentiation of patellar instability from a meniscus injury is a frequent diagnostic challenge after trauma. One condition may mimic the other. If there is tenderness about the patella, particularly medially, associated with an apprehension sign, patellar subluxation is suspect. Joint line tenderness associated with a palpable positive "clunk" or pain exacerbation on knee rotation points to a meniscal injury. The mechanism of injury may be similar for the two conditions, and repeated examination during subsequent visits may be necessary to fully elucidate the diagnosis.

11. **What is the difference between Osgood-Schlatter disease and the Sinding-Larsen-Johansson lesion?**
The lesion described by Osgood and Schlatter is pain in the area of the tibial tubercle caused by microfractures in the area of the apophysis that are associated with activity-related stress on this region. A similar condition occurs at the other end of the patellar ligament, which is the lower pole of the patella. Traction in this area may also be associated with pain and fragmentation of the bone. Both conditions are time limited and associated with rapid growth and immature bone maturation in the middle teenage years. What separates Osgood-Schlatter disease from Sinding-Larsen-Johansson lesion is the patellar ligament; the two conditions occur at opposite ends of the ligament.

12. **When should you place a patient with Osgood-Schlatter disease in a cast?**
Rarely should you use a cast for a child with Osgood-Schlatter disease, which is a developmental variation based on a stress reaction in the area of the tibial tubercle due to a relative overuse syndrome. In these individuals, the strength of the tibial tubercle can be exceeded by the activity of the individual's quadriceps, such as in vigorous sports activities. In the most extreme cases, a splint may be necessary, but it can be removed for active use of the joint and muscles to prevent atrophy and stiffness. The splint can be worn at night, with good relief of symptoms in the daytime. Use of a cast results in disuse and stiffness and tends to compound the situation more than it helps.

13. **Is arthroscopy ever indicated to evaluate chondromalacia patellae?**
The term *chondromalacia patellae* should probably be replaced in the literature by *patellofemoral pain*, or even by the more general term *anterior knee pain*, since the findings of softening of the patellar cartilage and pain do not correlate well. There are patients in whom arthroscopy demonstrates a softening of the articular cartilage under the patella, which may be an incidental finding when arthroscopy is performed for another reason. In contradistinction, patients with patellofemoral pain may have normal-appearing articular cartilage without softening. The mechanism of pain production is debatable but does not appear to be related to the anatomic abnormality of softened articular cartilage. In the past, the pathologic term had been applied to all anterior knee pain, but this led one away from a specific diagnosis. In each case, a specific diagnosis should be sought even if the therapy (such as stretching and strengthening) is nonspecific.

14. **What is an apprehension test?**
To perform the apprehension test, the examiner attempts to manually subluxate the patella laterally. The test is performed with the knee relaxed in an extended position. In a positive test, the patient suddenly becomes apprehensive and resists any further lateral motion of the patella.

The result of the apprehension test is commonly positive in patients with recurrent patellar instability (Fig. 53-1).

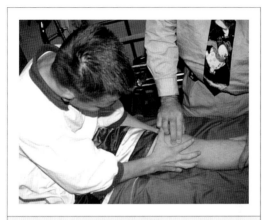

Figure 53-1. Positive apprehension test.

15. **What is a Q angle?**

The Q angle is a clinical measurement. A line from the anterosuperior iliac spine to the center of the patella is created. A second line is drawn from the center of the patella to the center of the tibial tubercle. The angle formed at the intersection of these two lines is the Q angle.

A normal Q angle ranges from 10–20 degrees. An increased Q angle creates a lateral force on the patella as the knee is extended and is a predisposing factor for patellar instability.

16. **What is the movie theater sign?**

Prolonged sitting classically exacerbates patellar pain. Patients with patellar pain from any cause often complain of pain on arising after prolonged sitting, such as in a movie theater.

17. **What produces the crepitus felt on examination of the patella while the knee is moved?**

A perception of grinding or crepitus can be palpated beneath the patella as the knee is flexed and extended. The crepitus may be caused by an irregularity of the articular cartilage or by synovial thickening or swelling.

18. **What imaging studies are most helpful in the evaluation of patellar pain and malalignment?**

Imaging does not often identify the specific cause of pain but can be useful for confirmation of a diagnosis of malalignment. Plain radiographs are useful for evaluation if the patient is carefully positioned, and magnetic resonance imaging is seldom necessary for diagnosis. The lateral radiograph shows the level of the patella relative to the femur where patella alta may exist, for example. The standard radiograph for measuring patellar tilt or subluxation is the Merchant's projection, taken with knee in 30 degrees of knee flexion.

KEY POINTS: PATELLOFEMORAL DISORDERS ✓

1. Patellar malalignment usually is present in cases of patellar dislocation.

2. Correct contractures about the knee in adolescents with anterior knee pain by a stretching program with physical therapy.

3. The vastus medialis obliquus (VMO) stabilizes the patella when it fires in the terminal 15 degrees of extension.

4. Dysfunction of the patellofemoral joint can be secondary to weakness of the VMO as well as malalignment.

5. Surgical realignment for the patellofemoral joint should be considered only after a trial of physical therapy since stretching and strengthening solve most pain problems.

19. **What characterizes congenital dislocation of the patella?**

In the first type of congenital dislocation, the patella is fixed and permanently dislocated laterally. These children present with a flexion contracture and delay in walking. The definitive diagnosis may require a magnetic resonance imaging scan (Fig. 53-2) because the patella is unossified and difficult to palpate.

In the second type, there is an obligatory dislocation of the patella as it shifts laterally from an underdeveloped trochlea with each flexion and extension cycle of the knee. More commonly, the patella is tethered laterally as the knee flexes and reduces in full extension, but the reverse may also be true. These children usually present at a later age because this condition does not usually delay walking. They have the striking physical finding of a "popping" patella that shifts laterally each time they flex and extend their knee.

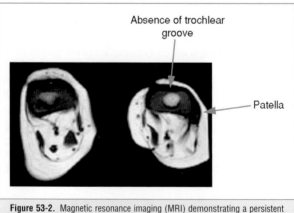

Figure 53-2. Magnetic resonance imaging (MRI) demonstrating a persistent (fixed) congenital lateral dislocation of the patella in a 1-year-old child.

20. **What is the significance of a bipartite patella?**

A bipartite patella is usually an asymptomatic, incidental radiographic finding (Fig. 53-3) that may be misdiagnosed as an acute fracture. The reported incidence ranges from 1–5%. The most common location is the superolateral patella.

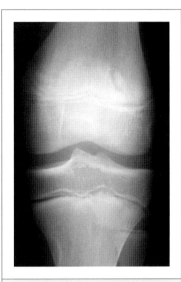

Figure 53-3. Note the smooth edges and contour of this bipartite patella, distinguishing it from an acute fracture.

BIBLIOGRAPHY

1. Baker RH, Carrol N, Dewar FP, Hall JE: The semitendinosus tenodesis for recurrent dislocation of the patella. J Bone Joint Surg Br 54:103–109, 1972.

2. Fulkerson JP: Disorders of the patellofemoral joint, 3rd ed. Baltimore, Williams & Wilkins, 1997.

3. Grelsamer RP: Current concepts review: Patellar malalignment. J Bone Joint Surg Am 82:1639–1645, 2000.

4. Merchant AC: Classification of patellofemoral disorders. Arthroscopy 4:235–240, 1988.

5. Micheli LJ: Patellofemoral disorders in children. In Fox JM, Del Pizzo W (eds): The Patellofemoral Joint. New York, McGraw-Hill, 1993, pp 105–122.

CHAPTER 54

CONGENITAL HYPEREXTENSION OF THE KNEE

N. M. P. Clarke, ChM, FRCS, and Klaus Parsch, MD

1. **Are there other terms that describe the problem of congenital hyperextension?**
   Synonyms include congenital genu recurvatum, congenital dislocation of the knee (CDK), and hyperextended knee.

2. **What is a hyperextension deformity?**
   In normal babies up to the age of 3 months, there is a knee flexion contracture of about 20–30 degrees (i.e., the knees do not straighten fully). In breech babies, the knees may hyperextend 20 degrees beyond the straight position (i.e., genu recurvatum). In such circumstances, the anterior articular surfaces of the tibia have continuous contact with the articular surface of the distal femur, distinguishing the physiologic deformity from congenital subluxation and dislocation of the knee (Figs. 54-1 and 54-2).

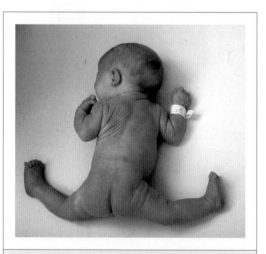

Figure 54-1. Bilateral hyperextension of the knees at 10 days of age.

3. **How often does one see hyperextended knees at birth?**
   About 2 in 100,000 children are born with a hyperextended knee. Only half have true subluxation or frank dislocation, whereas the majority show simple hyperextension without anterior tibial displacement. We see no more than one child with congenital genu recurvatum for every 100 with developmental dysplasia of the hip.

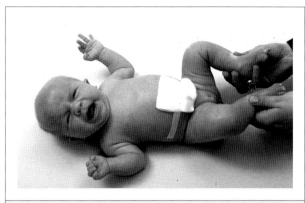

Figure 54-2. The same infant at 5 weeks of age after conservative treatment.

4. **What are the clinical types?**

Physiologic genu recurvatum is common in molded babies. Pathologic hyperextension deformities embrace a spectrum of anatomic displacements, from subluxation to dislocation. In congenital subluxation, there is some contact maintained between distal femoral and proximal tibial articular surfaces. Conventionally, the severity of deformity is graded from I to III, as follows:

- **Grade I:** The most common (50%); the joint can be passively flexed to 45–90 degrees.
- **Grade II:** Less common (30%); the tibia is displaced anteriorly on the femur, although there is still some retained articular contact. Clinically, there is perhaps 45 degrees of hyperextension and the knee will flex only to the neutral position.
- **Grade III:** Least common (20%), with total displacement of the proximal tibia and no contact between the articular surfaces. The knee is in severe hyperextension, with the toes often in contact with the face. There is often wrinkling of the skin over the patella, and there may be associated angular deformity of the knee.

5. **What are the causes?**

Intrauterine breech malposition is a common cause of genu recurvatum. It has been proposed that absence of the cruciate ligaments permits knee dislocation. Fibrosis of the quadriceps mechanism has also been incriminated. It is difficult, however, to differentiate primary causative factors from secondary adaptive changes.

6. **What is the pathology?**

In pathologic, as opposed to physiologic, displacement, the upper end of the tibia is anterior to the distal end of the femur. There may be associated lateral subluxation or angular deformity of the knee, and contraction of the lateral soft tissue structures may be encountered. As a consequence of the bony displacement, the hamstrings may be displaced anteriorly and may effectively function as extensors of the knee joint. The patellar tendon and quadriceps are usually contracted. Often, the patella is hypoplastic. The cruciate ligaments are elongated but always present. No associated neurovascular abnormalities have been reported.

7. **What imaging methods are used?**

Plain radiographs do not reveal very well the amount of subluxation present at birth because the femoral and tibial physes are not yet ossified. Arthrography has some value and was used in the past to identify the underlying disorder. Ultrasonography is very useful in identifying the position of the tibia against the femur and is also an efficient method of monitoring the reduction achieved during conservative treatment. It is probably the imaging modality of choice. Magnetic resonance imaging (MRI) has similar value but is more expensive and less available.

8. **What is the natural history?**
It is usual for simple genu recurvatum deformities to resolve spontaneously (in 50% of cases). Active treatment is necessary for subluxation and dislocation. In the most severe cases, surgical correction of the contracture of the quadriceps mechanism and relocation of the joint should allow the patient to walk normally and to retain reasonable knee function.

9. **What are the associated problems?**
Other congenital malformations. Hyperextension may be a component, for instance, of Larsen's syndrome, which is characterized by multiple joint dislocations. The most frequent association (45%) is with developmental dysplasia of the hip, perhaps as a consequence of the generalized molding deformity. Congenital foot deformities and congenital dislocation of the elbow are also recognized as associations, as are cleft palate and imperforate anus. Hyperextended knees are frequently seen in arthrogryposis. CDK can be associated with congenital dislocation of the patella, which is demonstrated by ultrasonography. If it is present, surgical management must include a patella tendon transfer medially. Finally, joint dislocations in general can be related to syndromes incorporating generalized joint laxity, such as Down or Ehlers-Danlos syndromes.

10. **What is the management in the newborn?**
It is not necessary to begin active treatment for simple congenital hyperextension deformities since they will resolve spontaneously. Gentle active physiotherapy may hasten resolution of the deformity. In congenital subluxation and dislocation, treatment is commenced as soon as possible. Reduction may be achieved by manipulation of the joint into flexion, held by plaster casts. Serial changing of the cast allows a gradual increase in the range of flexion. Joint stability is achieved by 6–8 weeks, after which the position is held by means of a Pavlik harness. The splint is primarily used for treatment of developmental dysplasia of the hip but does allow dynamic movement at the knee while maintaining flexion. It may be necessary to maintain harness treatment for 2–3 months. If reduction cannot be achieved by conservative means or if satisfactory flexion cannot be obtained, operative treatment is necessary. Open surgical reduction of the knee displacement is required.

11. **Are there alternative conservative methods of treatment?**
Traction in the prone position used on an inpatient has proved to be successful.

12. **What should be done with knees that cannot be reduced by conservative treatment?**
Knees that are irreducible after a course of conservative treatment require surgical reduction. Lengthening of the quadriceps tendon is performed in combination with a medial and lateral release of the patellar retinaculum. In cases with additional lateral dislocation of the patellar insertion, the patellar tendon is lengthened as well. The elongated cruciate ligaments are placed in their anatomic position. After reduction, the leg is held in a plaster cast for a period of 6 weeks. It may not be possible to hold the leg in 90 degrees of flexion owing to pressure on the skin anteriorly. If this is the case, the best possible position is obtained and the patient is brought back in 1–2 weeks for further manipulation until 90 degrees of flexion is obtained.

13. **What happens to the cruciate ligaments in congenital dislocation of the knee? Do these knees become stable?**

We have never seen a child with CDK without cruciate ligaments. The anterior and posterior cruciate ligaments can be elongated and thinned out. This is especially true for complete irreducible dislocations and children with Larsen's syndrome. It is obvious that after considerable cruciate ligament elongation, the knee will not have normal stability after reduction. Additional instability may be caused by the medial and lateral release necessary for otherwise irreducible knees. We have seen meniscal tears arising in adolescence as a late sequela of the initial instability.

KEY POINTS: CONGENITAL HYPEREXTENSION OF THE KNEE

1. Congenital hyperextension of the knee may be a part of other syndromes, such as Larsen's syndrome or arthrogryposis, in which there are multiple joint dislocations.

2. Many cases of congenital hyperextension of the knee resolve spontaneously or with minimal treatment.

3. For congenital dislocation or subluxation of the knee, active treatment and surgical reduction are often necessary.

14. **What is the final functional outcome in CDK?**

The functional outcome after conservative or surgical treatment is variable. Some children achieve full flexion with normal extension and show no further disadvantage. The majority will live with a restricted flexion of around 90 degrees. In addition, lack of stability may be seen in children who needed surgical reduction owing to the necessary medial and lateral releases. Quadriceps muscle power can be reduced in children who have had late reduction of the displaced knee. The majority, however, show normal motor power in their knee extensors.

15. **How is the knee treated in Larsen's syndrome?**

In Larsen's syndrome, there is a combination of knee dislocation and other malformations such as developmental dislocation of the hips and facial anomalies. Conservative treatment cannot reduce the knee joint. It seems wise to support the child's motor activity by stimulating exercises in the first 1–2 years of life. Open reduction with quadriceps lengthening is needed, most likely in combination with a realignment of the patellar tendon.

BIBLIOGRAPHY

1. Austwick DH, Dandy DJ: Early operation for congenital subluxation of the knee. J Pediatr Orthop 3:85–87, 1983.

2. Bell MJ, Atkins RM, Sharrard WJW: Irreducible congenital dislocation of the knee. J Bone Joint Surg Br 69:403–406, 1987.

3. Bensahel H, Dal Monte A, Hjelmstedt A, et al: Congenital dislocation of the knee. J Pediatr Orthop 9:174–177, 1989.

4. Curtis B II, Fisher RL: Congenital hyperextension with anterior subluxation of the knee: Surgical treatment and long term observations. J Bone Joint Surg Am 51:255–269, 1969.

5. Ghanem I, Wattincourt L, Seringe R: Congenital dislocation of the patella. Part II: Orthopaedic management. J Pediatr Orthop 20:817–822, 2000.

6. Katz MP, Grogono BJS, Soper KC: The etiology and treatment of congenital dislocation of the knee. J Bone Joint Surg Br 49:112–120, 1967.

7. Larsen LJ, Schottstaedt ER, Bost FC: Multiple congenital dislocations associated with characteristic facial abnormality. J Pediatr 37:1–8, 1950.

8. Laurence M: Genu recurvatum congenitum. J Bone Joint Surg Br 49:121–134, 1967.

9. Leveuf J, Pais C: Les dislocations congénitales du genou (genu recurvatum, subluxation, luxation). Rev Chir Orthop 32:313–350, 1946.

10. Niebauer JJ, King DE: Congenital dislocation of the knee. J Bone Joint Surg Am 42:207–225, 1960.

11. Nogi J, MacEwen GD: Congenital dislocation of the knee. J Pediatr Orthop 2:509–513, 1982.

12. Parsch K: Congenital dislocation of the knee. In Editions Scientifiques Médicales SAS (Paris). Duparc J (ed): Surgical Techniques in Orthopaedics and Traumatology 2001, 55-580-D-10. Paris, Elsevier, 2001.

CHAPTER 55

BOWLEG

Edilson Forlin, MD, MSc, PhD

1. **What is bowleg?**

   Bowleg (or tibial bowing) is the angulation of the leg, mainly the tibia, with the apex of the deformity directed anterolaterally, anteromedially, or posteromedially. Each type of bowing tends to have a classic etiology.

   Anterolateral bowing is associated with a presentation of pseudarthrosis of the tibia. **Anteromedial bowing** may be associated with congenital deformity such fibular hemimelia. These two conditions represent a more complex deformity, require treatment, and have a potential for clinical disability. **Posteromedial bowing** is associated with calcaneovalgus foot deformity. Both of these deformities tend to resolve, but a leg-length inequality commonly develops and may require treatment.

   For the orthopaedic surgeon, the term *bowleg* (or tibial bowing) refers to the varus angulation of the tibia or the knee, a more benign condition. It is associated with some degree of internal rotation of the leg.

2. **Is bowleg (i.e., tibia vara) always an abnormal finding?**

   No. Tibia vara is the pattern from 0–12 months (Fig. 55-1), and some degree of varus angulation is normal up to the age of 2 years. There are some families that present a pattern of genu varum in adulthood.

3. **What is the normal development of the leg in children?**

   We know that children are born with a varus tibial-femoral angle. Its value decreases with age. By 18–24 months of age, the knee is straight. At the age of 3–5 years, valgus angulation becomes more pronounced. From that point to the end of growth, there is a normal valgus angulation of the knee of around 5–10 degrees. Of course, development can vary in normal children; for example, the Japanese population has a higher percentage of varus knee in adulthood.

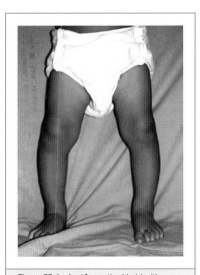

Figure 55-1. An 18-month-old girl with symmetric varus knees.

4. **How do I differentiate clinically physiologic tibia vara from other diseases with bowing legs?**

   In physiologic tibia vara, the child has no other findings and stature and development are within normal range. Also, bowing has to be symmetric, not intense, with the diaphysial apex of the varus. It improves up to the age of 18–24 months.

5. **When is radiography of a bowleg required?**
   Most children referred to an orthopaedic surgeon will not require radiography. There are some situations in which I find it necessary—for example, if there is unilateral bowing, if there is any feature not associated with physiologic bowing (like short stature), or if it progresses. In Blount disease, radiographic features are present only after the age of 18 months.

6. **What diseases are associated with marked tibia vara?**
   Blount disease, skeletal dysplasias (as the metaphyseal chondrodysplasias), rickets, fibrocartilaginous dysplasia of the tibia, and post-traumatic or bone infection at the proximal tibial epiphysis or metaphysis, leading to proximal tibial physeal arrest.

7. **What is the fibrocartilaginous dysplasia of the tibia?**
   Fibrocartilaginous dysplasia is a rare benign entity that affects the proximal tibia, leading to unilateral tibia vara at childhood. It can be present in other bones like the femur and the humerus. It was originally described in 1985 as a fibrocartilaginous defect at the medial side of proximal tibia. The imaging shows a radiotransparent defect with a distal sclerosis. As the child grows, the defect moves toward the diaphysis. Spontaneous resolution of the lesion with correction of the angular deformity has been reported.

8. **What is Blount disease? What is its pathogenesis?**
   It is growth disorder of the medial part of the proximal tibia physis, epiphysis, and metaphysis that causes a medial angulation and internal rotation of the tibia. Most histologic changes are localized at the zone of resting cartilage. It can be divided into three types according to the onset of the disease: infantile (with onset up to 3 years of age), juvenile (onset from 3–9 years of age), and adolescent (after the age of 9 years).

   The pathogenesis may be repetitive trauma to the medial and posterior physeal area due to walking on a varus knee. Obesity may play a major role in Blount disease.

9. **How do I differentiate clinically physiologic bowing from Blount disease?**
   Usually, patients with Blount disease are obese and walked early, before the age of 1 year. Also, black children are affected more often than white children. In Blount disease, deformity is progressive and restricted to the upper tibia, whereas physiologic varus may improve until 18–24 months of age, and the varus is present at the femur and the tibia diaphyses. We should be aware that differentiation may be difficult before the age of 24 months, and observation is required. The clinical control is done by the measurement of the intracondylar distance, the femoral tibial angle and the thigh-foot angle. Documentation with pictures can be very useful.

10. **What are the clinical risk factors for Blount disease?**
    Early walking, obesity, familial history, more intense varus up the age of 2 years, and some degree of varus angulation after 2 years of age.

11. **How does imaging help to differentiate physiologic bowing from Blount disease?**
    After the age of 18 months, imaging studies can be useful, but distinction between physiologic bowing and Blount disease is not obvious in young children. At the initial phase, Blount disease can show an irregularity of the medial aspect of the proximal tibia. The metaphyseal-diaphyseal angle, which is the angle formed by a line parallel to the top of the proximal tibial metaphysis and a line perpendicular to the lateral cortex of the tibial shaft, has been used (Fig. 55-2). If the angle is greater than 11 degrees, Blount disease is the probable diagnosis. Because difficulties of measurement may occur, I believe we should consider an angle greater than 15 degrees to suggest Blount disease. However, some reports found that neither the tibiofemoral angle nor the metaphyseal-diaphyseal angle were helpful to differentiate the two conditions in the young child (of around 2 years of age). In order to confirm the diagnosis, it is important to follow the patient for a time to assess the course of the disease.

12. **What is a useful radiographic classification for Blount disease?**

The most referred are the six stages of the Langenskiöld classification (Fig. 55-3). Stage I and II are hardly distinguishable from physiologic bowing. A small irregularity at the medial side of metaphysis became apparent. At stage III, a fragmentation and erosion at metaphysis is characteristic. Stage IV presents as a step at the metaphysis and the medial epiphysial deformity. A depression of the medial plateau and angulation of the medial epiphysis are present at stage V. At stage VI, the medial deformity is intense, with severe depression of the articular surface, and a bone bar is evident. Important for treatment is avoiding the progression to stage IV, which would occur at around the age of 5 years. This stage is associated with early bar formation across the deformed physis, although it may be difficult to identify. Problems with this classification are the lack of reproducibility and the fact that it is not intended for use in determining the prognosis or the type of treatment, as pointed out by the author.

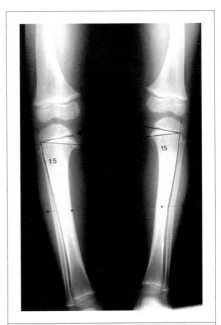

Figure 55-2. Metaphyseal-diaphyseal angle of 150 degrees. There is a deformity on the medial side of the epiphysis. These findings suggest Blount disease.

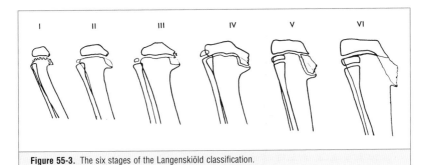

Figure 55-3. The six stages of the Langenskiöld classification.

13. **What is the natural history of Blount disease?**

In the infantile form (before the age of 3 years), spontaneous resolution is very uncommon and most cases progress to deformity with marked varus angulation and internal torsion. The medial part of the tibial epiphysis becomes depressed and fuses with the metaphysis by the age of 10–13 years. In the juvenile and adolescent types, these deformities are less pronounced.

14. **What is the conservative treatment for Blount disease?**
Although bracing is a classic recommendation for the initial stages, studies demonstrated that better results were found in unilateral cases. There are no sufficient data to confirm its effectiveness. The use of a Denis Browne night splint has been reported, but most authors recommend a nonarticulated knee-ankle-foot orthosis (KAFO). If the surgeon and the family decide to use an orthosis, it may have a system that forces valgus angulation at the knee and may be applied in children younger than 3 years old (i.e., Langenskiöd stage I or II). The brace treatment is continued until appropriated alignment and normal aspect of the proximal tibia (which would take 1–2 years of treatment).

The use of a brace is based on the idea that the splint corrects the deformity, but there is no consensus. We can point out some problems or questions regarding its use for Blount disease. Because the wearing during daytime is very difficult and uncomfortable for the child, many surgeons recommend its use during sleep along with a few hours of bracing by day. Also, the orthosis molding is difficult in a young child, especially at the calf, and the force to produce effective valgus angulation at the knee may be not tolerated. It locks the knee in extension, which is unphysiologic and uncomfortable, and stretches the ligaments. Its use also may affect the sleep pattern, causing an irritable child and behavior changes. The family should be informed about these topics prior to the prescription.

Exercises and physical therapy are of no value. Bracing also is not effective for treatment of late-onset tibia bowing.

15. **What are the indications and the recommendations for surgical correction for infantile Blount disease?**
Indications are an age older than 3 years at the initial visit, noncompliance with the brace, and marked obesity, especially for bilateral involvement. Valgus osteotomy should be performed before stage IV because, at this stage, a bone bridge may produce recurrence. Mechanical alignment should be checked intraoperatively (checking the center of the hip, knee, and ankle), clinically and by radiography.

16. **What type of surgery should be performed for initial Blount disease?**
In most instances, a single proximal osteotomy of the tibia is appropriate. The osteotomy is done distally to the tibial tubercle to avoid damage to the tibial apophysis. Osteotomy of the fibula is also performed to allow correction of the varus and internal rotation.

There are many techniques of osteotomy and fixation. Oblique wedge osteotomy is simple and safe. A dome osteotomy is simple and provides stability as well. An oblique osteotomy from anterior to posterior and inferior to superior has been described. We may remember that the internal torsion needs to be corrected simultaneously. Slight overcorrection is advised to effectively modify the support to the lateral compartment of the knee.

The corrected position can be held with a long-leg cast, but most authors recommend fixation. Options are the use of a Steinmann pin, a screw (when an oblique osteotomy is performed), a plate, or an external fixator.

I do not recommend a plate because it does not allow correction if we notice postoperatively that the position is not what was planned. In young child, a system with two Steinmann pins crossing the tibia transversally, proximally, and distally, incorporated with the cast, is simple, allows modification of the position if necessary, and is well accepted by the child. In an older child with juvenile or adolescent Blount disease, the Ilizarov device is a very good option.

17. **Is there another technique to be used in initial cases?**
Hemiepiphysiodesis may be an option for treatment if the physis are still open and the varus deformity is not severe. The staple hemiepiphysiodesis is recommended. The staple are placed extraperiosteally at the lateral proximal tibial physis. When complete correction is obtained, the staple may be removed to prevent overcorrection. Indication has to be carefully considered since the literature still has few data about the value of this procedure.

18. **What are the risk factors for recurrence?**
Black females, obesity, ligament laxity, Langenskiöld stage IV or more, presence of a bone bridge, and undercorrection.

19. **What are the surgical options for older children with more advanced disease?**
As children grow older and the deformity progresses (to stage IV, V, and VI), more complex procedures may be necessary. Bar resection and elevation of the medial plateau can be associated with the valgus osteotomy when there is an important medial depression with a physeal bar. When it is too large and cannot be identified or resected or when the procedure fails, epiphysiodeses of the lateral tibial physis and proximal fibula may be associated with the correction.
Femoral varus deformity has to be assessed. If it is present, lateral epiphysiodesis or osteotomy can be considered.

KEY POINTS: TIBIAL BOWING

1. Physiologic bowing is symmetrical, not intense, in a normal developed child.

2. Differentiation between physiologic bowing and Blount disease is difficult in a child younger than 2 years of age.

3. Conservative treatment has a better outcome in children under the age of 3 years.

4. Surgical treatment of Blount disease may be performed before stage IV.

5. To avoid compartment syndrome, percutaneous fasciotomy of the anterior compartment at the time of the tibial osteotomy is advised.

20. **What are the important aspects of late-onset juvenile and adolescent Blount disease?**
It is associated with severe obesity. Lateral knee laxity is an important factor. Medial knee pain is common. It can be associated with slipped capital femoral epiphysis (SCFE). Because of the patient's size and obesity, stable fixation without casting is recommended.

21. **What is the worst complication of the proximal tibial osteotomy?**
Compartment syndrome. To prevent it, I recommend percutaneous fasciotomy of the anterior compartment at the time of the osteotomy.

22. **What should I tell parents of children with probable physiologic tibial bowing?**
It must be made very clear to parents that physiologic tibial bowing carries an excellent prognosis and should not be considered a disease. Close follow-up every 3–6 months will rule out pathologic changes.

BIBLIOGRAPHY

1. Langenskiöld A: Tibia vara [editorial]. J Pediatric Orthop 14:141–142, 1994.

2. Levine AM, Drennan JC: Physiological bowing and tibia vara. The metaphyseal-diaphyseal angle in the measurement of bowleg deformities. J Bone Joint Surg 64A:1158–1163, 1982.

3. Morrissy RT, Weinstein SL (eds): Lovell and Winter's Pediatric Orthopaedics, 4th ed., vol. 1. Philadelphia, Lippincott-Raven, 1996, pp 322–329.

4. Salenius P, Vanka E: The development of the tibiofemoral angle in children. J Bone Joint Surg 57A:259–261, 1975.

CHAPTER 56

CONGENITAL PSEUDOARTHROSIS OF THE TIBIA

Edilson Forlin, MD, MSc, PhD

1. **What is congenital pseudoarthrosis of the tibia (CPT)?**
   Dysplasia of the bone and soft tissue of the half of the leg with failure of normal bone formation. There is a progressive apex anterolateral angulation; the tibia and fibula can present with medullary sclerosis and diaphyseal narrowing or cystic lesion. This leads to segmental weakening of the bone, developing pathologic fracture without bone reparation. The etiology is unknown. CPT is very rare (at 1:140,000), but it is the most common type of congenital pseudoarthrosis.

2. **Can we assume that the pseudoarthrosis is present at birth?**
   No. The term *congenital pseudoarthrosis of the tibia* is widely used among orthopaedic surgeons, but it is not correct. Usually, pseudoarthrosis is not present at birth. Some authors have proposed the term *infantile pseudoarthrosis*.

3. **What is the clinical picture?**
   Unilateral anterolateral bowing is noticed in the first year of life. The apex is middle to distal of the leg. In most patients, a nontraumatic fracture occurs by 2–3 years of age. Instability, ankle valgus, and leg-length shortening are progressive (Figs. 56-1 and 56-2). There is a slight predominance of boys affected.

4. **What is the other form of leg angulation in a newborn?**
   Posteromedial angulation. The prognosis is quite diverse from CPT. The correction is spontaneous, and there is no tendency to fracture. The only problem that may result is a mild leg-length discrepancy (of 3–6 cm). Anteromedial and angulations are associated with fibular hemimelia.

5. **What diseases are frequently associated with CPT?**
   The most common is neurofibromatosis. In published series, around 50% of children with CPT had a diagnosis of neurofibromatosis. On the other hand, among patients with neurofibromatosis type I (NF1), the incidence of CPT is 10%. The

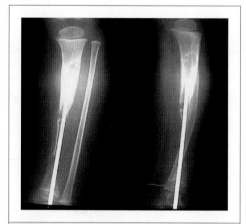

Figure 56-1. A female patient underwent two surgeries of intramedullary rod and grafting. One year after the last surgery there is reabsorption of the graft and no signs of consolidation.

second most common associated disease is fibrous dysplasia.

6. **What are the histologic findings?**
   Highly cellular, fibromatosis-like tissue was the common finding. The pseudoarthrosis gap can show histologic evidence of neurofibromatosis or fibrous dysplasia (less common), or it can be nonspecific.

7. **How is CPT classified?**
   There are three classifications, based on the radiographic features:
   Boyd and Anderson classification
   - **Dysplastic type:** Narrowing with sclerosis of the tibia (associated with neurofibromatosis, Fig. 56-3)
   - **Cystic type:** Resembles fibrous dysplasia and has a better prognosis
   - **Sclerotic type:** Sclerosis without narrowing
   - **Early type:** Pseudoarthrosis is present at birth

   Boyd classification
   - **Type 1:** Anterior bowing and a defect in the tibia present at birth
   - **Type 2:** Hourglass constriction and obliteration of the medullary canal; the most common type
   - **Type 3:** Congenital cyst, usually near the junction of the middle and distal thirds of the tibia
   - **Type 4:** Sclerotic without narrowing
   - **Type 5:** Dysplastic fibula
   - **Type 6:** Intraosseous neurofibroma or schwannoma

   Crawford classification
   - **Type I:** Cortical thickening with the medullary canal preserved
   - **Type II:** Cortical thickening, a thinned medullary canal, and tabulation defect
   - **Type III:** A cystic lesion that may be fractured
   - **Type IV:** Pseudoarthrosis is present, possibly with fibular nonunion

8. **Are there important limitations for the use of these classifications?**
   Yes. They are morphologic classifications, and the appearance of

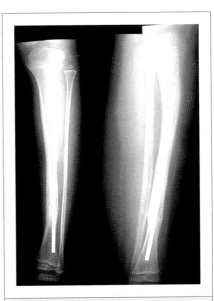

Figure 56-2. Three years post intramedullary rod and allograft from bone bank (a fibula from adult). The graft restored the length and consolidated. A KAFO for protection is still used.

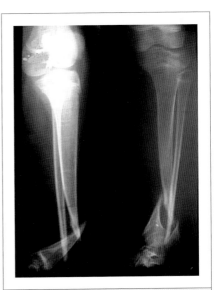

Figure 56-3. A dysplastic type of congenital pseudoarthrosis. This patient has neurofibromatosis as well.

CPT may change during the course of the disease. Also, some cases of CPT are difficult to classify; a definitive relationship between the classification and the prognosis has not been entirely proved, and the classification systems are not very helpful to guide treatment.

9. **What is the natural history of CPT?**
There is progressive anterolateral deformity of the leg, valgus ankle deformity, and shortening. The tibia presents a medullary canal sclerosis and diaphyseal narrowing or a cystic lesion. After the fracture has been apparent, there is no tendency to heal. The deformities, instability, and shortening make walking very difficult without an orthosis.

10. **Can we prevent a fracture? How?**
Most authors believe that we can prevent the fracture—or at least delay it for some years—by using a brace. There are two options: an above-the-knee brace or a below-the-knee brace with an anterior shell (usually a patellar tendon bearing). Prophylactic grafting is not recommended. Corrective osteotomy should be avoided, at least until maturity.

11. **What are the goals of treatment when pseudoarthrosis is established?**
   - Obtain union
   - Maintain the union
   - Correct the deformities
   - Obtain leg-length equality

12. **What is the best age for surgery?**
This issue is controversial. Most authors recommend delaying the surgery until at least after age 3 or 4 years because of the better prognosis for healing. Others suggest that there is no need to defer surgery until the child is older than 3 years as they believe that the healing prognosis is the same and that there are fewer secondary deformities. Surgery should not delay until older age, such as 10 years, because disuse atrophy and valgus deformity of the ankle joint will be aggravated.

13. **What are the principles and techniques of surgery?**
The principles of most techniques are resection of the dysplastic segment, correction of the deformity, and adequate apposition of the bone at the defect. Currently, three methods are considered the most successful, as follows:
   - **Intramedullary rod:** Corrects the deformity, prevents refracture, and is easily performed; does not provide correction of the leg-length inequality.
   - **Vascularized fibular graft:** Very specialized technique with high success rate but adds only a small amount of length
   - **Ilizarov technique:** Allows compression of the pseudoarthrosis and lengthening simultaneously but carries a high rate of refracture; demanding for the patients, especially young children

   Recent reports have suggested the combination of these procedures. An intramedullary rod has been used in the Ilizarov technique, protecting the tibia from refractures after device removal. Others have used the Ilizarov fixator in association with the vascularized fibular graft.

14. **What are the other surgical options?**
Coleman proposed the transfers of the ipsilateral fibula with the vascular pedicle left intact and secured to both fragments of the tibial pseudarthrosis by cerclage wires. His preliminary results were successful in five cases.

Some cases have been reported using structured allograft from a bone bank. After the resection of the pseudoarthrosis, a segment of long bone, usually a fibula from an adult, is placed under pressure, restoring the length. Fixation is done by the intramedullary rod. Early results seem to be positive.

15. **List some prognostic factors.**
   - **Associated with better prognosis:** Late onset, cystic type, or preserved medullary canal
   - **Associated with worse prognosis:** Early pseudoarthrosis, a more distal lesion, concomitant fibula pseudarthrosis, or hourglass constriction or dysplastic tibia

KEY POINTS: CONGENITAL PSEUDOARTHROSIS OF THE TIBIA (CPT)

1. Usually, the affected child is born with anterolateral angulation, and fracture will occur in the first 3 years.

2. Fifty percent of CPT is associated with neurofibromatosis type 1.

3. Better prognosis factors are late onset, a cystic type, and a preserved medullary canal.

4. The three main methods for treatment are the intramedullary rod, vascularized fibular graft, and the Ilizarov technique.

5. Complication are common. The most important are refracture, residual angular deformity, limb-length discrepancy, and ankle valgus.

16. **What are the complications of the treatment? How can we avoid or decrease their incidence?**
   The complications that can compromise the functional outcome include the following:
   - **Refracture:** This is the major complication and is associated with residual deformity, narrow bone diameter, or both. Protection with a brace for a long period of time and maintenance of the intramedullary rod can be effective preventative measures.
   - **Residual angular deformity:** The use of an intramedullary rod alone or in combination with other methods may result in a better alignment.
   - **Limb-length discrepancy:** This is a difficult situation. The option of external fixation allows an opportunity for concomitant treatment of the pseudoarthrosis and shortening. For the other options, a lengthening near the maturity or a contralateral epiphysiodesis, or both, may be effective.
   - **Ankle valgus:** Correction of fibular pseudoarthrosis, deformity, or insufficiency may decrease the incidence and amount of valgus, but this may not prevent it in all cases.

17. **When is amputation indicated? What type should be performed?**
   Amputation can be indicated in a patient with repeated surgical failures who has ankle stiffness or severe deformity and shortening. An ankle disarticulation (i.e., a Boyd or Syme procedure) is preferred rather than amputation through the lesion because it avoids problems such as spike formation, provides good end-bearing skin, and gives some length. It is important to remember the improvement of the prosthesis, which can provide excellent function.

18. **What is the present status of CPT treatment?**
   In prepseudoarthrosis, the use of a brace can delay the fracture and thus may improve the prognosis. Because of some disappointing results, some surgeons have recommended bracing without trying union. The problem with this option is that the shortening progresses, as do the valgus deformities of the leg and ankle.

Newer surgical techniques have improved the results of treatment. There is controversy about what is the best treatment: the Ilizarov technique, a vascularized fibular graft, or an intramedullary rod. Transfers of the ipsilateral fibula with its vascular pedicle and the use of an autologous diaphyseal shaft from a bone bank can be options, but longer follow-up is needed. In some instances, patients will need a permanent brace or a Syme or Boyd amputation.

Despite surgical improvements, CPT remains challenging. In most patients, several operations may be necessary, and the complication rate is still high. Even when union is obtained, additional surgery may be necessary because of residual deformity and refracture. Severe leg-length discrepancy and unsatisfactory ankle joint function are difficult to treat.

BIBLIOGRAPHY

1. Boyd HB: Pathology and natural history of congenital pseudoarthrosis of the tibia. Clin Orthop 166:5–13, 1982.
2. Dobbs MT, Rich MM, Gordon EJ, et al: Study of use of intramedullary rod for the treatment of congenital pseudoarthrosis of the leg: A long-term follow-up. J Bone Joint Surg 86A:1186–1197, 2004.
3. Grill F, Bollini G, Dungl P, et al: Treatment approaches for congenital pseudoarthrosis of tibia: Results of the EPOS multicenter study, European Paediatric Society (EPOS). J Pediatr Orthop 9(2):75–89, 2000.
4. Schoenecker P, Rich M: Congential pseudoarthrosis of the tibia. In Morrissy RT, Weinsstein SL (eds): Lovell and Winter's Pediatric Orthopaedics, 6th ed., vol. 1, Philadelphia, Lippincott Williams & Wilkins, 2006, pp 1189–1211.

HIP PAIN

John Charles Hyndman, MD

CHAPTER 57

1. **Where do you usually feel hip pain?**
   Hip pain can be experienced in the groin or in the anterior or anterolateral portion of the hip area. Not uncommonly, hip pain is felt in the knee or certainly in the distal thigh, usually medially.

2. **When is hip pain significant?**
   Hip pain is particularly significant when it is associated with other physical findings such as, most particularly, limp. Hip limps are usually seen as one of the earliest representations of hip pathology and are characterized by lateral translations or a trunk shift of the upper body toward the affected side during walking. This type of limp is a strategy that is automatically adopted by the patient because it decreases the force on the hip and thereby decreases the pain. Associated night pain that awakens the patient from sleep is a very significant historical feature and is frequently associated with a significant underlying pathologic condition.

3. **When is hip pain an emergency?**
   Hip pain associated with the inability of the child to walk is always a pediatric orthopaedic emergency. There are many pathologic lesions that must be defined urgently if the child is significantly affected as to be unable to bear weight. In those children who cannot walk, hip pathology is usually associated with a significant decrease in the range of motion (ROM).
   Commonly, and in children particularly, the range of motion can appear to be more than it is because of the flexibility of the adjacent lumbar spine. In quantifying the decreased range of motion, particularly in serial examinations, it is important to ensure that the lumbar spine is fixed, such as with the Thomas test. The ability to accurately assess whether the ROM is increasing or decreasing allows a definition of the longitudinal evaluation of the hip pathology and whether it is progressing or not.

4. **What is the most useful investigation in the evaluation of hip pain?**
   A single anteroposterior (AP) pelvis examination is essential in the evaluation of hip pain. It is inexpensive and will certainly define any significant pathology such as tumors, Perthes' disease, slipped epiphyses, or chronic inflammatory conditions such as osteoid osteoma. All patients who have a limp and hip pain should have, as a required minimum, an AP pelvis radiograph as part of the initial evaluation. Some early cases of slipped epiphysis will require a lateral examination to confirm this diagnosis, but the AP view is generally abnormal too.

5. **What other investigations are helpful in the evaluation of hip pain?**
   A complete blood cell count (CBC), sedimentation rate, and C-reactive protein are useful in defining infectious, nonspecific inflammatory conditions and, rarely, unusual and significant hematologic conditions such as granulocytic leukemia, which sometimes present as hip pain and arthritis. The absence of abnormality in the CBC and sedimentation rate, however, does not preclude a pathologic condition. Another investigation that is very helpful in the evaluation of hip pain is a bone scan. Bone scanning is nonspecific in terms of its ability to define pathology but is very sensitive in localizing abnormal foci of bone physiology.
   Less commonly, computed tomography (CT) is helpful in defining localized bony pathology and is particularly useful in preoperative planning. It is not particularly helpful in defining

pathology in patients who have normal plain radiographs. Magnetic resonance imaging (MRI) is particularly helpful in those circumstances in which soft tissue problems are the predominant issue. Further, MRI is very useful in the definition of the blood supply to the femoral head and may be the earliest indicator of abnormalities in such conditions as Perthes' disease.

Abnormalities involving the marrow cavity, such as other infection and tumor, are readily seen on MRI scans well before radiographic changes.

6. Is ultrasonography useful in hip pain evaluation?
Small quantities of fluid can be detected with ultrasonography. Whether the nature of the fluid (e.g., pus vs. blood) can be defined remains debatable. Prospective studies have not shown ultrasonography to be more sensitive than clinical evaluation. Careful clinical evaluation therefore remains the standard for detecting and following hip pain associated with fluid in the hip.

7. Can hip pain be psychologic?
In children, particularly young children, hip pain is rarely psychologic. It is true that in older children, and after careful evaluation with no evidence of pathology, hip pain can be found to have more of a psychogenic nature. It is important to remember, however, that this is a diagnosis of exclusion, and you must remember that hip pain, particularly hip pain associated with limp and objective physical findings, usually has a definable pathologic cause, and a careful history and physical examination, coupled with well-selected investigations, will usually easily define the nature of this pathology.

8. When should the patient with hip pain be referred?
It should be emphasized that those children who are unable to walk require careful and urgent determination as to the cause of this inability. Additionally, suspicion that the patient may have an early slipped epiphysis, as manifested by the typical clinical findings and the presence of a limp, even in the presence of a questionable radiograph, should be urgently referred because of the serious consequences of progressive slip. These patients should be protected from weight-bearing as soon as the question arises and referred promptly for further evaluation.

KEY POINTS: HIP PAIN

1. Hip pain is often referred to the anterolateral thigh. If a child presents with "knee pain," be sure to evaluate the hip.

2. The differential diagnoses for hip pain in children is age- and sex-dependent.

3. Hip pain with an inability to walk should be treated as a relative emergency, with rapid evaluation.

9. Do age and sex influence the pathologies that present with hip pain?
Many childhood hip pathologies definitely have predilections for both age and sex with respect to the conditions they reflect. For example, Perthes' disease is more common in boys and is usually found between the ages of 3 and 7 years. Slipped epiphysis typically affects a preadolescent, often obese, child, who is more commonly a male. Transient synovitis, on the other hand, follows a similar distribution to Perthes' disease, being found more commonly in boys and more commonly in the 3- to 7-year age group. Conditions such as osteoid osteoma are more commonly seen in the older child or in the young adolescent. Infectious diseases cover the whole age range of childhood, as do developmental abnormalities of the hip.

10. **What is the most sensitive indicator of pathology in patients with hip pain?**
In my experience, there is essentially no pathology that is not associated with limp. Frequently, the limp is not noticed, often because the patient's gait is not examined carefully in a hallway and rather is assessed in a small examining room. The presence of limp virtually always precedes pain and is always associated with thigh atrophy secondary to the limp. Careful evaluation for these clinical findings will strengthen your clinical suspicion that true pathology exists and should encourage a more aggressive investigation of the problem. On the other hand, if, on careful examination, there is no limp and no atrophy, questionable results on imaging studies are more usually benign in their interpretation.

CHAPTER 58

TRANSIENT SYNOVITIS

John Charles Hyndman, MD

1. **What is transient synovitis?**
   Transient synovitis is a condition that commonly affects children, particularly boys, between the ages of 3 and 7 years. It has had many names, including *observation hip* and *toxic synovitis,* among others, but the term *transient synovitis* perhaps best describes its natural history.

2. **How does transient synovitis present?**
   Generally, transient synovitis presents with acute pain, limp, and, sometimes, the inability to walk. Transient synovitis presents most commonly in the morning. There may be no prodrome. Generally, the patient is not sick, and nonspecific investigations such as complete blood count and sedimentation rate are either normal or show slight deviations. X-rays and bone scans are usually normal or show nonspecific signs.

3. **What causes transient synovitis?**
   The cause of transient synovitis is unknown. It may reflect a manifestation of a viral illness (although it is difficult to explain the strong male predilection), or it may relate to some form of trauma. The fact remains, however, that the cause is unknown.

4. **What is the differential diagnosis of transient synovitis?**
   The particular importance of transient synovitis lies in its confusion with more significant pathologic conditions such as septic arthritis. These conditions require urgent and aggressive treatment, whereas the treatment for transient synovitis is expectant. The clinician, therefore, must make a clear distinction between septic arthritis and transient synovitis. Other less acute conditions such as Perthes' disease can be confused, at least initially, with transient synovitis, and rarely osteomyelitis adjacent to the hip joint, in either the pelvis or the neck of the femur, may have an associated synovitis that is nonspecific. Bone tumors near the hip may also present with limp, although the range of motion of the hip is more likely normal.

5. **How do you distinguish septic arthritis from transient synovitis?**
   The very important distinction between transient synovitis and septic arthritis is in the first instance clinical. Specifically, the patient with transient synovitis is not sick, and, if there is a fever, it is usually of a low-grade nature. Similarly, investigations such as the white blood cell count (WBC) tend not to be elevated as much as they would be in the case of acute infection. Serial examination forms a very important part of the evaluation as it is not unusual for transient synovitis to be worse in the morning and better as the day progresses, whereas, in the case of infection, the patient will always get worse.

   In patients who appear in significant distress, who have marked restriction of range of motion, and who are unable to walk, it may be necessary to aspirate the hip in order to define whether or not pus is present. Transient synovitis usually has an amber-colored effusion, as opposed to a purulent one. Intra-articular pressure on occasion can be quite high and, in some instances, may be associated with a falsely positive bone scan, indicating the possibility of avascular necrosis or early Perthes' disease. Photopenia on bone scan is not diagnostic of avascular necrosis.

6. **Does transient synovitis cause Perthes' disease?**
   The association of transient synovitis and Perthes' disease has long been discussed, and historically many authors have felt that there was a relationship between transient synovitis and Perthes' disease. Currently, however, it is not generally believed that there is a relationship between transient synovitis and Perthes' disease. Occasionally, however, in less than 5% of cases, transient synovitis can be followed by Perthes' disease some months later. Whether or not this is cause and effect is unknown, but clinicians should be aware that there may be some soft relationship between the two. Parental education is prudent.

7. **How do you treat transient synovitis?**
   Once the diagnosis of transient synovitis is secure, it remains to follow the patient through the expected natural history of this condition. This is a benign process, and there will not generally be residua from transient synovitis. There is no good evidence that any of the more conventional forms of treatment, such as traction or anti-inflammatory drugs, will affect the natural history of this condition. Therefore, the treatment is expectant, with continued vigilance to ensure that the diagnosis indeed excludes pathologic conditions.

8. **Isn't traction commonly used?**
   Traction has been traditional, even though there is no good evidence to support its use. Several studies have pointed out that placing the hip in extension increases significantly the intra-articular pressure. Whether or not this has adverse consequences is unknown; theoretically, however, the knowledge that increased intracapsular pressure may be associated with avascular necrosis suggests that traction probably is unnecessary. More practically, I find that patients in traction are not examined as often or as well as those who are not in traction.

9. **When should a patient be hospitalized with transient synovitis?**
   In the past, it was not unusual that children with transient synovitis were admitted to the hospital fairly frequently. Currently, however, careful assessment on an outpatient basis, particularly of patients who can walk, albeit with a limp, allows safe expectant management. Parents can be instructed that if the inflammatory condition of the child has gets worse, it will be readily apparent in that the child will have an increased limp or indeed will not walk at all. It is our belief that the indication to admit patients with transient synovitis is limited to children who cannot walk and who must be urgently investigated and frequently reexamined.

10. **When does a child with transient synovitis return to normal activity?**
    Generally, return to normal activities, including gym, is restricted until such time as the presenting complaints, specifically the hip pain or limp, disappear. Furthermore, a full range of motion should be established prior to normal activities as occasionally the increasing activities will result in aggravation of the synovitis and subsequent confusion of the evolution of the natural history. This may result even in reinvestigation and readmission of the patient.

11. **What is the usual time frame for recovery?**
    Outpatient follow-up of these patients usually shows that the return to a completely normal range of motion is in the range of 2–3 weeks. Persistence, particularly of a significant restriction of motion beyond this time, should cause concern that the diagnosis is incorrect, and the possibility of some nonspecific inflammatory condition such as juvenile rheumatoid arthritis (JRA) should be entertained.

KEY POINTS: TRANSIENT SYNOVITIS

1. Transient synovitis commonly affects children, particularly boys, between the ages of 3 and 7 years. The cause is unknown.

2. Transient synovitis presents with acute pain, limp, and sometimes the inability to walk.

3. The very important distinction between transient synovitis and septic arthritis is in the first instance clinical. The patient with transient synovitis is not sick, and, if there is a fever, it is usually low-grade.

4. Serial examination forms a very important part of the evaluation as it is not unusual for transient synovitis to be worse in the morning and better as the day progresses, whereas, in the case of infection, the patient will always get worse.

5. Once the diagnosis is secure, it remains to follow the patient through the expected natural history. This is a benign process, generally without residua.

12. **Is transient synovitis a recurrent disease?**
    Recurrent bouts of transient synovitis are seen in less than 5% of cases. Children who experience repeated bouts of inflammatory arthritis of the hip should probably be investigated further, with the question of JRA or some other collagen vascular disease being entertained. JRA is an elusive diagnosis, occasionally taking months to define.

13. **Is transient synovitis bilateral?**
    Oddly, transient synovitis is rarely bilateral. Ultrasonography may suggest abnormality on the contralateral side, but practically bilateral transverse synovitis is extremely unusual—so unusual that the diagnosis should be highly suspected.

14. **Is aspiration of the hip beneficial?**
    Some studies have suggested that the course of the illness is shortened after aspiration. Given the cost benefit of aspiration, it is our belief that aspiration should be reserved for cases wherein the diagnosis is in doubt and significant concern regarding septic arthritis is apparent.

DEVELOPMENTAL DYSPLASIA OF THE HIP

Blaise A. Nemeth, MD, MS, and Kenneth Noonan, MD

CHAPTER 59

1. **What is developmental dysplasia of the hip (DDH)?**
   DDH encompasses the spectrum of hip disorders that involve an abnormal relationship between the acetabulum and femoral head, including subluxable, dislocatable, and dislocated hips. Previously termed *congenital dislocation of the hip*, the current terminology more accurately reflects that dislocation may not be present at birth and may evolve due to intrinsic and extrinsic factors, as well as including radiographic dysplasia without accompanying laxity.

2. **What is a teratologic dislocation of the hip?**
   A teratologic dislocation of the hip occurs *in utero* during the first trimester and is usually associated with neuromuscular diseases such as spina bifida or arthrogryposis. At birth, these hips have limited motion with severe dysplasia of the acetabulum and femoral head. Clinically, there are usually other neurologic or orthopaedic findings, and the hips are not able to be reduced without surgical intervention.

3. **What is the estimated incidence of hip dislocation at birth? Dysplasia?**
   Studies estimate that approximately 1 in 1000 children are born with a dislocated hip, whereas nearly 1 in 100 children are born with a dysplastic hip.

4. **When should the primary physician examine the child's hips?**
   Regular hip examinations should occur at each well child check until after the child has begun walking and demonstrates a normal gait for his or her age. The American Academy of Pediatrics (AAP) recommends these visits at 2–4 days with a second visit before 1 month, 2 months, 4 months, 6 months, 9 months, 12 months, and 15–18 months of age, until after the child has begun walking and demonstrates a normal gait for his or her age.

5. **What are the risk factors for DDH?**
   Given the baseline for decreased prevalence of DDH in the male infant; females, infants in the breech position during the last 4 weeks of pregnancy, and children with a family history of hip dysplasia are at known increased risk. Variable increased risk has been reported for children with findings of positional molding at birth (e.g., torticollis, metatarsus adductus, and calcaneovalgus foot). Idiopathic clubfoot is not associated with DDH.

6. **What role does prematurity play in DDH?**
   Premature infants have a disproportionate prevalence of late presentation of DDH. The cause is unclear, but it may be related to no or inadequate exam in a newborn with other distracting medical issues, decreased sensitivity of clinical examination or ultrasonography, or other unidentified factors inducing dysplastic development.

7. **What is the Ortolani maneuver? What is its significance in the evaluation of DDH?**
   For the Ortolani maneuver (Fig. 59-1A), the child is placed supine on an examination table with the pelvis level. Each hip is examined separately. One hand supports the pelvis and the hip that is not being examined. The other hand cradles the thigh of the leg to be examined, with the thumb on the medial side and the index or middle finger (or both) over the greater trochanter

and the hip, which is at 90 degrees of flexion. The hip is then abducted with slight elevation of the greater trochanter. The palpable reduction of the femoral head into the acetabulum constitutes a positive test (i.e., a dislocated hip). This sensation has commonly been referred to as a *clunk*.

Then, as the thigh is brought into slight adduction from the abducted position, with gentle pressure directed posteriorly (i.e., the **Barlow maneuver**), the hip will dislocate with the same sensation (Fig. 59-1B). The Barlow maneuver also assists in identifying hips that may not be dislocated but that have increased laxity and presumed underlying dysplasia.

8. **What is a hip click?**
   Clicks constitute palpable or audible sensations during the physical exam, primarily musculotendinous movements over bony prominences. Most adventitial clicks resolve by 2 weeks of life. The initial translation of Ortolani's maneuver described a positive test as a click, confusing the significance of this finding.

9. **What other physical findings may aid in the identification of a dislocated hip, especially in an older child or in a teratologic dislocation if the Ortolani maneuver is negative?**
   In nonteratologic dislocations, the muscles about the hip often tighten within the first few months, preventing clinical reduction and the ability of the Ortolani maneuver to detect dislocation in the older child. Thus, for both late presenting and teratologic dislocations, the dislocation is typically fixed. If unilateral, there may appear to be a leg-length discrepancy and a positive Galeazzi sign (i.e., a difference in the height of the knees and apparent length of the femur when the hips are flexed at 90 degrees in the supine position and adducted). Likewise,

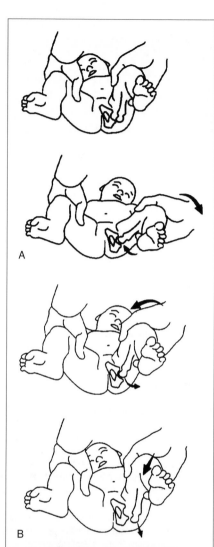

A

B

Figure 59-1. *A,* Ortolani test. This maneuver reduces a posteriorly dislocated hip. The affected hip is gently abducted while the femoral head is reduced with an anteriorly directed force provided by the fingers placed over the greater trochanter. *B,* Barlow test. This maneuver tests for dislocation or subluxation of a reduced hip. This is done by gently adducting the examined hip while directing a posterior force across the hip.

there may be asymmetry of the gluteal folds. In both cases, due to the muscle contractures, hip abduction is decreased. The pelvis must remain level as any tilting may mask subtle asymmetry in abduction in unilateral cases. In bilateral cases, limited abduction may be the only clinical finding.

10. **What are the common presentations of hip dislocation in the ambulatory child?**
    Often, children with a unilateral dislocation are referred for evaluation of an apparent leg-length discrepancy, as in the younger child or for toe walking (which is an accommodative maneuver for the functional shortening of the leg with a hip that is dislocated superiorly). In bilateral cases, children often walk with a waddling gait and have hyperlordosis of the lumbar spine.

11. **What work-up should be performed in a newborn with an Ortolani-positive hip?**
    A positive examination has identified a dislocated or dislocatable hip; therefore, no imaging is required. Examination should occur to detect other orthopaedic or neurologic abnormalities. Genetics evaluation may be appropriate, based on concomitant clinical findings. Referral to an orthopaedist should occur to initiate treatment.

12. **What is the role of ultrasound in the evaluation and treatment of DDH in the newborn?**
    Due to the primarily cartilaginous nature of the hip in children under 4 months of age, imaging of the acetabulum and proximal femur is best achieved with ultrasound. Ultrasonography provides information about both the development of the acetabulum as well as the stability of the hip by imaging during provocative maneuvers. Thus, ultrasound is recommended for the evaluation of newborns with equivocal or subtly positive examination findings or with historical risk factors for DDH.

13. **What is the primary limitation to ultrasound identification of hip dysplasia?**
    The presence of maternal relaxin generates hip laxity in the immediate newborn period. Early ultrasound imaging incurs a high rate of diagnoses of DDH, many of which will resolve by 4 weeks of age. As a result, ultrasonographic imaging is recommended at 4–6 weeks for equivocal or subtly positive examinations or if indicated by risk factors.

14. **What is the role of plain radiography in DDH?**
    Anteroposterior (AP, hips extended) and frog (hips abducted and externally rotated) views of the pelvis are useful in assessing bony development of the acetabulum and femoral head, which occurs primarily after 4 months of age (Fig. 59-2). Acetabular development is quantified by the measurement of the acetabular index (before closure of the triradiate cartilage) or the center-edge angle of Wiberg (for the skeletally mature patient). Development of the sourcil may also be assessed. Plain radiographs at 4–6 months are the preferred method of identification of dysplasia in a child with risk factors for DDH and a normal newborn exam or if signs or symptoms of DDH present after 4 months of age. The utility of plain radiographs in newborns is limited to identification of a stable, dislocated hip through the disruption of Shenton's line or through positioning of the medial femoral metaphysis outside of the inferomedial quadrant generated by the intersection of Perkin's and Hilgenreiner's lines if ultrasound (or a qualified ultrasonographer) is not readily available.

15. **What is the treatment for the newborn with DDH?**
    The Pavlik harness is the treatment of choice for the child with a dislocated, dislocatable, or subluxatable hip that is identified before 6 months of age and is reducible. The greatest success is achieved when treatment is begun before 7 weeks of age. The hip is allowed to stabilize for up to 4 weeks, and the harness is worn full-time for 6 weeks from the time of stabilization. The Pavlik harness is not indicated in the infant with teratologic dislocation of the hip.

16. **What is the Pavlik harness?**
    It is a hip flexion-abduction orthosis consisting of a chest strap, two shoulder straps, and an anterior flexion strap and a posterior abduction strap for each leg. The chest strap should be

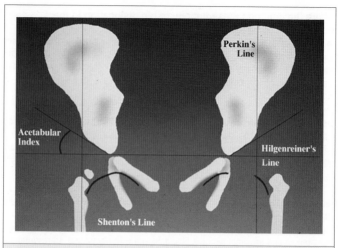

Figure 59-2. Radiographic findings in developmental dysplasia of the hip (DDH). The left hip with DDH shows delayed femoral head ossification, discontinuity of Shenton's line, and an increased acetabular index (the angle between Hilgenreiner's line and a line drawn parallel to the acetabulum) compared with the normal right hip.

at the level of the nipples: tighten the shoulder straps only to hold this position. The thighs are then positioned in 90–110 degrees of flexion using the anterior flexion straps, and the posterior abduction straps are tightened to prevent adduction beyond the point of dislocation.

17. **How successful is the Pavlik harness in managing DDH?**
    The Pavlik harness is successful in treating DDH in the newborn in 90–95% of cases. Children with a dislocatable hip that spontaneously reduces may have greater success than those who have a dislocated hip that spontaneously dislocates after reduction maneuvers. Bilateral hip dislocations may also have a higher failure rate for Pavlik harness treatment.

18. **What are the complications associated with the Pavlik harness?**
    Brachial plexopathy and femoral nerve palsy may occur when a tight harness results in shoulder depression and axillary impingement or in impingement under the inguinal ligament, respectively. If recognized early, both resolve quickly after proper repositioning of the harness. Avascular necrosis of the femoral head occurs rarely, most commonly due to continued use in an irreducible hip or a forced abduction.

19. **What is the treatment for the 6- to 24-month-old child newly diagnosed with DDH?**
    The older child requires closed reduction under anesthesia followed by hip spica casting. An arthrogram of the affected hip or hips aids in visualization of the acetabulum and any anatomic factors that may block reduction (i.e., pulvinar, dysplastic labrum or neolimbus, or redundant capsule) and require open reduction. Adductor tenotomy is widely used to aid in obtaining concentric reduction and to reduce compressive forces on the femoral head, which may induce osteonecrosis. The use of preoperative traction varies by surgeon and institutional preference. Hip spica casting maintains the reduction with the hip at 90–100 degrees of flexion and 45–60 degrees of abduction. Postreduction computed tomography (CT) confirms reduction within the cast. The cast may be changed after 6 weeks, allowing for repeat arthrography, but should be continued for a total of 8–12 weeks.

20. **What are the potential blocks to closed reduction that necessitate performing an open reduction?**

    Blocks to reduction that would necessitate open reduction can be considered intra-articular and extra-articular blocks. **Intra-articular blocks** to reduction include hypertrophic ligamentum teres, constricted transverse acetabular ligament fibrofatty tissue (pulvinar), an inverted labrum, or neolimbus. **Extra-articular blocks** include the adductor longus and the psoas tendon, which may lead to an hourglass constriction in the capsule, also preventing reduction of the hip.

21. **What are risks and benefits to the various surgical approaches to open reduction of DDH?**

    There are two well-accepted surgical approaches in developmental dysplasia of the hip: the anterior medial or medial approach to the hip and the anterior approach to the hip. In the **anterior medial approach,** the interval may be above or below the pectineus muscle. The adductor longus tendon and the psoas tendons are easily identified and sectioned. This approach allows direct exposure to the inferior medial capsule of the hip. Once the capsule has been opened, easy sectioning of the transverse acetabular ligament and resection of the ligamentum teres are possible. Pulvinar and inverted labrums may be dealt with equally from this approach. This medial approach is typically used in children up to 18 months of age. After 18 months of age, an **anterior approach** to the hip is performed through a bikini incision. This approach is more extensive and gains full exposure to the capsule, thus allowing for a capsulorrhaphy, which cannot be performed through the anterior medial approach. In addition, the anterior approach to the hip allows exposure and access to the superior acetabular region for performing concurrent acetabular procedures. Risks to the anterior medial approach include injury to the medial femoral circumflex vessels, which lie adjacent to the capsule and the psoas tendon. Potential injury to this vessel could lead to avascular necrosis. Problems with the anterior approach to the hip include extensive stripping of the gluteal musculature off of the iliac wing and capsule, which can lead to stiffness.

22. **What is the Salter innominate osteotomy? What are the indications for its use in the treatment of DDH?**

    The Salter innominate osteotomy is made by cutting through the superior acetabular region from the sciatic notch to the region above the anteroinferior iliac spine. This osteotomy is typically done in children who are less than 3 years of age who have deficient acetabular coverage. The acetabulum is hinged anteriorly and laterally. The inferior fragment pivots on the pubic symphysis. The displacement is maintained with a wedge of bone graft, which is transfixed with pins. The Salter innominate osteotomy can be done at the same time as an open reduction in an older child with acetabular instability or in a child who has had a previous open or closed reduction at a young age but has failed to develop adequate acetabular shape.

23. **Name and briefly describe indications and techniques for the Pemberton, Steel, Ganz, Chiari, and Shelf procedures used in the treatment of DDH.**

    There are basically three different types of pelvic osteotomies for the treatment of acetabular dysplasia, as follows:

    - **Redirectional osteotomies:** Cuts are made about the acetabulum, allowing the hyaline cartilage of the deficient acetabulum to be rotated over the femoral head. This category includes the Salter, Steel, and Ganz osteotomies.
    - **Volume-reducing osteotomies:** These involve periacetabular cuts that, with leverage, improve coverage but also tend to decrease the volume of the acetabulum. This category includes the Pemberton and Dega osteotomies.
    - **Salvage osteotomies:** These provide coverage of the capsule of the femoral head, leading to metaplasia into fibrocartilage. This category includes the Chiari and Shelf procedures.

In general, the redirectional osteotomies are performed for patients with residual acetabular dysplasia, the Pemberton and Dega osteotomies are used for patients with residual acetabular dysplasia and a capacious acetabulum, and the Chiari and Shelf procedures are used for patient with incongruent hip joints and sufficient hip coverage.

Indication for the **Pemberton osteotomy** is similar to that of the Salter innominate osteotomy. It is, however, intended to be used in children who are older and is performed with an osteotome cutting between the anteroinferior iliac spine and the anterosuperior iliac spine. The cut curves in a posterior-to-superior direction and then curves in an inferior direction down to the posterior limb of the triradiate cartilage. This bicortical cut is through the inner and outer tables of the ilium. A laminar spreader is then used to displace the distal segment, providing anterior and lateral coverage. The osteotomy is fixed with a tricortical piece of graft from the iliac crest.

The **Steel osteotomy** is performed with a Salter innominate cut through the superior acetabular region, connecting the sciatic notch to just above the anteroinferior iliac spine. Another cut is then performed in the pubis, and the final cut is performed in the ischium. This osteotomy is used in older children with more severe acetabular dysplasia and provides more significant coverage. The acetabular fragment can be rotated in almost any position and must be transfixed with screws for stability's sake.

The **Ganz osteotomy,** or periacetabular osteotomy, is used in patients with a closed triradiate cartilage. This osteotomy utilizes a cut in the superior acetabular region down through the posterior column into the sciatic notch, where another cut is then performed in the pubis. This osteotomy allows for excellent redirection of the acetabulum over the femoral head. The advantage of this osteotomy is that it is inherently stable because the posterior column of the pelvis is not violated. In addition, the acetabular center of head of rotation is not as laterally displaced as is often seen in triple-innominate or Steel-type osteotomies.

Chiari osteotomies are performed for those patients with an uncovered femoral head and who have an incongruous hip joint. The goal of the Chiari osteotomy is to provide lateral coverage to increase the surface area for weight transfer. This osteotomy is performed by making an oblique cut in the direct superior acetabular region, directing 20 degrees cephalad. The distal segment is then translated superomedially, allowing for coverage of the femoral head with the cut portion of the ilium.

The **Shelf** osteotomy is also a salvage procedure for those patients with an incongruous hip joint, and this is performed by cutting a slot over the superior acetabular region and harvesting an iliac crest graft from the lateral side of the ilium. These are then cut into strips and placed into the groove with autogenous bone over the cortical strips. Consolidation over the next several months then leads to a bony roof, which increases the femoral head surface. Both the Chiari and Shelf procedure are used in patients who have very severe acetabular dysplasia and a misshapen head, which may be a result of avascular necrosis.

24. **What is the natural history of untreated DDH?**

The natural history of DDH depends upon several factors, including the amount of acetabular dysplasia, the degree of displacement from the acetabulum, and whether the process is unilateral or bilateral. For instance, a dislocated hip may or may not develop a false acetabulum. A false acetabulum is defined as an area of remodeling in the ilium where the femoral head articulates. Some patients with dislocated hips will not develop a false acetabulum. The femoral head and capsule is suspended in the soft tissues of the gluteal musculature. Other hips may have partial displacement or subluxation. Subluxation should be defined as a break in Shenton's line. Some hips may be located without subluxation but have residual acetabular dysplasia.

Patients who have bilateral dislocated hips without development of false acetabuli can be expected to function well into their 60s without severe osteoarthrosis. They will typically ambulate with a waddling, hyperlordotic gait. They may have some fatigue in their muscles as they age. Patients who have a dislocated hip with a false acetabuli can be expected to develop osteoarthritis and disabling hip pain in 40–50 years of life. Patients who have partial subluxation of the hip as defined by Shenton's line have the worst natural history and are likely to develop osteoarthritis in their 30s. Patients with acetabular dysplasia have a variable rate of developing osteoarthritis and depend upon the severity of the osteoarthritis and demographic variables, including obesity and a family history for osteoarthritis. In general, patients who have a center-edge (CE) angle less than 10 degrees can be expected to develop osteoarthritis to a greater degree than those with less acetabular dysplasia.

KEY POINTS: DEVELOPMENTAL DYSPLASIA OF THE HIP

1. Developmental dysplasia of the hip (DDH) is a continuum of disorders, from radiographic dysplasia to frank dislocation.

2. Ortolani-positive hips in the newborn do not require imaging prior to initiation of treatment in the Pavlik harness.

3. Teratologic and late-presenting hip dislocations are usually "fixed" dislocations, requiring surgical reduction.

4. Pelvic osteotomies improve femoral head coverage, with the choice of osteotomy dependent on age and the severity of dysplasia.

25. What is the most serious complication associated with DDH?
Proximal femoral growth disturbance or avascular necrosis is the most significant complication and is seen only in patients who have been treated either with open or closed reduction. The exact etiology for growth disturbance is not known; however, it is felt to be due to altered blood supply to the proximal femoral epiphysis and apophysis, which results in necrosis and perturbations in normal growth and development. Patients with avascular necrosis may have small delays in ossification but still generate a spherical head. Others may develop injury to the growth plate, arrest resulting in coxa vara and a limb-length discrepancy. Yet others may have complete necrosis of the femoral head, resulting in very severe wear-and-tear arthritis of the hip.

26. What are treatment options for the painful hip in the adolescent or young adult with residual acetabular dysplasia and subluxation?
The treatment options for the painful hip in an adolescent with residual acetabular dysplasia include hip reconstruction with a femoral or acetabular osteotomy (or both). Acetabular osteotomies are best performed with periacetabular osteotomy or Ganz osteotomy, which tend to provide increased coverage. Occasionally, patients will have residual femoral valgus, which can be treated with a proximal femoral varus osteotomy. Patients with severe osteoarthritis are not good candidates for reconstructive procedures. Other procedures, such as femoral head resurfacing, total hip replacement, or hip fusion, are considered.

BIBLIOGRAPHY

1. American Academy of Pediatrics Committee on Quality Improvement, Subcommittee on Developmental Dysplasia of the Hip: Clinical practice guideline: Early detection of developmental dysplasia of the hip. Pediatrics 105(4 Pt 1):896–905, 2000.
2. Bond CD, Hennrikus WL, DellaMaggiore ED: Prospective evaluation of newborn soft-tissue hip "clicks" with ultrasound. J Pediatr Orthop 17:199–201, 1997.

3. Gardiner HM, Clarke NM, Dunn PM: A sonographic study of the morphology of the preterm neonatal hip. J Pediatr Orthop 10:633–637, 1990.

4. Gillingham BL, Sanchez AA, Wenger DR: Pelvic osteotomies for the treatment of hip dysplasia in children and young adults. J Am Acad Orthop Surg 7:325–337, 1999.

5. Grill F, Bensahel H, Canadell J, et al: The Pavlik harness in the treatment of congenital dislocating hip: Report on a multicenter study of the European Paediatric Orthopaedic Society. J Pediatr Orthop 8:1–8, 1988.

6. Malvitz TA, Weinstein SL: Closed reduction for congenital dysplasia of the hip: Functional and radiographic results after an average of thirty years. J Bone Joint Surg 76A:1777–1792, 1994.

7. Mubarak S, Garfin S, Vance R, et al: Pitfalls in the use of the Pavlik harness for the treatment of congenital dysplasia, subluxation, and dislocation of the hip. J Bone Joint Surg 63A:1239–1248, 1981.

8. Murphy SB, Reinhold G, Muller ME: The prognosis of untreated dysplasia of the hip. J Bone Joint Surg 77A:985–989, 1995.

9. Ramsey PL, Lasser S, Muller ME: Congenital dislocation of the hip. Use of the Pavlik harness in the child during the first six months of life. J Bone Joint Surg 58A:1000–1004, 1976.

CHAPTER 60

LEGG-CALVÉ-PERTHES DISEASE

J. A. Herring, MD

1. **What is Legg-Calvé-Perthes disease?**
   Legg-Calvé-Perthes disease is idiopathic avascular necrosis of the femoral head (also called the *capital femoral epiphysis*) that occurs in children.

2. **What ages of children are affected?**
   The most common ages are 5–9 years, but children as young as 18 months and as old as 18 years can develop the problem.

3. **How did the name originate?**
   It was discovered by Arthur Legg of Boston, Jacques Calvé of France, and Georg Perthes of Germany in 1909. Each worked at a hospital for children with tuberculosis, and each had a newfangled x-ray machine. With this magic machine, the authors found a subset of children who had mild symptoms and no tuberculosis. Actually, Dr. Waldenstrom of Sweden wrote about it in the preceding year, but he called it mild tuberculosis.

4. **Does it have another name?**
   It is commonly referred to as *Perthes' disease,* especially by the Germans, or as *LCP*.

5. **What causes it?**
   We are still not sure. One theory suggests that it occurs in children with abnormalities of thrombolysis. These children are deficient in either protein S or C or in thrombolysis. The femoral head changes may be due to arterial or venous infarction, the latter being most likely. There is some evidence relating the etiology to passive smoking.

6. **Is it a bad problem?**
   It is not the worst thing that can happen to a child. More than 50% will have a year or two of stiffness, a limp, and some pain in the hip and then will return to normalcy. Some children have continued disability. Early patterns of femoral head involvement are prognostic and help determine the likelihood of effectiveness of treatment.

7. **Which children are prone to develop it?**
   There is a typical patient profile. He (boys outnumber girls 4:1) is a wiry, thin, very active boy who is noticeably smaller than his agemates. Of course, some children who develop the symptoms do not fit this profile.

8. **How do I make the diagnosis?**
   The parent reports that the child limps and complains of occasional pain, either in the hip or in the knee. The patient often denies hurting but will point to the hip or knee when pinned down.

   These symptoms may have been going on for weeks or even months, and the parents often relate it to an injury. The examination shows a mild limp and decreased range of motion of the hip. Internal rotation is especially limited.

9. **What studies should be performed?**
The best initial study is anteroposterior (AP) and lateral pelvis radiographs. The early film will show an increase in the density of the femoral head compared with the asymptomatic side (Fig. 60-1). If that is negative and the symptoms are very recent, the radiograph should be repeated in a month. A technetium bone scan or even a magnetic resonance imaging (MRI) scan will yield an earlier diagnosis than a radiograph, but since there is no advantage to earlier treatment, these studies are not really necessary.

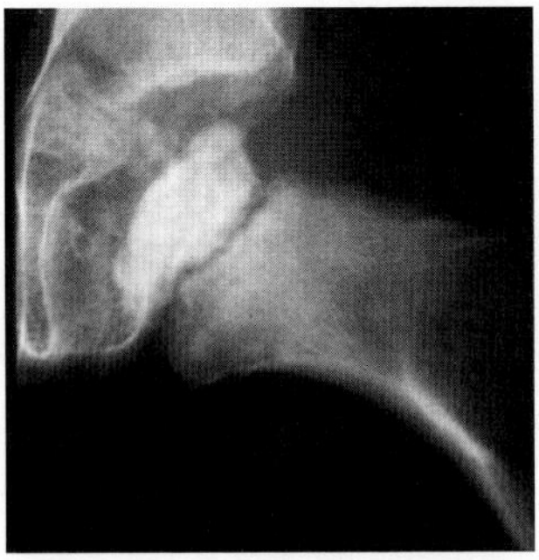

10. **How does the disease progress?**
There are four stages, as follows:
   - **Initial stage:** The femoral head is dense.
   - **Fragmentation stage:** The femoral head is soft and deforms (Fig. 60-2).
   - **Healing stage:** New bone grows into the femoral head (Fig. 60-3).
   - **Residual stage:** The femoral head is healed, with some deformity.

   Clinically, in the early stages, there is intermittent synovitis with pain, limp, and irritability of the hip. These symptoms increase with activity and diminish with rest. As the head fragments and deforms, there is more definite loss of motion, especially internal rotation and abduction. After about a year of symptoms, the patient gradually improves. After 2 years, he or she is usually back to normal activities with little in the way of complaints.

11. **What is the natural history?**
In the short run, the natural history is very favorable. Most patients go through adolescence and most of adulthood with either no symptoms or with mild transient aches and pains. By the fifth decade, half the patients will have developed degenerative arthritis and will be in need of hip replacement. The other half will remain asymptomatic through adulthood (as far as we know).

12. **How is the natural history influenced by the age at onset?**
The age at onset is the most important prognostic factor. The older the child, the worse the outcome. This is probably due to the ability of a mostly cartilaginous femoral head of a 3-year-old to remodel compared with the limited remodeling capacity of a 16-year-old's bony femoral head. Those with onset at less than 6 years of age do well in general and have not been shown to benefit from specific treatment. Those between 6 and 8 years of age at onset should have symptomatic treatment with emphasis on maintaining range of motion. Those with onset at 8 years of age and over have been shown to benefit from surgical containment in lateral pillar groups B and B/C border.

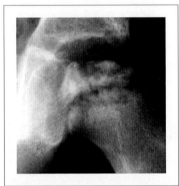

Figure 60-1. Radiograph of a child with early Legg-Calvé-Perthes disease, with symptoms present for 1 month. There is uniform increased density in the femoral head.

Figure 60-2. Radiograph of a child who has had Legg-Calvé-Perthes disease for 8 months. There is fragmentation of the femoral head, with lucency in the center of the head.

13. **How is the severity classified?**
    The current favorite classification method is the lateral pillar classification, as follows:
    - **Group A:** Femoral heads have no change in the lateral pillar (i.e., the lateral one third or so of the femoral head) and do well without treatment.
    - **Group B:** Heads have partial (up to 50%) collapse of the lateral buttress of the femoral head and have an intermediate prognosis.
    - **Group B/C border:** These are between B and C in their behavior.
    - **Group C:** Heads have more than 50% collapse of the lateral pillar and do not do well in general.

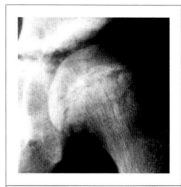

Figure 60-3. Radiograph of the same hip as in Fig. 60-2, now 3 years after onset. The hip has healed, and the roundness has gradually improved.

14. **What is the appropriate treatment?**
    The proper early approach is to observe the child and to restrict him or her from vigorous sports. If the symptoms continue or worsen, short periods of rest may help, along with anti-inflammatory medications. Crutches may be used if the symptoms are really severe. Children under 6 years of age at onset rarely require treatment. Those over age 8 years benefit from surgical treatment in groups B and B/C border.

15. **How soon should a patient be referred?**
    A reasonably early referral is appropriate, but this is not an emergency. The child can be seen by a pediatric orthopaedist in a week or two with no harm done.

KEY POINTS: LEGG-CALVÉ-PERTHES DISEASE

1. Legg-Calvé-Perthes disease is idiopathic avascular necrosis of the femoral head (also called the *capital femoral epiphysis*) that occurs in children.

2. The most common ages are 5–9 years, but children as young as 18 months and as old as 18 years can develop the problem. Boys outnumber girls 4:1.

3. In the short run, the natural history is very favorable. Most patients go through adolescence and most of adulthood with either no symptoms or with mild transient aches and pains.

4. By the fifth decade, half the patients will have developed degenerative arthritis and will be in need of hip replacement. The other half will remain asymptomatic through adulthood.

5. The proper early approach is to observe the child and to restrict him or her from vigorous sports. If the symptoms continue or worsen, short periods of rest may help, along with anti-inflammatory medications. Crutches may be used if the symptoms are really severe.

6. Older patients (onset at 8 years of age or older) usually benefit from containment surgery in lateral pillar groups B and B/C border.

16. **Can the other hip become involved?**
    Sequential involvement of the other hip happens in about 10% of children. When both hips are simultaneously involved, one should consider the diagnosis of epiphyseal dysplasia.

17. **Are there other diseases that could be confused with LCP?**
Multiple epiphyseal dysplasia, spondyloepiphyseal dysplasia, and the mucopolysaccharidoses have abnormalities in femoral head ossification that can resemble avascular necrosis. Hypothyroidism may mimic LCP, and other causes of avascular necrosis, such as steroid therapy and hemoglobinopathies, should be considered.

CONTROVERSIES

18. **How should LCP be treated?**
The treatment approach mentioned above has been substantiated in a long-term multicenter study. Treatment still varies widely from center to center.

19. **Is nonsurgical treatment better than surgical treatment?**
Nonsurgical treatment is better for the children who are young (i.e., less than 6 years of age) or who do not meet the surgical criteria outlined in Question 14. This usually amounts to activity reduction and the use of nonsteroidal anti-inflammatory drugs.

BIBLIOGRAPHY

1. Calvé J: On a particular form of pseudo-coxalgia associated with a characteristic deformity of the upper end of the femur. Clin Orthop 150:4–7, 1980.
2. Catterall A: The natural history of Perthes' disease. J Bone Joint Surg Br 53:37–53, 1971.
3. Glueck CJ, Crawford A, Roy, D, et al: Association of antiturmibotic factor deficiencies and hypofibrinolysis with Legg-Perthes disease. J Bone Joint Surg Am 78:3–13, 1996.
4. Hall DF: Genetic aspects of Perthes' disease: A critical review. Clin Orthop 209:100–114, 1986.
5. Herring JA: Legg-Calvé-Perthes disease: A review of current knowledge. In Barr JS Jr (ed): Instructional Course Lectures XXXVIII. Park Ridge, IL, American Academy of Orthopaedic Surgeons, 1989, pp 309–315.
6. Herring JA: Legg-Calvé-Perthes disease. In Monograph Series. Rosemount, IL, American Academy of Orthopaedic Surgeons, 1996.
7. Herring J, Kim HT, Browne R: Legg-Calvé-Perthes disease. Part I: Classification of radiographs with use of the modified lateral pillar and Stulberg classifications. J Bone Joint Surg 86A:2103–2120, 2004.
8. Herring J, Kim HT, Browne R: Legg-Calvé-Perthes disease. Part II: Prospective multicenter study of the effect of treatment on outcome. J Bone Joint Surg. 86A:2121–2134, 2004.
9. Herring JA: In Tachdjian's Pediatric Orthopaedics: From the Texas Scottish Rite Hospital for Children, 3rd ed. Philadelphia, W.B. Saunders, 2001, pp 655–709.
10. Herring JA, Neustadt JB, Williams, JJ, et al: The lateral pillar classification of Legg-Calvé-Perthes disease. J Pediatr Orthop 12:143–150, 1992.
11. Landin LA, Danielson LG, Wattsgard G: Transient synovitis of the hip: Its incidence, epidemiology, and relation to Perthes' disease. J Bone Joint Surg Br 69:238–242, 1987.
12. Loder RT, Schwartz EM, Hensinger RN: Behavioral characteristics of children with Legg-Calvé-Perthes disease. J Pediatr Orthop 12:598–601, 1993.
13. McAndrews MP, Weinstein SL: A long-term follow-up of Perthes disease treated with spica casts. J Pediatr Orthop 3:160–165, 1983.
14. Roy DR: Perthes-like changes caused by acquired hypothyroidism. Orthopedics 14:901–904, 1991.
15. Stulberg SD, Cooperman DR, Wallensten R: The natural history of Legg-Calvé-Perthes disease. J Bone Joint Surg Am 63:1095–1108, 1981.

CHAPTER 61

SLIPPED CAPITAL FEMORAL EPIPHYSIS

Randall T. Loder, MD

1. **What is slipped capital femoral epiphysis?**

   Slipped capital femoral epiphysis (SCFE) is a displacement, or so-called "slipping," of the proximal femoral epiphysis on the femoral metaphysis through the growth plate (Fig. 61-1). SCFE occurs during the adolescent growth spurt. The displacement usually is posterior and medial. However, SCFE is really a misnomer as the epiphysis cannot move relative to the acetabulum because it is fixed by the ligamentum teres. In reality, the proximal femoral metaphysis displaces anterior and laterally to the epiphysis.

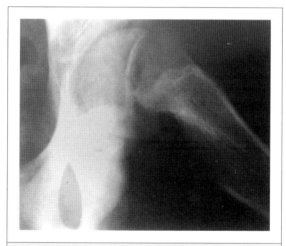

   Figure 61-1. Acute SCFE with moderate displacement.

2. **How frequently does SCFE occur? Who is most at risk?**

   SCFE is the most common hip disorder in adolescents, with a prevalence that varies greatly by geographic locale and the race of the child. In the United States, rates vary from approximately 2 in 100,000 to 10 in 100,000. Boys aged 9–16 years and girls aged 8–15 years are most at risk; the gender ratio is 60% boys to 40% girls. SCFE tends to be more common in African-American and Polynesian children. Most children with SCFE are obese, with at least half weighing more than 95th percentile of children in their age group.

3. **Is slipping of the epiphysis due to a traumatic event?**

   Rarely, extreme trauma may cause an acute physeal fracture, resulting in displacement of the epiphysis, but most children do not recall a specific traumatic event. The exact cause of SCFE is still unclear. On the other hand, chronic subclinical trauma may have a significant role in the etiology of SCFE. Since most children with SCFE are obese and a reduction in femoral anteversion is common in both obese children and children with SCFE, mechanical factors appear to play a significant role. When applied to a normal physis, the high shear forces in an obese adolescent who is simply running or walking and has a femur with decreased or 0 degrees of anteversion are adequate to cause an SCFE. In addition to trauma, other suggested causes are endocrine and renal disorders, irradiation therapy, physeal structural and chemical abnormalities, abnormalities in physeal chondrocyte apoptosis, and a subtle endocrine dysfunction as yet undescribed and undiagnosable using current laboratory methods.

4. **How is SCFE classified?**
   SCFE was traditionally classified by the duration of symptoms, grouped as **acute** (i.e., sudden onset of symptoms for less than 3 weeks), **chronic** (with symptoms for more than 3 weeks), **acute-on-chronic** (i.e., symptoms for more than 3 weeks with sudden exacerbation of pain), or **preslip** (essentially a radiographic finding of irregularity, widening, and fuzziness of the physis).
   Newer classifications depend upon the stability of the SCFE, which also imparts a prognosis regarding the potential risk of avascular necrosis. A child with a **stable** SCFE can walk, with or without crutches; a child with an **unstable** SCFE cannot walk, even with crutches. The risk of avascular necrosis is much higher in children with an unstable SCFE. Approximately 85–95% of patients have stable SCFEs.
   The amount of epiphyseal displacement relative to the metaphysis can be classified as **mild** (i.e., one third or less of the metaphyseal diameter), **moderate** (i.e., one third to one half of the metaphyseal diameter), or **severe** (i.e., more than one half of the metaphyseal diameter).

5. **What are the clinical features of SCFE?**
   The onset of symptoms may be sudden or, more typically, may occur insidiously over many months, with good and bad days. Symptoms are variable but usually include pain in the groin, medial thigh, or knee and limitation of hip motion, especially internal rotation. Patients with longstanding stable slips may have mild or moderate shortening and external rotation of the affected extremity. Red flags that should alert the physician to the possibility of SCFE include the following:
   - An older child or adolescent
   - Obesity
   - Limp
   - Pain in the hip, groin, thigh, or knee

6. **What imaging studies should be ordered in SCFE? What is seen on these studies?**
   Anteroposterior (AP) and lateral radiographs of **both hips** are the most important study for diagnosis and treatment. Since the slip is usually posterior, the earliest findings are on the lateral radiograph. Subtle, stable slipping is best appreciated on frog-leg lateral comparison views. The lateral radiographs will demonstrate posterior step-off and slipping of the capital epiphysis. The earliest radiographic finding on the AP view is usually a slight widening and irregularity of the physis. One may also see the metaphyseal blanch sign, which is a double-density shadow just inferior to the physis and represents double cortical shadows of both the metaphysis and the posteriorly slipping epiphysis. The central height of the epiphysis may be slightly less than in the contralateral hip, similar to a sunset when the sun is just beginning to sink over the horizon.
   In chronic slips, callus formation at the inferomedial metaphyseal-physeal junction and smoothing of the superior proximal edge of the metaphyseal-physeal junction can be seen on the lateral view. When acute slipping of a chronic slip occurs, the acute physeal separation can be superimposed on the osseous metaphyseal remodeling.
   In patients with unstable slips, frog-leg views should not be attempted because of the severe discomfort to the child and the risk of iatrogenic further displacement. Due to the approximately 33% incidence of bilaterality in SCFE, and also to the fact that the opposite hip

of a symptomatic SCFE may have an asymptomatic SCFE, radiographs of both hips must be performed. Ultrasonography, bone scanning, and computed tomography (CT) scanning have all been described and used in SCFE but are not necessary for routine diagnosis and treatment. Rather, they should be reserved for special circumstances.

7. **What is the most effective treatment?**
    The primary goals of treatment are to stop any further slipping and to incite closure of the physis. Currently, the most frequently used treatment for the stable SCFE is percutaneous *in situ* single-screw fixation under fluoroscopic control. A 6- or 7-mm cannulated screw, either partially or fully threaded, is inserted into the center of the epiphysis. Because the epiphysis is posterior, screw insertion begins on the anterior aspect of the femoral neck; the more severe the SCFE, the more anterior the screw insertion.

    The best treatment for an unstable SCFE is controversial and probably not yet known due to conflicting results in the literature of this relatively rare type. If fixation is performed, an unstable slip often spontaneously reduces simply with induction of anesthesia and patient positioning on the operating table. Open reduction rarely is required if closed reduction cannot be obtained. The timing of the surgery, the role of reduction, the type of reduction (closed vs. open), the need for decompressive arthrotomy, and the use of one versus two cannulated screws are all controversial points in the treatment of unstable SCFEs.

8. **If SCFE is present in one hip, will an SCFE develop in the contralateral hip? Is prophylactic fixation warranted?**
    The prevalence of bilateral SCFE has reportedly ranged from 21–80% and has been reported to be 37% in children with symptomatic slips; if asymptomatic slips are included, the prevalence rate is probably higher. Approximately 50% of the children with bilateral SCFE present with bilateral involvement, and the other 50% develop SCFE in the opposite hip at a later date. Nearly all patients who develop SCFE in the contralateral hip do so within 18 months of diagnosis of the first slip. Therefore, patients with unilateral SCFE should be followed closely to detect the development of SCFE in the opposite hip.

    Prophylactic fixation of the uninvolved hip in a child with a unilateral SCFE is controversial. Children with significant remaining growth (i.e., those of <10 years of age) will have a much higher chance of developing an SCFE in the opposite hip, and prophylactic fixation can also be considered. Bilateral SCFE is present in at least 60% of patients with endocrine disorders, and prophylactic treatment of the opposite hip should be strongly considered in this rare group.

9. **What are the complications of *in situ* fixation? How can errors be avoided?**
    Incorrect screw placement probably is the most common error. Either the screw may be passed obliquely toward the anterior surface rather than the center of the femoral head, or it may pass out the posterior neck and into the head. This can be avoided by selecting a starting point on the anterior femoral neck so that the device enters the center of the femoral head perpendicular to the physeal surface. The more posterior the slip, the more anterior the starting point. Screw penetration can be avoided by keeping the tip of the screw in the center of the epiphysis in both anterior and posterior views, advancing the screw tip to no more than 8 mm or to one third of the femoral head radius from subchondral bone, whichever projection is closest. While reaming over the guide pin in preparation for cannulated screw fixation, care should be taken so as not to bend the guide pin, which can result in breakage of the guide pin. Also, advancement of the guide pin deep into the acetabular bone, pelvis, or both should be avoided by multiple fluoroscopic spot views during reaming, tapping, and placement of the cannulated screw.

10. **When is realignment osteotomy indicated?**
    Although some surgeons will consider realignment osteotomy as the initial surgery in severe SCFEs (i.e., >60 degrees), most surgeons consider osteotomy only after *in situ* pin fixation and

complete physeal closure. Problems with gait, sitting, or cosmetic appearance after physeal closure are indications for osteotomy. Osteotomy may also be indicated to improve the normal relationship of the femoral head; however, its role in the delay of degenerative joint disease is much less known. The goals, risks, and benefits must be clearly discussed with the parents and patient as the risk of complications with osteotomy is not insignificant.

11. **What type of osteotomy is best to correct the deformity?**
This question is still controversial. The advantage of femoral neck osteotomy is correction of the deformity itself; however, postoperative avascular necrosis is extremely high in most surgeons' hands. This procedure is contraindicated when the proximal femoral physis is closed.

Osteotomy at the base of the femoral neck is safer since it is distal to the major posterior retinacular blood supply of the epiphysis; avascular necrosis and chondrolysis are infrequent after this osteotomy. The production of a compensatory deformity shortens the femoral neck.

Intertrochanteric or subtrochanteric osteotomies provide good reorientation of the capital physis with little risk of avascular necrosis. The compensatory deformity created by the osteotomy makes subsequent total hip replacement more difficult.

12. **What complications may occur after treatment?**
The most serious complication is **avascular necrosis**. Avascular necrosis almost never occurs in untreated slips or after *in situ* fixation of stable slips. In unstable SCFEs, the incidence of avascular necrosis is much higher: it has been reported to be as high as 50%. Reduction of stable SCFE by aggressive manipulation is contraindicated as it will disrupt the blood supply to the capital epiphysis. Although a number of risk factors for the development of avascular necrosis after SCFE have been suggested—adequacy, timing, and fixation of reduction; severity and chronicity of slip; and gender, age, and race of the patient—currently available data cannot substantiate any of these as definite predictive factors. Most authors now believe that vascular damage and the resulting avascular necrosis occur at the time of the acute, abrupt, fracture-like displacement, with subsequent obstruction or tearing of the posterior retinacular vessels.

Chondrolysis is a less frequent complication (about 1–2% in recent series).

Further slipping after pinning of SCFE has been described and seems to occur most often in children with underlying endocrinopathies and in those with unstable slips and antecedent knee and hip pain (i.e., acute-on-chronic slip).

KEY POINTS: SLIPPED CAPITAL FEMORAL EPIPHYSIS (SCFE)

1. Children with SCFE often do not present with hip pain but rather with groin, thigh, or medial knee pain or with a limp.

2. The incidence of avascular necrosis in children with unstable SCFE is as high as 50%.

3. Bilateral involvement in children with SCFE is common and requires frequent follow-up until physeal closure.

4. The most effective treatment for a stable SCFE is fixation with a single central screw.

13. **Does the development of avascular necrosis require early reconstructive surgery?**
The natural history of avascular necrosis after SCFE appears to be that of gradual degenerative changes, for which reconstructive surgery most often can be delayed until

adulthood. In a group of 22 patients (and a total of 24 involved hips) evaluated at an average of 31 years after treatment of SCFE, only 9 had undergone reconstructive surgery, 4 during adolescence and 5 during adulthood. The remaining 13 patients (with 15 involved hips) had no further surgery, but all showed degenerative changes on radiographs.

Early operative treatment of avascular necrosis has been advocated by some authors, but no long-term results of such treatment have been reported.

14. **How long should a child with SCFE be followed?**
As discussed earlier, a child with a unilateral SCFE may develop an SCFE on the opposite hip. Therefore, a child with SCFE should be followed until complete closure of the proximal femoral physis is seen radiographically. Similarly, in children with an initial bilateral SCFE, follow-up should also occur until complete physeal closure since progression of the SCFE or growing off the screw can rarely occur. Perform follow-up at 3–4 month intervals with AP and frog pelvis radiographs until complete physeal closure. Finally, any child with a unilateral SCFE should be counseled to call the physician immediately if symptoms develop in the opposite hip similar to those of the first hip, rather than waiting until the next scheduled follow-up appointment.

BIBLIOGRAPHY

1. Aronson DD, Carlson WE: Slipped capital femoral epiphysis: A prospective study of fixation with a single screw. J Bone Joint Surg Am 74:810–819, 1992.

2. Blanco JS, Taylor B, Johnston CE II: Comparison of single pin versus multiple pin fixation in treatment of slipped capital femoral epiphysis. J Pediatr Orthop 12:384–389, 1992.

3. Carney BT, Weinstein SL, Noble J: Long-term follow-up of slipped capital femoral epiphysis. J Bone Joint Surg Am 73:667–674, 1991.

4. Castro FP Jr, Bennett JT, Doulens K: Epidemiological perspective on prophylactic pinning in patients with unilateral slipped capital femoral epiphysis. J Pediatr Orthop 20:745–748, 2000.

5. Jerre R, Billing L, Hansson G, et al: The contralateral hip in patients primarily treated for unilateral slipped upper femoral epiphysis: Long-term follow-up of sixty-one hips. J Bone Joint Surg Br 76:563–567, 1994.

6. Kallio PE, Mah ET, Foster BK, et al: Slipped capital femoral epiphysis: Incidence and clinical assessment of physeal instability. J Bone Joint Surg Br 77:752–755, 1995.

7. Kennedy JG, Hresko MT, Kasser JR, et al: Osteonecrosis of the femoral head associated with slipped capital femoral epiphysis. J Pediatr Orthop 21:189–193, 2001.

8. Krahn TH, Canale ST, Beaty JH, et al: Long-term follow-up of patients with avascular necrosis after treatment of slipped capital femoral epiphysis. J Pediatr Orthop 13:154–158, 1993.

9. Loder RT: Current issues: Unstable slipped capital femoral epiphysis. J Pediatr Orthop 21:691–699, 2001.

10. Loder RT, Richards BS, Shapiro PS, et al: Acute slipped capital femoral epiphysis: The importance of physeal stability. J Bone Joint Surg Am 75:1134–1140, 1993.

11. Sanders JO, Smith WJ, Stanley EA, et al: Progressive slippage after pinning for slipped capital femoral epiphysis. J Pediatr Orthop 22:239–243, 2002.

X. SPINE AND NECK PROBLEMS

BACK PAIN
B. Stephens Richards, MD

CHAPTER 62

1. How common is back pain in children and adolescents?

In a review of several large community studies, it appeared that 10–30% of children (including adolescents) experience back pain. In the young child, the pain is typically located in the middle back, whereas in the adolescent, the pain is equally distributed between the middle and low back. In young children, underlying disease is frequently detectable by obtaining a careful history, by performing a complete examination, and, as needed, by using various imaging studies.

2. How often can the cause of back pain be identified in children?

Several older studies reported finding a definite diagnosis in 63–84% of children with back pain. A recent study, however, reported finding a definite diagnosis in only 22% of those who presented with pain. In general, if young children and toddlers, who are unlikely to exaggerate symptoms or physical findings, are thoroughly evaluated, an abnormality is likely to be found.

3. What should be asked when taking a history?

By emphasizing the initial onset and the duration of symptoms, the presence of trauma or infection, the location of the pain, and the frequency and intensity of the pain, enough information is often gained to form an initial impression.

4. What is looked for during the physical examination?

Initially, a general examination with the child gowned or in shorts should be done to rule out any associated abnormalities (systemic or neurologic). Once done, specific attention can be focused on the child's back to assess posture, alignment, and skin condition. The forward-bending test assesses for thoracic and lumbar asymmetry and flexibility. Underlying disease should be suspected with the presence of localized tenderness, exaggerated stiffness of the lumbar spine, pronounced thoracic kyphosis, midline skin defects (including sinuses, hemangiomas, or hair patches), excessive hamstring tightness, or neurologic abnormalities (i.e., asymmetric abdominal reflexes, clonus, gait disturbances, and motor or sensory deficiencies).

5. What types of imaging studies are helpful in the assessment of back pain?

Plain radiographs, technetium bone scans, single photon emission computed tomography (SPECT), computed tomography (CT) scans, and magnetic resonance imaging (MRI) scans are all valuable tools. Rarely would all be needed together.

6. When should plain radiographs be ordered?

These are consistently found to be the most helpful imaging studies in children with back pain. Anteroposterior and lateral radiographs of the thoracolumbar spine should be obtained during the initial evaluation in children who are age 4 years or younger, who have had pain longer than 2 months, who have pain that awakens them from sleep, or who have associated constitutional symptoms. Disk space narrowing, vertebral end-plate irregularities, vertebral scalloping, bone defects, and scoliosis are several detectable abnormalities. Additional oblique radiographs will provide further detail in areas of concern (e.g., spondylolysis). Adequate visualization of the pelvis is required because some conditions involving the pelvis, such as osteoid osteoma, may lead to complaints of back pain.

7. **When should bone scans be ordered?**
   If suspicion of an abnormality is high but the neurologic examination and the plain radiographs are normal, a technetium bone scan should be the next imaging study obtained. This should include the entire spine and pelvis, but a total body scan generally is not necessary. Although this test is not specific, it is quite sensitive for infection, benign and malignant neoplasms, and occult fractures. SPECT scans may be useful when the plain bone scan is equivocal since it is superior in precisely locating lesions within the spine (e.g., spondylolysis).

8. **When should an MRI scan be ordered?**
   If the neurologic examination finding is abnormal, then the spinal cord and canal should be evaluated with MRI. It is the optimal study for assessing the neural axis, particularly in the evaluation of spinal cord tumors, syringomyelia, and disk herniations. MRI scans must be carefully interpreted to avoid over-reading positive disk disease and thereby making the assumption that this is responsible for the back pain.

9. **When are CT scans helpful?**
   When a bone lesion has been identified on plain radiographs or a bone scan, a CT scan remains the best imaging study to clarify the extent of the disease. CT myelography may still provide additional useful information in adolescent patients with difficult-to-evaluate disk herniations.

10. **What are useful laboratory studies?**
    A complete blood cell count with differential, erythrocyte sedimentation rate, and C-reactive protein are the most useful screening tests. These should be obtained early in young children, those complaining of night pain, and those with constitutional symptoms in whom infection, lymphoma, or leukemia is suspected. If a rheumatologic disorder is suspected, further helpful tests include analysis of rheumatoid factor, antinuclear antibody, and HLA-B27.

11. **What is included in the differential diagnosis?**
    See Table 62-1.

12. **After muscle strain, what are the more common causes of back pain in the young?**
    Diskitis, spondylolisthesis, and Scheuermann's kyphosis.

13. **What can be done for back pain secondary to muscle strain?**
    Rest from activities that led to the back pain and the use of nonsteroidal anti-inflammatory medication are usually sufficient. Recovery should be expected within several weeks. If pain persists and further work-up has ruled out causes other than muscle strain, physical therapy instruction in back stretching and strengthening exercises may be helpful.

14. **What is diskitis?**
    This is thought to represent infection within the disk space, usually with *Staphylococcus aureus*. It is the most common cause of back pain in the very young child and occasionally can lead to osteomyelitis of the adjacent vertebrae.

15. **When should diskitis be suspected?**
    Diskitis typically affects children of 1–5 years of age. The child may complain of pain in the back or abdomen, may refuse to walk, or may present with a limp. Some children may appear ill, but fewer than half are febrile. Often, movement of the spine is limited and is accompanied by tenderness to palpation of the lower back. The child may refuse to bend over to retrieve a toy from the floor.

TABLE 62-1. DIFFERENTIAL DIAGNOSIS OF PEDIATRIC BACK PAIN

Developmental
Scheuermann's kyphosis
Painful scoliosis
Infectious
Diskitis and vertebral osteomyelitis
Tuberculous spondylitis
Traumatic
Muscle strain
Spondylolysis
Spondylolisthesis
Herniated disk
Slipped vertebral apophysis
Fractures
Neoplastic Benign
Osteoid osteoma
Osteoblastoma
Aneurysmal bone cyst
Histiocytosis
Malignant
Leukemia
Lymphoma
Sarcoma
Visceral
Renal abnormalities
Gynecologic abnormalities

16. **What kind of work-up is needed if diskitis is suspected?**
    A plain lateral radiograph of the thoracolumbar spine may demonstrate disk-space narrowing. The erythrocyte sedimentation rate and C-reactive protein will be elevated. Radiographic findings frequently lag behind the clinical picture, however. If it is early in the disease process, disk-space narrowing and subsequent adjacent vertebral end-plate erosions will not yet be evident. A bone scan, demonstrating increased uptake in the disk, will confirm the diagnosis. MRI also picks up the abnormalities in the disk and adjacent vertebrae but is not necessary if a positive bone scan has been obtained. A needle biopsy of the disk space should be considered only if the child does not respond to treatment.

17. **What treatment is needed for diskitis?**
    Intravenous antibiotics, first-generation cephalosporins (usually), and bed rest are recommended by most authors. The antibiotics can be changed to the oral route after 7–10 days and should be continued for 3–4 weeks. Immobilization in a brace or cast may provide some

comfort. Biopsy or debridement is reserved for those whose conditions do not improve with treatment or who are shown on imaging studies to have abscess formation.

18. **What is spondylolisthesis?**
Spondylolisthesis represents a forward slippage of part of one vertebra upon another. This occurs in the low back region, most commonly when the fifth lumbar vertebra slips forward on the sacrum. For this to happen, a stress fracture of the pars interarticularis (i.e., spondylolysis) is necessary, which weakens the structural support of the spine. Spondylolysis and spondylolisthesis are the most common causes of identifiable lumbar back pain in adolescents. Generally, the symptoms begin during the adolescent growth spurt.

19. **What causes the stress fracture of the pars to occur?**
Repetitive activities that involve an increased amount of lumbar lordosis lead to stress on the pars (a part of the posterior element of each vertebra). Several examples include gymnastics, dancing, diving, and weight lifting.

20. **What are the symptoms and signs of spondylolisthesis?**
Lower back or buttock pain is most common. Occasionally, this will be accompanied by pain radiating into the legs. The discomfort is associated with activity, particularly those activities that involve hyperextension or twisting of the lumbar spine. Flattening of the normal lumbar lordosis may be evident and probably is secondary to hamstring tightness.

KEY POINTS: PEDIATRIC BACK PAIN

1. Back pain is common in adolescents, occurring in 10–30%.

2. Plain radiographs, bone scans, computed tomography (CT) scans, and magnetic resonance imaging (MRI) are all valuable tools in the assessment of back pain but rarely are needed together.

3. Backpacks exceeding 15–20% of the carrier's body weight are associated with back discomfort, but rarely is it severe enough to warrant orthopaedic evaluation.

21. **How is spondylolisthesis diagnosed?**
Spondylolisthesis is readily recognized on a lateral radiograph of the lumbar spine (Fig. 62-1). If spondylolysis is suspected but there is no spondylolisthesis, then oblique radiographs of the lumbar spine will often provide a clear picture of the abnormality. If these radiographs are equivocal but suspicion remains high, then a bone scan is often helpful in identifying an occult pars fracture. SPECT offers superior visualization. Occasionally, CT is needed for confirmation. Recently, MRI has shown promising results in detecting and monitoring the early onset of spondylolysis.

22. **What treatment is needed for spondylolisthesis?**
If the abnormality has been noticed incidentally, the patient is asymptomatic, and the amount of slip is mild (i.e., less than 50%), then no active treatment is needed. If the adolescent is symptomatic, activity modification and nonsteroidal anti-inflammatory medication are used. Additionally, a lumbosacral corset may be used to provide minimal immobilization. In most adolescents, this will be sufficient. Some will continue to experience significant low back pain, however. These adolescents, along with those whose slips have been noted to worsen progressively on serial radiographs and those who on initial diagnosis have severe slips greater than 50%, require surgical fusion in the lower back. Excellent long-term results can be expected.

23. **Does scoliosis cause back pain in children?**

Generally, children and adolescents with scoliosis (the idiopathic type being the most frequently encountered) present for evaluation because of cosmetic concerns rather than for back discomfort. If discomfort is present in this group of children, it usually is mild, nonspecific, intermittent, and nonradiating. It resolves with rest and does not limit activities. Further investigation of the discomfort is usually not necessary. When persistent severe back pain is the prominent complaint and a scoliotic deformity is noted secondarily, however, a thorough investigation into the source of pain is needed. Painful scoliosis is not a specific diagnosis, but it is a physical finding that may be associated with many underlying abnormalities and can affect any age group.

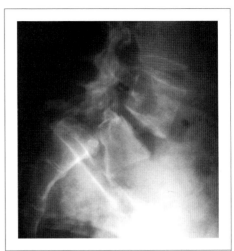

Figure 62-1. Lateral radiograph of a 15-year-old girl with spondylolisthesis of L5 onto the sacrum. The displacement measures approximately 50%. She underwent posterolateral fusion between L5 and the sacrum because of persistent symptoms.

24. **Do backpacks cause back pain?**

Backpacks weighing more than 15–20% of the carrier's body weight are associated with back pain, but there is no evidence that spinal deformity results from their use. However, school-age children with back pain severe enough to require orthopaedic evaluation rarely attribute their pain to wearing a backpack. Of backpack injuries, 89% do not involve the back; instead, the areas involved include the head or face, the hand, the wrist, the shoulder, and the foot.

BIBLIOGRAPHY

1. Brown R, Hussain M, McHugh K, et al: Discitis in young children. J Bone Joint Surg Br 83:106–111, 2001.

2. Cohen E, Stuecker RD: MRI in diagnosis and follow-up of impending spondylolysis in children and adolescents: Early treatment may prevent pars defects. J Pediatr Orthop B 14:63–67, 2005.

3. Dickson RA, Millner PA: The child with a painful back. Curr Orthop 14:369–379, 2000.

4. Kjaer P, Leboeuf-Yde C, Sorensen JS, et al: An epidemiologic study of MRI and low back pain in 13-year-old children. Spine 30:798–806, 2005.

5. Mackenzie WG, Sampath JS, Kruse RW, et al: Backpacks in children. Clin Orthop Relat Res 409:78–84, 2003.

6. Richards BS, McCarthy RE, Akbarnia BA: Backpain in childhood and adolescence. In Zuckerman JD (ed): Instructional Course Lectures. Rosemont, IL, American Academy of Orthopaedic Surgeons, 1999, pp 525–542.

7. Ring D, Johnston CE, Wenger DR: Pyogenic infectious spondylitis in children: The convergence of discitis and vertebral osteomyelitis. J Pediatr Orthop 15:652–660, 1995.

8. Siambanes D, Martinez JW, Butler EW, et al: Influence of school backpacks on adolescent back pain. J Pediatr Orthop 24:211–217, 2004.

9. Thompson GH: Back pain in children. In Schafer M (ed): Instructional Course Lectures 43. Rosemont, IL, American Academy of Orthopaedic Surgeons, 1994, pp 221–230.

10. Wall EJ, Foad SL, Spears J: Backpacks and back pain: Where's the epidemic? J Pediatr Orthop 23:437–439, 2003.

11. Wedderkopp N, Leboeuf-Yde C, Andersen LB, et al: Back pain reporting pattern in a Danish population-based sample of children and adolescents. Spine 26:1879–1883, 2001.

CHAPTER 63

IDIOPATHIC SCOLIOSIS

Kit M. Song, MD

1. **What is idiopathic scoliosis?**

   Scoliosis is defined by the Scoliosis Research Society (SRS) as a lateral curvature of the spine >10 degrees as measured on a frontal plane radiograph by the Cobb angle. The cause of the curvature is not identifiable, and affected children are otherwise typically developing individuals. It is characterized not only by the frontal plane lateral curvature but also by rotation of the spine and alteration of the normal kyphosis and lordosis of the spine in the sagittal plane. When present in the thoracic spine, there is generally loss of normal thoracic kyphosis; hence the term *lordoscoliosis*.

2. **What is the prevalence of scoliosis?**

   The incidence of spinal curvatures >10 degrees in the general population is 2–3%. The incidence of curves >20 degrees is 0.3–0.5%, >30 degrees is 0.1–0.3%, and >40 degrees is <0.1%. For curves of 10–20 degrees, the male-to-female ratio is 1.4:2.1. For curves of 20–30 degrees, it is 5.4:1. For curves >30 degrees, it is 10:1.

3. **How is idiopathic scoliosis classified? What implications do these classification systems have upon prognosis or treatment?**

   Idiopathic scoliosis can be classified according to age at the time of diagnosis. Historically, the age breakdown has been as follows:

   - **Infantile:** <3 years
   - **Juvenile:** 3–10 years
   - **Adolescent:** >11 years

   Though the age of detection is used, the time of onset of the scoliosis is often different. For example, an 11-year-old presenting with a 50-degree curve would be classified as having adolescent idiopathic scoliosis but most likely had onset of the curve as an infant or juvenile. Another classification scheme defining early-onset scoliosis as age <5 years and late-onset scoliosis as age ≥5 years has been used. For both classifications, the implication is that progressive curves at younger ages have a higher likelihood of progression. Idiopathic scoliosis can also be classified for descriptive purposes by the following:

   - **Location of the apex of the major curve:** An apex from T2–T11 would be thoracic, an apex from T12–L1 would be thoracolumbar, and an apex from T2 distal would be lumbar.
   - **Characteristics of the curve:** Curves can be called major or minor based upon their size and flexibility. Curves may also be called structural or compensatory based upon their flexibility and the degree of rotation.
   - **A combinations of the above:** The two most widely used classifications have been the King/Moe and Lenke classifications. Both have been used to describe curve patterns prior to surgery and to try to predict the behavior of segments of the spine that are not treated during selective spinal fusions.

4. **What is the genetic predisposition for scoliosis?**

   If one has a first-degree relative with scoliosis, the incidence of scoliosis has been reported to be 7%, versus 2–3% in the general population. Both an X-linked and an autosomal dominant pattern of inheritance have been suggested in the past. Recent studies suggest that there are multiple critical loci, with chromosomes 1, 2, 6, 8, 10, 16, 17, 19, and X being highlighted.

5. **What are the physical findings or signs of idiopathic scoliosis?**
The physical findings of scoliosis are related to the three-dimensional deformities seen with this condition. Spine and trunk rotation lead to a visible bump along the spine and asymmetry of both the anterior and posterior chest wall. This is best detected by the Adam's forward-bend test, in which the child leans forward in front of you and you sight along the child's back to see asymmetry. Increasing frontal plane curvature can present as apparent shoulder elevation or depression, waist asymmetry, and shift of the trunk. Loss of normal thoracic kyphosis leads to a flattening of the spine and may accentuate the rib deformity due to spinal rotation.

6. **What are the physical symptoms associated with scoliosis?**
For smaller curves, there are few if any symptoms. It is reported that up to 30% of teenage children with or without scoliosis may have mechanical back pain. This is often over the thoracic prominence if present or may be in the convexity of the lumbar compensatory curve. Idiopathic scoliosis is not associated with any neurologic or respiratory symptoms. The presence of either should prompt a search for other causes.

7. **What morbidity or increased mortality is associated with idiopathic scoliosis?**
The long-term morbidity associated with idiopathic scoliosis is related to progression to large curve magnitudes. Pulmonary dysfunction in the form of restrictive lung disease can be seen in larger curves. Significant alterations in lung volumes and airflow are seen in nonsmokers with thoracic curve magnitudes of approximately 90 degrees and in smokers with thoracic curve magnitudes of 60 degrees.

In the lumbar spine, a moderately large untreated lumbar curve followed for 40–50 years may show radiographic evidence of degenerative arthritis. As mechanical back pain is quite frequent in adults and is becoming more frequent in teenagers, it is unclear that the presence of a moderately large lumbar curve increases the incidence of low back pain compared to a control population. No impact of lumbar scoliosis upon visceral organs has been shown.

Mortality associated with idiopathic scoliosis has been shown only for very early onset curves that progress to a very large size during early growth. The mechanism for this appears to be poor alveolar development during early lung growth. The subsequent hypoventilation can, in severe cases, lead to pulmonary hypertension, secondary heart failure, and, ultimately, death. No increase in mortality has been demonstrated for progressive thoracic curves that have their onset in adolescence.

8. **Can one predict the natural history of curve progression for any individual patient?**
No. All studies looking at curve progression indicate that young age, female sex, a large amount of growth remaining, the rate of growth, the curve magnitude, and the curve location are important variables in assessing the risk of curve progression. Indicators of rapid growth are an immature Risser sign (i.e., ossification of the apophysis along the iliac crest; Fig. 63-1), onset of menses, and height velocity change. None is independently highly reliable. Most studies look at the risk of curve progression of 5 degrees but do not address the question of the risk of progression to surgery. Curves that are less than 20 degrees have an inherently low risk of progression. In general, curve progression stops once the child's spine growth stops. The exceptions to this are thoracic curves >50 degrees and lumbar curves >35 degrees with a moderate amount of rotation, in which there is a risk of progression of the curve into the adult years.

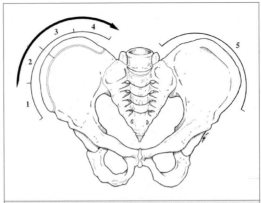

Figure 63-1. Indicators of rapid growth include the immature Risser sign (i.e., ossification of the apophysis along the iliac crest).

9. **How should one document the presence of scoliosis?**

Radiographs are the best way to demonstrate the presence of a curve. One should obtain an x-ray if there is a high index of suspicion of a curve being present. The scoliometer developed by Bunnell is a good screening tool. The device is a level that is placed upon the child's back while he or she is leaning forward and is used to measure rotation at different levels of the spine. If one uses trunk rotation of 5 degrees or greater, there will be little chance of missing a curve greater than 20 degrees, but there will be a high rate of false positives and many unnecessary x-rays. The use of 7 degrees of rotation appears to give an acceptable rate of false positives while maintaining a reasonable degree of sensitivity for detection of curves greater than 20 degrees.

Radiographs should be full-length films. It is recommended that the initial view be an anteroposterior (AP) and lateral view to give good bone detail. Follow-up radiographs are recommended to be posteroanterior (PA) views so as to decrease radiation exposure to radiosensitive breast tissue.

Measurement of the scoliosis is done using the Cobb method (Fig. 63-2).

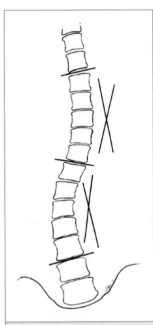

Figure 63-2. Cobb angle.

10. **What are the treatment options for idiopathic scoliosis?**

Many nonsurgical options have been tried, including physical therapy, exercises, manipulation, electrical stimulation, diet, and bracing. Although no long-lasting adverse effects of these treatments have been reported, only bracing has been shown to have some efficacy in decreasing the rate of curve progression.

Cast molding of the spine has been used successfully in younger children with very large progressive curves.

All current surgical options involve a spinal fusion unless the child is very young and there is a desire to preserve growth. In these cases, expandable systems are used to support the spine until growth is nearly completed, at which time a spinal fusion is performed.

KEY POINTS: IDIOPATHIC SCOLIOSIS

1. Idiopathic scoliosis is defined by a frontal plane curve >10 degrees.

2. The risk of curve progression is greater in immature females with moderately large curves.

3. Bracing is the only nonsurgical intervention for which evidence exists that it may arrest the progression of scoliosis.

4. Surgery should be considered only for curves greater than 50 degrees.

5. Surgical fusion of the spine does not leave the spine normal and does not eliminate the possibility of longer-term back problems.

11. **When should a brace be used? How effective is bracing?**
Only one small controlled study of bracing has been performed. For selected patients, using a worst-case scenario for the study, the treatment effect was a 20% less likelihood of curve progression >5 degrees when treated with a brace as compared to no brace. This was a statistically significant difference in outcome. Published brace studies of boys have not shown any effect of bracing. Current recommendations are as follows:
   - **Curve <20 degrees:** Observe
   - **Curve of 20–30 degrees, skeletally immature, and with progression:** Brace
   - **Curve >30 degrees, skeletally immature:** Brace
   - **Curve >45 degrees:** Consider surgery; no brace
   - **Mature patients who are growing slowly:** Indications for bracing are highly variable and should be considered on a case-by-case basis

12. **How is bracing done?**
There are over 15 different brace designs described in the literature. These range from computer-designed traction bracing to off-the-shelf thoracolumbosacral orthoses (TLSOs) and dynamic postural control braces. Brace wear has ranged from full time (i.e., 23 hours/day) to night time only or part time (i.e., 16 hours/day). Centers are highly variable in their prescribed braces and wear patterns. Compliance studies suggest that children are 60–75% compliant on average with the prescribed time of brace wearing.

13. **When should surgery be considered?**
Surgery should be considered for patients who have thoracic curves >50 degrees and lumbar or thoracolumbar curves >40–45 degrees. For skeletally mature patients who have borderline thoracic curves of 50–60 degrees, thoracolumbar curves of 40–45 degrees, or balanced double curves of 50–60 degrees that have not been demonstrated to be progressive, the indications for surgery are more controversial.

14. **What does the surgery for scoliosis involve?**
The primary goals of surgery are to stabilize the spine and to prevent progression to a very large deformity. The secondary goals are to correct some of the scoliosis and to balance the spine

in the frontal and sagittal planes. To do this, a spinal fusion is performed, through which joints are removed from between the vertebrae, injury is done to the vertebrae, and bone grafting is performed in order to promote growth of the vertebrae together into a single rigid segment.

The success of this operation has been greatly improved by the introduction of rigid, multilevel spinal instrumentation to stabilize and correct the spinal deformity. The surgery can be done from a posterior approach, wherein the spinal instrumentation is applied to the lamina or is introduced through the pedicles of the vertebrae. It can also be done through an anterior approach, in which an incision is made along the side to expose the vertebral bodies and instrumentation is applied directly to the vertebrae. Minimally invasive thoracoscopic methods exist for anterior procedures that are technically demanding and should be done only by experienced surgeons.

15. **What are the complications that can be seen with surgery? What are the long-term results of surgical fusion?**
Infections have been shown to occur in up to 2–4% of children who have undergone spinal surgery. Problems with bone healing (i.e., pseudoarthrosis) are much less common in children than in adults but have been seen in 1–3% of children. Paralytic injury rates due to surgery have been variable but are generally less than 0.5%. Pancreatitis has been reported in 0.5% of patients undergoing major spinal procedures and seems to be more common in children with neuromuscular scoliosis or who are having correction of kyphosis. Hardware prominence, back pain, and the above complications have a cumulative risk of hardware removal in as many as 10% of children who have spinal fusion.

Long-term (i.e., >20 year) follow-up of children undergoing current spinal instrumentation and fusion is not known. Studies of prior distraction instrumentation with longer-term follow-up suggest that patients who have had surgery extended into the lower lumbar spine or who have been left with a "flat-back," meaning they have lost normal lumbar lordosis and thoracic kyphosis, have a higher incidence of back pain than age- and sex-matched controls.

BIBLIOGRAPHY

1. Bunnell WP: An objective criterion for scoliosis screening. J Bone Joint Surg 66A:1381–1387, 1984.
2. Diraimondo CV, Green NE: Brace-wear compliance in patients with adolescent idiopathic scoliosis. J Pediatr Orthop 8:143–146, 1988.
3. Karol LA, Johnston CE, Browne RH, Madison M: Progression of the curve in boys who have idiopathic scoliosis. J Bone Joint Surg 75A:1804–1810, 1993.
4. Lonstein JE, Carlson JM: The prediction of curve progression in untreated scoliosis during growth. J Bone Joint Surg 66A:1061, 1984.
5. Nachemson AL, Peterson LE: Effectiveness of treatment with a brace in girls who have adolescent idiopathic scoliosis. J Bone Joint Surg 77A:815–822, 1995.
6. Noonan KJ, Weinstein SL, Jacobson WC, Dolan LA: Use of the Milwaukee brace for progressive idiopathic scoliosis. J Bone Joint Surg 78A:557–567, 1996.
7. Pehrsson K, Larsson S, Oden A, Nachemson A: Long-term follow-up of patients with untreated scoliosis. Spine 17:1091–1096, 1992.
8. Rowe DE, Bernstein SM, Riddick MF, et al: A meta-analysis of the efficacy of non-operative treatments for idiopathic scoliosis. J Bone Joint Surg 79A:664–674, 1997.
9. Weinstein SL, Ponseti IV: Curve progression in idiopathic scoliosis. J Bone Joint Surg 65A:447–455, 1983.

CHAPTER 64

KYPHOSIS AND LORDOSIS

Paul Connolly, MD, and Stuart L. Weinstein, MD

1. **What is kyphosis?**
   Kyphosis is a posterior curvature of the spinal column when viewed from the side (i.e., the sagittal plane). It originates from the Greek word *kyphos*, meaning *humpbacked*. It refers to a curve pointing backwards (i.e., the apex of the curve is posterior), as in a diver ready to dive into a swimming pool.

2. **What is lordosis?**
   Lordosis refers to a spinal curve pointing forward (i.e., the apex of the curve is anterior). The Greek word *lordos* means *curved forward*. This curve is in the opposite direction to kyphosis.

3. **What is a normal spinal curvature?**
   Normal spinal curvature varies with age. In the frontal plane, the normal pediatric and adult spines are relatively straight. In the sagittal plane, the neonate has a single kyphotic spinal curve. As the infant starts to gain head control, cervical lordosis develops. With progressive bipedal ambulation, the toddler starts to assume an upright position and develops a lumbar lordosis. As childhood progresses, a quadruple curve pattern is observed.

   By the age of 6 years, the single curve has become a quadruple one, with thoracic and sacral kyphotic curves and cervical and lumbar lordotic curves. The thoracic and sacral kyphosis curves are considered primary curves as they are present at birth. Lumbar and cervical lordosis are secondary curves and are related to upright posture. Structural wedging of the vertebral bodies contributes to most of the primary kyphotic curves. The lordoses of the cervical and lumbar curves, however, are created by the adjacent vertebrae being angulated with respect to each other. The disks, rather than the vertebral bodies, are wedged. In a normal school-aged child, kyphotic and lordotic curves seem to balance each other in that the head is well aligned over the pelvis in the lateral projection.

4. **How do I measure kyphosis and lordosis?**
   It is virtually impossible to measure these sagittal curves on a purely clinical basis. You can appreciate the sagittal alignment of a patient in a standing or sitting position, but only a standardized radiograph of the spine in the lateral projection allows you to quantify these parameters objectively. The radiograph is taken in the standing (and looking straight forward) position, with the patient's left side against the cassette. The patient should flex his or her elbows, placing knuckles in the supraclavicular fossae bilaterally. The knees and hips should be fully extended with the feet a shoulder width apart.

   The Cobb method of measurement is most commonly used to quantify kyphosis and lordosis. This technique requires a goniometer and a pencil. The vertebral end plates are used as reference points. You should include the most inclined end vertebrae in the measured curve (Fig. 64-1). There is some variability in measuring these angles; the interobserver range of measurement is 5–10 degrees. It is important to be aware of the three-dimensional aspect of some spinal deformities. A lateral radiograph supplies two-dimensional information. Therefore, a posteroanterior radiograph of the spine is also usually taken.

5. **What is normal kyphosis and lordosis?**

   Normal sagittal spinal alignment is not easily defined. The four curves (i.e., cervical and lumbar lordosis and thoracic and sacral kyphosis) vary significantly among individuals. Normal cervical sagittal alignment has been reported as 15–35 degrees, measured from C2–C7. The angular value for the thoracic kyphotic curve should be 20–40 degrees, measured from T5–T12.

   Kyphosis between 40 and 50 degrees is borderline normal. Values below 20 degrees are referred to as hypokyphosis and above 50 degrees as hyperkyphosis.

   Normal levels for lumbar lordosis fall between 20 degrees and 55 degrees, measured between L1 and L5. A line parallel to the end plates of L3 should point to 3 o'clock, and one drawn parallel to L4 should point to 4 o'clock.

   Normal sacral inclination, defined as the angle between a horizontal line and a line along the cranial sacral end plate, should measure between 20 and 60 degrees.

   Pelvic tilt refers to the angle between a vertical line and a line joining the middle of the sacral plate and the center of the femoral head. Normal values for this parameter range between −4 and 25 degrees.

   Pelvic incidence refers to the angle between a line perpendicular to the midpoint of the sacral end-plate line and the line joining the middle of the cranial sacral end plate to the center of the femoral head: this ranges from 35–80 degrees (Fig. 64-2). Normally, spinal curves tend to balance each other in that an increased pelvic tilt is accompanied by lumbar hyperlordosis. In a normal standing individual, a plumb line dropped from the middle of the C7 body falls within 2.5 cm of the posterosuperior corner of the first sacral body.

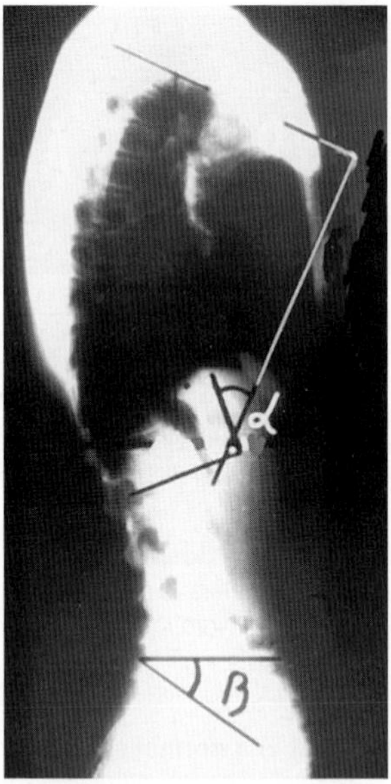

Figure 64-1. Lateral radiograph of the spine showing normal spinal curvature: the Cobb angle method of measurement. Draw lines parallel to the selected end plates. Measure the angles in the frame of the radiograph. The alpha (α) angle measures thoracic kyphosis. The beta (β) angle measures sacral inclination.

6. **What are the causes of kyphosis?**

   Kyphosis is a normal component of the human spinal curvature, but some pathologic conditions may lead to hyperkyphosis or hypokyphosis (Table 64-1).

7. **What are the causes of lordosis?**

   Lordosis is also a normal component of the human spinal curvature, but increased or decreased lordosis may be seen in some diseases (Table 64-2).

8. **What is the three-column spine concept?**

   A better understanding of sagittal deformities of the pediatric spine is possible by applying the biomechanical concept of three columns. The concept was originally described in 1983 by Dr. Francis Denis to study and classify acute thoracolumbar spinal injuries:

   - **Anterior column:** Formed by the anterior longitudinal ligament, the anterior annulus fibrosus, and the anterior half of the vertebral body
   - **Middle column:** Formed by the posterior half of the vertebral body, the posterior annulus fibrosus, and the posterior longitudinal ligament

■ **Posterior column:** Consists of the posterior bony complex (i.e., the posterior arch) alternating with the posterior ligamentous complex. (The ligamentous complex is formed by the supraspinous and interspinous ligaments, the facet joint capsule, and the ligamentum flavum.) Normal spinal growth requires many features. The balanced growth of each column of each vertebra adds to the overall increase in length and shape of the spine. Inadequate formation of and injury or damage to one or more segments of the columns can alter the development of normal spinal alignment.

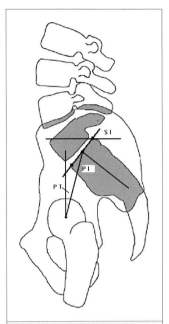

Figure 64-2. Diagram of sacral incidence (SI), pelvic incidence (PI), and pelvic tile (PT).

9. **What causes congenital kyphosis?**
   Two basic types of spinal abnormality can result in congenital kyphosis. Failure of formation of whole vertebrae or parts of them can result in deficient anterior and middle column support and congenital hyperkyphosis. If some vertebrae fail to separate (i.e., failure of segmentation) and the cell masses remain fused as in block vertebrae or in bar conditions, normal anterior column spinal growth may be impaired as well. Failure of formation of various portions of the posterior elements results in spina bifida, as in meningocele or meningomyelocele. If this happens at the cervical or thoracic level, the lack of stabilizing posterior column structures may result in congenital hyperkyphosis.

10. **Why can children with neuromuscular disease develop abnormal kyphosis?**
    In children with neuromuscular involvement, paraspinal muscle weakness and poor head, neck, and trunk control, together with gravity effects, may cause segmental instability, especially at the cervicothoracic and the thoracolumbar spinal junctions. Other factors such as diminished spinal muscle control and impaired spinal balance mediated by central pathways may also be involved.

11. **How can the balanced growth of the spine be altered so that hyperkyphosis develops?**
    Compression of the vertebral body may result in a segmental collapse of the anterior and middle columns of the spine and may thus result in a kyphotic deformity. This can occur with high-impact injuries (i.e., fractures) or with conditions in which the bony strength has decreased, as in osteolytic tumors, osteoporosis, infections, or osteogenesis imperfecta. Growth disturbances of the vertebral end plate can occur as sequelae of infections (pyogenic and tuberculous) or after irradiation of the spine for tumors such as neuroblastoma, Wilms' tumor, astrocytoma, or ependymoma. Any condition destabilizing the structures of the posterior column of the spine, however, can result in kyphotic deformities such as decompressive laminectomy, high-impact flexion-type spinal injuries, and collagen diseases. Severe spondylolisthesis at the lumbosacral junction may result in a clinical pseudohyperlordosis, but, radiographically, this is a kyphotic deformity that extends over the distal lumbar vertebrae and the sacrum.

12. **What is Scheuermann's disease?**
    Scheuermann's disease is named after Dr. Holger Scheuermann, who in 1921 described "a typically juvenile (i.e., >10 years of age) kyphotic vertebral disorder that could be

TABLE 64-1. PATHOLOGIC CONDITIONS LEADING TO HYPERKYPHOSIS OR HYPOKYPHOSIS

Kyphosis	Hyperkyphosis	Hypokyphosis
Physiologic (thoracic or sacral)	**Congenital Conditions**	Scoliosis
	Failure of formation	
	Failure of segmentation	
	Neuromuscular Conditions	Iatrogenic (i.e., spinal fusion)
	Static encephalopathy	
	Neurofibromatosis or arthrogryposis	
	Poliomyelitis	
	Spina bifida (e.g., myelomeningocele)	
	Postural conditions	
	Scheuermann's disease	
	Juvenile rheumatoid arthritis or ankylosing spondylitis	
	Post-traumatic conditions	
	Metabolic Conditions	
	Osteopenia or osteoporosis	
	Osteogenesis imperfecta	
	Collagen diseases	
	Sponydylolisthesis at the lumbosacral junction	
	Postinfectious (from tuberculosis)	
	Tumor or irradiation	
	Iatrogenic (from laminectomy)	

TABLE 64-2. CAUSES OF LORDOSIS

Lordosis	Hyperlordosis (Swayback)	Hypolordosis
Physiologic causes	Flexible lumbar curve in late childhood (a normal condition)	Post-traumatic (e.g., whiplash injury)
	Skeletal dysplasia (e.g., achondroplasia)	Iatrogenic causes (i.e., flat back syndrome)
	Spina bifida (e.g., myelomeningocele)	
	Hip joint contractures	
	Juvenile rheumatoid arthritis	
	Congenital hip dislocation (bilateral)	

distinguished from postural kyphosis on the basis of peculiar rigidity." This condition is radiographically characterized by anteriorly wedged vertebrae and irregularities of the vertebral end plates. To make the diagnosis, at least three wedged (5 degrees) adjacent vertebrae should be seen on the lateral radiograph of the axial skeleton. Scheuermann's kyphosis affects boys more often than girls.

13. **What are Schmorl's nodes?**
In adolescents with Scheuermann's disease, small rounded radiolucent erosions can sometimes be seen in the vertebral end plate. These erosions are called Schmorl's nodes, and they represent herniations of the discal nucleus pulposus into the vertebra. Related pressure phenomena may cause pain.

14. **What is the clinical difference between postural kyphosis and Scheuermann's disease?**
The main clinical difference is the rigidity of the curve. Both conditions occur in prepubertal and adolescent children. The otherwise healthy teenager presents with a cosmetically apparent round-back deformity or with vague back pain. Often, the parents may be affected as well.
   Voluntary or forced correction of the curve is not possible in Scheuermann's kyphosis. Furthermore, the forward-bending test reveals a more-or-less acute angulation of the back if observed from the side (Fig. 64-3). In postural kyphosis, the test shows normalization of the lateral spine profile (Fig. 64-4). Finally, patients with Scheuermann's disease often present with tight hamstrings or contracted pectoral muscles.

15. **How do I manage a teenager with Scheuermann's disease?**
The parents are most often concerned about the cosmetic deformity and the potential for future problems. It is important to determine the skeletal maturity of the teenager and the flexibility of the kyphosis.
   - If pain is the major complaint and if the kyphosis of the immature spine measures less than 45 degrees but is correctable to the normal range (with hyperextension in the supine position), a short course of nonsteroidal anti-inflammatory medication taken on a regular basis (for 10–14 days) may be sufficient.
   - If there is no pain and if the kyphosis is mild, clinical follow-up at 6-month intervals until skeletal maturity is recommended.
   - If the deformity progresses to more than 50 degrees, brace treatment is indicated. The most effective is the Milwaukee brace, worn 23 hours a day. If this is unacceptable to the patient and family, try an underarm thoracolumbosacral orthosis (TLSO).
   - Surgery is indicated for progression despite bracing. Many authors recommend surgery for curves of

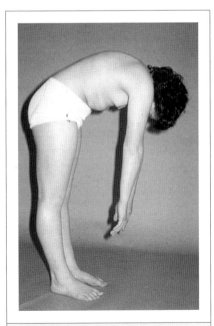

Figure 64-3. Adam's forward-bend test: an angulated spine profile, as seen in Scheuermann's disease.

more than 75 degrees. In the absence of documented progression, continued careful follow-up should be recommended.

16. **What can be done to maintain a good posture?**
Many factors play a role in determining the posture of each individual child, including puberty, height relative to peers, beginning breast development, self-consciousness, and genetic factors. The patient should be approached directly and engaged in an adult-to-adult dialogue about any postural problems. A full-length mirror can be used to provide feedback. Home exercise programs are often doomed to failure. Engaging in such activities as regular swimming (20 minutes, three to four times per week) is a good option. The value of exercises that strengthen the shoulder girdle or the back muscles in preventing adult back pain is not scientifically proven. Exercises supervised by a physical therapist are not cost effective unless paraspinal muscle weakness induced by pain is present.

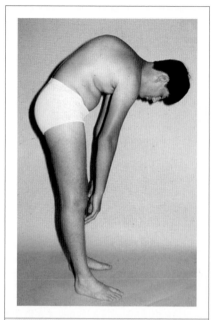

Figure 64-4. Adam's forward-bend test: a normal spine profile.

17. **When does hypokyphosis develop?**
Hypokyphosis of the thoracic spine is usually present in idiopathic scoliosis, the most common type of scoliosis. It is unclear whether the more vertical alignment of the shingle-type facet joints precedes or accompanies the characteristic vertebral rotation or deformity in the frontal plane. Thoracic hypokyphosis, however, may also be an unintentional feature of posterior column fusion owing to the continued growth of the anterior and middle spinal columns. It is important for the spine surgeon to acknowledge the sagittal spinal alignment of the patient before surgery. It has been shown that the use of straight rods to correct scoliotic deformities may lead to the so-called "flat back syndrome" in the lumbar spine (i.e., hypolordosis).

18. **Can juvenile rheumatoid arthritis change the sagittal alignment of the spine?**
Juvenile rheumatoid arthritis has one of the most devastating effects on normal spinal growth. The inflammatory synovitis may decrease the height and diameters of the vertebral bodies and of the intervertebral disks. Muscle spasm, fibrous tissue contractures or ruptures, gradual facet joint destruction, and enhanced blood flow alter the growth patterns of the spine significantly. High-dosage steroid use depletes bone stock, with the potential for compression fractures. Clinically, this may result in a child of short stature with a short hyperlordotic neck, thoracic hyperkyphosis, and compensatory overgrowth of lumbar vertebrae.

19. **How does lumbar hyperlordosis relate to contractures about the hip joint?**
Excessive lumbar lordotic posture can be due to tight hip flexor muscles. The psoas muscle originates from the proximal lumbar vertebrae. Tight rectus femoris and sartorius muscles may increase the pelvic tilt and can influence the sacral inclination. These muscular and tendinous

contractures can be seen in children with skeletal dysplasia or with lumbar meningomyelocele (i.e., muscular imbalance).

20. **What is the clinical relevance of rigid lumbar lordosis?**
The lordosis will not reverse on the forward-bending test or with the hips hyperflexed. This may suggest an intrathecal mass. A full work-up is warranted.

KEY POINTS: KYPHOSIS AND LORDOSIS

1. Kyphosis and lordosis refer to sagittal plane alignment of the spine. Many conditions can lead to abnormalities of spinal alignment in this plane. A careful history and physical examination, along with the use of appropriate investigations, will lead to accurate diagnosis in most cases.

2. Considering the spine as a three-column structure helps in understanding kyphotic and lordotic deformities. Derangement in one or more of these columns by a disease process may cause sagittal plane malalignment.

3. Kyphosis and lordosis are most commonly quantified using the Cobb method of measurement on standardized lateral radiographs of the spine.

4. For cervical lordosis, values between 15 and 35 degrees measured between C2 and C7 are considered normal. Thoracic kyphosis measured between T5 and T12 usually ranges between 20 and 40 degrees. Normal values for lumbar lordosis L1–L5 are between 20 and 55 degrees, whereas 20–60 degrees of sacral inclination is considered normal.

5. Postural kyphosis and Scheuermann's disease are two conditions most often seen in prepubertal and adolescent children causing increased kyphosis in the thoracic spine.

21. **What type of imaging is useful in abnormal kyphosis or lordosis?**
Radiography remains the mainstay of diagnostic imaging, but radiographs should not be routinely taken for every child with minor deviations of the normal sagittal balance found on physical examination. In a 35-kg child, a posteroanterior or lateral radiograph of the spine requires a radiation exposure of 200 milliroentgens (mR). A chest radiograph exposes the child to 15 mR. One receives a yearly radiation exposure of 100–300 mR from the earth itself, depending on the geographic location. It is preferable to allow the consulting orthopaedic surgeon to order any imaging studies. Spine radiographs should be taken in the upright position on 36-inch film using shielding and techniques that avoid excessive radiation exposure. The film must include the entire spine, from C1 to the coccyx.

22. **What does the sagittal spinal alignment on radiography reveal?**
The complete or partial loss of the four physiologic curvatures may be pathologic, even in neonates, suggesting a spectrum of conditions ranging from tumors to ordinary muscle spasms. Flexion or extension views may help in determining the flexibility of an abnormal curve.

23. **In a conscious patient with neck pain, what is a radiographic feature of a whiplash injury?**
An abrupt deceleration of the human body as in a frontal collision may result in a forceful thrust of the head and neck. Painful contractures of muscles can produce flattening of the normal cervical lordosis.

24. **Should I order laboratory tests?**

    In the setting of a general practice, a laboratory work-up is only occasionally necessary to rule out infections or inflammatory diseases in children with significantly abnormal sagittal alignment.

25. **How do I screen children with abnormal sagittal alignment of the spine?**
    - Have the child participate actively in the inquiry about the onset and duration of complaints, the presence of cosmetic concerns and disability, and the progression of the deformity. The family history can be helpful in cases of Scheuermann's disease.
    - A proper clinical examination should be done with the child wearing underwear, a swim suit, or a hospital gown that opens in the back.
    - The chest must be examined. Be aware that obesity can mask abnormal kyphosis or lordosis.
    - Observe the body habitus in the standing position from the front, the back, and the side. Ask the child to look straight forward (preferably away from the parents) and to stand with the knees fully extended.
    - Note any shoulder asymmetry, scapular prominence, rib hump, trunk shift, pelvic tilt, or asymmetry.
    - Note any skin lesions such as dimples, hairy patches, and hemangiomata, which are often associated with intraspinal lesions or dysraphism.
    - In the case of a leg-length discrepancy, use a small wooden block of appropriate size to correct the imbalance.
    - Look for abnormalities of the feet, knowing that cavovarus deformities suggest spinal dysraphism or neuromuscular disorders.
    - Palpate the prominences of the spinous processes and the paraspinal muscles.
    - Drop a plumb line from the C7 prominence. It should fall between the gluteal creases.
    - Assess spinal flexibility in the sagittal plane by asking the child to hyperextend.
    - Perform Adam's forward-bend test. Ask the child to assume the diving position with the feet placed together, the knees fully extended, and the palms opposed. Limited forward bending (above the midshin level) because of pain in the back or hamstrings, hesitation, or trunk shift to one side is abnormal. These may be associated with general body stiffness, diskitis or disk herniation, spinal column or cord tumors, or spondylolisthesis. The back should curve smoothly and evenly. Sharp segmental angulation as seen in congenital kyphosis or Scheuermann's disease should be noted. Evaluate the spine in the Adam's position from the bottom, from the head, and from the side.
    - Palpate the spine in the prone position. If local tenderness over the midline can be elicited, ask the child to hyperextend (i.e., the instability test). Note any decrease or increase in pain.
    - Do a careful neurologic examination. Do not forget to assess the abdominal reflexes.

26. **What do I look for in children with neuromuscular disease?**
    - Evaluate head-neck and trunk control and motor strength in the sitting position.
    - Look for pressure sores and skin breakdown.
    - Assess the flexibility of the curvature.
    - Examine the child in the prone position, with the pelvis balancing on the edge of the table. Extend the hip. An increase in the lumbar lordosis suggests a hip flexion contracture.
    - Note any documented change in or asymmetry of neurologic integrity. Increased intracranial pressure, tethered cord syndrome, or spinal dysraphism may be present.

27. **What are the pitfalls in common practice when assessing the sagittal balance of a child?**

    Underestimating back pain in a child with abnormal sagittal balance can lead to the major diagnostic error of missing a spinal tumor or an infection. Most back pain is related to muscle strain, and a wait-and-see period of 7–10 days will resolve most complaints. Over-the-counter nonsteroidal anti-inflammatory drugs can be taken on a regular basis with food. If pain persists or if the sagittal deformity is fixed or progressive, we would recommend referral to an orthopaedic surgeon, preferably one interested in pediatric conditions.

BIBLIOGRAPHY

1. Bernhardt M: Normal spinal anatomy: Normal sagittal plane alignment. In Bridwell KH, DeWald RL (eds): The Textbook of Spinal Surgery, 2nd ed. Philadelphia, Lippincott-Raven, 1997, pp 185–191.

2. Propst-Doctor L, Bleck EE: Radiographic determination of lordosis and kyphosis in normal and scoliotic children. J Pediatr Orthop 3:344–346, 1983.

3. Stagnara P, de Mauroy JC, Dran G, et al: Reciprocal angulation of vertebral bodies in a sagittal plane: Approach to references for the evaluation of kyphosis and lordosis. Spine 7:335–342, 1982.

4. Vialle R, Levassor N, Rillardon L, et al: Radiographic analysis of the sagittal alignment and balance of the spine in asymptomatic subjects. J Bone Joint Surg 87A:260–267, 2005.

5. Voutsinas SA, MacEwen GD: Sagittal profiles of the spine. Clin Orthop 210:235–242, 1986.

6. Weinstein SL (ed): The Pediatric Spine: Principles and Practice, 2nd ed. Philadelphia, Lippincott Williams & Wilkins, 2001.

XI. SHOULDER PROBLEMS

TORTICOLLIS

Peter Pizzutillo, MD

CHAPTER 65

1. **What is torticollis?**
   Tilt of the head with rotation to one side.

2. **What is the most common type of torticollis?**
   Congenital muscular torticollis.

3. **What are the causes of torticollis?**
   - Response to fracture of the clavicle
   - Congenital muscular torticollis
   - Congenital absence of the sternocleidomastoid and trapezius muscles
   - Congenital anomalies of the base of the skull
   - Plagiocephaly without synostosis of the skull
   - Congenital anomalies of the upper cervical spine
   - Imbalance of extraocular muscles
   - Rotary subluxation of the atlantoaxial joints
   - Neoplasm of the posterior fossa, brain stem, cervical spinal cord, and atlas or axis
   - Dystonia
   - Pseudotumor cerebri
   - Benign paroxysmal torticollis of infancy
   - Dissecting vertebral artery aneurysm

4. **Describe the pathophysiology of congenital muscular torticollis.**
   Intrauterine positioning may result in compartment syndrome of the sternocleidomastoid muscle with resultant fibrosis, which restricts normal motion of the cervical spine.

5. **What are the presenting clinical signs of congenital muscular torticollis?**
   Persistent tilt and rotation of the head and neck.

6. **What physical findings are associated with congenital muscular torticollis?**
   Limited lateral rotation and lateral side-bending of the neck, flattening of the occiput on the same side as the tilt, and facial asymmetry. Occasionally, a firm, nontender mass is palpable in the substance of the sternocleidomastoid on the side of the tile. The mass spontaneously resolves in a matter of months.

7. **What conditions are associated with congenital muscular torticollis?**
   Hip dysplasia occurs in 20% of children with congenital muscular torticollis. Although infrequent, congenital muscular torticollis may occur in association with congenital anomalies of the cervical spine.

8. **What other types of physical examination are required in the patient with torticollis?**
   Neurologic examination is required to rule out an underlying neurologic cause. If indicated, obtain an ophthalmologic or neurologic consultation.

9. **What imaging studies are indicated?**

Routine radiographs of the cervical spine frequently rule out congenital anomalies of the cervical spine and rotary subluxation of the atlantoaxial junction. Anteroposterior radiographs of the hips and pelvis detect subluxation or dysplasia of the hip joint.

More precise evaluation of the upper cervical spine and the base of the skull is accomplished with computed tomography (CT). Magnetic resonance imaging (MRI) is most effective in detecting neoplasms of the neurologic system.

10. **What is the treatment for congenital muscular torticollis?**

When other forms of torticollis have been eliminated, stretching of the sternocleidomastoid muscle of the neck to increase lateral rotation and lateral side-bending has been successful in infants younger than 2 years of age. Exercises are usually performed on the child by the child's parent; only rarely is formal physical therapy needed. If exercises have not significantly improved motion after 9 months of stretching, a botulinum toxin (i.e., Botox) injection of the sternocleidomastoid, followed by stretching exercises, has successfully improved more than 75% of refractory patients. When this program does not result in increased range of motion of the neck, surgical intervention is indicated.

11. **What factors suggest a neurologic cause?**

The presence of ophthalmologic dysfunction, the *de novo* development of torticollis after the newborn period, and recurrent torticollis in the older child suggest a neurologic cause. Benign paroxysmal torticollis of infancy, which begins in the first 12 months of life, presents with recurrent head tilt, vomiting, pallor, and ataxia and resolves in a matter of hours or days. Although recurrence is likely, permanent resolution is noted by 5 years of age.

12. **What factors suggest rotary subluxation of the atlantoaxial junction?**

Previous normal alignment and motion of the neck, history of recent upper-respiratory infection preceding the onset of torticollis, normal neurologic examination, and spasm of the sternocleidomastoid muscle on the side opposite the head tilt. Radiographs and CT scans of the upper cervical spine will confirm the diagnosis of rotary subluxation of the atlantoaxial junction.

13. **What treatment is required for rotary subluxation of the atlantoaxial junction?**

If the disorder is detected within the first week of symptoms, many children respond to the use of a soft cervical collar and limitation of activities. If the subluxation does not respond to early interventions or if it is not treated until after 1 week of symptoms, inpatient treatment with halter traction is usually successful in restoring normal range of motion of the neck. Following restoration of alignment and motion, immobilization in a Minerva cast or a halo cast is usually required. When subluxation has been present more than 4 weeks, maintenance of alignment may require surgical fusion of the upper cervical spine.

14. **What is the treatment of torticollis due to congenital dysplasia of the base of the skull?**

Observation is indicated to establish whether the condition is static or progressive. When head alignment is unacceptable or when the clinical condition is progressive, use of the halo vest with posterior occipitocervical fusion is indicated.

15. **What is the treatment of torticollis due to congenital anomalies of the cervical spine?**

Most congenital anomalies of the cervical spine are right and not progressive. Intervention is rarely indicated. When congenital fusion of the cervical vertebrae is present, it is important to evaluate hearing acuity and to rule out the existence of renal anomalies.

KEY POINTS: TORTICOLLIS

1. Torticollis indicates the presence of persistent tilt of the head with rotation of the head to one side.

2. The coexistence of congenital muscular torticollis and hip dysplasia is reported in older series to be as high as 17–20% and suggests the need for careful evaluation of the development of the hip.

3. Nonoperative stretching of the contracted sternocleidomastoid muscle is successful in restoring head and neck alignment and motion of the neck in more than 90% of infants younger than 2 years of life.

4. Partial resection of the sternocleidomastoid muscle is most successful in individuals less than 10 years of age but does offer significant, if incomplete, correction in those older than 10 years of age.

5. Congenital muscular torticollis remains the most common cause of torticollis in infants.

16. **When is helmet treatment indicated?**
In the infant who displays plagiocephaly without cranial synostosis, the use of a helmet has been successful in resolving the plagiocephaly and preventing the development of secondary torticollis.

17. **What are the results of surgical resection of the sternocleidomastoid in the child older than 10 years?**
Whereas surgical treatment of individuals less than 10 years of age yields 97% excellent or good results, treatment of those older than 10 years of age will result in 82% excellent or good results, with improved neck motion and head tilt but less improvement in remodeling of facial asymmetry.

BIBLIOGRAPHY

1. deChalain TM, Park S: Torticollis associated with positional plagiocephaly: A growing epidemic. J Craniofacial Surg 16:411–418, 2005.

2. Giffin NJ, Benton S, Goadsby PJ: Benign paroxysmal torticollis of infancy: Four new cases and linkage to CACN1A mutation. Develop Med Child Neurol 44:490–493, 2002.

3. Oleszek JL, Chang N, Apkon SD, Wilson PE: Botulinum toxin type a in the treatment of children with congenital muscular torticollis. Am J Phy Med Rehabil 84:813–816, 2005.

4. Shim JS, Noh KC, Park SJ: Treatment of congenital muscular torticollis in patients older than 8 years. J Pediatr Orthop 24:683–688, 2004.

CHAPTER 66

NEWBORN BRACHIAL PLEXUS PALSY

Marybeth Ezaki, MD

1. **What is newborn brachial plexus palsy (NBPP)?**
   NBPP is a stretch injury to the brachial plexus that occurs during the birth process.

2. **What is the incidence of NBBP?**
   About 3 per 1000 live births.

3. **What are the risk factors for NBPP?**
   - Increased birth weight
   - Gestational diabetes
   - Maternal obesity
   - Difficult vaginal delivery and shoulder dystocia
   - Prior delivery of a large baby or one with shoulder dystocia

4. **Can anything be done to prevent NBPP?**
   The vast majority of babies, even large babies, are born without NBPP. The development of shoulder dystocia is not predictable. Prenatal ultrasounds are not accurate enough to predict birth weight.

5. **Can NBPP occur with cesarean section delivery?**
   NBPP has been reported following cesarean section delivery, but it is not as common as in vaginal births.

6. **What nerve roots are involved in NBPP?**
   Some or all of the nerves arising from C5, C6, C7, C8, T1, and sometimes those from C4 if it contributes to the upper plexus.

7. **How can you tell if a baby has NBPP?**
   The limb will appear to be palsied or paralyzed.

8. **How can you tell what part of the plexus is injured?**
   The typical posture of the upper limb in a neonate with an upper (i.e., C5 or C6) NBPP will be internal rotation of the shoulder, extension of the elbow, and flexion of the wrist, the so-called "waiter's tip" position. A lower or complete plexus injury will be flail at first.

9. **What other diagnoses must be considered in an infant who presents with a unilateral paralytic upper limb?**
   - Fracture of the clavicle or humerus
   - Septic arthritis of the shoulder or osteomyelitis of the humerus

10. **Can NBPP be bilateral?**
    Yes, in up to 2% of cases. Breech birth is a risk factor.

11. **What initial investigation should be performed for a neonate who presents with a motionless or paralytic upper limb?**
    Plain x-ray, looking for fractures about the shoulder girdle or upper limb.

12. **What are good prognostic signs for NBPP?**
Limited plexus involvement and early recovery of arm function.

13. **What clinical signs are indicative of a lower plexus or pan plexus injury and are associated with a poorer prognosis?**
Horner syndrome (including constricted pupil, drooping eyelid, and hemifacial dryness) and paralysis of hand muscles.

14. **How is NBPP classified?**
Narakas classified plexus injuries by the pattern of involvement, as follows:
 - **Group 1:** C5 and C6
 - **Group 2:** C5, C6, and C7
 - **Group 3:** Near complete paralysis, but with finger flexion present neonatally
 - **Group 4:** Complete paralysis and Horner's syndrome present

15. **What percentage of infants with an NBPP can be expected to recover completely?**
 - **Group 1:** About 90%
 - **Group 2:** About 65%
 - **Group 3:** <50%
 - **Group 4:** None

16. **What should be done in the first weeks to months for an infant with NBPP?**
The arm should be protected from further injury. Gentle range-of-motion exercises should be started to keep the joints in good condition.

17. **Is there anything that can be done for the infant who does not recover neurologic function?**
Most children will spontaneously recover some function. Surgical exploration of the brachial plexus and nerve surgery have the potential to improve recovery but not to restore the limb to normal.

18. **What type of surgery can be done on the plexus?**
Direct nerve repair is rarely possible. Surgical options include nerve grafts using sural nerves as an interposition graft across a damaged area or nerve transfers to bring in nerve function from outside the plexus.

19. **Are there risks for this type of surgery?**
Any surgery carries risks. In addition to the risk of bleeding and anesthetic complications in an infant, there is a risk of damaging nerves that would recover if given more time.

20. **What are the results of surgery on the brachial plexus in a baby?**
Recovery of some function in some cases has been reported after surgery to reconstruct the brachial plexus. The limbs are not normal after surgery.

21. **When will you know the results of nerve surgery?**
The nerve must heal from the cell body outward. This occurs at a speed of about an inch a month. It takes many months to know the results of nerve surgery.

22. **When should microsurgical treatment be considered in NBPP?**
The decision to operate on a baby with NBPP must be individualized. In general, if a baby has not had recovery of elbow flexion by 5–8 months, plexus surgery can be considered.

23. **What complication can occur with regard to the shoulder joint in infants with NBPP?**
Posterior subluxation, or dislocation of the shoulder. This is caused by muscle imbalance between the strong internal rotators and the still-nonfunctional or weak external rotators.

KEY POINTS: NEWBORN BRACHIAL PLEXUS PALSY

1. Brachial plexus injuries are related to the birth of big babies or breech babies.
2. Not all recover completely, but most children recover to a functional level.
3. Shoulder muscle imbalance causes deformity in the shoulder joint.
4. Nerve surgery does not result in normal limbs.
5. The treatment of these brachial plexus injuries continues to evolve.

24. **How early can shoulder subluxation happen?**
Shoulder subluxation and dislocation can occur early, by 3–4 months of age.

25. **How can this complication be diagnosed clinically? What investigation should be performed?**
Lack of external rotation beyond neutral is the cardinal clinical sign (Fig. 66-1). An ultrasound shows the displaced position of the humeral head relative to the glenoid.

26. **How is it treated?**
Closed or open reduction and casting. Open reduction, if required, is usually combined with tendon transfer surgery.

27. **What tendon transfer is most commonly used to try to improve this function?**
Latissimus dorsi to infraspinatus or supraspinatus.

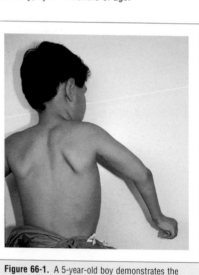

Figure 66-1. A 5-year-old boy demonstrates the inability to abduct and externally rotate his shoulder independently of the scapula due to paralysis of deltoid and shoulder external rotator musculature.

28. **What happens if the shoulder subluxation is not recognized and reduced?**
Persistent muscle imbalance causes abnormal forces on the shoulder joint and also causes deformity in the shape, alignment, and congruency of the joint, which limit passive and active range of motion.

29. **In patients with upper-root brachial plexus (i.e., Erb's) palsy, which upper limb muscles are affected?**
Supraspinatus, infraspinatus, teres minor, biceps, and wrist extensors.

30. **In patients who have recovered elbow flexion and wrist extension, what is the major residual deficit?**
    External rotation of the shoulder.

31. **Is there treatment for the older child who has a deformed shoulder joint?**
    The position of the limb can be changed by orthopaedic procedures such as osteotomy.

BIBLIOGRAPHY

1. Jackson ST, Hoffer MM, Parrish N: Brachial plexus palsy in the newborn. J Bone Joint Surg 70A:1217–1220, 1988.
2. Laurent JP, Lee RT: Birth-related upper brachial plexus injuries in infants: Operative and nonoperative approaches. J Clin Neurol 9:111–117, 1994.
3. Narakas AO: Obstetrical brachial plexus injuries. In Lamb DW (ed): The Paralysed Hand. Edinburgh, Churchill Livingstone, 1987, pp 116–135.
4. Phipps GJ, Hotter M: Latissimus dorsi and teres major transfer in rotator cuff in Erb's palsy. J Shoulder Elbow Surg 4:124–129, 1995.
5. Waters PM, Smith GR, Jaramillo LA: Glenohumeral deformity secondary to brachial plexus birth palsy. J Bone Joint Surg 80A:668–677, 1998.

CHAPTER 67

NECK AND SHOULDER DEFORMITIES

Chris Reilly, MD, and Stephen J. Tredwell, MD

1. **What is an os odontoideum?**

   An os odontoideum is a separate rounded ossicle of variable size in the anatomic location of the dens. It is separated from the body of C2 by a transverse radiolucent gap. A mobile os lesion effectively disables the transverse ligament, which destabilizes the C1-C2 segment and may give rise to instability that threatens the spinal cord. The os lesion may be difficult to visualize on plain radiographs. It typically has a very sclerotic border and is easily distinguished from an acute fracture on computed tomography (CT) imaging, which may be required to confirm the diagnosis.

2. **What is the etiology of an os odontoideum?**

   It appears that early trauma can lead to the development of an os odontoideum, presumably through a fracture nonunion. The odontoid blood supply in a young child is precarious and may place the child at increased risk for nonunion. Os lesions are commonly seen in patients with skeletal dysplasias and Down syndrome. It is unclear whether the os lesion represents a fracture nonunion, a failure of primary ossification of the odontoid ossification center, or a true congenital lesion in these patients. Tranverse radiolucent cartilaginous bands can persist postnatally. It is possible that patients with ligamentous laxity or vertebral dysplasia might subject this chondral band to excessive load, leading to failure of ossification and, ultimately, an os odontoideum lesion.

3. **What is the clinical significance of an os odontoideum?**

   The os may be attached to the body of the axis through fibrocartilage, or a formal pseudoarthrosis may exist. A mobile pseudoarthrosis destabilizes the C1-C2 articulation, potentially allowing the posterior arch of C1 to impinge the back of the spinal cord in flexion and the dens or clival base to impinge on the anterior aspect of the spinal cord in extension. Movement of the os odontoideum with the base of the clivus and C1 seen on flexion-extension films is an indication of significant risk of neurologic injury. Stable os lesions in asymptomatic patients may not require surgical management.

4. **What is the appropriate work-up and treatment for an os odontoideum?**

   The patient with an os odontoideum often presents with neck discomfort and may even present with the so-called Lhermitte's sign, transient electric-shock-like feelings in hands or feet on sudden jerky movement. Occasionally they may present with a spinal cord injury. Plain x-rays plus flexion-extension lateral films will often reveal the deformity and the amount of displacement. The os lesion is best visualized on sagittal CT images, which aid in discussion of the lesion with the family. If the os is mobile, a magnetic resonance imaging (MRI) scan will establish the presence or absence of spinal cord signal changes and may demonstrate cord impingement. Stable, asymptomatic lesion should be observed in most patients. Patients with symptoms, spinal cord impingement, or signal change, as well as those with significant instability, should be managed with C1-C2 fusion. Primary repair of the os lesion is not indicated.

5. **What other clinical conditions can compromise the room available for the spinal cord at C1 and C2?**

   The hyperlaxity seen in children with Down syndrome may produce abnormal movement at this level. Abnormalities in the room available for the cord are also seen in patients with seropositive and seronegative arthropathies. Underdevelopment of the dens and possible spinal cord compromise can be seen with spondylodysplasias and the mucopolysaccharidoses. The posterior arch of C1 may play a role in compression of the posterior aspect of the spinal cord seen in patients with achondroplasia.

6. **What percentage of patients with Down syndrome are at significant risk for spinal cord compromise at C1 and C2?**
Although in almost 20% of children with Down syndrome there will be 5 mm or more between the anterior arch of the atlas and the dens on forward flexion, only 5% will show enough instability to suggest cord compromise. As a result, although modification of activity may be required in some children, surgical intervention is not common.

7. **What other abnormal relationships may exist in the upper cervical spine in Down syndrome?**
Children with Down syndrome may have significant anatomic and functional abnormalities of the upper cervical spine. In addition to a high rate of os odontoideum lesions, these children may have hypoplasia of the posterior arch of C1 and the occipital condyles. The C1 posterior and anterior arches may be incomplete. An incomplete posterior arch is not protective in the presence of anterior C1 instability because the defect is spanned by a tight band of fibrous tissue. The anatomic and soft tissue abnormalities lead to a high rate of instability of C1 on C2, either anteriorly or posteriorly. In addition, the occiput-C1 articulation may be unstable, usually with excessive posterior roll back of the condyles and potential impingement of the anterior cord by the base of the clivus.

8. **Describe the concept of the room available for the spinal cord and its relationship to the atlantodens interval. Which is more important?**
In the upper cervical spine, at the C1 level, the spinal canal at age 3 is 18–23 mm in its sagittal diameter, and at age 8 it is 21–24 mm. The spinal cord is 7–10 mm at age 3 and 8–14 mm in diameter at age 8. As a rule of thumb, about one third of the volume of the total ring of C1 is for the dens, one third is for the spinal cord, and one third is empty space to allow for movement without cord compromise. If the room available for the spinal cord falls below 12 mm, the spinal cord is at risk.

Because the atlantodens interval is visible on plain radiographs, it is often an easily acquired measurement. In the normal child, on forward flexion, there should be no more than 3 mm between the anterior arch of C1 and the dens. More than 5–6 mm difference should cause clinical concern, and more than 9 mm is usually accompanied by a significant reduction in room available for the spinal cord. Although the atlantodens interval is a more easily acquired measurement, the room available for the cord is a more specific and clinically relevant value, especially when it is used as a surgical indicator. Patients with hypoplasia of the posterior arch of C1 may be at risk of cord injury at a much lower atlantodens interval measurement than those with a large posterior arch.

9. **When and how often should one order x-rays of the cervical spine in the patient with Down syndrome?**
Many children with Down syndrome are involved in active sports programs. Orthopaedic clinicians must evaluate these children's cervical spine and assure both the parent and the sponsors that the child is not at risk and can continue to participate. Although a small percentage of children with Down syndrome are at risk, it is recommended that flexion-extension lateral films be done at or around age 4, when the child can cooperate (Figs. 67-1, 67-2). There is controversy as to whether these films should be repeated if normal. It is reasonable to repeat the flexion-extension lateral films at approximately 10 years of age in the children who were normal at 4 years.

10. **What are the common chondrodystrophies that may include compromise of C1 and C2?**

The chondrodystrophies that involve the axial skeleton are spondyloepiphyseal dysplasia and the storage diseases. In these disorders, dens hypoplasia may lead to C1-C2 instability and put the spinal cord at risk. The underdeveloped dens in Morquio's syndrome may also be accompanied by stenosis at C1; therefore, an MRI work-up is essential. Fusion of C1 and C2 in these syndromes is not necessarily indicated unless the cord is at risk.

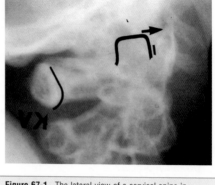

Figure 67-1. The lateral view of a cervical spine in extension in a child with Down syndrome shows an atlantodens interval of 1 mm.

11. **What is the cause of the C1-C2 instability in juvenile ankylosing spondylitis or in juvenile rheumatoid arthritis?**

There is a synovial joint between the transverse ligament and the dens. This may become involved in the seropositive and seronegative arthropathies. A build-up of pannus can erode the odontoid or attenuate the transverse ligament, resulting in instability. The pannus can also act as a space-occupying lesion, further reducing the space available for the cord. As in all the other syndromes, the reduction of that room below 12 mm is an indication for surgical intervention.

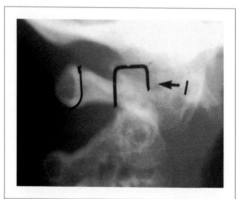

Figure 67-2. In a radiograph of the same child as in Fig. 67-1, the atlantodens interval increases to 10 mm with flexion of the spine.

12. **What is the clinical triad in Klippel-Feil syndrome?**
    - Short neck
    - Low posterior hairline
    - Marked limitation of range of motion of the neck
      See Figure 67-3.

13. **What is the anatomic anomaly in Klippel-Feil syndrome?**
    Congenital fusion of the cervical spine. This varies from as few as two segments to the entire cervical spine.

14. **What is the medical importance of Klippel-Feil syndrome?**
    Because the cervical spine develops in the embryo at or around the same time as many other organ systems, patients with this anomaly often display congenital anomalies of the genitourinary system (25–35% of patients), cardiovascular anomalies (5–10%), and

sensorineural hearing loss (15%). Neurologic abnormalities of movement and cord decussation within the cervical spine have been seen. The most common is termed *synkinesis*. This is a mirroring movement, an unconscious mimicking of the movement of the hand or foot on the other side. Miscellaneous anomalies of formation of the gastrointestinal tract are reported in a small number of cases.

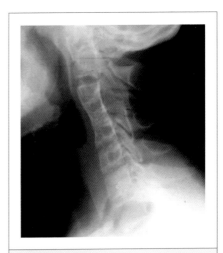

Figure 67-3. Multiple-level cervical spine fusions in Klippel-Feil syndrome.

15. **What other skeletal anomalies can be associated with the Klippel-Feil syndrome?**
Other fusions or malformations of the vertebral column are common in the Klippel-Feil syndrome. Scoliosis occurs in up to 60% of patients. Failure of descent of the scapula, called *Sprengel's deformity*, is also seen in up to 20–30% of patients, as are cervical ribs (in up to 15%).

16. **Given the wide range of anomalies in this syndrome, what is an appropriate work-up?**
Ultrasonography should be completed to exclude genitourinary anomalies. Competent medical examination can be sufficient to evaluate for potential cardiovascular anomalies. Preschool children should have an audiology assessment.

If a congenital cervical fusion is identified, dynamic stability should be evaluated with neutral, flexion, and extension radiographs. Radiographs should also be evaluated for evidence of stenosis and the potential for future deformity. Recent reports of stenosis of the cervical canal and decussation abnormalities of the spinal cord at the cervical level would also suggest that the more severely involved patients should have an MRI of the brain stem and the cervical and upper thoracic spinal cord. Families should be counseled about the risk of instability and cervical injury; activity modifications may be required in some cases. Patients with fusion patterns at high risk for future instability, such as atlanto-occipital fusion associated with subaxial fusion, should be followed longitudinally for instability. Progressive instability is an indication for cervical fusion.

17. **Are there other syndromes than can mimic Klippel-Feil syndrome?**
Children with fetal alcohol syndrome may have congenital cervical vertebral fusions; however, the associated anomalies are quite different. These children very often have microcephaly and very rarely have renal anomalies.

18. **What is the significance of absence of the clavicle?**
Symmetric clavicular absence is one of the clinical hallmarks of cleidocranial dysostosis; there may be complete absence or absence of a variable amount of the lateral clavicle. In addition to the absent or underdeveloped clavicles, these children have delayed ossification of the fontanelles, delayed and abnormal dentition, absence of the pubic rami, coxa vara, and short stature.

19. **What is the role of the orthopaedist in the management of the patient with cleidocranial dysostosis?**

The orthopaedic clinician should make the family aware of the dangers of the exposed fontanelle and the advantages of protective headgear in some situations. Early pediatric dental referral is necessary. Coxa vara can be managed with a valgus osteotomy. Scoliosis associated with syringomyelia has been reported in this group of patients. They should be checked at the time of presentation and followed through their growth peak.

KEY POINTS: NECK AND SHOULDER DEFORMITIES

1. Os odontoideum is a significant finding that should be carefully evaluated.

2. A wide variety of conditions can lead to upper cervical instability.

3. Patients with congenital cervical fusions may have a variety of associated abnormalities, as well as cervical instability, requiring a detailed work-up.

4. Clavicle hypoplasia or absence should prompt the physician to consider the underlying diagnosis.

20. **What is the significance of an asymmetric clavicular defect?**

Unilateral absence of the central third of the clavicle is termed *congenital pseudarthrosis*. Of interest, it is almost always seen on the right side (although up to 10% of cases may be bilateral).

21. **What is the clinical significance of pseudarthrosis of the clavicle?**

Congenital pseudarthrosis of the clavicle is primarily a cosmetic deformity. Most children are able to function normally but present with asymmetry of the shoulder.

In some patients, the shortening of the shoulder girdle may be very significant, leading to a very visible asymmetry. If the cosmetic appearance is very objectionable, grafting of the central third of the clavicle can be attempted. However, the family must be aware that there is a significant failure rate, and the surgical scar may be equally objectionable from a cosmetic point of view.

22. **What is the rhomboid fossa of the clavicle? Why is it important?**

The rhomboid fossa is an indentation of the clavicle at its medial end on its undersurface. It represents the insertion of the rhomboid ligament that runs between the first rib and the clavicle. Its importance is that, when pronounced, it can simulate a destructive lesion and, if the clinician is unaware of the entity, can precipitate a decision to biopsy.

23. **What is Sprengel's deformity? What is the major functional difficulty encountered by patients with this problem?**

Sprengel's deformity is a failure of scapular descent. From the 9th through the 12th week of gestation, the scapula normally descends from a paramidline structure in the neck oriented in the sagittal plane to a posterior thoracic structure oriented in the coronal plane. Failure of descent leaves the scapula abnormally elevated and the acromion laterally rotated, limiting apparent glenohumeral abduction. Scapulothoracic motion is also often markedly restricted, further restricting global shoulder abduction.

24. **What are the classic clinical findings in Sprengel's deformity?**

The scapula is usually smaller and is high-riding, and the interior pole is rotated medially. Patients stand with shoulder asymmetry, higher on the affected side. The clinical appearance may mimic a high thoracic scoliotic deformity. Shoulder abduction may be severely restricted. (Figs. 67-4, 67-5)

25. **What treatment options are available for patients with Sprengel's deformity?**
   In patients who have functional shoulder range of motion and in whom the high elevation presents a cosmetic difficulty or causes pain, resection of the medial corner of the scapula will often produce a satisfactory shoulder contour. If shoulder abduction is severely restricted, scapular repositioning may be considered.

26. **What are the hazards of repositioning the scapula?**
   Repositioning the scapula may lead to compression of the thoracic outlet by the clavicle, resulting in brachial plexus injury. Clavicular osteotomy and plexus monitoring can be used during scapular repositioning surgery to try to reduce the risk of neurologic injury.

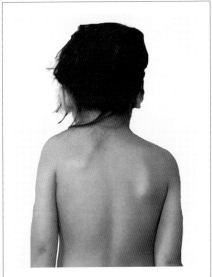

Figure 67-4. Sprengel's deformity on the left side.

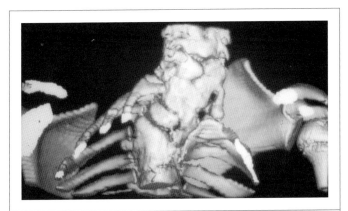

Figure 67-5. The three-dimensional computed tomographic reconstruction in a child with Sprengel's deformity shows the elevated and hypoplastic scapula.

27. **What is the omovertebral bone?**
   The omovertebral bone is an abnormal bony and cartilaginous structure extending from the upper medial border of the scapula to the spinous processes and laminae of the cervical spine. It is present in up to one third of patients with Sprengel's deformity and can contribute to the decreased motion. It also can contribute to pain. Excision is indicated when it is symptomatic.

BIBLIOGRAPHY

1. Herring JA (ed): Tachdjian's Pediatric Orthoapedics. Philadelphia, Saunders, 2002, pp 171–209.
2. Weinstein SL (ed): The Pediatric Spine: Principles and Practice. Philadelphia, Lippincott Williams & Wilkins, 2001, pp 219–252.

UPPER LIMB PAIN

CHAPTER 68

Charles Douglas Wallace, MD

1. **In evaluating a child with a painful extremity, what is the single most important part of the work-up?**

   Obtaining a thorough history. This will provide valuable insight into potential causes for the discomfort. There may clearly be a traumatic event to account for the pain or evidence of infection or overuse. Familial patterns or other involved areas of the body may aid in diagnosis.

   The next step is a careful physical exam to determine the exact location of tenderness, the presence of warmth or redness, inciting manipulations, and the range of motion of the joints. Detailed consideration must be given to the anatomic structures beneath the area of pain and tenderness.

2. **I have a patient in her teens with symptoms suggestive of carpal tunnel syndrome. Does this occur in children?**

   Yes, carpal tunnel syndrome can occur in children and teens, although it is most frequently seen in women older than 40 years of age. Many of the potential causes of carpal tunnel syndrome seen in adults also may be found in children. These include tumors, (juvenile) rheumatoid arthritis, oral contraceptive use, pregnancy, and repetitive use and trauma. In general, treatment is conservative, utilizing activity modification, splints, nonsteroidal anti-inflammatory medications, and, occasionally, steroid injections into the carpal canal. Operative release of the transverse carpal ligament is reserved for cases resistant to nonoperative treatments.

3. **What may cause concern in a patient who seems to have hypersensitivity to touch or manipulation after even a trivial injury?**

   Reflex sympathetic dystrophy, or complex regional pain syndrome (CRPS) type I, as it is being renamed, is a concern. This is a poorly understood, painful condition that may be progressive and debilitating following even minor trauma. In children, the upper extremity is affected only one sixth as often as the lower, and there is a striking female predominance of 7:1. The pathophysiology is not well delineated but is felt to be related to sympathetic reflex pathways. Management is difficult, with results often slow to attain. Successful outcome should be expected in the child, although it requires early diagnosis, a high index of suspicion, and prompt aggressive treatment.

4. **What are the elements of CRPS?**

   Pain, impaired function, and dystrophic changes with autonomic dysfunction. There is hyperalgesia, in which normal, generally nonpainful stimuli elicit an exaggerated sensation of pain. The dystrophic changes include stiffness of the involved joints, local edema, dermal atrophy, and osteopenia. The combination of hyperalgesia with dystrophic skin and bone changes leads to significant impairment of function. The autonomic abnormalities may be expressed as asymmetric thermal changes, sweating of the affected area, and vasomotor activity, yielding skin discoloration.

5. **For a patient in whom one suspects the diagnosis of CRPS, medical intervention, as well as intensive occupational therapy, is often recommended. In these days of containing medical costs, is all this really necessary?**

Yes! Early aggressive treatment of suspected reflex sympathetic dystrophy is the key to a successful outcome. Delay in diagnosis or in instituting treatment may allow progression of the symptom complex, making a good result less likely or much more difficult to attain. A relatively small area of involvement of the hand can easily progress to debilitate an entire extremity!

6. **What are the steps in managing a patient with CRPS?**

Management of this difficult problem is multifaceted. Pharmacologic intervention may include the use of tricyclic antidepressants such as amitriptyline, anticonvulsants, α-antagonists, calcium channel blockers, and local anesthetics given as regional or ganglionic blocks. Early involvement of a pain specialist will aid in balancing the effects of the many medicines involved. In addition to these angles of attack, occupational and (possibly) physical therapy to maintain or gain joint motion, to prevent contractures, to attempt systematic desensitization, and to teach strengthening exercises are critical. Therapy should involve not only the hand but also the arm and shoulder. Modalities such as transcutaneous electrical nerve stimulation (TENS), desensitization, massage, and temperature baths are often utilized. Continuous peripheral nerve blocks with 0.2% ropivacaine administered through an indwelling catheter has yielded excellent success in acute pain relief and enhanced therapy participation, thereby lowering the recurrence rate in CRPS. Acupuncture has also been shown to enhance outcomes and to reduce the need of potentially addictive narcotic agents. The role of psychotherapy cannot be downplayed. Both individual and family psychologic issues have a major impact on the perpetuation of this condition. Surgery is indicated only if a specific triggering lesion such as a neuroma can be identified. Management of reflex sympathetic dystrophy clearly involves an intensive team approach.

Despite a good outcome of therapy in the management of CRPS, recurrences are common. In fact, there is a variant in which recurrent episodes of CRPS are seen in different locations over time. This recurrent migratory form can be treated successfully with both therapy and pharmacologic intervention; however, it can be somewhat frustrating nonetheless. Long-term follow-up of children who have been successfully treated has shown residual symptoms in up to 25% of the children despite an overall successful outcome.

7. **If a patient who has been successfully treated for CRPS comes to require surgery in the ipsilateral extremity, is this ill advised, or should I be particularly concerned?**

When operating on a patient who has experienced CRPS in the past, extra care needs to be paid to management of that extremity. A recent study compared the recurrence rate of CRPS in patients who received a postoperative stellate ganglion block versus no intervention. The recurrence rate of CRPS was 10% in the patients who received a postoperative ganglion block compared with 72% in those who received no intervention. If a patient's history clearly demonstrates management for CRPS in the past, a postoperative stellate ganglion block should be planned at the time of surgery to minimize the risk of recurrence. Regional anesthetic blockade should also be utilized intraoperatively to prevent the nociceptor afferent barrage of the surgical procedure from inducing a central hyperexcitable state. In addition to this, the possibility of recurrence should be included in the preoperative counseling for this patient.

8. **How do you approach the toddler with a limp arm?**

There are many conditions that may lead to a toddler's not wanting to use an arm. The first step is to rule out any history of trauma to the extremity, although a negative history does not preclude injury in this active age group. Also, determine the presence or absence of any recent fevers or infections of the ear, throat, or other areas. The next step is to attempt to identify the location of the painful area (e.g., the shoulder, elbow, or wrist) by first gaining the child's confidence, if possible, and then manipulating only one area at a time. Plain films are taken of any areas in question. If there is no clear history of trauma, obtain a complete blood count with differential, erythrocyte sedimentation rate, and C-reactive protein level.

Diagnoses to consider include septic arthritis of the shoulder, elbow, or wrist. Fractures of the clavicle, the humerus (most frequently in the supracondylar region), or along the radius or ulna may also lead to a limp arm, as may a nursemaid's elbow from a pulling injury. Look critically at the plain films. A fat pad sign or a minor wrinkle in the bone may be the only evidence of a fracture. A suspected nursemaid's elbow should resolve several minutes following a gentle flexion-supination maneuver of the elbow with pressure over the radial head. Certainly, tumors are possible, although they are extraordinarily rare.

9. **A child presents with medial elbow pain with activity, as well as radiating pain to the hand. What should be considered?**
The symptoms are suggestive of ulnar nerve irritation. This may result from a previous injury to the area, such as a lateral condyle fracture malunion with a resultant fishtail deformity of the distal humerus and a tardy ulnar nerve palsy. It may also be caused by injury to the nerve from a direct blow with neuroma formation. Ongoing reinjury in the area may also lead to these symptoms. The patient may have medial epicondylitis or ulnar collateral ligament strain from repetitive throwing stress (such as in a pitcher) or a snapping ulnar nerve that subluxates out of a hypoplastic trochlear groove upon flexion of the elbow. The latter tends to be related to an anomalous portion of the triceps pushing the nerve out of the cubital tunnel, with symptoms caused by the resulting neuritis. Compression of the nerve adjacent to the cubital tunnel (such with a hypertrophied flexor carpi ulnaris), the ligament of Struthers, or the arcade of Struthers should also be considered.

10. **A teen presents with a radial-side wrist pain. What should you consider?**
De Quervain's stenosing tenosynovitis is one of the most common causes of radial-side wrist pain and has been known to occur in children and adolescents. The first dorsal compartment of the wrist contains the abductor pollicis longus and the extensor pollicis brevis, which may become inflamed and painful. The classic provocative test to evaluate for this condition is ulnar deviation of the thumb in a hand clenched into a fist, known as the Finkelstein test.

Management begins with application of a Velcro strap on splint and use of nonsteroidal anti-inflammatory medications. Steroid with lidocaine injection into the first dorsal compartment of the wrist may be both therapeutic and diagnostic. Surgical release of the sheath, which has a high success rate, may be indicated if conservative measures fail.

Some other causes of radial-side wrist pain include radial nerve compression, as well as injury to the scaphoid, trapezium, or trapezoid.

11. **What is the best way to manage a painful wrist ganglion in a child?**
As in adults, dorsal wrist ganglia are more common than volar ganglia. The most common site of origin is the area of the scapholunate interval. Ultrasonography provides a quick, noninvasive way to confirm the diagnosis in cases in which there may be a question as to the cause of the mass.

Conservative care with rest and splinting is the first step. This should decrease the discomfort and, in a fraction of the cases, may result in partial or complete resolution of the cyst. Needle aspiration should be offered to the family, with the proviso that recurrence is seen in adults in approximately 60% of cases. No good series in the pediatric population treated with aspiration alone is available for more age-specific recommendations. I do not advise steroid injection of the cyst. Surgical excision is the most reliable method to eliminate the cyst permanently, although there is still approximately a 5–15% recurrence rate despite careful removal of the cyst and its base off the capsule. I utilize a transverse incision over the mass when it is dorsal for cosmetic reasons, with care to avoid injury to the dorsal sensory branches of the radial nerve. Postoperatively, the wrist is placed in a cast, flexed and extended away from the side of resection to reduce stiffness.

12. **In evaluating the patient with midline wrist pain, other than a ganglion, what condition should be considered?**

Midline wrist pain can be associated with a number of pathologic conditions. Certainly, the most common in the pediatric population other than simple strains and sprains of trauma would be a painful wrist ganglion. Other diagnostic considerations can include scapholunate ligament injuries. Carpal instability is extremely rare in children; however, carpal dissociation has been described in the skeletally immature patient. This tends to be in the adolescent age group, either by nature of skeletal maturity or by the mechanics of the injury.

Another finding in the adolescent age group is pain associated with a lunotriquetral coalition. The incidence of lunotriquetral coalition is not well defined; however, it is a well-known entity. Various degrees of coalition, ranging from a fibrous coalition to a complex solid osseous coalition, are seen; treatment begins with routine care, including wrist immobilization, ice, and, once the pain has resolved, therapeutic exercises. A partial or fibrous (or both) coalition may proceed on to a complete condition over time. The management of a fibrocartilaginous coalition, which is resistant to conservative care, may include lunotriquetral arthrodesis to complete coalition.

Another rare contribution to wrist pain in the region includes a condition known as *os styloideum*. This is another form of a fibroosseous protrusion and partial coalition in the region of the trapezoid capitate and the index and long metacarpal bases. This generally presents in the older population, when degenerative changes have occurred; however, this has been seen and described in the adolescent population. A fine-cut computed tomography (CT) scan through this region appears to be the best modality for confirmation of diagnosis. The treatment for this condition has not been well delineated; however, it should be based upon the degree of involvement of the articular surfaces in the region. Minor articular involvement could be treated with resection of the involved fibroosseous structures with an interposition graft of fat versus completion of the arthrodesis if a significant amount of the joint is involved.

13. **How should I approach a patient with pain along the ulnar side of the wrist?**

Ulnar-side wrist pain is a distinct diagnostic challenge. One must visualize the structures beneath the skin to delineate the origins of the discomfort. Tenosynovitis of the extensor carpi ulnaris, flexor carpi ulnaris, or extensor digiti quinti may be an element of the pain. Disease in the triangular fibrocartilaginous complex due to an old injury must be considered. Lunotriquetral instability can also lead to ulnar-side wrist pain. Patients who have sustained a perhaps-forgotten forearm fracture in the past may have experienced physeal arrest of either the distal radius or the ulna, which can dramatically alter wrist biomechanics. A distal radius physeal arrest may lead to relative ulnar positivity with ulnocarpal abutment. Similarly, a distal ulnar physeal arrest can cause severe relative shortening of the distal ulna, resulting in pain and limited radial deviation of the wrist. A supinated anteroposterior (AP) film of both distal forearms should indicate either of these conditions. In addition, ganglia are rarely found in this area. Ulnar nerve compression at Guyon's canal may occur (although it is extremely rare in children), as may bony injuries to the carpus and distal ulna.

Evaluation should include a detailed history and a careful physical exam. Diagnostic studies should start with plain radiography but may include arthrography or magnetic resonance imaging (MRI), depending on your specific suspicions. Recent studies have evaluated the efficacy of magnetic resonance (MR) arthrography, compared with standard MRI utilizing wrist arthroscopy as the gold standard. The diagnostic accuracy, sensitivity, and specificity all are dramatically enhanced when contrast is added to the wrist prior to performing the MRI.

KEY POINTS: UPPER LIMB PAIN

1. Thorough and complete patient evaluation, which is always appropriate, can prove the most valuable tool in evaluation and management of a child with upper-extremity pain, especially if chronic in nature.

2. Complex regional pain syndrome type I is a described and not uncommon diagnosis in children and adolescents.

3. Birth brachial plexus palsy patients are not known to have chronic arm pain from the perinatal nerve injury.

4. Patients with rheumatologic diagnoses can present with upper-extremity pain, stiffness, and swelling.

5. Vigorous extremity overuse in sports can lead to physeal injury in addition to muscle strains and chronic tendinitis.

14. **What is thoracic outlet syndrome? How is it diagnosed and treated?**
Thoracic outlet syndrome is neurovascular compression secondary to unique individual anatomy at the thoracic outlet, affecting the upper extremities. The symptoms, even in adults, tend to be somewhat vague and nondescript. Most frequently, they include pain and paresthesias along the medial arm, although they may include the neck, chest, and lateral shoulder or arm. In children, the symptoms more frequently include aches, fatigue, and heaviness. Differential diagnosis includes any form of median or ulnar nerve compression, shoulder tendinitis, reflex sympathetic dystrophy, inflammation or tumor in the region of the brachial plexus, or cervical spine disease. This condition is rare in children, although it certainly does exist.
   Anatomic sites of neurovascular compression include a cervical rib, the interscalene interval, and the area beneath the clavicle or coracoid process. Diagnosis is based on detailed physical exam and provocative clinical maneuvers as well as plain films of the cervical spine, chest, and shoulder on the involved side. Electromyography has not proven helpful. Angiography is reserved for those with vascular alteration on provocative testing.
   Management begins with a progressive shoulder-strengthening program and postural reeducation. Avoiding overhead and other provocative activities has also been advocated. A 2-year trial of conservative therapy is advocated unless symptoms are progressive. Surgical intervention is considered after failure of conservative therapy and is based on decompression of the neurovascular elements at the site of proven or suspected compression.

15. **An active youth presents with shoulder pain and trouble abducting or flexing the shoulder. Does this indicate impingement syndrome or a rotator cuff tear?**
The answer is most likely "no." True impingement syndrome and rotator cuff tears are extraordinarily rare in children and adolescents. Examine the patient carefully for evidence of multidirectional instability of the shoulder, as well as generalized ligamentous laxity. Shoulder pain in a ligamentously lax active young person can easily be due to a new backstroke technique, a change in throwing patterns or frequency, or new exercises recently introduced into a physical training program. An additional consideration of diagnostic entities that contribute to pain in this region includes proximal humeral physeal damage secondary to repetitive trauma. This can be seen in competitive throwing athletes with open physis. Careful attention to the lateral aspect of the proximal humeral physis should be directed when evaluating plain films

of this region. Comparison with the asymptomatic proximal humerus may be necessary in an attempt to discern widening of the physis in this region.

The first step in attacking this problem is to identify and reduce provocative activities. Nonsteroidal anti-inflammatory drugs, rest, and ice can all be used, followed by physical therapy to address shoulder mobility and rotator cuff muscle strength and tone. The offending activity is then gradually reintroduced, with modifications in technique as necessary to prevent recurrence.

16. **What is of concern with lateral elbow pain in the active adolescent?**
The most frequently seen condition of greatest concern in general is an overuse syndrome. Many children are in organized activities at a high level of competition. Some join multiple teams in different leagues to pursue their interest in sports. They and their parents need to be aware of the risks involved in overuse of growing and developing limbs.

Although simple lateral epicondylitis can possibly be treated with nonsteroidals, rest, and stretching, a more severe condition is osteochondritis dissecans of the capitellum, with possible loose-body formation and collapse and fragmentation of the capitellum. MRI can be quite useful in delineating the extent of lesion found on plain radiographs, as well as suggesting the integrity of the articular surface and the presence of loose bodies. Drilling of the lesion, as well as removal of loose bodies, may be indicated. Prevention of reinjury is also important, necessitating analysis of both activity participation and environmental factors that may predispose the patient to injury.

BIBLIOGRAPHY

1. Arner S: Intravenous phentolamine test: A diagnostic and prognostic use in reflex sympathetic dystrophy. Pain 46:17–22, 1991.
2. Gellman H: Reflex sympathetic dystrophy: Alternative modalities for pain management. Instr Course Lect 49:549–557, 2000.
3. Leffert RD: Thoracic outlet syndrome. J Am Acad Orthop Surg 2:317–325, 1994.
4. Reuben SS: Preventing the development of complex regional pain syndrome after surgery. Anesthesiology 101:1214–1224, 2004.
5. Reuben, SS, Rosenthal EA, Steinberg RB: Surgery on the affected upper extremity of patients with a history of complex regional pain syndrome: A retrospective study of 100 patients. J Hand Surg Am 25:1147–1151, 2000.
6. Scheck RJ, Romagnola, A, Hierner R, et al: The carpal ligaments in MR arthrography of the wrist: Correlation with standard MRI and wrist arthroscopy. J Magn Reson Imag 9:468–474, 1999.
7. Tong HC, Nelson VS: Recurrent and migratory reflex sympathetic dystrophy in children. Pediatr Rehabil 4(2):87–89, 2000.
8. Wilder RT, Berde CB, Wolohan M, et al: Reflex sympathetic dystrophy children: Clinical characteristics and follow-up of seventy patients. J Bone Joint Surg 74A:910–919, 1992.
9. Yang J, Letts M: Thoracic outlet syndrome in children. J Pediatr Orthop 16:514–517, 1996.

CHAPTER 69

CONGENITAL HAND ANOMALIES

Donald S. Bae, MD, and Peter M. Waters, MD

1. **When does the upper extremity form *in utero*?**
   The limb bud first appears at 26 days after fertilization and continues to develop through the 47th day of development, by which time the joints of the hand appear. By day 56, development of all the structures of the upper limb has occurred.

2. **What is the apical ectodermal ridge (AER)?**
   The AER is a thickened ridge of dorsal and ventral ectodermal tissue that forms at the tip of the developing limb bud. It plays a critical role in proximal-to-distal limb development as well as in interdigital apoptosis required for individual digital formation. A number of fibroblast growth factors (FGFs) are specifically expressed by the AER, contributing to longitudinal limb growth and development.

3. **What are homeobox genes?**
   Homeobox (HOX) genes are a group of genes encoding transcription factors critical for limb development. There are four clusters, or groups, of HOX genes—HoxA, HoxB, HoxC, and HoxD—each of which resides on a different chromosome, collectively accounting for a total of 38 known transcription factors. It is believed that each type of HOX gene is responsible for a different component of limb development. The HoxD group genes, for example, have been shown to affect radioulnar differentiation of the hand; mutations in the HoxD locus have been identified in several types of synpolydactyly.

4. **How are congenital hand anomalies classified?**
   Although many different classifications have been proposed, the most widely accepted classification system of congenital limb anomalies is based upon the clinical and morphologic appearance of the affected extremity. The seven different classes of congenital anomalies are as follows:
   - Failure of formation
   - Failure of differentiation
   - Duplication
   - Undergrowth
   - Overgrowth
   - Congenital constriction band syndrome
   - Generalized skeletal anomalies

5. **What are the most common congenital hand differences?**
   Syndactyly and polydactyly occur in approximately 1 out of 3000 live births and are generally thought to represent the most common types of congenital hand differences.

6. **What other organ systems are commonly affected in patients with congenital hand anomalies?**
   Congenital hand anomalies may be accompanied by congenital abnormalities in other organ systems developing at the same time. These include the following:
   - Cardiac (e.g., atrial and ventricular septal defects and Holt-Oram syndrome)

- Hematologic (e.g., thrombocytopenia and Fanconi's anemia)
- Craniofacial (e.g., Apert's syndrome)
- Other musculoskeletal anomalies (e.g., vertebral abnormalities, anal atresia, cardiac abnormalities, tracheosophageal fistula, renal, and/or radial limb defects [VACTERRL association])

7. **How is syndactyly classified?**

Syndactyly is classified according to the extent and complexity of digital involvement and is described in two ways:

- **Complete versus incomplete:** Complete syndactyly extends to the tips of the fingers, whereas incomplete syndactyly does not.
- **Simple versus complex:** Simple syndactyly (Fig. 69-1) refers to situations in which only skin joins the affected digits. Complex syndactyly describes shared or conjoined bone, joints, tendons, or a combination thereof.

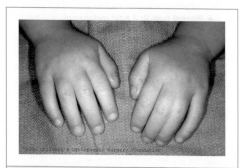

Figure 69-1. Simple syndactyly involving the third web space of the left hand.

8. **How is syndactyly treated?**

In general, syndactyly release is performed by separating the skin with the use of zig-zag incisions or Z-plasties to prevent subsequent longitudinal scar contracture. The interdigital commissure is usually reconstructed using a dorsally based flap of skin. In cases of simple complete syndactylism, full-thickness skin grafting is typically required to provide adequate skin coverage. In cases of complex syndactyly releases, the phalanges must be separated as well. Distal bifurcation of the digital artery, nerve, or both, may limit the extent of digital separation.

9. **What is the difference between preaxial and postaxial polydactyly?**

Preaxial polydactyly refers to radial-side, or thumb, duplications. Postaxial polydactyly refers to ulnar-side duplications (Fig. 69-2).

10. **What is the difference between camptodactyly and clinodactyly?**

Both terms are used to describe angular deformities of the digits of varying etiologies. **Camptodactyly** refers to angulation in the flexion-extension plane, whereas **clinodactyly** refers to angulation in the radioulnar plane.

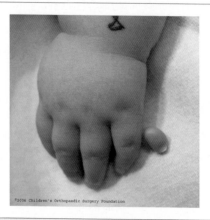

Figure 69-2. Postaxial polydactyly. In this case, the supernumerary digit is rudimentary and pedunculated.

11. **How are thumb duplications classified?**

The Wassel classification is used to describe preaxial polydactyly based upon the level of thumb duplication, from distal to proximal:

- **Wassel type I:** A bifid distal phalanx
- **Wassel type II:** A duplication at the level of the interphalangeal joint
- **Wassel type III:** A bifid proximal phalanx
- **Wassel type IV:** A duplication at the level of the metacarpophalangeal joint (most common, occurring in approximately 40% of cases)
- **Wassel type V:** A bifid metacarpal
- **Wassel type VI:** Duplication at the level of the carpometacarpal joint
- **Wassel type VII:** Thumb duplication, in which the supernumerary thumb is triphalangeal

12. **How is thumb duplication treated?**

Simple resection of the more hypoplastic of the two thumbs will not suffice as each of the thumbs contain anatomic elements critical for successful thumb reconstruction. Surgical treatment, therefore, typically comprises excising the skeletal elements of the more hypoplastic thumb, reconstructing the collateral ligaments and tendons, preserving the digital arteries and nerves, and fashioning soft tissue flaps to allow for appropriate skin reapproximation.

13. **What are the characteristic clinical features of thumb hypoplasia?**

In general, thumb hypoplasia has four characteristic clinical features:

- Stiff interphalangeal joint
- Unstable metacarpophalangeal joint
- Tight first web space
- Weak or absent thenar muscles

KEY POINTS: CONGENITAL HAND ANOMALIES

1. Homeobox genes have been found to be critical for limb development, and mutations have been found to be associated with congenital upper-limb abnormalities.

2. Some congenital hand abnormalities can be accompanied by congenital abnormalities of other organ systems.

3. The use of full-thickness skin grafts should be considered in the release or reconstruction of syndactyly.

4. Reconstructions of thumb abnormalities are generally attempted since functional gains can be significant.

5. Prosthetic fitting may be considered in children with congenital below-elbow amputations as they approach sitting age.

14. **What are the treatment options for thumb hypoplasia?**

Thumb hypoplasia is typically treated in one of two ways, depending upon its severity. In patients with stable carpometacarpal joints, surgical reconstruction is typically performed by stabilization of the metacarpophalangeal joint, first–web-space deepening, and tendon and muscle transfers to improve thumb opposition. In patients with unstable or absent carpometacarpal joints—including patients with floating or absent thumbs—pollicization is recommended.

15. **What is pollicization?**
    Pollicization refers to the surgical procedure in which an index finger is converted to a thumb (Fig. 69-3). By removing the index metacarpal, transposing the index finger, deepening the intervening web space with skin flaps, and transferring muscles and tendons, a new "thumb" may be fashioned.

16. **What is radial dysplasia, and how is it treated?**
    Radial dysplasia (also referred to as *radial clubhand*) refers to abnormal growth and development of the radius, often accompanied by deficiencies of the radial carpus and thumb. Clinically, there is a broad spectrum of presentations, ranging from patients with slightly smaller arms and hands with minimal limitations in function or appearance to patients with complete absence of the radius, radial carpus, and thumb. In general, the muscles and nerves of the arm in question are affected in addition to the bony skeleton (Fig. 69-4).

    At birth, stretching and corrective splinting or casting is initiated. Between 6 to 12 months of age, surgical centralization or radicalization is performed to place the hand and wrist over the ulna. Shortly thereafter, surgery may be undertaken to reconstruct a hypoplastic thumb or to perform a pollicization. External fixation devices have also been used to gradually lengthen or correct the radial deviation of the forearm, wrist, and hand in more complex cases.

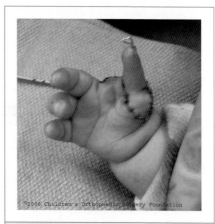

Figure 69-3. Intraoperative photo after pollicization of the index finger.

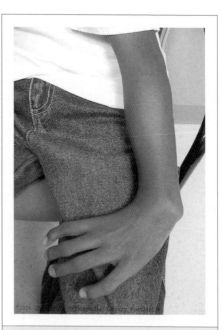

Figure 69-4. Radial deviation of the wrist with absence of the thumb in a patient with radial dysplasia.

17. **What is the most common type of congenital upper-limb amputation?**
    Congenital below-elbow amputations are thought to be the most common congenital amputation of the upper limb, with an estimated incidence of 1 in 20,000 live births (Fig. 69-5).

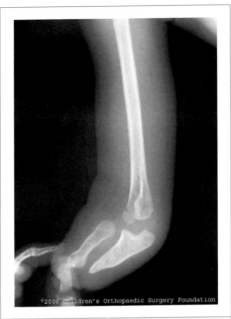

Figure 69-5. Radiograph depicting a congenital forearm-level amputation.

18. **When is prosthetic fitting for congenital upper-limb amputations recommended?**
    Traditionally, passive-hand prostheses are fitted in patients with congenital forearm-level amputations at around the age of 6 months. This coincides with the development of truncal balance and the ability to sit independently (hence the expression, "sit to fit").

BIBLIOGRAPHY

1. Buck-Gramcko D: Pollicization of the index finger. Method and results in aplasia and hypoplasia of the thumb. J Bone Joint Surg 53A:1605–1617, 1971.
2. Jain S: Rehabilitation in limb deficiency II. The pediatric amputee. Arch Phys Med Rehabil 77:S9–S13, 1996.
3. Johnson RL, Tabin CJ: Molecular models for vertebrate limb development. Cell 90:979–990, 1997.
4. Light TR, Ogden JA: The longitudinal epiphyseal bracket: Implications for surgical correction. J Pediatr Orthop 1:299–305, 1981.
5. Manske PR, McCarroll HR: Reconstruction of the congenitally deficient thumb. Hand Clin 8:177–196, 1992.
6. Morgan BA, Tabin CJ: The role of homeobox genes in limb development. Curr Opin Genet Dev 3:668–674, 1993.
7. Swanson AB: A classification for congenital limb malformations. J Hand Surg Am 61A:8–22, 1976.
8. Wassel HD: The results of surgery for polydactyly of the thumb. Clin Orthop 64:175–193, 1969.
9. Watson BT, Hennrikus WL: Postaxial type-B polydactyly: Prevalence and treatment. J Bone Joint Surg 79A:65–68, 1997.

CHAPTER 70

ACQUIRED HAND PROBLEMS

Terri Bidwell, MD, FRACS, and Marybeth Ezaki, MD

1. **What are causes for a tight thumb in an infant?**
   A thumb that is tight or held in the palm may be a normal finding, or it may be a trigger thumb, a clasped thumb, or an early sign of cerebral palsy.

2. **How can you tell if the thumb is normal?**
   A normal thumb has normal anatomy and can be passively extended fully at all joints. The child will open the thumb if a startle reflex (i.e., the Moro reflex) is elicited.

3. **What is trigger thumb?**
   Trigger thumbs are common and usually develop between about 3 and 6 months of age. They are not congenital. The thumb is most commonly locked in flexion at the interphalageal joint; however, it can rarely be snapping (i.e., triggering) or locked in extension. (Be sure to differentiate this from the congenital absence of the flexor tendon, indicated by a stiff joint, an absent flexion crease, and no passive or active motion.)

4. **What causes trigger thumb?**
   Thickening of the flexor pollicis longus tendon where it enters the flexor tendon sheath, just proximal to the A1 pulley. It is probably due to irritation at the opening of the flexor sheath. This thickening can be felt as a nodule (called *Notta's nodule*) at the level of the metacarpophalangeal joint (Fig. 70-1).

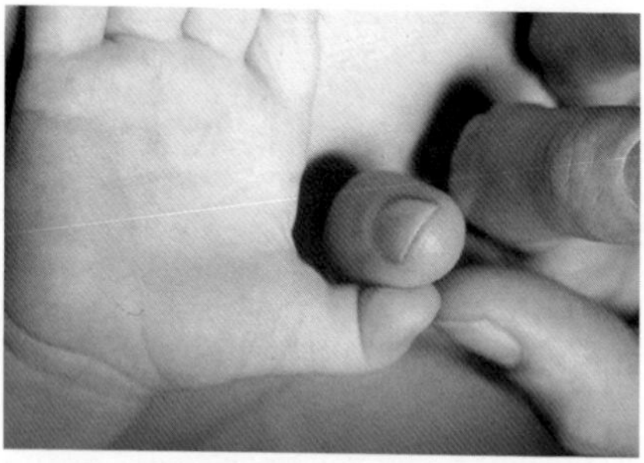

Figure 70-1. Trigger thumb. Photograph shows the limitation of extension of the thumb. This is caused by a thickening, or Notta's node, in the tendon, which prevents excursion of the tendon into the flexor sheath.

5. **What is the treatment of trigger thumb?**
   Some trigger thumbs may resolve with no treatment. If there is no improvement, surgery after about 1 year of age will correct the problem. Surgical treatment involves release of the A1 pulley. Recurrence after adequate release is rare.

6. **What is a clasped thumb?**
   The thumb is held flexed into the palm at the metacarpophalangeal joint and lacks active extension. The anatomy is abnormal and does not allow passive extension. The child will not open the thumb during a startle response.

7. **What is the underlying problem?**
   There is a spectrum of deficiency, from hypoplasia of the extensor mechanism to absence of the extensor tendons and deficiencies of the thenar muscles, web space, and soft tissues.

8. **What is the treatment?**

There are two types of clasped thumb, known as *supple* and *complex*. Initially, the treatment is splinting for both. In the more deficient or complex thumbs, surgery may be required later. This may include soft tissue release, web-space deepening, opponensplasty, and ligament reconstruction.

9. **Are trigger fingers the same as trigger thumbs?**

No, trigger fingers in childhood are more complex than trigger thumbs.

10. **What are the causes of trigger finger in children?**

Trigger fingers may be caused by anatomic abnormalities of the flexor tendons or a functional imbalance between the profundus and superficialis tendons such as that related to nerve injury. This causes a bunching up of the tendons as they enter the finger. Trigger fingers may also be associated with arthritic conditions and storage diseases such as the mucopolysaccharidoses.

11. **What is the treatment of trigger finger?**

Adequate treatment of a trigger finger requires a more extensive exploration of the flexor mechanism as well as release of the A1 pulley. Sometimes a portion of the superficialis must be removed. Incisions must be planned to reflect this possibility.

12. **What is camptodactyly?**

A nonpainful flexion deformity of the proximal interphalangeal joint unrelated to trauma.

13. **How does camptodactyly present?**

There are two major forms. One presents in infancy with an equal male-to-female ratio of frequency. It may be associated with syndromes that have multiple contractures. The other form presents in adolescence and is more common in females. The ulnar fingers are generally the most affected in both forms.

14. **What is the cause of camptodactyly?**

Abnormalities in the insertion of extrinsic or intrinsic flexor tendons and a presumed imbalance between flexor and extensor forces in the digit.

15. **What is the treatment for camptodactyly?**

Treatment must balance the need to correct the deformity with the need for further function of the digit. Night-time splinting with dynamic or static adjustable splints for a prolonged period of time is the standard treatment. Daytime passive stretching and maintenance of the range of motion is also important. A hand therapist should be involved in care whenever possible. Nonoperative treatment must be used exhaustively, but surgery may offer some improvements in severe cases.

16. **What is clinodactyly?**

An abnormal radial or ulnar angulation of a finger. Most commonly, it is seen in the little finger as an angulation toward the ring finger. It may appear to worsen with growth.

17. **With what condition is clinodactyly of the little finger associated?**

Most commonly, clinodactyly is a familial condition and is a normal variant. It may be associated with other syndromes, especially when it occurs in other fingers.

18. **What is Kirner's deformity?**

Kirner's deformity is a radial and palmar angulation of the distal phalanx caused by a disruption of the radial and palmar part of the distal phalangeal growth plate.

19. **What is the treatment of Kirner's deformity?**
Since there is usually no pain or functional deficit, often no treatment is needed. Splinting is ineffective. If the cosmetic deformity is displeasing, then corrective osteotomy of the distal phalanx may improve the appearance.

20. **What is macrodactyly?**
Macrodactyly is a focal gigantism with a disproportionately big digit or digits (Fig. 70-2). It is thought to be a hamartomatous enlargement of soft tissue and underlying bone.

21. **What are the clinical features of macrodactyly?**
It may be present at birth or during infancy. The classic form of macrodactyly is nerve-territory oriented and occurs in association with a lipofibroma, usually of the median nerve and its branches in the hand and digits. Macrodactyly may also occur in association with other syndromes such as neurofibromatosis, Klippel-Trénaunay-Weber syndrome, and vascular malformations, although the enlargement in these disorders may be more generalized.

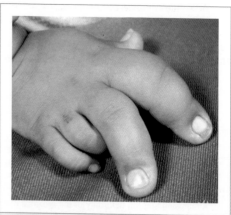

Figure 70-2. Macrodactyly with massive enlargement of the fingers in an infant. The digits involved are within a nerve territory.

22. **What can be done to treat macrodactyly?**
There is no effective nonoperative treatment. Surgical treatment is aimed at debulking the affected digits and trying to preserve function. Debulking of the abnormal nerve, corrective osteotomy, and epiphysiodesis may all improve the appearance of the digit. In the case of the grossly enlarged nonfunctional digit, amputation may improve cosmesis and function.
    In cases of median nerve territory macrodactyly, compression can occur in the carpal tunnel. This must be examined for and treated with carpal tunnel release if necessary.

23. **What are the common masses in children's hands?**
The most common masses in children's hands are benign. They include ganglion cysts, giant cell tumors of tendon sheath, epidermoid inclusion cysts following trauma, and retained foreign bodies. There are other rare lesions that include some malignancies.

24. **What should be done if a child has a mass in the hand?**
If the mass is clearly a ganglion cyst, observation is the best treatment. All others should be referred to a specialist who can diagnose and treat the mass. Do not attempt to aspirate a mass in the hand.

25. **What is a ganglion cyst?**
A fluid-filled cyst that arises from a synovial-lined space. It most commonly occurs over the wrist joint or in the flexor tendons of the fingers.

26. **How is the diagnosis made?**
The cyst will transilluminate if a penlight or otoscope is placed against the side of it. Ultrasound can also be used. If there is any doubt about the diagnosis or if the mass is thought to be solid, then further evaluation is necessary.

27. **What is the treatment of a ganglion cyst in children?**
Observation is the best treatment. Splinting can be used if the cyst grows. Aspiration can be performed in the large or symptomatic cyst. Most spontaneously resolve without any treatment. Surgery is rarely required.

28. **How do ganglion cysts in children differ from those in adults?**
A ganglion cyst in a child is rarely symptomatic, often regresses spontaneously, and has a very high likelihood of recurrence with any kind of treatment. Adult ganglion cysts are often trauma-related, are more likely to cause discomfort, and recur less often after treatment.

KEY POINTS: ACQUIRED HAND PROBLEMS

1. Most masses in the hand of a child are benign, easily recognized, and can be treated. There are some lesions that are worrisome, and these should be further evaluated by someone skilled in treatment as well as diagnosis.

2. Trigger fingers are very different from trigger thumbs. The former are difficult to resolve, whereas the latter are straightforward.

3. Ganglion cysts in children will resolve on their own in the majority of cases. Surgery is usually not necessary.

4. Refer hand masses to a specialist.

29. **What is a giant cell tumor of tendon sheath?**
A giant cell tumor of tendon sheath is a form of localized pigmented villonodular synovitis. The lesions are a reddish-brown color. The lesions can cause bony change from a pressure phenomenon but are not invasive or malignant. After ganglions, this is the second most common lesion in the hand.

30. **How is a giant cell tumor of tendon sheath treated?**
Surgical resection to remove all the abnormal tissue is needed. The reported recurrence rates after resection are between 5% and 50%.

31. **What is Madelung's deformity?**
Madelung deformity is a characteristic deformity of the distal radius that presents during adolescence with prominence of the distal ulna, loss of forearm rotation, and discomfort at the wrist joint (Fig. 70-3). It is most common in females.

32. **What causes Madelung's deformity?**
Madelung's deformity is a complex lesion that involves disorganization of the growth plate at the palmar and ulnar parts of the distal radius. There is a soft tissue thickening, known as *Vicker's ligament,* associated with the palmar radio-carpal capsule that tethers the carpal bones into the space between the radius and the ulna.

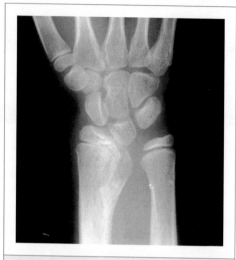

Figure 70-3. Madelung's deformity. Radiograph showing the disruption of the ulnar and palmar aspect of the distal radial growth plate. This results in progressive deformity and loss of rotation in the forearm.

33. **What is the treatment of Madelung's deformity?**

    In the past, the recommended treatment was to wait until the patient reached skeletal maturity and then to attempt a corrective surgical procedure. It has been shown in some cases that growth can be realigned by doing an epiphysiolysis when the skeleton is still immature. A corrective osteotomy may still be necessary but can be done before the end of growth.

BIBLIOGRAPHY

1. Colin BT, Shall L: Idiopathic bilaterally symmetrical brachymetacarpia of the fourth and fifth metacarpals. J Hand Surg 11A:735–737, 1986.
2. Colon F, Upton J: Pediatric hand tumors: A review of 349 cases. Hand Clin 11:223–243, 1995.
3. Dell PC: Microdactyly: Symposium on congenital deformities of the hand. Hand Clin 1:511–524, 1985.
4. Engber WM, Flatt AE: Camptodactyly: An analysis of sixty-six patients and twenty-four operations. J Hand Surg 2A:216–224, 1977.
5. Flatt AE: The Care of Congenital Hand Anomalies. St. Louis, Quality Medical Publishers, 1994.
6. Ger E, Kupcha P, Ger D: The management of trigger thumb in children. J Hand Surg 16A:944–946, 1991.
7. http://www.emedicinehealth.com/juvenile_rheumatoid_arthritis/article_em.htm.
8. Poznanski AK, Pratt GB, Manson G, Weiss L: Clinodactyly, camptodactyly, Kirner's deformity, and other crooked fingers. Radiology 93:573–582, 1969.
9. Rodgers WB, Walters P: Incidence of trigger digits in newborns. J Hand Surg 19A:264–268, 1994.
10. Vickers D, Nielsen G: Madelung deformity: Surgical prophylaxis (physiolysis) during the late growth period by resection of the dyschondrosteosis lesion. J Hand Surg 17B:401–407, 1992.

CHAPTER 71

HAND INFECTIONS

Charles Douglas Wallace, MD

1. **What are the hallmark signs of flexor tenosynovitis?**

   Kanavel's four cardinal signs of flexor tenosynovitis include the following:
   - The digit is held in a slightly flexed posture
   - Fusiform uniform swelling along the finger (not localized)
   - Intense pain on passive extension of the finger
   - Tenderness that tracks along the course of the flexor tendon sheath, from the level of the distal interphalangeal joint down to the palm

   The earliest and most sensitive sign is pain on passive extension of the finger. The most frequently found organisms include *Staphylococcus aureus*, *Streptococcus* species (sp), and *Pseudomonas* sp.

2. **Children in pain can be difficult to examine. If I suspect flexor tenosynovitis, are there any tests that can help to confirm the diagnosis?**

   High-resolution ultrasonography can be quite helpful in the diagnosis and management of hand infections. Fluid within the tendon sheath can be visualized, as can retained foreign bodies, which may confound the diagnosis or contribute to the infection.

3. **What are the most common organisms isolated from infections of the hand?**

   In one study, the most common organisms cultured from hand infections were *Streptococcus* sp, followed by *Staphylococcus aureus*, *Staphylococcus epidermidis*, *Haemophilus parainfluenzae*, *Eikenella corrodens*, *Bacteroides melaninogenicus*, and *Peptostreptococcus* sp.

4. **What is the best antibiotic coverage for a cat bite?**

   Bites from cats and dogs require coverage for an organism known as *Pasteurella multocida*, found in 50–70% of cat bite wounds. This gram-negative anaerobe can lead to rapid onset of signs and symptoms only 12–24 hours after inoculation. Penicillin is the agent of choice for these bites, coupled with a first-generation cephalosporin for improved staphylococcal coverage. In patients with dog bites to the hand, *Pasturella* sp have been identified in up to 30% of the cases, although polymicrobial infections are common, with *Staphylococcus aureus* cultured in 10%.

5. **What is the best antibiotic coverage for a human bite?**

   The bite from a human can lead to infection with streptococci, staphylococci, *Eikenella*, *Neisseria*, *Bacteroides*, *Peptostreptococcus*, *Fusobacterium*, and *Veillonella* species. *Eikenella corrodens* is resistant to cephalosporins and aminoglycosides, requiring penicillin for management. Because of frequent resistance to penicillin in some components of these polymicrobial infections, a semisynthetic penicillin plus clavulanic acid (i.e., Augmentin) is the drug of choice. Tetanus prophylaxis must be considered in every case and updated as indicated.

6. **What are the deep spaces of the hand? What is their significance in hand infections?**

   There are two deep bursal pockets in the hand that may become infected by direct inoculation, hematogenous seeding, or proximal extension of flexor tenosynovitis. One is the thenar space, which is deep to the index flexor tendons and adjacent to the flexor pollicis longus tendon sheath. The other deep space is the midpalmar space (Fig. 71-1), which is deep to the flexor tendons of the long, ring, and small fingers. A fibrous septum extending from the palmar fascia to the long-finger metacarpal separates these two spaces into distinct compartments. An infection of thenar space leads to pain and swelling over the thenar eminence and may abduct the thumb. A midpalmar space infection may cause swelling on the dorsum of the hand in addition to swelling on the palmar aspect.

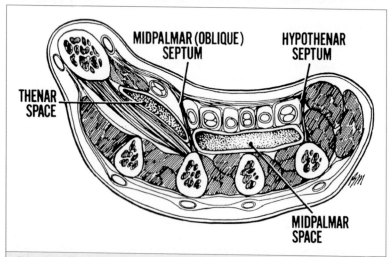

MIDPALMAR (OBLIQUE) SEPTUM

HYPOTHENAR SEPTUM

THENAR SPACE

MIDPALMAR SPACE

Figure 71-1. The potential midpalmar space. (From Nevasier RJ: Infections. In Green DP [ed]: Operative Hand Surgery. New York, Churchill Livingstone, 1993.)

7. **What is the best way to drain a felon surgically?**
Although fishmouth incisions have been advocated in the past, these leave a potentially painful scar on the tip of the finger. A better approach is the midlateral incision, with care to disrupt intentionally the fibrous septae that anchor the skin to the distal phalanx to assure adequate decompression of the abscess cavities.

8. **Does flexor tenosynovitis (FTS) always require open drainage?**
Confirmed, established flexor tenosynovitis must be decompressed surgically to prevent progressive tendon destruction or extension of the infection to the deep spaces of the hand. Elevation of the hand and prompt intravenous administration of high-dose antibiotics may be instituted for managing a child with a hand infection with some findings consistent with FTS who presents very early in the clinical course. Close clinical follow-up with serial examinations is critical if this path is chosen.

9. **What is the best way to decompress FTS?**
I prefer to use the two-incision technique. This involves feeding an irrigation catheter into the flexor tendon sheath proximal to the A1 pulley in the palm (a #10 pediatric feeding tube is a good first try) and opening the flexor tendon sheath distally for flow-through irrigation. Saline (15–20 mL) is flushed through manually every 2–4 hours postoperatively for 36–72 hours (until the tenderness along the sheath abates, Fig. 71-2).

10. **With the enhanced vascularity of the hand, can septic joints of the hand be treated with antibiotics alone?**
No, some form of decompression of the purulent fluid is necessary to allow adequate antibiotic penetration into the confined space. The gold standard is surgical arthrotomy with irrigation and drainage. Needle aspiration and decompression can be utilized only if serial aspiration is performed to document declining white blood cell concentration and to repeatedly decompress the joint. Needless to say, children tend not to tolerate this well.

11. **Does a septic wrist require open drainage?**
The management of septic arthritis is controversial. Most surgeons feel that it is of great surgical urgency to decompress and lavage the joint. The literature also supports needle aspiration and effective antibiotic coverage. Needle aspiration may be successful in cases with low-viscosity fluid, early diagnosis, and a patient willing to undergo as many serial aspirations as needed, as often as needed, to ensure clinical improvement. Herein lies the difficulty with needle aspiration of infected joints in children. This is the impetus to perform open irrigation of the joint, which also flushes away the neutrophil proteases and collagenases, followed by several days of suction drainage.

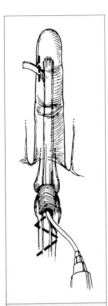

Figure 71-2. Closed tendon-sheath irrigation technique. (From Nevasier RJ: Infections. In Green DP [ed]: Operative Hand Surgery. New York, Churchill Livingstone, 1993.)

12. **What are the sequelae of unrecognized septic arthritis of the wrist and hand?**
As with septic arthritis of other joints, septic arthritis in the hand leads to proteoglycan loss, cartilage degeneration, and joint-space narrowing or total loss. Pain and potential joint instability or stiffening and arthrodesis may result from unrecognized infection.

13. **Does osteomyelitis occur in the hand?**
Yes, generally secondary to an open fracture, rarely because of hematogenous seeding. Biopsy of the infection to determine the responsible organisms and to plan antibiotic choice and dosing is indicated. Remember the high incidence of *Salmonella* (80%) in the young patient with sickle cell anemia and lytic changes in the bone.

14. **What other conditions may mimic an infection in the hand?**
Collagen vascular disease, foreign body reaction, inflammatory tenosynovitis, and neoplasms (very rarely). In the adult, one should also include gout and acute soft tissue calcification in the differential diagnosis.

15. **What unusual infections can be seen in an infant's hand?**
Herpetic whitlow can be found on the thumb or other digits frequently suckled by a child with herpes simplex infection of the mouth. In one review, 11 of 14 patients with herpetic whitlow had oral lesions. The most common age is 5 months to 6 years. The appearance of the affected digit is fairly characteristic, with multiple vesicles, some with clear fluid. Open vesicles are highly infectious. A Tzanck smear should provide a diagnosis. Treatment is the application of dry dressings and isolation of the digit until the open vesicles close. Spontaneous resolution within 1–3 weeks is the norm. Recurrence is anticipated, and superinfection of the whitlow with *Staphylococcus* may occur, indicating the need for oral antibiotic administration.

16. **Are there any particular concerns in patients with varicella infections?**
    Recently, patients with chickenpox have been noted as have a surprising incidence of necrotizing fasciitis and deep soft tissue abscesses, which may extend distally to involve the forearm and hands, as well as septic arthritis and osteomyelitis. Group A β-hemolytic streptococcus and *Staphylococcus aureus* are the primary causative organisms. Early aggressive management with debridement and lavage as well as appropriate antibiotic coverage are key to a successful outcome.

KEY POINTS: HAND INFECTIONS

1. Pain with passive extension of a finger is the most sensitive and earliest sign of flexor tenosynovitis.

2. *Pasteurella multocida* is highly prevalent in hand infection secondary to cat and dog bites.

3. Herpetic whitlow should resolve spontaneously and requires supportive treatment.

4. Septic arthritis of the wrist in infants may present as a swollen, painful hand.

5. Due to the high vascularity of the hand, many infections respond rapidly to proper antibiotic management.

17. **What is the best approach to drain a septic metacarpophalangeal joint?**
    An infection of the metacarpophalangeal (MCP) joint may occur owing to hematogenous seeding or direct inoculation, such as from a splinter or a bite. Because of concerns regarding potential extensor tendon subluxation, the MCP joint should be approached from the dorsoulnar side, if possible.

18. **Is there such a thing as extensor tenosynovitis?**
    This is arguable. A confined space containing the tendon and tenosynovioma (i.e., the flexor sheath, volarly) is required for this condition to occur. Certainly, infections of the dorsum of the hand and fingers can and do occur but would not be considered true extensor tenosynovitis. The passage beneath the extensor retinaculum is the only area in which a true tenosynovitis may occur, although this quite rare. Be wary of wrist sepsis in a child with swelling on the dorsum of the hand and pain on wrist motion or digital excursion.

19. **What is a horseshoe abscess?**
    An infection that originates in either the radial bursa (along the flexor pollicis longus) or the ulnar bursa (along the small finger flexors) may spread to the other bursae, where they closely approximate each other at the wrist. The result is tenosynovitis of the thumb and small finger, which are connected near the carpal tunnel and thus form a horseshoe.

20. **What is a collar-button abscess?**
    A collar-button abscess is in the region of the web space and often begins palmarly, spreading dorsally through the region of the transverse metacarpal ligament. The resulting dumbbell-shaped dual abscesses with a connecting stalk inspired the name. These can progress to deep-space infections in the palm if they are not adequately decompressed. Dorsal and volar incisions are necessary to address both areas.

21. **What are the current treatment options for fungal infections of fingernails in a child?**

There are two potential treatment options, which were recently described. One involves treatment of the infection with bifonazole-urea ointment. The ointment is placed on the nail under an occlusive dressing until the nail sloughs off. This is then followed by a 4-week course of bifonazole cream. This resulted in a 68% cure rate, with an additional 24% of cases showing improvement. Another approach involves oral administration of itraconazole. The patients are treated with daily to twice-daily pulses of itraconazole for 1 week per month for a 3–5 month course. There is 94% cure rate with this treatment modality, with a low relapse rate. The authors note an increased risk of recurrence of other family members having an ongoing infection. Familial treatment was recommended in these cases.

BIBLIOGRAPHY

1. Burkhalter WE: Deep space infections. Hand Clin 5:553–559, 1989.

2. Fette A, Mayr J: Hand and finger sonography in suppurative flexor tenosynovitis in children. Eur J Plastic Surg 25(3):139–142, 2002.

3. Freeland ARE, Senter BS: Septic arthritis and osteomyelitis. Hand Clin 5:533–552, 1989.

4. Huang PH, Paller AS: Itraconazole pulse therapy for dermatophyte onychomycosis in children. Arch Pediatr Adolesc Med 154:614–618, 2000.

5. Neviaser RJ: Closed tendon sheath irrigation for pyogenic flexor tenosynovitis. J Hand Surg 3:462–466, 1978.

6. Neviaser RJ: Tenosynovitis. Hand Clin 5:525–531, 1989.

7. Schreck P, Schreck P, Bradley J, Chambers H: Musculoskeletal complications of *Varicella*. J Bone Joint Surg 78A:1713–1719, 1996.

8. Walker LG, Simmons BP, Lovallo JL: Pediatric herpetic hand infections. J Hand Surg 15A:176–180, 1990.

ARTHRITIS

David D. Sherry, MD

CHAPTER 72

1. **What is arthritis?**
   Arthritis is inflammation of the joint lining (i.e., the synovium). The signs of inflammation include pain, warmth, swelling, redness, and a limitation of function. Generally, two signs need to be present to define arthritis. Inflammatory synovial fluid is defined as that containing more than 2000 white blood cells/mm^3. The presence of pain alone is the definition of arthralgia.

2. **How common is arthritis in childhood?**
   By various estimates, approximately 2 in 1000 children have arthritis. Arthritis is the second most common chronic condition in childhood. It is less frequent than epilepsy but more frequent than diabetes and cystic fibrosis.

3. **What are some pitfalls in the initial evaluation of children with arthritis?**
   Frequently, physicians will think that a swollen joint is due to trauma (even without a history of injury). They will splint or cast the limb and wait for weeks for the swelling to subside. Recognizing the fact that young children get inflammatory joint disease is key. Also, physicians often will focus on the presenting joint and will not examine all the joints. Many children presenting with a single swollen joint will, on examination, have multiple-joint involvement. It is important to recognize that involved joints may have only subtle symptoms and signs of inflammation and may be painless. Many physicians also do not realize that migratory or episodic arthritis and arthralgia are features of childhood leukemia.

4. **What are some tip-offs that indicate subtle joint inflammation?**
   Important symptoms include morning stiffness and stiffness after a nap or prolonged sitting (i.e., gelling). On examination, guarding is usually present even though, in some children, the complete range of motion may be preserved. Swelling may be minimal, so knowing the spectrum of what normal joints feel like is imperative.

5. **What about painless arthritis?**
   The arthritis of children with juvenile rheumatoid arthritis (JRA) can be painless. Twenty-five percent of children with pauciarticular JRA may have absolutely no pain in their joints and are fully active. A few children with polyarticular or systemic-onset JRA have no pain. Sarcoidosis can also be painless and may involve multiple joints; therefore, in some patients, synovial biopsies are indicated.

6. **Does painless arthritis need to be treated?**
   Yes. Children with painless arthritis can still develop joint contractures, muscle atrophy, and bony erosions, leading to destruction of the joint.

7. **What is juvenile chronic arthritis?**
   Chronic arthritis, by definition, is inflammation of the joint lasting longer than 6 weeks. *Juvenile* is defined as younger than 16 years old.

8. **What kinds of chronic arthritis are seen most frequently in children?**

   JRA (pauciarticular, polyarticular, and systemic), spondyloarthropathies (i.e., reactive arthritis, juvenile-onset ankylosing spondylitis, and arthritis associated with inflammatory bowel disease), and psoriatic arthritis.

9. **How do I classify JRA?**

   Pauciarticular JRA involves four or fewer joints in the first 6 months of the illness. Polyarticular JRA involves five or more joints during the first 6 months of illness. Systemic JRA can involve any number of joints but is characterized by high spiking fevers, above 103°F.

10. **What is the most common kind of JRA?**

    Pauciarticular (50%) is most common, followed by polyarticular (30%) and then systemic-onset (20%) arthritis.

11. **What is the cause of JRA?**

    The cause is not known. Genetic factors seem to be closely associated with pauciarticular JRA (namely, human leukocyte antigen, DR subregion [HLA-DR] 5 and 8) and with rheumatoid-factor-positive polyarticular JRA (HLA-DR 4). Various infectious agents have been implicated, but proof of a causal relationship is lacking. Systemic JRA has many hallmarks of being an infection, but no one single agent has been identified.

12. **What is the typical presentation of pauciarticular JRA?**

    Pauciarticular JRA commonly affects girls (80%); most are between the ages of 1 and 4 years. The most commonly involved joint is the knee, followed by the ankle and then the fingers. In 70% of these children, the antinuclear antibody (ANA) test will have positive results; almost all are rheumatoid-factor negative. In 20%, there will be asymptomatic iritis, which can lead to blindness if untreated.

13. **In the child with monoarticular arthritis, how can one be sure it is pauciarticular JRA?**

    Clues to pauciarticular JRA include a positive ANA test or the presence of chronic asymptomatic iritis. Other conditions have to be considered, especially Lyme disease, pigmented villonodular synovitis, and foreign body synovitis.

14. **Can children with pauciarticular JRA present with hip or shoulder disease?**

    Only extremely rarely will children with pauciarticular JRA present with hip disease. Many of these children require full antibiotic coverage so to prevent failure of treating a septic hip. Isolated shoulder disease virtually never occurs in pauciarticular JRA.

15. **How should I look for iritis?**

    There are two kinds of iritis: chronic and acute. Chronic iritis is seen in JRA, and acute iritis in those with spondyloarthropathy. Acute iritis is hard to miss—the child will have a very painful, red, photophobic eye and will seek help long before seeing an orthopaedist. Children with JRA, especially those with pauciarticular JRA, are at risk for developing chronic iritis that is totally painless and does not cause a red eye. When you see a child with arthritis, closely examine the eyes in a darkened room to make sure the pupils are round. If there is any suggestion of irregularity, immediate ophthalmologic consultation for a slit-lamp examination is indicated.

16. **How frequently does a patient with JRA need to see an ophthalmologist?**

    It depends on the child's age, the type of onset, and the ANA test results. Children with systemic-onset JRA need a slit-lamp examination of their eyes yearly. Children who are younger than 7 years old and are ANA positive need an examination every 3–4 months for 4 years, then every 6 months for 3 years, and yearly examinations thereafter. If the ANA test is negative, they need an examination every 6 months for 7 years, with yearly examinations thereafter. If the child is older than 7 years at the onset, regardless of ANA result, an examination is needed only every 6 months for 4 years, with yearly examination thereafter.

17. **What is the difference among iritis, iridocyclitis, and uveitis?**
Many authors use these terms interchangeably. The uveal tract consists of the iris, the ciliary body, and the choroid. By strict definition, iritis is inflammation of the iris, iridocyclitis is inflammation of the iris and the ciliary body, and uveitis is inflammation of the entire uveal tract.

18. **How is iritis treated?**
Usually with steroid eyedrops, with or without a mydriatic agent. Occasionally, steroid injection or immunosuppressant therapy, with methotrexate, for example, is required.

19. **What is the typical presentation of a patient with polyarticular JRA?**
There are two typical groups of children who develop polyarticular JRA. The first group are young girls of 1–4 years of age with multiple small- and large-joint involvement. Usually, the joint involvement is symmetric. In 50%, ANA results are positive, and most are rheumatoid-factor negative. Less frequently, this is complicated by asymptomatic iritis. The second group are adolescent girls, again with large and small joints involved in a symmetric pattern. Up to half of these girls are rheumatoid-factor positive, and few are ANA positive. Rarely will these children develop asymptomatic iritis.

20. **What is the typical presentation of a patient with systemic JRA?**
Both boys and girls get systemic-onset JRA in equal numbers, usually between the ages of 3 and 10 years. They have high spiking fevers that start in the evenings, peak at night, and return to normal or below normal in the morning. When these children are febrile, they are very toxic-appearing, have severe myalgias and arthralgias, and develop a fleeting small, red macular rash, generally on the trunk. They may have sore throats and stiff necks, causing one to suspect meningitis. Other symptoms include enlarged lymph nodes (especially the axillary nodes), an enlarged liver and spleen, pericarditis, myocarditis, and disseminated intravascular coagulation.
These children are rarely seen by the orthopaedist since they tend to develop arthritis later in the course of illness (and may never get chronic arthritis).

21. **What is the typical presentation of a patient with spondyloarthropathies?**
These usually occur in older children (6 years of age or older) who present with predominantly lower-extremity arthritis. Both large and small joints of the legs and feet may be involved. Enthesitis is a frequent finding and most commonly occurs at the plantar fascial insertion, metatarsal heads, and sacroiliac joints. It is slightly more common in boys. Often, there is a family history of low back pain, although the parents may not readily identify back spasms or back pain that they think is due to injury as being significant. Also, ask about a family history of heel pain or spurs or of bursitis.

22. **What is the cause of spondyloarthropathies?**
Both genetic and infectious agents have been very closely associated with the development of spondyloarthropathies. The HLA-B27 gene (or a closely linked allele) is a strong marker for the disease. In children, reactive arthritis frequently follows gastrointestinal infections by *Campylobacter, Salmonella, Shigella,* and *Yersinia* species. In adults, there has been an association with *Klebsiella* sp and ankylosing spondylitis.

23. **What blood tests should I order for a child with arthritis?**
It is useful to obtain a complete blood cell count, erythrocyte sedimentation rate (or C-reactive protein), ANA, and rheumatoid factor. The vast majority of children are rheumatoid-factor negative, so this test is generally more useful in older girls with polyarticular involvement who

may have early-onset adult rheumatoid arthritis. Testing for HLA-B27 is helpful in children suspected of having spondyloarthropathy since it is associated with a poorer outcome (and thus requires early aggressive treatment) and may also help confirm the diagnosis. Urinalysis can be helpful if reactive arthritis is suspected since the child may have sterile pyuria without dysuria.

24. **Should I get a serum uric acid level?**
No. Gout and other crystal diseases are almost unknown in childhood.

25. **How is the arthritis portion of JRA treated?**
The aim is to control the synovitis. In children with a limited number of joints involved, directly treating the joint with an intra-articular corticosteroid injection (i.e., triamcinolone hexacetonide) is most useful, and the effect usually lasts over a year. Generally, 1 mL (i.e., 20 mg) is used in large and medium joints and lesser amounts in the smaller joints. As much as 1 mg/kg can be used in bigger children. Children with more widespread joint involvement require early treatment with methotrexate. Anti-tumor necrosis factor (TNF) agents are next used, and they may be able to halt erosions. There is insufficient evidence to strongly support the use of sulfasalazine or hydroxychloroquine. Nonsteroidal agents are given for symptomatic relief. If a few joints continue to be inflamed, intra-articular injections can be helpful.

   Children with systemic JRA may require oral or parenteral corticosteroids and aggressive anti-inflammatory and immunosuppressive therapy. These children require the services of a pediatric rheumatologist.

26. **How do I treat spondyloarthropathies?**
If there are a limited number of involved joints, intra-articular corticosteroid injections can be used. More widespread disease can be controlled with disease-modifying agents such as sulfasalazine, methotrexate, or an anti-TNF drug. Anti-TNF drugs are preferred for psoriatic arthritis. Nonsteroidal medications are used for symptomatic relief.

27. **How do I treat enthesitis?**
I prefer to use indomethacin, sulindac, diclofenac, or piroxicam. Other nonsteroidal agents may be useful as well. Some patients will respond to one and not another, so several may need to be tried. Shoe inserts or heel cups to redistribute weight around tender entheses can be of great help. Injections of the entheses are fraught with difficulties and should be done only as a last resort (if at all). Occasionally, the enthesitis is severe enough to require therapy with methotrexate or sulfasalazine.

28. **Are there any differences among nonsteroidal agents?**
Yes. A given child may respond nicely to one and not another. I prefer to use once- or twice-daily medications for most children, although liquid preparations (like ibuprofen) are useful in younger children. A piroxicam capsule can be emptied into a single bite of food and has very little taste, thus making it very useful for older children who cannot swallow a pill. I rarely use naproxen, especially in fair-skinned children, owing to its association with facial scarring. I prefer indomethacin, sulindac, diclofenac, or piroxicam for the spondyloarthropathies and for enthesitis. An adequate therapeutic trial for each agent is 3–4 weeks at a full therapeutic dose.

29. **What laboratory tests are indicated for children on nonsteroidal medication?**
Complete blood cell count (for anemia and leukopenia), aspartate aminotransferase (for hepatotoxicity), and creatinine along with urine analysis (for nephrotoxicity). These should be checked after the first month or two of therapy and then every 6–12 months (but more frequently for younger children).

30. **What are the side effects of intra-articular steroid injections?**
The most common side effect is subcutaneous atrophy and hypopigmentation at the site of injection. This can be minimized by placing the medication well within the joint and, perhaps, limiting activity for a day or two afterward. The subcutaneous fat regrows, but this may take several years. Occasionally, the medication is irritating to the joint and the child will have increased pain starting on the day of injection. The pain lasts 2–3 days, but the arthritis usually still subsides. Rarely (in an estimated 1:50,000 injections), septic arthritis can occur. This would manifest a few days postinjection, with typical symptoms and signs of infection. Juxta-articular calcifications, incidentally noted on radiographs, can occur but usually do not interfere with joint function. After a joint injection, the child will be steroid suppressed for about a month; if general anesthesia is required, appropriate stress doses of corticosteroids are prudent.

31. **How do I inject a joint in a small child in the office?**
A single joint or two can be down with local anesthesia and quiet distraction. A topical anesthetic agent such as LMX or EMLA is placed over the injection site for 30–60 minutes. The joint is cleaned three times, twice with povidone-iodine and once with alcohol. While spraying ethyl chloride at the site, I place 1 mL of buffered lidocaine (i.e., 2 mL of sodium bicarbonate in a 10-mL vial of lidocaine) under the skin as deep as a 30-gauge needle will go. Then, a 1.5-inch 20- or 22-gauge needle is placed in the knee. Synovial fluid is aspirated and placed in an ethylenediamine tetraacetic acid (EDTA, purple top) tube. The syringe is changed to the one with medication, and the medication is injected. It should flow with ease. More joints should be done under conscious or deeper sedation.

KEY POINTS: ARTHRITIS

1. Arthritis in children is not uncommon and can take several forms.

2. In young children, trauma is virtually never the cause of joint swelling.

3. Pauciarticular juvenile rheumatoid arthritis is associated with asymptomatic iritis that, if untreated, may lead to visual impairment.

4. Intra-articular triamcinolone hexacetonide is the treatment of choice in children with arthritis in just a few joints.

32. **How frequently should I inject a joint?**
We do not like to reinject the same joint more than 3 or 4 times within 12 months or 8–10 times in total. The response to the first injection does not predict the response to the second. Rarely, the synovitis will recur quickly. If so, reinjection is indicated since its effect may last more than a year.

33. **What tests are useful on the synovial fluid that is aspirated?**
Put the synovial fluid in an EDTA (purple top) or heparinized (green top) tube for cell count and differential analysis. Most children with JRA have synovial fluid cell counts of 5000–25,000. Children with systemic-onset JRA, however, can have joint-fluid white blood cell counts exceeding $100,000/mm^3$, as can children with acute rheumatic fever. Synovial fluid protein is not helpful, nor is glucose, unless infection is suspected. Culture and Gram staining are indicated if you are concerned about possible infection. Crystal analysis is rarely indicated since crystal disease is virtually absent in childhood.

34. **What is the outcome of chronic childhood arthritis?**

The arthritis can be controlled in most children. The majority (about 70%) with pauciarticular JRA generally do well but may need treatment for many years. Older children with polyarticular JRA, especially if they are rheumatoid-factor positive, tend to have long-lasting disease and are at higher risk for developing erosive joint disease. Systemic JRA is both the best and the worst kind to have. In many of these children, all systemic and arthritic problems resolve after a few months to a year or so. Others have continuing destructive arthritis and frequently require joint replacement or fusion. Although systemic JRA accounts for only 20% of all cases of JRA, 90% of those requiring wheelchairs and joint replacements have systemic JRA. A few children with spondyloarthropathies will do poorly. These generally are boys with early-onset hip disease who are HLA-B27 positive.

35. **In spondyloarthropathy, what (besides HLA-B27) portends a worse outcome?**

Early hip disease is a poor prognostic sign. Boys tend to fare worse than girls.

36. **What are the orthopaedic complications of chronic childhood arthritis?**

Younger children, especially those with unilateral knee involvement, can develop overgrowth and leg-length discrepancy with an ipsilateral long leg. In older preadolescent patients who have unilateral knee involvement, the epiphysis can prematurely fuse and the patient can end up with a contralateral long leg. Rarely, joint involvement can lead to subluxation. A few patients have destructive arthritis and degenerative joint disease and will require a soft tissue release, synovectomy, joint replacement, or fusion.

37. **What is the role of synovectomy?**

It is rarely indicated, although early synovectomy of the wrist may be helpful. On the whole, synovectomy does not lead to improved joint function or long-lasting remission. However, there are a few patients with a very recalcitrant joint who may benefit from synovectomy.

38. **What should the family be told?**

Initially, the family needs to be reassured that the child will do well and that most children with arthritis will not end up crippled. Let them know that there are numerous treatments and that most of the time the arthritis can be controlled. Prompt referral to a specialist on a multidisciplinary team who can care for both the child and the family is indicated.

39. **Who should manage the problem?**

Most children with chronic arthritis are best managed by a pediatric rheumatologist along with a host of pediatric health care specialists, depending on the need, including ophthalmologists, orthopaedic surgeons, physical therapists, occupational therapists, nurse specialists, social workers, psychologists, nutritionists, and others. If a pediatric rheumatologist is not available in the area, an adult rheumatologist with experience in childhood arthritis should be consulted.

40. **What are danger signs?**

Red joints are extremely rare in JRA and should alert you to think of infection or another disease (such as rheumatic fever, reactive arthritis, lupus, leukemia, Kawasaki disease, or polyarteritis nodosa). A marked degree of disability is also rarely due to arthritis and should lead the physician to consider such possibilities as subtle fractures, osteomyelitis, leukemia, amplified pain, and tumor.

41. **What are the tip-offs in distinguishing leukemia from JRA?**

Most children with leukemia fall outside the typical spectrum of presentation of JRA. Specifically, they are disproportionately sick or disabled and have bone pain, episodic or migratory arthritis, hip arthritis, and nocturnal waking due to pain (especially waking after midnight). Look for discordant laboratory tests that suggest leukemia such as a high erythrocyte sedimentation rate with a normal or low white blood cell count or a normal-to-low platelet count. Disproportionate anemia is also suggestive. Children with arthritis and Down syndrome are especially worrisome.

BIBLIOGRAPHY

1. Cassidy JT, Petty RE, Laxer RM, Lindslel CB: Textbook of Pediatric Rheumatology, 54th ed. Philadelphia, W.B. Saunders, 2005.
2. Weiss JE, Ilowite NT: Juvenile idiopathic arthritis. Pediatr Clin North Am 52:413–442, 2005.

XIV. TUMORS

INITIAL EVALUATION OF MUSCULOSKELETAL TUMORS IN CHILDREN

Ernest U. Conrad III, MD

1. Pediatric bone and soft tissue tumors are extremely unusual. Why is this an important topic?

Although malignant tumors of bone and soft tissue are unusual, they are not rare. The typical orthopaedist will see several primary sarcomas of bone or soft tissue and many benign tumors in his or her lifetime. The significance of these abnormalities is enhanced by the importance of early diagnosis and effective treatment, which is curative in 70% of children. In addition to malignant tumors or sarcomas of the musculoskeletal system, there are a large number of benign tumors of bone and soft tissue that are relatively common and are a source of great morbidity because of a high local recurrence rate and a high fracture rate in the bone tumors. When these tumors occur in children, they suffer multiple osseous recurrences; the consequences are dramatic. Early appropriate treatment is very effective. A late diagnosis or ineffective treatment will result in the loss of life or limb, deformity, the risk of multiple procedures, prolonged rehabilitation, and significant morbidity.

2. What are the four most common musculoskeletal tumors in children?

The most common tumors in children are benign. The most common benign bone tumors include the unicameral bone cyst, the aneurysmal bone cyst, and exostoses of the skeleton. Another common benign bone tumor is the nonossifying fibroma (NOF), which involves the cortex of bone and is associated with a relatively high incidence of fractures. Benign tumors of the soft tissues most commonly involve lipomas, hemangiomas, or lymphangiomas. These benign soft tissue tumors are also a source of significant diagnostic challenge, morbidity, and treatment failure. Hemangioma is a common soft tissue tumor that is difficult to resect. Another soft tissue tumor, sometimes referred to as benign, is desmoid tumor, or fibromatosis, which behaves like a low-grade malignancy and has the highest rate of local recurrence of all musculoskeletal tumors. The most important message to convey to parents is the relatively high risk of local recurrence (10–20%) for benign soft tissue and bone tumors. These so-called "benign" soft tissue and bone tumors are also a source of significant diagnostic challenge.

Malignant soft tissue sarcomas may be recognized by the following clinical characteristics: most soft tissue sarcomas are larger than 5 cm in diameter, are firmer or denser than normal muscle, are nontender, and are deep to the superficial fascia. Tumors with those characteristics should be evaluated with a magnetic resonance imaging (MRI) scan. Approximately half of all soft tissue sarcomas involve a diagnosis of rhabdomyosarcoma, whereas other soft tissue sarcomas require similar treatment (i.e., chemotherapy, surgery, and radiation-therapy protocols).

3. Are there pediatric age groups at risk for certain tumors?

Clearly, adolescents are most at risk for malignancies of the musculoskeletal system. Osteosarcoma has a peak age of 14 years, and Ewing's sarcoma has a peak age of 12 years. Young children (less than 10 years of age) are at less risk for a sarcoma, although they are at greater risk for a benign bone tumor, a benign soft tissue tumor, or an infection. When these tumors are located adjacent to an active physeal growth plate, then the risk of growth-plate injury becomes a potentially significant problem. Because they are at greater risk, adolescents should be evaluated with greater caution when presenting with persistent extremity pain, especially pain around the knee or pain that has lasted longer than several months.

4. **What is the typical history for a child presenting with an osteosarcoma?**
A child with an osteosarcoma will typically have deep-seated pain that is worse at night. Such pain is not typically related to physical activity. Other benign tumors may also be associated with night pain, such as the pain associated with osteoid osteoma. The typical history of pain for a child with osteosarcoma involves a 3- to 4-month interval. Children or adolescents with bony pain or so-called "injuries" lasting 6 weeks or longer should be evaluated with a bone scan, an MRI, or both.

   Teenagers with persistent knee pain are the highest-risk group for an osteosarcoma. Patients presenting with knee pain should be evaluated with a careful clinical exam and plain radiographs. Determining specifically where the pain is located is an important and challenging part of the initial evaluation. The distal femur is the most common location for osteosarcoma and many other tumors. If the plain x-ray is nondiagnostic and bony pain persists, then an MRI should be obtained for patients without a diagnosis.

   Patients with persistent pain and an equivocal MRI should be reevaluated clinically and with repeat x-rays every 2–3 weeks. Although MRI is not the best initial screening x-ray, it is a good study for osteosarcomas in determining the exact extent of bony and soft tissue involvement. As a general rule, a computed tomography (CT) scan is the preferred imaging technique for benign bony abnormalities and MRI is the best imaging study for soft tissue tumors or malignancies.

5. **How do you distinguish a simple bone cyst from a malignant bone tumor on plain x-rays?**
I evaluate three x-ray characteristics for bony abnormalities: the location, the margin, and the density of the lesion.
   - **Location:** The location of the lesion refers to its bony location (i.e., metaphyseal, epiphyseal, or diaphyseal) and whether the abnormality is centrally located or eccentric.
   - **Margin:** The margin, or bony interface, refers to whether or not the tumor is surrounded with reactive bone.
   - **Density:** The density of the center of the abnormality refers to the radiographic appearance of the content of the lesion (i.e., lucent, empty, calcified, or osteoblastic).

   The anatomic location of the tumor will give some indication of which diagnosis is most likely (e.g., an eccentric cortical-metaphyseal lesion with a sclerotic margin is suggestive of nonossifying fibroma). The bony margin is the most important and predictive characteristic. It reflects the interaction of the tumor with adjacent host bone. Slow-growing or inactive tumors will be surrounded by a sclerotic margin.

   Fast-growing or malignant tumors will have little to no surrounding bony margin or reaction because the tumor's growth rate is faster than the bony reaction. The density of the abnormality will give some indication of the contents of the tumor by the ability to identify osseous tumors (i.e., osteoblastic), cartilage (i.e., calcified) lesions, and empty or cystic lesions (i.e., aneurysmal bone cysts [ABCs] or cystic lesions). Evaluating these characteristics will assist with establishing a differential diagnosis from the plain x-rays.

6. **What is staging of musculoskeletal tumors?**
Staging is a term that refers to the assessment of the growth rate of a tumor and the extent of disease. For benign tumors, that refers to the local anatomic containment of a benign aggressive tumor or its degree of cellular activity. For malignant tumors, staging refers to the tumor's containment by adjacent tissues, its degree of histologic activity (i.e., the histologic grade), and whether or not there is metastatic disease.

Unlike adult sarcomas, the vast majority of pediatric malignancies are high grade, so grading is not a major issue. Whether or not a child presents with lung metastasis is an extremely important topic because the occurrence of metastatic disease cuts that child's survival in half. Thus, all children with an apparent sarcoma should have an initial chest CT scan to rule out lung metastasis at presentation.

7. **What lab tests are useful for making the diagnosis of osteosarcoma?**
Blood laboratory studies are an essential part of the work-up of bone infections but not of bone tumors. This is particularly true for children under the age of 10 years with bony abnormalities that includes osteomyelitis in the differential diagnosis. Studies such as complete blood cell count (CBC), erythrocyte sedimentation rate (ESR), and C-reactive protein are important in the assessment of possible osteomyelitis.

The most helpful blood test for bone tumors is alkaline phosphatase, which is elevated in more than half of all osteosarcoma patients. New molecular studies are receiving attention as diagnostic studies for some sarcomas, such as reverse transcriptase polymerase chain reaction (RT-PCR) values for Ewing's sarcoma, and will no doubt play a significant diagnostic role in the future for diagnosis and the assessment of treatment response.

8. **How should I evaluate a child with a soft tissue mass?**
Most soft tissue masses in children are benign. Benign soft tissue masses are usually small, soft, and superficial. Soft tissue masses that are larger than 5 cm (in diameter), firmer than muscle, and deep are more likely to represent a sarcoma and should be evaluated with an MRI and a biopsy. Small (i.e., < 5 cm), soft, superficial soft tissue tumors are usually benign and may be excised with or without preoperative imaging.

All masses that are 5 cm in diameter or larger should be evaluated with an MRI prior to biopsy or resection. Incisional or needle biopsy by a surgeon with experience in tumors is recommended prior to excision of these larger masses.

Soft tissue cysts are one of the more common soft tissue tumors in children under the age of 10 years. These cysts typically occur behind the knee or in the calf. They should be transilluminated to confirm that they are fluid-filled. Masses that truly contain clear fluid are rarely malignant. These cysts will frequently rupture spontaneously and may or may not recur. MRI is not required to image a cyst that transilluminates.

KEY POINTS: INITIAL EVALUATION OF MUSCULOSKELETAL TUMORS IN CHILDREN

1. Persistent extremity pain beyond 4–6 weeks and night pain in teenagers are concerning symptoms that should raise suspicion about an occult malignancy.

2. When evaluating bone neoplasms, carefully consider what the lesion is doing to the bone and what the bone is doing to the lesion. Rapidly growing and potentially malignant lesions do not allow the bone enough time to form a mature reactive ring around them.

3. Large or deep (subfascial) soft tissue masses in the extremity should undergo biopsy and possibly excision.

4. Most benign neoplasms in children have a high recurrence rate after resection.

9. **A patient has an MRI demonstrating a large (10-cm) soft tissue tumor. How should the patient be managed?**

The patient should be managed with an open biopsy in the operating room by a surgeon with experience with soft tissue tumors. If that biopsy is diagnostic for a high-grade soft tissue sarcoma, preoperative chemotherapy prior to resection of the mass should be the preferred management. The most common location for soft tissue sarcomas is the thigh, and teenagers are at greater risk to develop soft tissue sarcomas than younger children. Benign or low-grade soft tissue tumors are appropriately managed with a resection after a frozen-section biopsy. Careful resection of benign soft tissue masses is important as the risk of local recurrence is also high.

10. **What are the most common errors in diagnosing an osteosarcoma?**

The most common diagnostic problems involve three areas:
- Failure to recognize the need for MRI
- Failure to get good plain x-rays that are interpreted properly in a teenager with persistent pain
- Failure to follow all patients with persistent pain for reassessment

As a famous surgical quote implies, your eyes see what your mind knows. Be aware of the risk of malignancies in all children with undiagnosed bony pain. Be careful with regard to the initial history and exam and the clinical follow-up. They are probably the most important first steps, leading to an accurate and early diagnosis.

BIBLIOGRAPHY

1. Downing JR, Khandekar A, Shurtleff SA, et al: Multiplex RT-PCR assay for the differential diagnosis of alveolar rhabdomyosarcoma and Ewing's sarcoma. Am J Pathol 146:626–634, 1995.
2. Mankin HJ, Lange TA, Spanier SS: The hazards of biopsy in patients with malignant primary bone and soft-tissue tumors. J Bone Joint Surg 64A:1121–1127, 1982.
3. Schmale GA, Conrad EU, Raskind WH: The natural history of hereditary multiple exostoses. J Bone Joint Surg 76A:986–992, 1994.
4. Simon MA: Current concepts review. Causes of increased survival of patients with osteosarcoma: Current controversies. J Bone Joint Surg 66A:306–310, 1984.

CHAPTER 74

BONE TUMORS

John P. Dormans, MD

1. **What factors or clues help one establish a differential diagnosis for a lesion of bone in a child?**
   - The age of the child
   - The specific location of the bone involved (i.e., the geographic location of the lesion within the bone—epiphyseal? metaphyseal? diaphyseal? central? eccentric?)
   - The radiographic characteristics of the lesion, as determined by Enneking's classic questions

2. **What are the classic questions of Enneking with regard to the radiologic evaluation of any bone tumor?**
   - What is the lesion doing to the bone?
   - What is the bone doing to the lesion?
   - What is the periosteal response?

3. **Which bone tumors in children typically occur in the diaphysis?**
   These can be remembered by the mnemonic **FAHEL:**
   - **F:** **F**ibrous dyplasia
   - **A:** **A**damantinoma (and the similar tumor-like condition osteofibrous dysplasia, also known as *ossifying fibroma* or *Campanacci disease*)
   - **H:** **H**istiocytosis (also known as *Langerhans cell histiocytosis* or *eosinophilic granuloma*)
   - **E:** **E**wing sarcoma
   - **L:** **L**ymphoma or leukemia of bone

   Parenthetically, a unicameral bone cyst and osteoid osteoma can sometimes occur in the diaphysis of bone.

4. **What are the typical clinical presentation, classic radiographic features, and treatment of a patient with an aneurysmal bone cyst (ABC)?**
   A typical clinical presentation is usually a painful (caused by micro or macrofracture) radiolucent expansile lesion occurring in almost any bone. A thin rim of reactive bone is often seen. Treatment consists of meticulous removal of the contents of the cyst with curettage, high-speed burring, and electrocauterization of the cyst wall lining; the use of adjuvants such as dilute phenol; and packing reconstruction with autograft or allograft bone graft.

5. **What pathologic features distinguish an ABC from a simple bone cyst?**
   ABCs are expansile and contain blood-filled loculations (i.e., cystic spaces containing blood) with thin septae of bone covered with thin soft tissue with hemorrhagic, fleshy, hemosiderin and giant-cell-laden fibrous tissue. Simple or unicameral bone cysts contain very little tissue (just lining the peripheral shell or rim) and are often filled with clear yellow fluid if they are untreated or have had no previous fracture.

6. **What are the typical clinical presentation and treatment of a unicameral (i.e., simple) bone cyst?**
A well-marginated, lucent lesion of bone occurring most commonly in the metaphysis of the proximal humerus or femur in a child between the ages of 5 and 20. The lesions are painless unless a pathologic micro- or macrofracture has occurred. A large number of surgical and nonsurgical treatments have been employed for this lesion in the past. Regardless of the treatment selected, local persistence and recurrence rates are high. Up until recently, the most popular treatment was dual-needle cyst aspiration and steroid injection. Current surgical treatment of a child with a simple bone cyst is percutaneous curettage with intramedullary decompression and grafting with allogeneic cancellous bone or, alternatively, bone substitutes such as calcium sulfate pellets.

7. **What are the typical clinical presentation, classic radiographic features, and treatment of osteofibrous dysplasia in the child?**
Osteofibrous dysplasia is also known as *Campanacci's disease* and *ossifying fibroma*. A typical clinical presentation is usually pain and swelling in the leg in a child younger than age 10 years, occasionally associated with anterior bowing of the tibia.. The classic radiographic features include an intracortical diaphyseal tibial or, less commonly, a femoral lesion associated with expansion and thinning of the cortex and multiple radiolucencies with intervening regions of sclerosis. Treatment for osteofibrous dysplasia includes the observation for asymptomatic lesions or curettage (with or without adjuvants) and bone grafting of the radiolucent cystic lesions. Grafting with autologous or allogeneic cancellous bone is used to fill the defects. Local recurrence rates are 20–30% with intralesional resection, compared with 5–10% with marginal resection. Some think osteofibrous dysplasia may transform into a more aggressive lesion known as *adamantinoma*. The presence of an associated soft tissue mass is the distinguishing feature, and treatment of adamantinoma is *en bloc* excision.

8. **Describe the typical clinical presentation, classic radiographic features, and treatment of osteoid osteoma.**
A typical clinical presentation is a characteristic history of osseous pain, usually pain at rest and at night, that is relieved by aspirin or nonsteroidal anti-inflammatory medication. The classic radiographic features include fusiform cortical thickening and sclerosis with a tiny central lucency (the nidus). Nonsurgical treatment requires regular nonsteroidal anti-inflammatory use. Percutaneous minimally invasive CT, radiofrequency ablation, or mechanical removal is becoming the preferred surgical treatment, especially for difficult anatomic sites. Alternatively, open excision of the radiolucent nidus with bone grafting may be used.

9. **Describe the clinical presentation and treatment of a patient with osteoblastoma.**
With osteoblastoma, the nidus is larger than that seen with osteoid osteoma (it is usually greater than 2 cm) and may contain a central density. This lesion is common in the posterior elements of the spine. It usually occurs in older teenagers or young adults. Usually, extended curettage with adjuvants (i.e., curettage, high-speed burring into adjacent normal bone, cauterization, and use of dilute phenol) is used for treatment when possible. Grafting the defect with cancellous bone graft is done after reconstruction. *En bloc* resection can also be considered for more aggressive lesions or for tumors involving expendable sites.

10. **Describe the typical clinical presentation, principal pathologic features, diagnostic radiographic features, and treatment of an osteochondroma.**
Osteochondromas are first noted during childhood, usually being first noticed in children older than age 6–8 years. These children usually present with a juxta-articular firm mass. The most common locations are the distal femur, the proximal humerus, and the proximal tibia. Pain may be present as a result of irritation of overlying tendons or muscles. The principal pathologic features are eccentric cortical and cancellous bone structures with a thin cartilaginous cap. The radiographic features include a pedunculated or sessile projection of bone from the metaphysis

of a long bone. There is continuity of cortical and cancellous bone of the lesion with that of the underlying metaphysis. This radiographic feature will distinguish exostosis from myositis ossificans and parosteal osteosarcoma. Treatment often involves reassurance with observation unless the lesion is symptomatic. Lesions that are irritating overlying muscles or tendons may be treated by simple excision. Local recurrence is rare but might occur if the lesion is immediately adjacent to the abnormal physis that is producing additional osteochondroma. In these very young children, lesions occur very near the growth plate from which they arise. The cartilage cap may be in continuity with the growth plate. Injury to the growth plate must be avoided, and local recurrence rates are higher.

11. **Describe the typical clinical presentation, diagnostic radiographic features, characteristic histologic features, and treatment of chondroblastoma.**
A typical clinical presentation is usually in a child older than the age of 10 years, or occasionally a young adult, presenting with a painful lesion located in the epiphysis or apophysis of a long bone, most commonly the proximal humerus (Codman's tumor), distal femur, proximal tibia, or proximal femur. These lesions can also arise in the trochanteric apophysis and triradiate cartilage. The diagnostic radiographic features include a well-marginated geographic radiolucent lesion with a thin sclerotic rim, occasional expansion of the epiphysis or apophysis, and matrix calcification in less than 25% of children. Histologic features are numerous ovoid polyhedral chondroblasts with multinucleated giant cells, islands of chondroid, and a characteristic pattern of matrix production by the chondroblasts, which gives rise to the so-called "cobblestone appearance." Mineralization of this matrix will lead to the observation of "chicken-wire calcification." Treatment, then, involves an extended curettage with local adjuvant therapy such as high-speed burring, cauterization of the remaining wall, and phenolization, followed by bone grafting. Local recurrence rates range from 10–20%.

12. **What primary benign bone processes occur in the epiphysis or apophysis of the growing child?**
Chondroblastoma and subacute epiphyseal osteomyelitis (also known as Brodie's abscess of epiphysis).

13. **Describe the typical clinical presentation and treatment of a nonossifying fibroma.**
A typical clinical presentation is usually between the ages of 6 and 20 years with an asymptomatic, often incidentally found, metaphyseal eccentric lucent lesion, most likely in the distal femur, distal tibia, or proximal tibia. Multiple lesions may be present. There is usually a thin, sclerotic rim. Lesions may present in various stages of healing. Pathologic micro- or macrofractures can occur if lesions are large enough. Treatment for most nonossifying fibromas is observation if they are asymptomatic. Large lesions occupying more than 30% of the diameter of the bone involved, particularly if they are elongated and show no evidence of healing, can be considered at risk for pathologic fracture and can be treated. Treatment consists of curettage and grafting with autologous or allogeneic cancellous bone. In some instances, this can be done percutaneously.

14. **Describe the typical clinical presentation and appropriate initial evaluation of a patient presenting with an apparent eosinophilic granuloma.**
A typical clinical presentation includes one or more painful radiolucent lesions of bone involving any bone of the body in any location in the bone. Initially, the lesions will have less reactive healing bone, but, with time, they heal with an adjacent maturing bone reaction. The skull is commonly affected. Lesions are polyostotic in 5–15% of cases. They are most common in the first and second decades but can be seen up to age 60 years. The appropriate initial evaluation involves a complete blood count, sedimentation rate, and C-reactive protein. A technetium bone scan or skeletal surveys can be done to look for other lesions, and you should make a

careful physical examination for evidence of hepatosplenomegaly or signs or symptoms of diabetes insipidus.

15. **What classic histologic features are seen in eosinophilic granuloma?**
One sees characteristic histiocytes (i.e., large cells with a characteristic coffee-bean-like indented or folded nucleus). Eosinophils and Langerhan giant cells are also seen.

16. **Describe the differential diagnosis of vertebra plana and the treatment of eosinophilic granuloma in a child.**
The differential diagnosis includes eosinophilic granuloma, lymphoma of bone, osteosarcoma, and Ewing sarcoma. The characteristic feature of eosinophilic granuloma causing vertebra plana is that no soft tissue mass is seen on MRI. If symptoms are minimal, observation is indicated and spontaneous resolution is the rule for treatment. Bracing may be used for comfort and for protection of the involved spine, especially early in the process.

17. **Describe the typical clinical presentation, classic radiographic features, and treatment of enchondroma.**
Enchondromas usually are first diagnosed in older teenagers and young adults. They may be found incidentally or in association with pathologic fractures. The most common sites are the small bones of the hands and feet, the distal femur, and the proximal humerus. The classic radiographic features are a central geographic intramedullary radiolucent lesion and, sometimes (in older patients especially), intralesional calcifications. The lesion calcification pattern has been described as punctuate and popcorn-like, with rings and arcs. Treatment usually involves observation. In the adult, these lesions must be distinguished from low-grade chondrosarcoma. This distinction is made based on evidence of lesion growth (which should not occur in adulthood) that is marked by increasing lucency in a previously mineralized tumor, cortical erosion, a soft tissue mass, and pain. Biopsy is generally not helpful in distinguishing low-grade chondrosarcoma from enchondroma.

18. **What is the difference between Ollier disease and Maffucci syndrome?**
Ollier disease is described as multiple enchondromatosis typically occurring in a unilateral distribution, whereas **Maffucci syndrome** is described as multiple enchondromatosis associated with multiple soft tissue hemangiomas. Malignant degeneration of enchondromas into chondrosarcomas in adulthood is much more common in Ollier disease and Maffucci syndrome than in solitary enchondromas.

KEY POINTS: BONE TUMORS

1. When assessing a lesion in the bone of a child, consider what the lesion is doing to the bone, what the bone is doing to the lesion, and the periosteal response.

2. It is important when describing a lesion of the bone to note the specific portion or location of the bone involved and the age of the child.

3. Rest pain or night pain in older children is a concerning history when associated with a bone lesion.

4. Bone tumors with multiple sites of involvement (i.e., multifocal), such as multiple enchondromatosis and multiple hereditary exostosis, have a low but real potential for malignant transformation when the patient reaches adulthood.

19. **Describe the typical clinical presentation and treatment of Ewing sarcoma.**
The typical clinical presentation involves a painful extremity, is usually associated with night pain or rest pain, and occurs between the ages of 5 and 20 years. There may be associated fever or an elevated erythrocyte-sedimentation rate. An associated soft tissue mass is common. Diaphyseal long bones are commonly affected. Involvement of the pelvis is common. Radiographically, a permeated, poorly defined diaphyseal lesion associated with periosteal reaction and a soft tissue mass is seen. Treatment includes neoadjuvant chemotherapy followed by resection of the tumor with wide margins, followed by adjuvant chemotherapy, radiation therapy, or both. Limb-sparing surgery is possible in most cases. Alternatively, chemotherapy and radiation therapy for local control may be employed for unresectable lesions such as extensive lesions of the spine.

20. **What is the 5-year survivorship of Ewing sarcoma?**
Survival rates are currently 60% or more for those with nonmetastatic disease. Late osseous and pulmonary metastases are not uncommon.

21. **What are the typical clinical presentation and treatment of classic high-grade osteogenic sarcoma?**
A typical clinical presentation is usually pain, often associated with a soft tissue mass, most commonly about the knee. Radiographs reveal a destructive lesion with a variable amount of malignant immature bone formation and a soft tissue mass. Treatment includes neoadjuvant chemotherapy followed by wide surgical resection (usually limb salvage reconstruction), followed by more adjuvant chemotherapy.

22. **How is myositis ossificans differentiated from parosteal osteosarcoma?**
The ossification associated with myositis ossificans is more peripheral than central, whereas the ossification of parosteal osteosarcoma is more dense centrally than peripherally.

23. **What are the typical clinical presentation and treatment of fibrous dysplasia in the child?**
A typical clinical presentation is usually a child older than the age of 10 years presenting with a metaphyseal or diaphyseal radiolucent bone lesion characterized by cortical expansion, sharp margination, and, occasionally, deformity or pathologic micro- or macrofracture. Metaphyseal and diaphyseal long bones are commonly involved. Rib lesions are common. Polyostotic disease is common. In fact, Albright syndrome is a polyostotic fibrous dysplasia associated with cutaneous pigmentation and precocious puberty. Treatment for fibrous dysplasia involves observation for most asymptomatic lesions. Symptomatic lesions or those associated with deformity may be treated by curettage and grafting, usually with a cortical allograft. Extensive involvement of long bones may be successfully treated with intramedullary stabilization.

24. **What are the classic histologic findings in osteofibrous dysplasia? How do they differ from fibrous dysplasia?**
Osteofibrous dysplasia is a hypocellular tumor with a storiform pattern of spindle cells and scattered bony trabeculae. There is prominent osteoblastic rimming about the bony trabeculae. This contrasts with fibrous dysplasia, in which the moderately cellular spindle-cell background is associated with a dense collagenous matrix and metaplastic bone formation in a pattern characteristically termed "alphabet soup" or "Chinese letters," seen under low-power magnification.

BIBLIOGRAPHY

1. Copley L, Dormans JP: Benign pediatric bone tumors. Evaluation and treatment. Pediatr Clin North Am 43:949–966, 1996.

2. Dormans JP, Pill SG: Fractures through bone cysts: Unicameral bone cysts, aneurysmal bone cysts, fibrous cortical defects, and nonossifying fibromas. Instr Course Lect 51:457–467, 2002.

3. Himelstein BP, Dormans JP: Malignant bone tumors of childhood. Pediatr Clin North Am 43:967–984, 1996.

4. Pierz KA, Womer RB, Dormans JP: Pediatric bone tumors: Osteosarcoma, Ewing's sarcoma, and chondrosarcoma associated with multiple hereditary osteochondromatosis. J Pediatr Orthop 21:412–418, 2001.

CHAPTER 75

SOFT TISSUE TUMORS

Mark C. Gebhardt, MD

1. **What are the most common causes of death in childhood?**
   Trauma is the most common cause and cancer is the second most common cause of death in children up to the age of 15 years.

2. **How common are soft tissue sarcomas in children?**
   Soft tissue sarcomas are an important, but not a common, cause of cancer in children. Surveillance, Epidemiology, and End Result (SEER) data indicate that soft tissue sarcomas occur in 11.3 per million children, which represents about 7% of childhood (under the age of 20) cancer.

3. **Which are more common: benign or malignant lesions?**
   Benign lesions are much more common than malignant ones, but it may be difficult to distinguish between the two.

4. **How frequent are pediatric soft tissue sarcomas in the United States?**
   There are about 850–900 new soft tissue sarcomas reported each year in the United States in children younger than the age of 20 years, and 350 of these are rhabdomyosarcomas. In contrast, about 650–700 cases of bone sarcomas are reported per year in the same age group. Of these bone sarcomas, about 400 are osteosarcomas and 200 are Ewing's sarcomas.

5. **How many deaths per year are due to soft tissue sarcomas?**
   Soft tissue sarcomas account for 153 deaths per year; bone sarcomas account for 179 deaths per year.

6. **What is the cause of soft tissue sarcomas?**
   We do not know. Genetic alterations have been found in many, but not all, soft tissue sarcomas. They include clonal karyotype abnormalities such as translocations of parts of one chromosome to another, which in some instances are specific for a given histologic subtype. Recently, the fusion products of many of these newly formed genes have been sequenced and are believed to be related to the pathogenesis of the lesions. Genetic alterations in specific tumor suppressor genes (p53 and retinoblastoma [RB]) have been identified in soft tissue sarcomas and may be correlated with outcome. Chemical carcinogens and trauma have also been implicated in the development of sarcomas, but the exact mechanism is unknown.

7. **What are the different types of benign lesions of soft tissue in children?**
   The most common lesions are ganglions (including popliteal cysts), lipomas, and vascular malformations. Perhaps the most difficult to manage is the desmoid tumor, or aggressive fibromatosis. In addition to presenting in teenagers as large masses that may mimic a soft tissue sarcoma, they may present in an infantile form or as plantar fibromatosis. Synovial chondromatosis, pigmented villonodular synovitis, and nerve sheath tumors are also seen. In addition, it is important to recognize that nonmalignant soft tissue lesions, such as myositis ossificans, can mimic soft tissue tumors.

8. **What are the different types of malignant tumors?**

   Rhabdomyosarcoma is the most common malignant soft tissue sarcoma in children, accounting for more than half of all soft tissue sarcomas. Nonrhabdomyosarcoma soft tissue sarcomas also occur—most commonly, synovial sarcomas, malignant peripheral nerve sheath tumors, fibrosarcoma, and malignant fibrous histiocytoma. Finally, Ewing's sarcoma and peripheral primitive neuroectodermal tumors (PNETs) may present as soft tissue sarcomas.

9. **What are the pathologic features of these lesions?**

   Rhabdomyosarcomas are round cell tumors, meaning that, under the microscope, they appear as sheets of homogeneous cells with large hematoxylin-staining nuclei and varying amounts of eosinophilic cytoplasm. Two subtypes occur in the extremity and trunk: embryonal (more common in young children) and alveolar (usually in the adolescent age group). Differentiation usually requires special studies such as immunohistochemistry, electron microscopy, and, at times, karyotype analysis. The t(2;13) translocation is specific for alveolar rhabdomyosarcoma. Other round cell sarcomas (i.e., Ewing's sarcoma and PNET) are part of the differential diagnosis and are distinguished from rhabdomyosarcoma by the findings on immunohistochemistry and electron microscopy. Ewing's sarcoma and PNET share a clonal t(11;22) translocation and are positive for the MIC2 antibody. The nonrhabdomyosarcomas are spindle cell neoplasms of either low or high grade. Again, immunohistochemistry is helpful in the differential diagnosis. It is essential that the pathologist be familiar with the clinical and radiographic presentation of all these lesions so that biopsy tissue can be properly processed.

10. **What happens if these lesions are not treated?**

    Certain benign lesions such as a popliteal cyst may regress spontaneously. Others, such as lipomas and vascular malformations, remain relatively constant in size and are usually asymptomatic. Lesions such as pigmented villonodular synovitis and synovial chondromatosis continue to enlarge and become painful if not treated. Malignant lesions are to be taken much more seriously. Most sarcomas grow progressively and ultimately metastasize. The lung is the most frequent site of metastasis, but certain lesions, such as rhabdomyosarcoma and synovial sarcoma, may also spread to lymph nodes in about 15% of cases. Less commonly, they may spread to bone or bone marrow and, rarely, to other organs as well. Without treatment, they are invariably fatal. For reasons that are not well understood, synovial sarcoma may be present as an asymptomatic mass for a year or more before enlarging and becoming painful.

11. **What are the clinical features of soft tissue lesions?**

    The sign that alerts the patient or parent to the problem is usually a mass of the involved extremity. In benign and some malignant lesions, the mass may be asymptomatic. Often, the recognition of the mass is preceded by an injury that may call attention to the lesion. Benign lesions are usually asymptomatic, but they may also be painful, especially if bumped or touched. Vascular malformations are painful, presumably because of venous stasis and thrombophlebitis within the vascular channels of the lesion. Popliteal cysts have smooth borders and are located most frequently near the medial gastrocnemius origin. Diagnosis can be confirmed by transillumination or ultrasonography. Lipomas have a characteristic doughy feel on palpation and have smooth lobular borders. Pigmented villonodular synovitis and synovial chondromatosis usually present with pain, limitation of motion, and swelling or effusion of a joint. It may be extremely difficult to distinguish a benign from a malignant mass. In general, benign lesions are small and superficial and malignant ones are large and deep, but malignant ones may also be tiny and located in the subcutaneous tissue. A mass larger than 5 cm that is deep to the fascia should be presumed to be malignant until proven otherwise!

12. **What should be asked regarding the history?**

    The patient's age and the location of the mass are important. Embryonal rhabdomyosarcomas usually present in young patients (i.e., <5 years of age), and alveolar rhabdomyosarcoma presents in older children. Infantile fibromatoses and fibrosarcomas present in the first year of life. The extremity and pelvis are common sites for soft tissue sarcomas. One should ascertain the nature of the pain and the length of time that symptoms have been present. Find out if symptoms began following an injury. Most benign lesions do not cause pain at rest or at night but hurt mainly following aggravation or with activity. The pain of a malignant lesion is usually constant, steadily worsens, and may cause symptoms at rest or at night. It is important to learn whether the lesion is enlarging. Are there predisposing conditions such as neurofibromatosis or familial cancer syndromes (e.g., Li-Fraumeni syndrome) that may alert the physician to the possibility of malignancy?

13. **What are the physical findings with an extremity soft tissue lesion?**
It is difficult to distinguish benign from malignant lesions with history and physical examination alone. A small, smooth-bordered lesion on the wrist or in the popliteal fossa that transilluminates is almost certainly a ganglion or popliteal cyst. A smooth-bordered, doughy, subcutaneous mass is most likely a lipoma. Vascular malformations of the extremity often present as an ill-defined fullness that increases in size in the dependent position. At times, skin discoloration may be present. Bruits are seldom noted since the majority of these are low-flow venous lesions. Schwannomas and neurofibromas present as smooth, mobile masses aligned along nerves; these lesions are more likely in patients with café au lait markings and other findings of neurofibromatosis. There are no pathognomonic findings of an extremity or pelvic soft tissue sarcoma. At times, they may present as an asymptomatic superficial mass. Lesions that are painful to palpation, large (i.e., >5 cm), and deep to the deep fascia should be presumed to be malignant, however (Fig. 75-1). Enlarging, painful "neurofibromas" in patients with neurofibromatosis should also be viewed with suspicion.

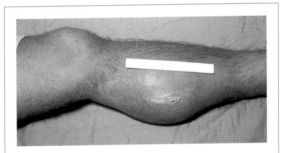

Figure 75-1. This 15-year-old boy had a mass on his thigh that was initially thought to be due to an athletic injury. Myositis ossificans was the provisional diagnosis because a radiograph showed calcifications of the posterior calf. He presented 6 months later with this large posterior compartment mass, which was firm and tender.

14. **Which type of imaging is useful?**
The most useful test for evaluating a questionable soft tissue lesion in an extremity or in the pelvis is magnetic resonance imaging (MRI). Although it will not give a definitive diagnosis, it does provide important clues such as the size, the depth, and the relationship of the mass to surrounding muscle and neurovascular structures. Certain lesions can be diagnosed with a degree of certainty. Lipomas can be distinguished by their signal characteristics, which are identical to those of fat. Vascular malformations can be distinguished from solid lesions and may demonstrate slow (venous) or fast (arterial) flow. Malignant lesions are characterized by a

location deep to the fascia and generally have well-defined borders with respect to the surrounding muscle (Fig. 75-2). It is not usually possible to distinguish one tumor type from another or to determine benign or malignant status with assurance, but in combination with other historic and physical findings, the physician can usually identify worrisome lesions. Ultrasound is excellent for defining cystic and vascular lesions but, in the author's experience, is of little other value. Computed tomography (CT) scans provide information similar to that seen on MRI but with less distinction from normal tissues. It is essential to obtain CT scans of the chest for lesions suspected to be malignant. Plain films are of value in distinguishing lesions with mineralization (e.g., myositis ossificans and synovial sarcoma). Bone scans are obtained in children with soft tissue sarcomas to look for bony metastases.

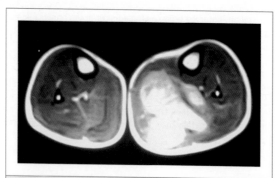

Figure 75-2. An axial T1-weighted magnetic resonance imaging (MRI) scan shows the extent of this mass in the musculature of the posterior calf. A biopsy showed synovial sarcoma, and chest computed tomography (CT) scan showed multiple pulmonary metastases. Wide excision and radiotherapy achieved local control, but, despite initial response with chemotherapy, he died 3 years later.

15. **What type of laboratory studies are useful?**
Other than excluding infection or hematopoietic malignancy (which rarely presents as a soft tissue mass) by means of a complete blood count and an erythrocyte sedimentation rate, laboratory studies are not of diagnostic importance in the work-up of patients with a soft tissue mass.

16. **Which lesions require treatment?**
Lipomas, popliteal cysts, ganglions, and vascular malformations can be observed unless they are symptomatic. Pigmented villonodular synovitis and synovial chondromatosis require synovectomy and are associated with a relatively high local recurrence rate. Malignant lesions require biopsy to establish the diagnosis and the appropriate local and systemic treatment.

17. **Who should manage the malignant lesions?**
These highly lethal tumors should be treated by a multidisciplinary team consisting of pediatric surgeons, orthopaedic surgeons, pediatric oncologists and radiotherapists, and pathologists and radiologists with expertise in this area. The biopsy should be performed by the surgeon who is capable of carrying out the definitive local treatment. The pathologist must be knowledgeable in handling the specimen for appropriate histology, immunohistochemistry, electron microscopy, and molecular studies. The multidisciplinary team makes the treatment decision relative to the combination of surgical resection, radiotherapy, and chemotherapy,

depending on the diagnosis and stage. Since these are rare lesions, they should be treated in clinical protocols so that advances in our ability to treat these patients can continue.

KEY POINTS: SOFT TISSUE TUMORS

1. Soft tissue sarcomas are rare, and less than 1000 are diagnosed in the United States in children each year. Over one third are rhabdomyosarcomas.

2. Benign soft tissue lesions are much more common than malignant ones, but at times it may be difficult to distinguish between them, leading to surgical excisions with inadequate margins.

3. Soft tissue lesions that are small and superficial are more likely to be benign, whereas large lesions deep to the fascia are more likely to be malignant, but there are exceptions to both rules.

4. Advances in the adjuvant treatment of rhabdomyosarcoma have improved the outcome of these patients in the recent decades so that nearly 75% of patients can be expected to survive. It is important to keep this in mind and to not frighten parents too much when a new soft tissue mass is discovered.

18. **What is the prognosis?**
The prognosis will vary with the grade, size, and clinical stage of the lesion, but tremendous advances have been made in our ability to achieve long-term survival in childhood soft tissue sarcomas. The third Intergroup Rhabdomyosarcoma Study demonstrated a 76% overall progression-free survival. Nonrhabdomyosarcomas that can be completely resected have an even better prognosis. It is important to note, however, that improper biopsy technique and delay in the diagnosis of these lesions can have a detrimental effect on the eventual outcome.

19. **What should I tell the family?**
It is important not to frighten the patient and parents unnecessarily. It is best to tell them that you are concerned about this mass and would like to seek the opinion of an expert to decide whether a biopsy is indicated. You can point out that the likelihood of a benign mass is much greater than that of a malignant one but that it is best to check it out. Most major medical centers have expertise in evaluating these lesions, so it is generally possible to quickly schedule a referral to an orthopaedic or pediatric surgeon with expertise in oncology.

20. **What are the complications?**
The complications of the untreated malignancy have already been discussed. The complications of surgical resection and chemotherapy are complex and are related to the location of the primary tumor and the specific treatment regimen. An unplanned excision (i.e., a shell out) or an improperly done biopsy can be devastating and in many cases can lead to unnecessary amputation or poor disease outcome.

BIBLIOGRAPHY

1. Christ WM, Kun LE: Common solid tumors of childhood. N Engl J Med 324:461–471, 1991.

2. Conrad EU III, Bradford L, Chansky HA: Pediatric soft tissue sarcomas. Orthop Clin North Am 27:655–664, 1996.

3. Letson GD, Greenfield CB, Heinrich SD: Evaluation of the child with a bone or soft tissue neoplasm. Orthop Clin North Am 27:431–452, 1996.

4. Miller RW, Young JL, Novakovic B: Childhood cancer. Cancer 75:395–405, 1995.

5. Parker SL, Tong T, Bolden S, Wingo PA: Cancer statistics, 1997. CA Cancer J Clin 47:5–27, 1997.

6. Pizzo PA, Poplack DG: Principles and Practice of Pediatric Oncology. Philadelphia, J.B. Lippincott, 2006.

7. Rao BN, Santana VM, Parham D, et al: Pediatric nonrhabdomyosarcomas of the extremities: Influence of size, invasiveness and grade on outcome. Arch Surg 126:1490–1495, 1991.

8. Ries LAG, Smith MA, Gurney JG, et al (eds): Cancer Incidence and Survival among Children and Adolescents: United States SEER Program 1975–1995. National Cancer Institute, SEER Program. NIH Pub. No. 99–4649. Bethesda, MD, 1999 (Chapter VII, Malignant bone tumors; Chapter IX, Soft tissue sarcomas; Chapter XIV, Childhood cancer mortality).

9. Smith JT, Yandow SM: Benign soft tissue lesions in children. Orthop Clin North Am 27:645–654, 1996.

10. U.S. Cancer Statistics Working Group: United States cancer statistics: 1999–2002 Incidence and mortality web-based report. Atlanta: U.S. Department of Health and Human Services, Centers for Disease Control and Prevention and National Cancer Institute, 2005. Available at: www.cdc.gov/cancer/npcr/uscs.

11. Young JL Jr, Gloeckler R, Silverberg BS, et al: Cancer incidence, survival, and mortality for children younger than age 15 years. Cancer 58:598–602, 1996.

OSTEOMYELITIS

Walter B. Greene, MD

CHAPTER 76

1. Can I skip this chapter?

Absolutely not. Although a missed diagnosis does not harm most pediatric orthopaedic conditions, that is not the case in osteomyelitis. Indeed, even a 24- to 48-hour delay in diagnosis will allow spread of the bacterial infection and significantly increase treatment requirements and the risk of complications such as contiguous or distant spread of the infection, pathologic fracture, or the dreaded chronic osteomyelitis. Furthermore, it is important that primary care physicians and orthopaedic surgeons work together in the evaluation and management of osteomyelitis.

2. What is important and changing in the microbiology of osteomyelitis in children?

Age is an important factor in determining initial antibiotic therapy. At all ages, *Staphylococcus aureus* is the most common bacteria causing osteomyelitis. In neonates, group B streptococci and gram-negative bacteria also should be covered until culture results are determined. In infants and young children, group A streptococci (particularly after varicella), *Streptococcus pneumoniae,* and *Kingella kingae,* a pathogen of emerging prevalence and understanding, are relatively common; however, *Haemophilus influenzae* type B is now very uncommon in this age group due to the universal introduction of vaccination against this organism. After 4 years of age, *S. aureus* accounts for > 90% of acute osteomyelitis, and, in this age group, initial antibiotic coverage is limited to this organism.

Even with blood and bone cultures, approximately 40% of children with acute osteomyelitis do not demonstrate the etiologic pathogen. The incidence of a culture-negative pathogen is higher with subacute osteomyelitis. Empirical antibiotic therapy is universally required during initial treatment and in the child with negative cultures.

Unique situations are associated with other pathogens. *Pseudomonas aeruginosa* is the most common organism associated with puncture wounds of the foot and subsequent osteomyelitis or septic arthritis. *Salmonella* is associated with osteomyelitis in children with sickle cell disease. Chronic osteomyelitis is associated with *S. aureus* and gram-negative pathogens. Similar to adults, in children, multiple microbial organisms are linked with osteomyelitis associated with trauma or spread from infected contiguous soft tissues.

The increasing prevalence of community-acquired methicillin-resistant *S. aureus* (MRSA) as a cause of pediatric infections has resulted in an evolving and less-clear indication for initial antibiotic coverage. MRSA accounts for approximately 50% of soft tissue infections in children. Although the prevalence is lower in osteomyelitis, MRSA is increasingly noted in this clinical situation.

3. How does osteomyelitis in children differ from that observed in adults?

In children, osteomyelitis is most often acute and develops hematogenously in the metaphysis of long bones, particularly the femur, tibia, and humerus. In adults, osteomyelitis most often is chronic and most often develops following direct penetration (e.g., open fractures, diabetic ulcers, or surgical procedures).

4. **What is the pathophysiology of hematogenous osteomyelitis in children?**

The growth plate or physis is an avascular barrier to the terminal branches of the metaphyseal arteries. Therefore, these vessels must make a U-turn at the physis. The resultant sluggish circulation, in combination with transient bacteremia, creates a set-up for bacteria to gain a foothold. The columns of primary and secondary spongiosa also limit access of reticuloendothelial cells from the adjacent medullary canal.

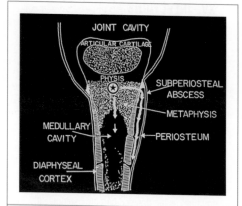

Figure 76-1. Spread of osteomyelitis in typical metaphysis.

The resultant infection spreads from its metaphyseal crypt (Fig. 76-1). Because pus under pressure takes the path of least resistance, the infection travels in two directions: down the medullary canal and through the relatively thin metaphyseal bone. The cartilaginous growth plate, however, is a barrier. Therefore, the physis and adjacent epiphysis are typically spared.

In certain locations, the insertion of the joint capsule is below (i.e., distal to) the physis. At these sites, osteomyelitis perforating the metaphyseal cortex will cause concomitant septic arthritis (Fig. 76-2). This most commonly occurs with spread of osteomyelitis from the proximal femur to the hip joint.

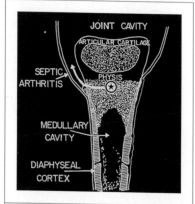

Figure 76-2. Spread of osteomyelitis when the joint capsule inserts distal to metaphysis.

5. **What determines the natural history of untreated disease?**

The extent and nature of osteomyelitis depend on the duration of the infection and the virulence of the infecting organism. Even with aggressive bacteria, if the infection is only of 24–48 hours' duration, the osteomyelitis is most likely confined to the medullary canal of the metaphysis. In this stage of the infection, recruitment of polymorphonuclear leukocytes is observed, but thrombosis of terminal vessels and necrosis of bone are limited. In essence, the early acute stage can be likened to a cellulitis of bone.

Left untreated, **acute osteomyelitis** progresses, with spread of the infection down the medullary canal and through the thin cortex of the metaphysis. Histologically, necrosis of osteocytes and hordes of acute inflammatory cells are observed. Bone resorption is dramatic in acute osteomyelitis, progressing at a rate far surpassing the most aggressive malignancy. Radiographic evidence of bone resorption is demonstrated 8–12 days after onset of symptoms by irregular patches of radiolucency in the metaphysis.

When pus perforates cortical bone, the periosteum is elevated and a subperiosteal abscess develops. Periosteal elevation is radiographically demonstrated 10–14 days after onset of symptoms by an outside rim of reactive new bone formation.

Similar to other conditions, bone formation follows osteonecrosis and bone resorption. The initial bone formed is woven, or immature, bone, which is not as dense as lamellar bone. Therefore, new bone formation also contributes to radiolucent changes that may be observed in the healing phase of osteomyelitis.

Chronic osteomyelitis develops with a delay or failure of therapy. As a result, a sequestrum (i.e., osteonecrotic bone surrounded by fibrous tissue) forms. Continued purulent drainage from the infected bone leads to formation of a sinus tract. These pathologic changes limit spread of the osteomyelitis, but the fibrous tissue is also a barrier to antibiotics and inflammatory cells. Therefore, eradicating chronic osteomyelitis requires resection of the sequestrum and the sinus tract.

Subacute osteomyelitis is secondary to infection by a less-virulent bacterium and a more effective response of the immune system. Histologically, subacute osteomyelitis is characterized by a greater proportion of granulation tissue, chronic inflammatory cells, and new bone formation. Two types of subacute osteomyelitis occur. Cavitary or cystic lesions are observed in the metaphysis or epiphysis. Subacute osteomyelitis can also simulate an aggressive, neoplastic-like lesion with periosteal elevation and new bone formation. This pattern is most often observed in the diaphysis.

6. **What are the different types of osteomyelitis?**
   - **Acute osteomyelitis:** Generally defined as infection diagnosed within 2 weeks of the onset of symptoms. The boundary between early acute and late acute is less precise, but most agree that patients presenting 4–5 days after the onset of symptoms should be placed in the late-acute category. A typical patient with early-acute osteomyelitis presents within 24–48 hours of symptom development. Osteomyelitis in this situation responds readily to antibiotic therapy. On the other hand, children who present 4–5 days after onset of symptoms are more likely to have a subperiosteal collection of pus and to require surgical drainage. Because the history is not always reliable and because bacterial strains are different, it is not possible to determine optimal treatment solely from the duration of symptoms.
   - **Subacute osteomyelitis:** Presents after 2 weeks of symptoms, but generally the duration of symptoms is 1 to several months. Subacute osteomyelitis is categorized as either a cavitary or an aggressive lesion.
   - **Chronic osteomyelitis:** Represents a delay in diagnosis or a failure of treatment. In third-world countries, chronic osteomyelitis in children is relatively common and typically follows inadequate treatment of hematogenous osteomyelitis. In industrialized countries, chronic osteomyelitis in children is uncommon and most often is a sequela of an open fracture.

7. **What happens if the condition is not treated?**
   The infectious process spreads, causing more destruction. The risk of complications is significantly increased. Even a few hours' delay may be detrimental. Laboratory studies, radiographs, and cultures should be obtained expeditiously and intravenous antibiotics started promptly, using a maximum or near-maximum dosage.

8. **What are the clinical features of the different categories of disease?**
   Acute osteomyelitis is more common in males (2:1), is most often monostotic (94%), and most often involves the lower extremity (90%). A limp or a refusal to walk is a common complaint voiced by the parents.

   Early acute osteomyelitis is characterized by a febrile illness of 24–48 hours' duration, generalized signs of acute infection, and limping, refusing to walk, or an avoidance of using the extremity.

   Late acute osteomyelitis is more likely to occur in three groups of children: infants who are not walking, children who are in the older age group, and premature neonates. Osteomyelitis that develops in infants who are not talking and not walking is not as obvious. Therefore, the diagnosis is more often delayed in this age group, and, at presentation, these children are more likely to have obvious swelling and severe pain on attempted movement of the involved extremity. In older children, the diagnosis may be delayed because this age group has better coordination; therefore, difficulty in walking is less obvious during the early stages of the infectious process. Premature infants who are in a neonatal intensive care unit are relatively immobile and are undergoing invasive procedures. In these children, the appearance of a mass may be the initial sign of osteomyelitis. Multifocal sites of osteomyelitis may be present in premature infants.

Children who develop **subacute** osteomyelitis are typically older, ranging in age from 2–16 years. In addition, the sex ratio in this category is more equivalent. The history is often vague, with neither the parents nor the child being able to pinpoint the onset of symptoms. Systemic signs such as fever are either mild or absent, and the physical exam either is within normal limits or demonstrates mild localized tenderness and swelling.

Likewise, children with **chronic** osteomyelitis may present with ill-defined symptoms or may only seek medical attention after spontaneous purulent drainage occurs.

9. **What questions should be asked in the history?**
Inquire about recent illnesses such as otitis media, pharyngitis, stomatitis, and impetigo. The vaccination status to *Haemophilus influenzae* type B, as well as recent temperature elevation, should be noted. The onset of symptoms and the duration of limping should be recorded.

10. **What are the physical findings?**
These depend on the location, duration, and severity of the infection. Osteomyelitis in locations that are relatively superficial (e.g., the distal femur and proximal tibia) causes swelling and localized tenderness. In deeper locations such as the proximal femur and the proximal humerus, physical findings are limited to the restriction of hip or shoulder motion, but this is not as severe as that observed in septic arthritis. A fever of 38–39°C is typical in late acute osteomyelitis, but the temperature may be normal or only slightly elevated in early acute, subacute, and chronic osteomyelitis.

11. **What laboratory studies should be obtained?**
Routine studies include a complete blood count, erythrocyte sedimentation rate, C-reactive protein, anteroposterior (AP) and lateral radiographs of the affected area, blood culture, and aspiration of the affected area. The **white blood cell count** is most often elevated in late acute osteomyelitis but may be within normal limits in all groups. **Sedimentation rate** and **C-reactive protein** are sensitive but nonspecific parameters of an inflammatory process. These studies are routinely elevated in late acute osteomyelitis but may be within normal limits in early acute and subacute osteomyelitis. The C-reactive protein is better than the erythrocyte sedimentation rate in monitoring early response to treatment. Initial radiographs in acute osteomyelitis are usually normal but may demonstrate contiguous soft tissue swelling. **Radiographs** are useful in excluding fractures and osseous tumors.

Blood cultures identify the offending organism 40–50% of the time in acute osteomyelitis. Obtaining a positive blood culture is less likely in subacute and chronic osteomyelitis; in these situations, blood cultures are only requested when there is evidence of systemic toxicity (i.e., a fever). **Aspiration of the bone** should be attempted. In patients with late acute osteomyelitis who have developed a subperiosteal abscess, the yield from aspiration will obviously be greater. Ultrasound guidance may enhance localization of a subperiosteal abscess. After sterile preparation of the skin, a spinal needle is inserted into bone at the suspected area of infection. If aspiration does not yield diagnostic material (i.e., pus) in the subperiosteal space, the needle is inserted, if possible, into the metaphysis, and aspiration is repeated. With **blood culture plus aspiration**, the offending organism can be identified approximately 60% of the time in acute osteomyelitis. Direct inoculation of aspirates into an aerobic blood culture bottle improves recovery of *K. kingae*. In subacute osteomyelitis, cultures are less likely to grow or to identify the infecting organism. In chronic osteomyelitis, surface swabs of sinus tract drainage are often contaminated by skin-surface contaminants. Therefore, obtaining a specimen of bone is often indicated to identify the bacteria responsible for the osteomyelitis.

12. **What special imaging studies are useful?**
A **technetium-99m bone scan** is a sensitive (reported range: 84–100%) and specific (70–90%) test for acute osteomyelitis; however, the test is not infallible (overall positive-predictive values approximate 85%).

The use of **single photon emission computed tomography (SPECT)** increases sensitivity and specificity. It should be noted that, in most cases, a bone scan is not needed because results of this study do not alter treatment. A bone scan is useful when the diagnosis is unclear, as frequently occurs with an infection in atypical locations such as the clavicle, pelvis, or fibula and when multifocal sites of infection are possible (i.e., in neonates).

Indium and gallium scans are more sensitive but have the disadvantage of causing higher radiation exposure and requiring 24–48 hours for completion.

Magnetic resonance imaging (MRI) is the best special study. Compared to a technetium-99m scan, MRI provides information concerning soft tissue spread, a more precise localization of the bony site of infection, better sensitivity, and similar specificity. Due to its cost and the frequent need for general anesthesia in children, it should be reserved for diagnostic purposes in unusual cases and to identify sequestrum and to map out chronic osteomyelitis.

Ultrasonography can demonstrate a subperiosteal abscess and has the advantage of low cost and ease of test administration, but its limited specificity and sensitivity preclude frequent usage in bone infections.

13. **What new laboratory studies may play an increasingly important diagnostic role in osteomyelitis?**
Polymerase chain reaction has proven useful for identifying cases caused by *K. kingae* and *Bartonella henselae*. In the future, this technique may be expanded to determine the cause of osteomyelitis when blood and bone cultures are negative.

14. **What other conditions may be confused with osteomyelitis?**
 - **Cellulitis:** May restrict movement and cause the child to limp, but, in most cases, swelling and erythema of the skin are obvious. If the infected bone is close to the skin (i.e., the proximal tibia or first metatarsal), osteomyelitis may cause erythema of the adjacent skin; however, the changes in the skin are considerably less than those observed in cellulitis.
 - **Septic arthritis:** A consideration in locations such as the hip. In this situation, aspiration of the joint may be required to define the site or sites of infection.
 - **Fractures:** Also cause swelling and increased warmth of the extremity. The history and radiographs usually differentiate these two conditions; however, in occult fractures or in children with insensate lower extremities due to myelomeningocele or other paralytic conditions, fractures may create a clinical picture similar to osteomyelitis.
 - **Neoplasms:** These, especially leukemia and Ewing's sarcoma, may be confused with osteomyelitis. Children with leukemia have neoplastic infiltrates of the hematopoietic marrow and may present with pain in the spine or extremity accompanied by a limp, lethargy, and even a fever. Radiographs in acute leukemia may also demonstrate osteopenia and lucent lesions. The diagnosis is made by the more gradual onset of symptoms in leukemia and other signs such as easy bruisability, night pain, pain at multiple sites, and a low leukocyte count. Subacute osteomyelitis in the diaphysis causing periosteal elevation may simulate Ewing's sarcoma. A biopsy will provide the correct diagnosis.
 - **Bone infarction:** In conditions such as sickle cell anemia and Gaucher's disease, this causes pain in the extremity, fever, and an elevated white blood cell count and sedimentation rate. Frequently, there is enough difference in these signs and symptoms to differentiate osteomyelitis from a sickle cell or Gaucher's crisis, but sometimes a biopsy is required.

KEY POINTS: OSTEOMYELITIS

1. Osteomyelitis is different between children and adults, primarily because the physis serves as a structural barrier to metaphyseal circulation in long bones.

2. Age is an important factor regarding which bacterial organism is most likely to cause hematogenous osteomyelitis in children.

3. Early diagnosis and treatment are the keys to efficient and successful treatment.

4. Community-acquired methicillin-resistant *Staphylococcus aureus* is increasingly prevalent and problematic in pediatric osteomyelitis.

5. Optimal treatment of pediatric osteomyelitis is most often achieved by cooperative and combined efforts of primary care and orthopaedic surgeon physicians.

15. **Does the condition require treatment?**
Yes! Furthermore, if acute osteomyelitis is suspected, treatment with intravenous antibiotics should start immediately. To do otherwise permits spread of the infection and increases complications. Aspiration of the bone does not affect the bone scan, at least for 24–72 hours. Therefore, if osteomyelitis is suspected, do not delay therapy to obtain special imaging studies.

16. **Pending a positive culture, what antibiotics should be prescribed?**
Initial selection of antibiotics is empirical. In **acute osteomyelitis**, the choice depends on the age of the child (see question 2). At all ages, *S. aureus* should be covered. In the past, nafcillin or cephalexin was the routine empiric choice. The emergence of MRSA has complicated the decision for initial antibiotic therapy. If the local rate of MRSA of community-acquired *S. aureus* osteomyelitis is > 10%, some experts recommend vancomycin for initial treatment. If MRSA is identified, treatment can be changed to clindamycin if the organism is susceptible and the D-test is negative for inducible macrolide-licosamide-streptogramin resistance. Vancomycin and clindamycin are also effective against *S. pyogenes* and *S. pneumoniae*; however, neither is routinely effective against *K. kingae*.
   For **subacute cavitary osteomyelitis**, a 6-week trial of oral antibiotic therapy effective against *S. aureus* should be initiated. Pending culture and biopsy results of an aggressive-appearing lesion, antibiotic therapy should be a drug effective against *S. aureus*. If cultures show no growth, then oral antibiotics should be continued for 6 weeks.
   A bone biopsy for culture should be obtained in children with **chronic osteomyelitis**. Because gram-negative bacteria are more common in chronic osteomyelitis, these organisms, as well as *S. aureus*, should be covered pending culture results.

17. **What are the indications for surgical treatment?**
Surgical intervention is rarely, if ever, needed for early acute osteomyelitis. In late acute osteomyelitis, most children can be treated with intravenous antibiotics for 24–48 hours before determining whether surgical drainage is indicated. If the child has persistent fever and swelling, the bone should be explored and the subperiosteal abscess decompressed. Some children with late acute osteomyelitis, particularly those diagnosed more than 1 week after the onset of symptoms, present with an obvious subperiosteal abscess. These patients should be treated with immediate surgical decompression. To minimize the risk of avascular necrosis, septic arthritis of the hip secondary to osteomyelitis of the proximal femur should be treated with immediate surgical drainage.

Cavitary subacute osteomyelitis used to be treated with surgical exploration. It is now recognized that most of these children can be treated with a trial of antibiotics. If the cavitary lesion does not respond, operative debridement and curettage should be done. Aggressive-appearing subacute osteomyelitis requires biopsy to rule out a neoplastic process.

Chronic osteomyelitis requires surgical biopsy for culture and removal of all necrotic bone and surrounding fibrous tissue.

18. **How long should antibiotics be continued?**

Generally, antibiotics are continued for 6 weeks. A longer course of therapy may be needed if the infection has not completely resolved. In acute osteomyelitis, antibiotics are discontinued when there is no tenderness and when radiographs demonstrate an appropriate healing response. Lucent areas due to new bone formation and bone remodeling may still be present at 6 weeks; however, if the radiographic changes are consistent with a healing response and if the child is asymptomatic, the antibiotics may be discontinued. Likewise, in subacute and chronic osteomyelitis, the radiographs may not be normal after 6 weeks of therapy, but if the picture is consistent with a resolving process, therapy can be discontinued.

C-reactive protein levels and erythrocyte sedimentation rates may also be used to monitor response to therapy. C-reactive protein levels decline more rapidly than erythrocyte sedimentation rates, and, therefore, this test is a better marker of therapeutic response in the first week of therapy.

19. **What are the complications?**

- **Distant seeding:** Hematogenous spread of infection to another location. This complication is more likely in late acute osteomyelitis. Pneumonia and septic pericarditis are the most likely consequences of distant seeding, but any location is vulnerable, and the physician should continue to examine the child for a possible secondary infection.
- **Septic arthritis:** Occurs in locations where the joint capsule inserts "below" the metaphysis, and, therefore, direct perforation of the metaphysis seeds the joint. This is most likely in the proximal femur but may also occur in the proximal humerus, proximal radius, or distal lateral tibia. When this occurs, the child typically presents with symptoms and signs more consistent with septic arthritis. The diagnosis of concomitant osteomyelitis is often made when lytic areas are observed on follow-up radiographs.
- **Pathologic fractures:** Occur because the bone is weakened by osteonecrosis, bone resorption, and subsequent bone formation and remodeling. During the last process, the infection, with its associated local and systemic symptoms, largely resolves. As a result, the child feels good and resumes normal activity. Unless the affected bone is protected, a fracture may occur through the site of osteomyelitis. This is most problematic with osteomyelitis involving the proximal femur. If the infection was diagnosed expeditiously, activity modifications such as carrying the child or using a wheelchair for 2–4 weeks may be sufficient. A spica cast is often necessary to protect the proximal femur if the osteomyelitis is a late acute type with extensive osteonecrosis.
- **Physeal bars:** More common with severe late acute osteomyelitis. Damage to the growth plate with subsequent partial closure may not be apparent for several months. Therefore, I recommend follow-up exams for 2 years after the onset of osteomyelitis. If the bar is central, growth is symmetrically tethered and a leg-length discrepancy develops. If the bar has a peripheral location, asymmetric growth and an angular deformity develop.
- **Recurrent infection:** This, along with resultant chronic osteomyelitis, may not be apparent for several months. This problem most often results when a sequestrum (i.e., a foci of necrotic bone) develops.

20. **Who should manage the problem?**

A primary care physician and an orthopaedic surgeon should work together. A primary care physician usually initiates the diagnostic evaluation, selects the initial antibiotic, monitors the child for distant seeding, and works with the orthopaedic surgeon to determine whether surgical drainage is indicated. The orthopaedic surgeon should assist in the diagnostic evaluation and should aspirate the bone for culturing. The orthopaedic surgeon should also apply appropriate forms of immobilization to minimize the risk of pathologic fracture and should determine when and if surgical drainage should be done. Both physicians work together to determine when intravenous antibiotics can be changed to oral therapy. The primary care physician monitors the child for possible antibiotic complications, and the orthopaedic surgeon determines when satisfactory resolution of infection and bone remodeling have occurred.

BIBLIOGRAPHY

1. Hamdy RC, Lawton L, Carey T, et al: Subacute hematogenous osteomyelitis: Are biopsy and surgery always indicated? J Pediatr Orthop 16:220–223, 1996.
2. Jaramillo D, Treves ST, Kasser JR, et al: Osteomyelitis and septic arthritis in children: Appropriate use of imaging to guide treatment. AJR 165:399–403, 1995.
3. Juhn A, Healey JH, Ghelman B, Lane JM: Subacute osteomyelitis presenting as bone tumors. Orthopaedics 12:245–248, 1989.
4. Kaplan SA: Osteomyelitis in children. Infect Dis Clin North Am 19:787–797, 2005.
5. Mah ET, LeQuesne GW, Gent RJ, Paterson DC: Ultrasonic features of acute osteomyelitis in children. J Bone Joint Surg 76B:969–974, 1994.
6. Pelota H, Unkila-Kallio L, Kallia MJ: Simplified treatment of acute staphylococcal osteomyelitis of childhood. The Finnish Study Group. Pediatrics 99:846–850, 1997.
7. Ross ERS, Cole WG: Treatment of subacute osteomyelitis in childhood. J Bone Joint Surg 67B:443–448, 1985.
8. Song KM, Sloboda JF: Acute hematogenous osteomyelitis in children. J Am Acad Orthop Surg 9:166–175, 2001.
9. Wong M, Isaacs D, Howman-Giles R, Uren R: Clinical and diagnostic features of osteomyelitis occurring in the first three months of life. Pediatr Infect Dis J 14:1047–1053, 1995.
10. Yagupsky P: Kingella kingae: From medical rarity to an emerging paediatric pathogen. Lancet Infect Dis 4:358–367, 2004.

CHAPTER 77

SEPTIC ARTHRITIS

Scott J. Luhmann, MD, and Perry L. Schoenecker, MD

1. **What are the joints most commonly affected by septic arthritis?**
   The most common site is the knee (41%), followed by the hip (23%), ankle (14%), elbow (12%), wrist (4%), and shoulder (4%). The remaining joints (of the hands and feet, as well as the sacroiliac and acromioclavicular joints) comprise the remaining 2%. Classic suppurative septic arthritis involves a single joint in 94% of the cases.

2. **Describe the basic pathophysiology of septic arthritis.**
   Bacteria can be introduced into the joint through transient bacteremia, direct inoculation (i.e., a puncture wound), or local extension (of osteomyelitis). Once a sufficient inoculum has been introduced into the joint, the bacteria colonize the vascular synovium and the culture-tube-like environment of the joint. Some bacteria (e.g., *Staphylococcus* and *Pseudomonas* species) have an affinity for cartilage and directly attach to the chondral surface. Bacterial proliferation is possible owing to the relatively nonimmunogenic environment of the normal joint.

3. **What is the causal relationship between osteomyelitis and septic arthritis?**
   The most common site of osteomyelitis in the skeletally immature patient is the metaphyses of long bones. Advanced metaphyseal osteomyelitis can directly decompress into (1) the hip joint, from metaphyseal involvement of the proximal femur; (2) the shoulder, from the proximal humeral metaphysis; (3) the elbow, from the proximal radius; and (4) the ankle joint, from the distal lateral tibia.

4. **What is the most common age group to be affected by septic arthritis?**
   The peak age for presentation is younger than 3 years, but it can present in patients of any age.

5. **What might be the clinical findings in septic arthritis in a 6-day-old child in the neonatal unit?**
   The 6-day-old might exhibit irritability, lethargy, difficulty in feeding, and limb disuse or pseudoparalysis. Fever is an inconsistent finding in this age group. The inability to communicate makes rapid diagnosis difficult, often resulting in a delay in diagnosis.

6. **What are the clinical hallmarks in a 15-month-old with septic arthritis?**
   Typically, the 15-month-old will be irritable and may go limp with weight-bearing or may refuse to use the involved extremity. Fever is an inconsistent finding. In subcutaneous joints, one should be able to detect an effusion, increased warmth, soft tissue swelling, and possibly erythema. To a variable degree, all septic joints will have a painful, limited range of motion and will be tender to palpation. The joints will be held in the position of maximal comfort (e.g., a hip will be in flexion, abduction, and external rotation; a knee will be in slight flexion; and an ankle will be plantarflexed).

7. **What studies should one obtain in the work-up of septic arthritis?**
   Hematologic studies, plain radiographs, and joint aspiration are all mandatory for a complete work-up. The peripheral white blood cell count (WBC) with differential is not a reliable index in an early infection but usually will be elevated ($>12,000/mm^3$) with a left shift after 24 hours.

Erythrocyte sedimentation rate (ESR) is elevated only after 48–72 hours of symptoms, with 90% of those tested showing an ESR between 50 mm/hr and 90 mm/hr. ESR will typically peak at 3–5 days. Be careful since ESR is unreliable in the neonate, in patients with hematologic disorders (e.g., sickle cell anemia), and in patients on steroids. C-reactive protein (CRP) is used in the detection of early septic arthritis. It will be elevated 6 hours after onset (with a mean at 90 mg/dL) and peaks on day 2. Blood cultures are essential and will be positive in 30–50% of cases. Plain radiographs may show (especially in the hip) joint-space widening, effusion, soft tissue swelling, or subluxation or dislocation of the joint. Comparison views of the contralateral joint may be useful. Normal hematologic and radiologic studies do not rule out septic arthritis.

8. **How do you make a definitive diagnosis of septic arthritis?**
The diagnosis is made by either joint aspiration or surgical identification of purulent effusion (WBC >40,000–50,000/mm^3, >90% segmented neutrophils), with or without identifiable pathologic organism (there are positive cultures only 50–60% of the time).

9. **Does the history of trauma to the extremity rule out septic arthritis?**
No, it is not infrequent for the caregivers to relate the child's complaints to a traumatic event. Minor trauma and falls are common in the peak age for septic arthritis and are frequently reported by parents.

10. **Are there any systemic conditions that are important to consider in the work-up and treatment of septic arthritis?**
One must consider any factors that may make the child more susceptible to the development of bacteremia. Recent systemic illness (chickenpox), infections (i.e., upper respiratory, urinary tract, or otitis media), indwelling intravenous catheters, and a positive exposure history have all been implicated in septic arthritis. In addition, suppression of the child's immune system, such as with steroid use or chemotherapy, must be noted since this will have an impact on the choice of antibiotic therapy.

11. **Why is the identification of a septic joint important?**
The presence of bacteria and inflammatory mediators in the joint space elicits a proliferative response by the host immune system. Cartilage damage occurs secondary to the enzymes (proteases, peptidases, collagenases, elastoses) released from both the endogenous cells (leukocytes and synovial cells) and the infecting organism. The initial damage is leaching of glycosaminoglycans (within 8 hours) from the cartilage, with eventual degradation of collagen in advanced cases. The cartilaginous destruction that occurs even after destruction of live organisms not only is due to the release of enzymes but also is secondary to the immune response by an Arthus-type reaction.

12. **Are magnetic resonance imaging (MRI) or bone scans useful?**
Neither MRI nor bone scans are useful initially in the diagnosis of acute septic arthritis. However, if the clinical findings are more suggestive of an inflammatory process in the bony tissue immediately adjacent to a suspected joint infection (either epiphyseal or metaphyseal) or if the patient's temperature remains elevated after irrigation and debridement, a bone scan, an MRI, or both can be helpful in evaluating possible involvement of the bone.

13. **Is ultrasonography helpful?**
Ultrasonography is an effective, safe, noninvasive imaging modality for the evaluation of a painful hip joint. It is the study of choice for assessing the presence or absence of an effusion and can be used to compare the affected joint to the unaffected contralateral hip joint. In the work-up of septic arthritis, the presence of an effusion warrants hip arthrocentesis. It should be

noted, however, that false negatives can occur: early in the course of disease, a relatively small effusion may not be readily detectable on ultrasound exam.

14. **Should aspiration of a suspicious joint ever be delayed?**
No, one should not delay arthrocentesis of suspected septic arthritis. It will not affect the results of further imaging studies (e.g., bone scan) if the arthrocentesis is dry.

15. **Can the joint aspiration be done bedside?**
Joint aspiration is a meticulous procedure that must be performed in a controlled environment with adequate sedation. Use of a sufficient needle caliber (i.e., 20 gauge) will optimize the possibility of a successful aspiration. Aspiration of a knee, an ankle, or an elbow would be predictably done at bedside. On the other hand, aspiration of a hip joint must be done in either a radiology suite or an operating room under fluoroscopic guidance, with needle position confirmed by arthrography.

16. **What studies of the joint aspirate should be performed?**
One should order a Gram stain, aerobic and anaerobic cultures, and WBC with differential for all joint fluid aspirates (Table 77-1). Visually, the fluid is opaque, varying from a cloudy yellow to creamy white in color. Gram stains will have positive findings in 30–40% of aspirates and can be helpful in diagnosing the gram-negative intracellular diplococci in gonorrheal septic arthritis. The WBC will be elevated within 24 hours of the onset of symptoms and will typically be greater than 40,000–50,000/mm^3. It is often greater than 100,000/mm^3, with a differential of more than 90% polymorphonuclear leukocytes.

17. **Are there any special technical considerations in the handling of fluid from a suspected septic joint?**
Fluid should be immediately transported to the laboratory and plated on the appropriate medium (i.e., agar). Several milliliters should also be injected into blood culture bottles, which may increase the possibility of positive identification of the pathogen. Joint aspirates of suspected cases of gonococcus need to be plated on chocolate agar to optimize yield. *Haemophilus influenzae* (now an unlikely organism because of the successful vaccination program against the same) type B and gonococcus need to incubated in a CO_2 environment.

18. **What is the likelihood of a positive culture of the joint aspirate?**
Typically it is in the 60–80% range. For *Neisseria gonorrhoeae,* it is around 50%.

19. **What are the most likely organisms causing septic arthritis?**
- **Neonate:** *Staphylococcus aureus,* enteric gram-negative organisms, and group B streptococci
- **Child < 5 years old:** *S. aureus,* group A streptococci, and *Streptococcus pneumoniae* (*H. influenzae* type B is now uncommon)
- **Child > 5 years old:** *S. aureus* and group A streptococci
- **Adolescent:** *S. aureus* and *N. gonorrhoeae*
  Other less-common organisms include *Kingella kingae, Salmonella* species (sp), *Neisseria meningitidis,* and anaerobic bacteria.

20. **What are the clinical and laboratory guidelines for differentiating toxic synovitis from acute septic arthritis?**
Toxic synovitis is an acute inflammatory process typically seen in the 2- to 10-year-old patient. Findings on physical exam can include painful and limited hip range of motion, muscle spasm, refusal to bear weight on the limb, and low-grade fever. Overall, the physical signs are not as dramatic in toxic synovitis. Typically, the ESR is greater than 30 mm/hr in only 14% of patients with toxic synovitis (compared with 71% in septic arthritis). WBC and differentials are not

TABLE 77-1. EVALUATION OF JOINT FLUID

	Appearance	WBC	PMNL (%)	Gram Stain	Culture
Normal	Clear or straw-colored	<200	<25%	Negative	Negative
Traumatic arthritis	Bloody	<5000, many red blood cells	<25%	Negative	Negative
Septic arthritis	Turbid or yellow-white	>50,000	>90%	Positive in 30–40% of cases	Positive in 50–70% of cases
JRA	Slightly cloudy or straw-colored	15,000–80,000	>60%	Negative	Negative

JRA = juvenile rheumatoid arthritis, PMNL = polymorphonuclear leukocytes, WBC = white blood cell count.

usually elevated. Ultrasonography of the affected hip will show no effusion in most patients and a slight increase in the minority of patients.

21. **What are the three main therapeutic interventions?**
Joint decompression and debridement, antibiotics, and initial joint immobilization (to decrease local irritation) followed by mobilization to decrease the development of fibrous adhesions and to improve cartilage nutrition.

22. **When should antibiotics be initiated?**
Intravenous antibiotics should be started after the arthrocentesis. If started prior to joint aspiration, the chance of obtaining a positive culture is lessened. Recent antibiotic use for otitis media or upper respiratory infection should not dissuade one from performing an arthrocentesis, however.

23. **What should the initial antibiotic regimen be?**
  - **Neonate:** Oxacillin plus either cefotaxime or gentamicin
  - **Child < 5 years old:** Oxacillin and cefotaxime, or cefuroxime alone
  - **Child > 5 years old:** Oxacillin
  - **Adolescent:** Ceftriaxone plus either oxacillin or first-generation cephalosporin

KEY POINTS: SEPTIC ARTHRITIS

1. Septic arthritis should be considered as a possible etiology for many of the pediatric musculoskeletal complaints in the outpatient and inpatient setting.

2. Arthrocentesis is advocated for any suspected septic arthritis.

3. Normal laboratory values do not rule out septic arthritis.

4. Early irrigation and debridement are optimal for any joint with nongonococcal septic arthritis.

5. Due to the difficulty in accurately identifying all septic arthritis, it is accepted that some patients may unnecessarily undergo surgical irrigation and debridement in order to capture all patients with true septic arthritis.

24. **What should the route of delivery of antibiotics be? How long should they be continued?**
Initial delivery should be intravenous for a minimum of 1 week, with conversion to oral antibiotics, if possible, for another 2–5 weeks. Oral antibiotics can be used if there is positive clinical improvement, the organism has been identified and is sensitive, the serum antibiotic level is adequate, the parents are reliable, there is no vomiting or diarrhea, and there is adequate surgical debridement. ESR or CRP levels can be used to monitor therapy. Antibiotics should be continued until ESR and CRP values normalize.

25. **What is the surest method of decompressing and debriding a septic joint?**
Open arthrotomy with debridement is the surest way to irrigate and debride the joint. Arthroscopy and arthrocentesis have their supporters but tend to be associated with higher recurrence rates, do not allow vigorous debridement of potential loculi and thick fibrinous exudates, and have been shown to predispose to more long-term joint-space narrowing.

26. **How quickly does treatment need to be done?**

    In general, treatment of most joints should proceed as soon as it is safe for general anesthesia, which may take 6 hours if the child has recently eaten. Infection of the hip joint is a surgical emergency, however. Prolonged elevated intracapsular pressure in the hip can tamponade blood flow to the femoral head and increase the possibility of developing avascular necrosis. Additionally, intracapsular septic emboli may further compromise critical proximal femoral blood flow.

27. **Is there a role for intra-articular antibiotic infusion as definitive management?**

    No, this has not been found to alter the course of septic arthritis. It has been implicated as being irritating to synovium and could exacerbate the inflammatory process. Antibiotics are delivered into the joint in sufficiently high bacteriocidal concentrations intravenously through the joint synovium.

28. **What are the complications of missed septic arthritis?**

    Aggressive surgical treatment of suspected septic arthritis might result in the occasional unnecessary arthrotomy of joints suspected of being infected; however, the potentially disastrous results of improperly diagnosed or inadequately treated septic arthritis make occasional overtreatment acceptable and a relative low morbidity risk for the child. Occurrence of avascular necrosis of the femoral head with secondary severe growth abnormalities of the hip joint can result in significant long-term functional disability and pain.

29. **What are the most important factors in determining long-term prognosis?**

    There are four main factors: (1) time from onset to irrigation and debridement, (2) the joint involved, (3) the presence of associated osteomyelitis, and (4) the age of the patient. The goal of diagnosis and treatment is rapid clearance of the intra-articular chondrocytic process; delays of more than 5 days lead to uniformly poor long-term results. Involvement of the hip can lead to avascular necrosis because the main blood supply to the femoral head is intra-articular. Effusions of the hip can impair blood flow to the femoral head, leading to total head necrosis. Associated osteomyelitis (in 10–16% of children with pyogenic arthritis) that has decompressed into the hip implies extensive involvement of the proximal femur with sequestrum. This can lead to significant pain and functional problems for the patient. Neonates often have a worse prognosis due to a delay in diagnosis. The morbid sequelae of septic arthritis may not be obvious until years after the occurrence of the acute infection. Therefore, long-term follow-up (>10 years) is necessary to assess the effect of other surgical or medical treatment.

30. **What are the characteristic findings in gonococcal (GC) septic arthritis?**

    This typically afflicts the teenager or preteenager who is sexually active. GC arthritis involves multiple joints (the average is 2.6 joints) in 60% of cases and is the most common cause of polyarthritis in this age group. In 80%, there will be a history of migratory polyarthralgia. Fever is present 60% of the time, and skin lesions 45% of the time. Genitourinary symptoms are present in 80% of males and 50% of females. GC arthritis occurs in 5% of patients with gonorrhea. This is most commonly seen in the hands (especially the dorsum), wrists, ankles, and feet. Joint aspirates usually average 48,000/mm^3. One needs to culture all orifices if GC arthritis is suspected, owing to the growth of gonococcus in culture in only 50% of cases. If one is suspicious of GC arthritis, the pharynx, anorectal areas, and blood and skin lesions need to be cultured.

31. **What is definitive treatment for GC septic arthritis?**

    Antibiotics. Specific antibiotic treatment depends on patient age and the chronicity of symptoms. Joint irrigation and debridement are not necessary owing to the rapid response of the infection to antibiotics. In addition, the gonococcus has a less damaging effect on joints; long-term cartilage damage is not seen until late in the process.

BIBLIOGRAPHY

1. Gordon JE, Huang M, Dobbs M, et al: Causes of false negative ultrasound in the diagnosis of septic arthritis of the hip in children. J Pediatr Orthop 22:312–316, 2002.

2. Kocher MS, Zurakowski D, Kasser JR: Differentiating between septic arthritis and transient synovitis of the hip in children: An evidence-based clinical prediction algorithm. J Bone Joint Surg 81A:1662–1670, 1999.

3. Luhmann SJ, Jones A, Schootman M, et al: Differentiation between septic arthritis and transient synovitis of the hip in children with clinical prediction algorithms. J Bone Joint Surg 86A:956–962, 2004.

4. McCarthy JJ, Dormans JP, Kozin SH, Pizzutillo PD: Musculoskeletal infections in children: Basic treatment principles and recent advancements. Instr Course Lect 54:515–528, 2005.

CHAPTER 78

ATYPICAL INFECTIONS

Dalia Sepúlveda, MD

1. **How often do we have to deal with atypical infections affecting bone in children?**

   Osteomyelitis is an infection of the bone and its bone marrow, generally generated by a bacterial origin. The main involved agent is *Staphylococcus aureus*, present in 70–90% of cases. Other common agents in older infants and children are β-hemolytic group A streptococci and *Streptococcus pneumoniae*. Other agents are found in about only 10% of cases.

   Bradley JS, Kaplan SL, Tan TQ, et al, for the Pediatric Multicenter Pneumococcal Surveillance Study Group (PMPSSG): Pediatric pneumococcal bone and joint infections. Pediatrics 102:1376–1382, 1998.

   Dich VQ, Nelson JD, Haltalin KC: Osteomyelitis in infants and children. Am J Dis Child 129:1273–1278, 1975.

   Frank G, Mahoney HM, Eppes SC: Musculoskeletal infections in children. Pediatr Clin North Am 52:1083–1106, 2005.

   Ibia EO, Imoisili M, Pikis A: Group A β-hemolytic streptococcal osteomyelitis in children. Pediatrics 112:22–26, 2003.

   Unkila-Kallio L, Kallio M, Eskola J, et al: Serum C-reactive protein, erythrocyte sedimentation rate, and white blood cell count in acute hematogenous osteomyelitis of children. Pediatrics 92:800–804, 1993.

2. **What are the main risk factors related to atypical bone infections?**

   The causes of atypical bone infections in children are mostly due to direct inoculation (for surgery, penetrating trauma, puncture wounds, or complex fractures) or in immune depressive states (e.g., cancer and human immunodeficiency virus [HIV]). Children who have sickle cell disease are at increased risk for bacterial infections because of functional asplenia and a defect in the alternate complement pathway. They are also at increased risk for osteomyelitis due to vaso-occlusive episodes that can result in bone necrosis and form a nidus for infection. Also, emergent agents should be taken into consideration.

   Gutierrez K: Bone and joint infections in children. Pediatr Clin North Am 52:779–794, 2005.

   Ladrón de Guevara D, Lobo G, Miranda M, Wu E: Atypical form of cat-scratch disease: Osseous involvement in two children detected by bone scan. Rev Chil Infect 20(3):202–209, 2003.

   Murray SJ, Lieberman JM: *Fusobacterium* osteomyelitis in a child. Pediatr Infect Dis J 21:979–980, 2002.

   Rasool MN: Osseous manifestations of tuberculosis in children. J Pediatr Orthop 21:749–755, 2001.

   Tager M, Zamorano J: Osteomyelitis, an uncommon involvement of cat scratch disease. Rev Chil Infect 17(4):326–331, 2000.

3. **Which are the most frequent atypical pathogens infecting children's bones?**

   Salmonella species (sp) is predominant in individuals with sickle cell disease. *Pseudomonas aeruginosa* is often identified in children with late infections of the foot following puncture wounds (Fig. 78-1). *Kingella kingae* is a common cause of osteomyelitis in the Middle East and tends to occur in children from 6 months to 2 years after upper respiratory tract infections and stomatitis. *Bartonella henselae* appears in patients with cat-scratch disease, causing axial skeleton lesions. In neonates, group B streptococci and *Escherichia coli* are other possible causative agents. *Mycobacterium tuberculosis* should be considered in immune depressive states as the rate of tuberculosis infections in major cities has increased dramatically.

   Kiang KM, Ogunmodede F, Juni BA, et al: Outbreak of osteomyelitis/septic arthritis caused by *Kingella kingae* among child care center attendees. Pediatrics 116:206–213, 2005.

   Lawson AB: Musculoskeletal infection in children. Curr Opin Orthop 16:445–450, 2005.

   Mankin HJ: Tuberculosis of bone and joints: The Red King lives! Curr Opin Orthop 12:489–498, 2001.

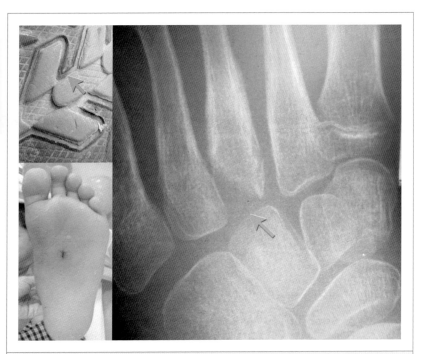

Figure 78-1. 12-year-old boy with a puncture wound through the tennis shoe. Radiograph shows lytic lesions after 6 weeks.

4. **Which other pathogens should be suspected?**
   In recurrent disease and inconsistent responses to antimicrobial agents, osteomyelitis attributable to *Actinomyces* sp should be considered, especially if located on the mandible. Chronic filamentous fungus infections are very rare but do appear in the literature. In those cases, biopsy and culture give the diagnosis. *Fusobacterium nucleatum* has been reported in children with sickle cell disease. Q-fever osteomyelitis (caused by *Coxiella burnetii*) should be considered in cases of chronic relapsing or multifocal osteomyelitis, especially if there is a history of exposure to farm animals or if granulomatous lesions are demonstrated on histologic analysis of bone specimens.

   Leggiadro RJ: Three cases of Q fever osteomyelitis in children and a review of the literature. Clin Infect Dis 39:e61–e66, 2004.
   Llinas L, Olenginski TP, Bush D, et al: Osteomyelitis resulting from chronic filamentous fungus olecranon bursitis. J Clin Rheumatol 11:280–282, 2005.
   Robinson JL, Vaudry WL, Dobrovolsky W: Actinomycosis presenting as osteomyelitis in the pediatric population. Pediatr Infect Dis J 24:365–369, 2005.

5. **How should we study a patient with a suspected atypical bone infection?**
   Imaging studies should include magnetic resonance imaging (MRI), which is considered the most useful supplemental study in any child with osteomyelitis. Bone scan has proved to be useful in detecting osteolytic damage in the axial skeleton in the cases of osteomyelitis due *B. henselae*. New special culture techniques allow more reliable detection of *K. kingae*, otherwise difficult to isolate, and should be ordered if this is suspected.

   Gene A, Garcia-Garcia J-J, Sala P, et al: Enhanced culture detection of *Kingella kingae*, a pathogen of increasing clinical importance in pediatrics. Pediatr Infect Dis J 23:886–888, 2004.

6. **How useful is MRI in atypical bone infection?**

   It allows a thorough delineation of the anatomic and spatial extent of the infection and may detect abscesses that require surgical drainage. It may also identify toothpick remnants that lead to osteomyelitis due to *Pseudomonas aeruginosa* and may result in inadequate debridement. It also helps to identify pyomyositis, which develops in children with immune compromise, and helps differentiate it from other bacterial infections in the pelvic area. MRI of the spine may show the changes of Pott's disease quite clearly and definitively.

   Imoisili MA, Bonwit AM, Bulas DI: Toothpick puncture injuries of the foot in children. Pediatr Infect Dis J 23:80–82, 2004.

7. **How useful is the needle aspiration culture in diagnosing atypical bone infections?**

   Aspiration of the subperiosteal space and metaphyseal bone at the site of maximum tenderness in an attempt to isolate the causative organism is highly recommended in order to ensure adequate antibiotic treatment. Biopsy and culture remain the gold standard for the identification of atypical infections and therapy guidance.

8. **What are the main risk factors for osteoarticular sequelae?**

   The main risk factor for sequelae is delay in diagnosis, which prevents accurate and appropriate treatment.

9. **What is brucellosis?**

   It is an infection caused by bacteria of the genus *Brucella,* mainly involving the reticuloendothelial system. This condition is characterized by fever, weakness, malaise, and weight loss. The disease is transmitted from domestic or wild animals to humans by contact with contaminated meats or unpasteurized lacteous products.

10. **How can brucellosis present as an osteoarticular infection?**

    Osseous infection is the most common complication of brucellosis in countries in which this pathogen is endemic. The clinical presentation of brucellosis is nonspecific. *Brucella* osteomyelitis can produce lytic lesions on radiographs that resemble neoplasms. Diagnosis can therefore be difficult unless a high index of suspicion is maintained.

    Colmenero JD, Reguera JM, Martos F, et al: Complications associated with *Brucella melitensis* infection: A study of 530 cases. Medicine (Baltimore) 75:195–209, 1996.

    Fowler TP, Keener J, Buckwalter JA: Brucella osteomyelitis of the proximal tibia: A case report. Iowa Orthop J 24:30–32, 2004.

11. **What studies should be ordered if brucellosis is suspected?**

    Conventional *Brucella* spp serology and an immunoagglutination test such as Brucellacapt.

    Benito R, Duran ME, Gil J, Rubio MC: Brucella bacteremia with negative conventional serology. Enferm Infecc Microbiol Clin 19(7):348–349, 2001.

12. **What is the treatment for brucellosis?**

    Antibiotic therapy with doxycycline combined with rifampicin or another aminoglycoside is recommended for treatment and prevention of recurrence.

13. **What is Lyme disease?**

    It is an infectious disease caused by *Borrelia burgdorferi*, a spirochete that is transmitted chiefly by *Ixodes dammini* and *Ixodes pacificus* ticks in the United States and *Ixodes ricinus* in Europe. It has early and late cutaneous manifestations, plus involvement of the nervous system, heart, eye, and joints in variable combinations.

14. **When should Lyme disease be suspected? What test should be ordered?**
It should be suspected in a clinical case characterized by the presence of a red, flat, or slightly raised lesion in the place of a tick bite, in association with fever, headache, myalgia, and inflammation of the larger joints. It can also be associated with intense pruritus and unusual behavior. Physical examination in advanced disease shows anomalies of the heart, joint, and brain. An antibody study for *B. burgdorferi* (i.e., an immunofluorescent assay [IFA] or an enzyme-linked immunosorbent assay [ELISA]) should be ordered. The ELISA test is confirmed with a Western blot test.

15. **What is a mycobacterium?**
Microorganisms from the *Mycobacterium* genus are aerobic, acid-fast bacilli. There are around 50 different species. Most of them are environmental and can be found in soil, water, and minerals, but the main habitat is the damaged tissue of warm-blooded hosts. There are mainly two types, *M. tuberculosis* and nontuberculous mycobacterial (NTM), or atypical mycobacteria. The atypical or nontuberculous bacteria have a lower incidence; these include *M. buruli, M. chelonae, M. duvalii, M. flavescens, M. fortuitum, M. gilvum, M. gordonae, M. kansasii, M. marinum, M. obuense, M. scrofulaceum, M. szulgai, M. terrae, M. ulcerans,* and *M. xenopi,* among others. Most of the infections caused by this type of pathogen are opportunistic, with an increasing incidence due to the larger number of immunosuppressed patients. Transmission from animals to humans is rare, and transmission from human to human is even rarer for NTM.

Meissner G, Anz W: Sources of *Mycobacterium avium*-complex infection resulting in human disease. Am Rev Resp Dis 116:1057–1064, 1977.

Ostroff S, Hutwagner L, Collin S: Mycobacterial species and drug resistance pattern reported by state laboratories 1992 [abstract U9]. In Program and Abstracts of the 93rd General Meeting of the American Society for Microbiology, Atlanta, GA. Washington DC: American Society for Microbiology, 1993, p 170.

Petitjean G, Fluckiger U, Schären S, Laifer G: Vertebral osteomyelitis caused by non-tuberculous mycobacteria. Clin Microbiol Infect 10:951–953, 2004.

16. **Which mycobacterial infections are more common?**
M. tuberculosis is the etiologic agent of tuberculosis (TB), a disease that primarily produces lesions in the lungs and can cause death if not treated correctly. TB is the most important presentation of infections due to mycobacteria. Other mycobacteria are also capable of causing disease in humans. *M. bovis* also causes tuberculosis, whereas infections due to *M. avium, M. kansasii, M. fortuitum,* and *M. chelonei* are considered opportunistic nontuberculous diseases. Leprosy is caused by *M. leprae,* an intracellular parasite that multiplies slowly in mononuclear phagocytic cells such as skin histiocytes and Shwann cells of the nerves.

17. **What mycobacterial infections can be found in osteoarticular disease?**
Mycobacterial pathogens are known to cause chronic infection of bone and articulations. Transverse myelopathy and vertebral osteomyelitis are typical presentations of direct infection due to *M. tuberculosis* and can be associated with arachnoiditis and medullar compression as a parallel process to pulmonary disease. Vertebral osteomyelitis caused by NTM is a very rare disease. The clinical presentation in most cases is indistinguishable from a pyogenic osteomyelitis. Chronic granulomatous infections of bursae, articulations, tendons, and bones can be found after direct inoculation of the pathogen through trauma, surgery, and penetrating injuries or injections. *M. ulcerans* disease, or Buruli ulcer, causes significant morbidity in West Africa. The disease presents in the skin as either nonulcerative or ulcerative and often invades bones either subjacent to the skin lesion (in contiguous osteomyelitis) or remote from the skin lesion (in metastatic osteomyelitis).

Portaels F, Aguiar J, Debacker M, et al: *Mycobacterium bovis* BCG vaccination as prophylaxis against *Mycobacterium ulcerans* osteomyelitis in Buruli ulcer disease. Infect Immunol 72(1):62–65, 2004.

Sarria JC, Chutkan NB, Figueroa JE, Hull A: Atypical mycobacterial vertebral osteomyelitis: Case report and review. Clin Infect Dis 26:503–505, 1998.

White VLC, Al-Shahi R, Gamble E, et al: Transverse myelopathy and radiculomyelopathy associated with pulmonary atypical infections *Mycobacterium*. Thorax 56:158–160, 2001.

18. **Who has the higher risk for osseous infections?**
Osseous infections caused by mycobacteria are generally associated with immunosuppressive status, including patients infected with HIV with an HIV helper cell count (CD4) less than 40 (they are rare with CD4 higher than 100) and patients under immunosuppressive treatment (e.g., for neoplasia or lupus), often in association with other opportunistic infections.

Klein JL, Corbett EL, Slade PM, et al: *Mycobacterium kansasii* and human immunodeficiency virus co-infection in London. J Infect 37:252–259, 1998.

Toll A, Gallardo F, Ferran M, et al: Aggressive multifocal Buruli ulcer with associated osteomyelitis in an HIV-positive patient. Clin Exp Dermatol 30:649–651, 2005.

19. **What are the most common locations for osteoarticular TB in orthopaedics?**
TB of joints remains the most common presentation of the disease in orthopaedic practice. It is most frequent in the hip or knee but can occur in any synovial-lined articulation. Tuberculous osteomyelitis is less common than skeletal TB involving the spine and synovial joints.
In children, the metaphyses of long bones, especially of the lower limbs, appear to be common sites of involvement, compared with the axial skeleton and pelvis in adults.

20. **Which location of osteoarticular TB infection is most severe in terms of future sequelae?**
In most cases, all lesions heal radiologically between 3 and 6 months, without relapse or recurrence. Evidence of avascular necrosis has been seen in the femoral head and the navicular bone.

KEY POINTS: ATYPICAL INFECTIONS

1. Atypical infections are rare but should always be suspected with failure of standard treatment.

2. A magnetic resonance imaging (MRI) study is the best image study for bone infection.

3. Biopsy and culture should always be performed during surgical exploration for bone infections. The results determine treatment in cases of atypical pathogens.

4. Always ask an infectious diseases specialist for advice about the most recent antibiotic treatments for atypical pathogens.

5. An accurate and in-depth history should be done in order to obtain useful information.

21. **What is the most recently proved medical treatment for TB?**
The antimicrobial treatment should be managed by an infectious disease specialist and currently includes an array of antituberculous medication, which usually should be continued for 1 year or, often, longer. Isoniazid is currently the best choice of a single agent, but it has some side effects, including peripheral neuritis. Rifampin is a good second choice with minimal side effects. Pyrazinamide is an excellent antituberculous drug but has a high risk of hepatitis. Ethambutol and streptomycin may also be used. Occasionally, the antituberculotic therapy is combined with surgical debridement; however, it is infrequently indicated.

Tristano AG, Willson ML, López A, De Abreu F: Sternal osteomyelitis caused by *Mycobacterium tuberculosis:* Case report and review of the literature. Am J Med Sci 319(4):250–254, 2000.

22. **Is the skin test important for TB diagnosis?**

The tuberculin test is positive in 90% of immunologically competent patients with skeletal TB; however, it can be negative in a small percentage of immunologically competent patients and in a greater percentage of patients with immunodeficiency. Therefore, a negative test does not rule out the diagnosis of TB. The test is not helpful in patients with HIV infection.

23. **Why have we failed to eradicate TB in the world?**

HIV infection and the other immune deficiency states, which resulted in a sharp increase in the rate of TB infections in major cities, are the main cause. TB has developed its own modification of gene structure so that in some cases it is no longer responsive to the drugs that had controlled it in the past. Also, physicians and managed care organizations have to take part of the blame in the sense that they reduced the length of time of administration (and the cost) of the drugs that controlled the disease, thus allowing the organism to develop some forms of immunity.

Hadley M, Maher D: Community involvement in tuberculosis control: Lessons from other health care programmes. Int J Tuberc Lung Dis 4:401–408, 2000.

Hall S: The return of tuberculosis—In a new, more menacing form. In The Race Against Lethal Microbes. Chevy Chase, MD, Howard Hughes Institute, 2000, pp 6–21.

Woods GL: Generalized tuberculosis in the acquired immunodeficiency syndrome. Arch Pathol Lab Med 124:1267–1274, 2000.

Woss AR, Hahn JA, Tulsky JP, et al: Tuberculosis in the homeless. Am J Respir Crit Care Med 162:460–464, 2000.

24. **What is the physiopathology of vertebral osteomyelitis due to atypical mycobacteria?**

Unlike other osteoarticular infections caused by NTM, this infection is rarely due to direct inoculation. A genetic defect in the interferon-γ receptor with reduction of the macrophage response *in vitro* has been described in patients with multifocal osteomyelitis. Another recent hypothesis postulates a minor locus resistance after nonpenetrating trauma. The macrophages containing NTM migrate from the traumatized region and then release the mycobacteria to initiate a new infectious center. A similar pathogenesis has been described for TB spondylitis.

Arend SM, Janssen R, Gosen JJ, et al: Multifocal osteomyelitis caused by nontuberculous mycobacteria in patients with a genetic defect of the interferon-γ receptor. Neth J Med 59:140–151, 2001.

Chan ED, Kong PM, Fennelly K, et al: Vertebral osteomyelitis due to infection with nontuberculous mycobacterium species after blunt trauma to the back: Three examples of the principle of locus minoris resistentiae. Clin Infect Dis 32:1506–1510, 2001.

Weir WR, Muraleedharan MV: Tuberculosis arising at the site of physical injury: Eight case histories. J Infect 7:63–66, 1983.

25. **How do we diagnose NTM infections?**

Because of the slow growth of the infectious center caused by NTM, early diagnoses is a challenge. Multiple cultures of osseous biopsies are necessary to confirm the definitive diagnosis. Blood cultures are generally negative. Only 28% of vertebral osteomyelitis episodes are diagnosed during the first month after the onset of symptoms. Late diagnosis is an independent risk factor for an unfavorable result. Routine radiologic studies should be made to assess the evolution of disease, ideally with computed tomography (CT), and to differentiate NTM infections from other causes of atypical infections.

McHenry MC, Easley KA, Locker G: Vertebral osteomyelitis: Long-term outcome for 253 patients from seven Cleveland-area hospitals. Clin Infect Dis 34:1342–1350, 2002.

26. **What microbiologic study detects mycobacteria?**

Pathogens of the *Mycobacterium* genus are characterized by a cell walls with a high lipid content that makes them impenetrable to hydrophilic agents. For this reason, mycobacterial pathogens do not stain properly with reactives used in Gram stain. Mycobacteria are stained properly with the Ziehl-Neelsen method (i.e., acid-fast stain), which uses as a bleaching agent a solution of ethanol and chloridic acid. This pathogen, once colored, is resistant to acid-alcohol bleaching; hence, it is called *acid-fast resistant*.

Lazzarini L, Amina S, Wang J, et al: *Mycobacterium tuberculosis* and *Mycobacterium fortuitum* osteomyelitis of the foot and septic arthritis of the ankle in an immunocompetent patient. Eur J Clin Microbiol Infect Dis 21:468–470, 2002.

27. **When should fungal infections be suspected?**
When there is no response to conservative or typical treatments, you should always suspect an infection of atypical agents. Patients with chronic granulomatous disease, in whom phagocytes fail to generate oxidant antimicrobial action because of an inherited failure in reduced nicotinamide adenine dinucleotide phosphate (NADPH) oxidase, comprise one of the more common situations associated with fungal infections, primarily caused by *Aspergillus* spp (e.g., *A. nidulans* and *A. fumigatus*). Patients with diabetes have a higher incidence of osteomyelitis due to fungus, mainly caused by superinfection of the typical lesions of the diabetic foot. Foot ulcers may suffer superinfection by pathogens such as *Blastomyces dermatitidis*, which generates osteomyelitis associated with inflammatory signs of soft tissues and abscess. In patients with foot ulcers but no antecedent diabetes, neither venous stasis nor lymphedema is highly suspicious for fungal infections. In chronic bursitis with poor response to normal treatment, a fungus should be suspected as the causal pathogen. Candidal osteomyelitis is an unusual but known entity. However, due to the increasing number of conditions that predispose to candidemia and invasive candidiasis, this situation is now more common.

Arias F, Mata-Essayag S, Landaeta ME, et al: *Candida albicans* osteomyelitis: Case report and literature review. Int J Infect Dis 8:307–314, 2004.

Dotis J, Roilides E: Osteomyelitis due to *Aspergillus* spp. in patients with chronic granulomatous disease: Comparison of *Aspergillus nidulans* and *Aspergillus fumigatus*. Int J Infect Dis 8:103–110, 2004.

Lerch K, Kalteis T, Schubert T, et al: Prosthetic joint infections with osteomyelitis due to *Candida albicans*. Mycoses 46(11–12):462–466, 2003.

Llinas L, Olenginski TP, Bush D, et al: Osteomyelitis resulting from chronic filamentous fungus olecranon bursitis. J Clin Rheumatol 11:280–282, 2005.

28. **What studies should be ordered when fungal infections are suspected?**
The serial radiologic study would be useful to identify an atypical lesion, especially with a CT scan. Most of the reports of fungal infections describe a dystrophic calcification of soft tissues with osteopenia and periostia reaction. Always take culture samples and ask for a microbiologic study, which will give the definitive diagnosis. In cases of joint infections, aspiration and analysis of synovial fluid cultures are essential to differentiate causes of atypical bursitis.

29. **What is the suggested treatment for fungus infections?**
Therapy should be initiated as soon as possible after diagnosis with antifungal agents such as amphotericin B and other azole agents, but some cases will require surgical debridement.

Embil JM, Wiens JL, Oppenheimer M, Trepman E: Foot ulcer and osteomyelitis. Can Med Assoc J 174(1):35–36, 2006.

Steinbach WJ, Schell WA, Miller JL, Perfect JR: *Scedosporium prolificans* osteomyelitis in an immunocompetent child treated with voriconazole and caspofungin, as well as locally applied polyhexamethylene biguanide. J Clin Microbiol 41:3981–3985, 2003.

Acknowledgments

The author gratefully acknowledges the support of Juan Carlos Hernández, MD, Pediatric Orthopedic Unit, Roberto del Río Hospital; Matías Sepúlveda, MD, University of Valdivia; and Estefanía Birrer, MD, University of Valdivia.

XVI. NEUROMUSCULAR DISORDERS

CHAPTER 79

CEREBRAL PALSY

H. Kerr Graham, MD, FRCS (Ed), FRACS

1. **What is cerebral palsy (CP)?**
   Cerebral palsy is a convenient term to describe neurodevelopmental conditions that are recognized in childhood and persist throughout life. The 2005 International Committee definition is as follows:

   Cerebral palsy (CP) describes a group of disorders of the development of movement and posture, causing activity limitation, that are attributed to nonprogressive disturbances that occurred in the developing fetal or infant brain. The motor disorders of cerebral palsy are often accompanied by disturbances of sensation, cognition, communication, perception, and/or behavior, and/or by a seizure disorder.

2. **What causes CP?**
   CP can be the result of a malformation, injury, or infection of the developing brain *in utero,* at the time of birth, or in very early childhood. The majority of cases have antenatal antecedents, and many cases are multifactorial. A minority are the result of birth trauma or asphyxia. Knowledge about the type and timing of the brain lesion or injury is developing rapidly because of the increasing availability and utilization of imaging, especially magnetic resonance imaging (MRI). Prematurity and low birth weight are the leading associations with CP in developed countries. Maternal birth canal infections and viral infections of mother and child are increasingly implicated in the etiology of CP; these include toxoplasmosis, rubella, cytomegalovirus, and herpes simplex (TORCH). Kernicterus as a cause of CP has fallen dramatically owing to the widely used prophylaxis with anti-D immune globulin G in the Rh-negative mother, intrauterine transfusion of the fetus, and phototherapy.

3. **How is CP diagnosed?**
   CP is suspected from the clinical history and confirmed by physical examination and brain imaging. Common factors are prematurity, low birth weight, and perinatal difficulties. Delay in achieving motor milestones is one of the most consistent and useful diagnostic and prognostic parts of the history. The physical findings range from mild and subtle to severe and overt.

4. **How is CP classified by motor disorder type?**
   Motor type is classified using terms to describe muscle tone and abnormal movements. Hypertonic types are spastic, dystonic, and mixed.
   - **Spastic:** (60–80%) Characterized by increase in velocity-dependant stretch reflexes; the most common, most predictable, and most amenable to intervention; all hypertonic CP types (except pure athetosis) develop contractures and deformities
   - **Dyskinetic:** (10–20%) Includes many terms and subtypes (e.g., dystonia and athetosis); dystonia may develop over time in children thought to be spastic in infancy; the most variable and least predictable motor type
   - **Mixed:** (5–15%) The most frequent combination is spasticity and dystonia
   - **Hypotonic:** (2–5%) Common in infancy; most become hypertonic with time
   - **Ataxic:** (2–5%) Characterized by poor balance and coordination, but no contractures and few deformities

5. **How is CP classified by topographical distribution?**
   - **Monoplegia:** One limb only; most cases are found to be hemiplegia if examined carefully
   - **Hemiplegia:** One side of the body affected
   - **Triplegia:** Three limbs affected
   - **Diplegia:** Both lower limbs affected, minimal involvement of the upper limbs
   - **Quadriplegia:** All four limbs affected. A better term may be *whole body involvement*
     Hemiplegia, diplegia, and quadriplegia each make up about one third of CP in population-based studies. Monoplegia and triplegia are uncommon. When a child appears to have a lower-limb monoplegia, ask him or her to run. Mild, hemiplegic posturing is frequently seen during running and is absent at rest.

6. **How is CP classified according to gross motor function?**
   Gross motor function in CP is best classified using the Gross Motor Function Classification System (GMFCS). This is a five-level ordinal grading system that can be applied to children, in three different age bands (Fig. 79-1). It classifies children according to posture, sitting, standing, and walking ability, with particular reference to the need for assistive devices. The GMFCS has been shown to be valid, reliable, and (relatively) stable over time. It is prognostic and predictive of musculoskeletal complications such as hip displacement.

7. **What are the most important priorities for the child with CP, who will become an adult with CP?**
   Parents and therapists often rate walking as their primary goal, but communication, which impacts socialization and education, is much more important than walking. Independence in activities of daily living is the second key issue. Functional mobility (which includes assistive devices and wheelchairs) is more important than walking.

8. **How can functional goals be implemented?**
   Assistive technology is available to improve all aspects of life for children and adults with CP. Additionally important are communication devices for the nonverbal child, motorized wheelchairs with electronic hand controls, wheelchair access in public and private spaces, adaptive toilet and bathroom equipment, and adaptive clothing, shoes, and sports equipment and programs. With the right equipment, funding, and support, children with severe CP can enjoy bicycle riding, horse riding, sailing, and skiing.

9. **What are the associated impairments and comorbidities in children with CP?**
   Included are seizure disorders, hearing and visual impairments, cognitive and learning difficulties, and emotional and behavioral difficulties. Associated medical comorbidities include aspiration and reflux, respiratory disease, feeding difficulties and nutritional deficits, the need for a feeding tube, osteopenia, and insufficiency fractures.

10. **Who are involved in the care of children with CP?**
    The most important caregivers are the parents. Health professionals can be effective only when they work in a partnership with parents. Therapists (including physical therapists, occupational therapists, and speech pathologists) are key confidants, educators, service providers, and supporters of parents and their children with CP. Pediatricians and neurologists may make the diagnosis and provide a range of medical and psychosocial support for the child with CP in the diagnosis, evaluation, and management of the medical comorbidities. Physiatrists and rehabilitation specialists offer management of hypertonia and mobility requirements. Neurosurgeons may be involved in surgical management of hypertonia by selective dorsal rhizotomy (SDR) or intrathecal baclofen (ITB) pump insertion. Orthopaedic surgeons offer reconstructive surgery for upper- and lower-limb deformities, gait-correction surgery, prevention and management of hip displacement, and scoliosis surgery.

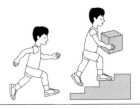

GMFCS Level I

Children walk indoors and outdoors and climb stairs without limitation. Children perform gross motor skills including running and jumping, but speed, balance and coordination are impaired.

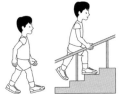

GMFCS Level II

Children walk indoors and outdoors and climb stairs holding onto a railing but experience limitations walking on uneven surfaces and inclines and walking in crowds or confined spaces.

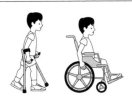

GMFCS Level III

Children walk indoors or outdoors on a level surface with an assistive mobility device. Children may climb stairs holding onto a railing. Children may propel a wheelchair manually or are transported when traveling for long distances or outdoors on uneven terrain.

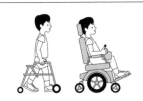

GMFCS Level IV

Children may continue to walk for short distances on a walker or rely more on wheeled mobility at home and school and in the community.

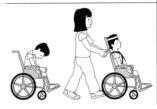

GMFCS Level V

Physical impairment restricts voluntary control of movement and the ability to maintain antigravity head and trunk postures. All areas of motor function are limited. Children have no means of independent mobility and are transported.

Figure 79-1. The Gross Motor Function Classification System (GMFCS) for children aged 6–12 years: descriptors and illustrations. (From Palisano RJ, Walter S, Russell D, et al: Development and reliability of a system to classify gross motor function in children with cerebral palsy. Dev Med Child Neurol 45:113–120, 1997; illustrations by Kerr Graham and Bill Reid, The Royal Children's Hospital, Melbourne.)

11. **What is the upper motor neuron syndrome (UMN)?**
    The UMN syndrome is a constellation of positive and negative features that result from an UMN lesion due to any cause. CP is by far the most common cause of the UMN syndrome in childhood. The positive features are spasticity, clonus, hyper-reflexia, and co-contraction. The negative features are weakness, impaired selective motor control, poor balance, and

sensory impairment. It is much easier to intervene to modify the positive features of the UMN syndrome than to correct the negative features. In spastic quadriplegia, spasticity can be reduced effectively using an ITB pump. However, the child may still not walk because of weakness, impaired selective motor control, and poor balance. In the hemiplegic upper limb, spasticity can be reduced by injections of Botox®, but the child may choose not to use the limb because of poor sensation (i.e., learned non-use).

12. **Is there a role for strength training in CP?**
   CP means weakness originating from the brain. Strengthening was historically considered to be unpredictable and possibly dangerous in CP because it might increase spasticity. Recent studies have established that weakness is pervasive in bilateral CP and is a more important factor than spasticity in determining gait and function. Strength can be reliably measured in children with CP using torque dynamometers and can be increased using various strengthening programs.

13. **What is meant by progressive musculoskeletal pathology?**
   Infants with CP do not have deformities at birth unless there is an associated congenital anomaly such as a congenital hip dislocation. The musculoskeletal pathology is acquired during growth because of the effects of hypertonia and reduced activity. The most common deformities are contracted muscle-tendon units, joint contractures, torsional deformities in long bones, hip displacement, and spinal deformities. Physical therapy, medications for spasticity, splinting, and positioning may slow the progress of contractures in many children. In severely involved children, contractures develop despite nonoperative management. Surgical correction is usually required.

14. **What is meant by a dynamic contracture?**
   A dynamic contracture describes spastic muscle shortening, which causes abnormal posturing, is reversible, and is not present when the child is relaxed under general anesthesia. Dynamic contractures may respond favorably to spasticity management such as injection of botulinum toxin (i.e., Botox®). The most common examples are toe-walking because of spastic equinus and scissoring because of spastic hip adductors.

15. **What is meant by a fixed contracture?**
   A fixed contracture means shortening of a muscle-tendon unit, resulting in restricted joint range of motion, which may impair function. The shortening is present under anesthesia, does not respond to spasticity management, and requires lengthening for correction. Muscles that cross two joints and that have their principal action in the sagittal plane are more commonly affected by contracture including gastrocnemius (i.e., equinus), medial hamstrings (i.e., flexed knee), and psoas (i.e., flexed hip).

16. **What are the most effective methods of spasticity management in children with CP?**
   Spasticity management refers to interventions to reduce spastic hypertonia with the aim of correcting spastic posturing, preventing progression to fixed contracture, and improving function. Spasticity management can be classified by whether the intervention is temporary or permanent and whether its effects are focal, regional, or generalized (Table 79-1).

17. **What is the role of oral medications for spastic hypertonia?**
   The most commonly used medications in the management of spastic hypertonia are diazepam (i.e., Valium), baclofen (i.e., Lioresal), and tizanidine. Oral medications are very useful for acute exacerbations of spastic hypertonia, such as may result after operations, injury, or anxiety or stress from any cause. They are much less useful in the management of chronic spasticity because of sedation and other unwanted side effects.

TABLE 79-1. MANAGEMENT OF SPASTICITY IN CHILDREN WITH CEREBRAL PALSY

Description	Temporary vs. Permanent	Focal vs. Regional vs. Generalized
Oral medications	Temporary	Generalized
Neurolytic injection (i.e., Botox®)	Temporary	Focal or regional
Neurolytic block (i.e., Phenol)	Temporary	Focal
Selective dorsal rhizotomy	Permanent	Regional (lower limbs)
Intrathecal baclofen pump	Semipermanent	Generalized

18. **What is the role of ITB?**
Baclofen is an effective drug in the management of spasticity in children with CP, but its usefulness is limited because of poor lipid solubility and the inability to achieve adequate concentrations of the drug in the cerebrospinal fluid without unwanted side effects. The delivery of baclofen directly to the intrathecal space by an implanted pump and catheter overcomes the problem of delivery of the drug. The concentration and timing of the delivery of the drug can be adjusted by programming the pump's computer. The pump is refilled at intervals but can be replaced or removed as necessary.

The **advantage** of ITB is effective spasticity reduction in the lower limbs and, to a lesser degree, in the upper limbs, depending on the positioning of the tip of the catheter.

The **disadvantages** of the ITB pump are its size, the invasive nature of the implantation procedure, and a high risk of both local and systemic complications, including infection around the pump or catheter, disconnection of the catheter, and potential overdosing or underdosing of baclofen. Despite the significant morbidity (and potential mortality) associated with the use of the ITB pump, it is one of the most effective tools in the management of severe spastic hypertonia in children and adolescents with CP.

19. **Which children may benefit from an ITB pump?**
Children with severe generalized spasticity, dystonia, or mixed movement disorders may benefit from tone reduction using an ITB pump. These individuals usually have quadriplegia and function at GMFCS levels IV or V. The goals of ITB therapy are to improve comfort, to relieve pain, to improve function, and to ease the burden of care. Improvements in gross motor function are small, but patients are frequently more comfortable, happier, and easier to care for.

20. **What is the role of SDR?**
Spasticity is, in part, the result of the loss of inhibition of the lower motor neurons. SDR is a neurosurgical procedure in which 20–40% of the lumbar dorsal rootlets are sectioned to interrupt the reflex arc and permanently reduce tone. The ideal candidate for SDR is usually a child aged 3–6 years with spastic diplegia who is GMFCS level II, with moderate to severe spasticity in the lower limbs but without significant fixed deformity. There should be good underlying strength and selective motor control. After SDR, children are weak and hypotonic. Intensive rehabilitation is required for up to a year to gain the maximum benefit, and the majority of children will still need orthopaedic procedures later in childhood, such as foot stabilization and femoral derotation osteotomy.

21. **What are neurolytic blocks?**
Neurolytic blocks refer to the injection of phenol, alcohol, or botulinum neurotoxin A (BoNT-A) for the focal relief of spasticity. Phenol and alcohol are cheap and widely available drugs that were extensively used in the past but have the disadvantage of causing tissue necrosis, scarring,

and painful dysesthesias in some children. Their use has largely been replaced by BoNT-A, which results in a temporary chemodenervation of muscle.

22. **How does Botox® work? What is it used for?**
BoNT-A is a highly purified preparation of a neurotoxin produced by *Clostridium botulinum* that binds with great affinity to the postsynaptic nerve terminal, interrupts the release of acetylcholine, and results in chemodenervation of muscle for 3–6 months. With time, normal nerve conduction is restored and full recovery of normal nerve conduction occurs. Side effects are dose-related and include weakness, temporary incontinence, and production of antibodies against the toxin. The principal use of botulinum toxin A in CP is for focal and temporary management of spasticity. The most common indication is to relieve spastic equinus. However, the majority of children will still develop an equinus contracture and ultimately will need orthopaedic surgery.

Botox® can also be used as a regional intervention in which multiple muscles at multiple levels are injected, including the gastrocsoleus, hamstrings, hip flexors, and hip adductors. Increased numbers of muscles mean increased doses and an increased risk of side effects. Other indications for Botox® include spastic muscle imbalance in the hemiplegic upper limb, postoperative protection of tendon transfers, and analgesia.

23. **What is the role of orthotic management in CP?**
The most commonly used orthosis in CP is the ankle-foot orthosis (AFO), which comes in a number of alignments providing variable degrees of support to the foot and ankle with different biomechanical principles. The more flexible AFOs (i.e., dynamic AFOs and hinged AFOs) are used in younger children in combination with injections of Botox® in the management of spastic equinus, equinovarus, and equinovalgus. The more rigid AFOs (i.e., solid AFO and ground-reaction AFO) are more frequently used in older children, especially after multilevel surgery. More extensive lower-limb bracing (i.e., knee-ankle-foot orthosis [KAFO] and hip-knee-ankle-foot orthosis [HKAFO]) are not effective in CP.

24. **What are assistive devices? What is their role in CP?**
Poor balance is one of the most important negative features of the UMN syndrome. When children with CP pull to stand, many require a walker, of which the wheeled posterior walker is the most popular and effective. With time and improvements in balance reactions, many children can graduate to a lesser level of support, and many learn to walk independently. A variety of crutches and walking sticks may help in the transition from the use of the posterior walker to independence. These devices are also very important in rehabilitation after major interventions for spasticity (in SDR and ITB) and also after multilevel orthopaedic surgery. In general, the child will want to use the least level of support consistent with not falling over and sustaining injury.

25. **When should a wheelchair be prescribed?**
Functional mobility is the ability to move safely and efficiently in the physical environment and to interact with the environment. For some children, this means an assistive device (i.e., a posterior walker or crutches), but for many it means a manual or powered wheelchair. Children with whole-body involvement (i.e., GMFCS levels IV and V) require a wheelchair for efficient interaction in the community and ease of transport by their parents. The acquisition of skills to control a powered wheelchair can be a significant milestone in achieving partial or complete independence for the more involved child.

26. **Is there a unified treatment or cure for CP?**
The central nervous system lesion in CP is by definition permanent and therefore incurable. However, the condition is variable in severity, and many children make rapid progress in the early years as part of the natural history. These improvements are often attributed to

various forms of early intervention and systems of therapy, including the Bobath method, neurodevelopmental treatment (NDT), Vötja, or educational systems such as conductive education (from the Peto Institute). All of these systems have their merit, but none of them have been shown in controlled trials to be superior to natural history or to each other. Curing CP will be achieved only when it is possible to replace lost neurons by tissue engineering. Stem cells can be induced to form neurons, but there is still a long way to go to engineer the complex circuits to repair extensive brain lesions. This will be the principal direction of future research, but, as yet, there are no convincing approaches for the direct repair of the brain lesion in CP. In the meantime, prevention of CP is clearly the most humane and cost-effective strategy.

27. **In spastic hemiplegia, what is the prognosis for function?**
Children with spastic hemiplegia are usually mildly involved, and the majority walk independently by 12–18 months. Many are so mild that diagnosis can be delayed until later in childhood (in GMFCS I and II).

28. **What are the upper-limb problems in spastic hemiplegia?**
Problems include astereognosis, weakness, impaired selective motor control hypertonia, and co-contraction. The most typical posturing in the upper limb includes adduction and internal rotation at the shoulder, elbow flexion, pronation of the forearm, wrist flexion, digital flexion, and flexion and adduction of the thumb (i.e., thumb-in-palm deformity).

29. **What is the role of spasticity management in the hemiplegic upper limb?**
Spastic posturing can be relieved by injection of spastic agonists with Botox®, including the biceps and brachialis for elbow flexion, pronator teres for pronation, flexor carpi ulnaris (FCU) and flexor carpi radialis (FCR) for wrist flexion, and the adductor pollicis, flexor pollicis longus (FPL), and flexor pollicis brevis for thumb-in-palm deformity. Improvement in joint range of motion and short-term functional gains can be achieved.

30. **What surgical procedures are useful in the hemiplegic upper limb?**
Surgical procedures are most useful for spastic hemiplegia and should rarely be used in patients with dystonia The most useful and reliable procedures are those designed to relieve elbow flexion (i.e., lengthening of biceps and brachialis), correction of pronation deformity (i.e., pronator teres release or rerouting), correction of wrist flexion deformity (i.e., the Green transfer of FCU to extensor carpi radialis brevis [ECRB] or FCR lengthening), and correction of the thumb-in-palm deformity by releasing the adductor pollicis and reinforcing thumb abduction by tendon transfers.

31. **Is upper-limb surgery in spastic hemiplegia of functional or cosmetic benefit?**
Surgery is effective in deformity correction, but functional gains are often limited by astereognosis, sensory deficits in the affected limb, and learned nonuse. However, improvements in cosmesis are extremely important for children with spastic hemiplegia, who are mostly in mainstream schooling and will later be in full-time employment. This is the main reason why the majority of adolescents are enthusiastic about the outcome of surgical reconstruction in the upper limb, whereas their parents see little change in the use of the limb or improvements in function.

32. **What are the gait problems seen in children with hemiplegia?**
Gait patterns can be classified according to the system described by Winters, Gage, and Hicks (Fig. 79-2). Types I and II involve the ankle only. In type III, involvement extends to the knee, and type IV, to the hip.
- **Type I:** Characterized by a drop foot during swing phase; an AFO can be useful

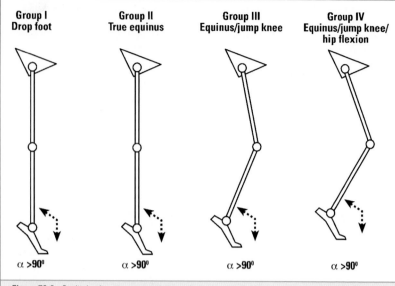

Figure 79-2. Sagittal gait patterns: spastic hemiplegia.

- **Type II:** Fixed equinus at the ankle; can be managed by gastrocsoleus lengthening (usually an Achilles tendon lengthening [TAL]) combined with an AFO
- **Type III:** Fixed equinus and a flexed stiff-knee gait
- **Type IV:** Similar to type III but includes involvement at the hip with hip flexion, adduction, and internal rotation. (Types III and IV can benefit from unilateral multilevel surgery.)
  These four types can be most accurately differentiated using instrumented gait analysis, but observing gait and clinical examinations identify most of these problems.

33. **What are the most common foot and ankle deformities in spastic hemiplegia?**
Equinus, equinovarus, and equinovalgus are the most common deformities in spastic hemiplegia. Spastic equinus can be managed by injection of Botox® and the use of an AFO. Fixed equinus results in toe walking and can be managed by lengthening of the Achilles tendon and the use of an AFO. Equinovarus is the result of imbalance between the inverters (i.e., the tibialis posterior and tibialis anterior) and the everters of the foot and ankle (i.e., the peroneals). The most reliable combination for fixed equinovarus is lengthening of the gastrocsoleus aponeurosis or Achilles tendon and intramuscular recession of tibialis posterior, combined with split anterior tibial tendon (SPLATT) transfer.

34. **What problems are associated with equinovalgus foot in spastic hemiplegia?**
Because children with spastic hemiplegia walk independently and are very active, equinovalgus deformities may result in excessive forefoot loading or hallux valgus and are difficult to brace. The valgus deformity is a passive phenomenon and is rarely related to spasticity in the peroneals, although adaptive shortening of peroneus brevis is common. The abducted-valgus foot deformity can be corrected by os calcis lengthening in combination with lengthening of the gastrocsoleus.

35. **Is there a role for multilevel surgery in spastic hemiplegia?**
Instrumented gait analysis has shown involvement at the knee and hip level in some patients with spastic hemiplegia that is amenable to a unilateral, multilevel surgical approach. Unilateral

multilevel surgery usually consists of correction of fixed equinus by lengthening of the gastrocsoleus, medial hamstring lengthening, and rectus femoris transfer for flexed stiff-knee gait, as well as lengthening of psoas over the pelvic brim and adductor longus combined with an external rotation osteotomy of the proximal femur.

36. **Does hip dislocation or scoliosis occur in spastic hemiplegia?**
Hip displacement is very uncommon in children with spastic hemiplegia. However, a number of children with the type IV involvement, according to Winters, Gage, and Hicks, develop hip displacement, usually between the ages of 6 and 12 years, which can lead to a painful subluxated hip and, rarely, to dislocation. Because hip displacement is uncommon in hemiplegia, it is not expected and often is diagnosed too late for optimal management. Early surgical correction is very effective (including lengthening of the adductor longus, lengthening of the psoas at the pelvic brim, and varus derotation osteotomy of the proximal femur). Scoliosis is uncommon in children with spastic hemiplegia. Most curves are postural and are due to shortening of the involved side and to limb length inequality.

37. **What is the difference between spastic diplegia and spastic quadriplegia?**
Spastic diplegia and spastic quadriplegia are bilateral types of CP. In spastic diplegia, the involvement is mainly in the lower limbs. However, there is usually some upper-limb involvement, with impairment of fine motor skills. In spastic quadriplegia, the upper-limb involvement is more severe and sometimes more pronounced than the lower-limb involvement. There is no clear separation between spastic diplegia and spastic quadriplegia. It is more important to categorize bilateral CP by gross motor function. Most children with spastic diplegia function at GMFCS levels I, II, or III. Most children with spastic quadriplegia function at GMFCS levels IV or V.

38. **What is the level of gross motor function in children with spastic diplegia?**
The majority of children with spastic diplegia can walk independently (GMFCS I or II), but a significant number require an assistive device (i.e., a walker or crutches) and use a wheelchair for longer distances in the community (GMFCS III).

39. **What gait patterns are seen in spastic diplegia?**
(Fig. 79-3). The principal patterns are jump gait and crouch gait; the other patterns are transitional. In jump gait, the child looks as if he or she is about to jump off a diving board. The child stands on tip-toes with hips and knees flexed. In crouch gait, the child looks as if he or she wants to avoid being seen by standing with reduced height, calcaneus (i.e., excessive dorsiflexion) at the ankle, and excessive flexion at the hip and knee.

40. **What musculoskeletal deformities are commonly found in spastic diplegia?**
Contractures of the main sagittal plane and muscles that cross two joints are common, including the gastrocnemius, the (medial) hamstrings, and the psoas. Contractures of single-joint muscles (i.e., the soleus, biceps femoris, and iliacus) are less common. Medial femoral torsion (with excessive or persistent femoral anteversion), lateral tibial torsion, and pes valgus are very common.

41. **Does hip dislocation or scoliosis occur in spastic diplegia?**
Hip displacement and dysplasia are common in children who need crutches or frames to walk but less common in those who walk unaided. Frank dislocation is less common because hip displacement is often detected during evaluation of gait dysfunction and is treated appropriately. Scoliosis is uncommon, is usually mild, and rarely requires intervention.

42. **What is the role of spasticity management in spastic diplegia?**
These patients walk on their toes because of spastic equinus and can be helped by Botox®, AFOs, serial casting, and physical therapy. A small number of children with severe, generalized lower-limb spasticity may be helped by SDR (see above).

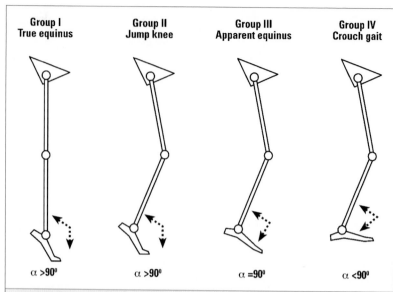

Figure 79-3. Sagittal gait patterns: spastic diplegia.

KEY POINTS: CEREBRAL PALSY

1. CP is a descriptive term for a large number of movement disorders that occur in infants. It is not a diagnosis.

2. Children with cerebral palsy can be managed but not cured. Management decisions for the child need to include consideration that physically disabled adults report that communication skills, activities-of-daily-living skills, and mobility skills rank higher than walking as important factors in their independence.

3. Children with cerebral palsy can have many health and cognitive issues that affect their management. Treatment of severely involved children is best done in a multidisciplinary setting, where all of these issues can be managed.

4. With increasing severity of cerebral palsy, more musculoskeletal abnormalities are present and indications for intervention and evidence for outcomes of treatment become less clear.

43. **Which is better for spastic equinus—Botox® injections or serial casting?**
Serial casting and Botox® injections are equally effective in the management of spastic equinus. The treatment effect is small and lasts for only 3–6 months. The main advantage is delaying surgery until multilevel surgery is an appropriate option.

44. **What is meant by single-level surgery and multilevel surgery?**
Surgery to correct gait deviations in children with CP was historically practiced at a single level, usually starting with the correction of equinus contractures at the ankle by lengthening of the

Achilles tendons. This usually resulted in crouch gait and had to be followed by distal hamstring lengthening a year or two later and then by lengthening of the psoas and transfer of the rectus femoris. The functional results were so poor that the patient or the surgeon simply gave up. Mercer Rang named this sequence the *birthday syndrome:* these children spent most of their birthdays in the hospital recovering from surgery.

It is now widely recognized that single-level surgery is the least efficient and most dangerous way to correct gait in CP. The principal risk is conversion of a functional toe-walking gait to a much less functional crouch gait. The effects of repeated operations, hospitalization, and periods spent in rehabilitation run counter to socially and developmentally appropriate pediatric care.

45. **What are the most important risk factors for crouch gait?**
    Crouch gait is part of the natural history of bilateral CP, spastic diplegia, and spastic quadriplegia. Iatrogenic factors are any intervention that weakens the gastrocsoleus, including any form of surgery for equinus, with percutaneous TAL as the worst offender. SDR, injections of Botox®, and the ITB pump can also increase the severity of crouch gait.

46. **What soft tissue and bony procedures are useful in gait correction surgery?**
    The principal muscle-tendon units, which work in the sagittal plane, are often contracted and may benefit from careful lengthening. These include the gastrocnemius, the medial hamstrings, and the psoas. In gait-correction surgery, muscle-tendon units are carefully lengthened in continuity; complete tenotomy is not appropriate, and aponeurotic or fascial lengthening is preferable to tendon lengthening. In hamstring lengthening, the lateral hamstrings rarely need to be lengthened. The most useful bony procedures are external rotation osteotomy of the femur for intoed gait and stabilization of the valgus foot by os calcis lengthening or subtalar fusion.

47. **What is the malalignment syndrome?**
    About one third of children with spastic diplegia who have medial femoral torsion of such severity to benefit from correction also have lateral tibial torsion. The combination of medial femoral torsion and lateral tibial torsion is sometimes called *malalignment syndrome* and, when severe, *malignant malalignment.* External rotation osteotomy of the femur alone will result in severely out-toed gait. Full correction requires four osteotomies: bilateral *external* rotation osteotomy of the *femurs* and bilateral *internal* rotation osteotomy of the *tibiae.* The supramalleolar region of the distal tibia is the best site for a rotational osteotomy of the tibia. Fixation can be achieved with crossed Kirschner (K) wires, a straight plate, or a "T" plate. Each option has advantages and disadvantages.

48. **How can the valgus foot be corrected?**
    Pes valgus commonly contributes to out-toed gait in spastic diplegia and may also be a major factor in the progression of severe crouch gait. Pes valgus can be managed effectively in most children using an AFO until age 6–8 years. After this age, AFOs are not effective and are not tolerated by most children. Surgical correction can be achieved by os calcis lengthening or subtalar fusion. Os calcis lengthening is effective for mildly involved children with mild foot deformities. Subtalar fusion is more effective and more durable for severely involved children with severe foot deformities. Autograft and allograft are equally effective for os calcis lengthening and subtalar fusion. Precise technique and stable fixation to permit early weight bearing are important.

49. **When are casts required after multilevel surgery?**
    Casts have been used too often and for too long. After lengthening of the psoas at the pelvic brim, casting is not required; prone positioning helps maintain correction of hip flexion deformity. Casting is usually not required after hamstring lengthening and rectus transfer surgery. Early mobilization using a removable knee extension splint is better than casting. Most foot and ankle surgery requires casting for about 6 weeks. However, early mobilization and

weight-bearing should be possible at 1–2 weeks after surgery. Femoral and tibial osteotomies should have stable internal fixation to avoid the need for prolonged casting and to permit early weight-bearing.

50. **Is the correction achieved by gait correction surgery permanent?**
Several long-term studies suggest that the results of multilevel surgery deteriorate between 1 and 5 years but that most of the correction is maintained.

51. **Does multilevel surgery in spastic diplegia improve function?**
There are no controlled clinical trials, but cohort studies suggest that walking speed and many gait parameters are improved by multilevel surgery.

52. **What is the level of gross motor function in spastic quadriplegia?**
Walking ability is very limited by weakness, poor balance, impaired selective motor control, spasticity, and musculoskeletal deformities. Some individuals can stand for transfers and can take a few steps with maximum help (GMFCS IV). Many lack head control and sitting balance (GMFCS V).

53. **What is the most efficient method of achieving mobility in the community in spastic quadriplegia?**
Wheeled mobility is very important in spastic quadriplegia at all ages. Younger children are transported in strollers or buggies. Many enjoy supportive walkers during childhood. Customized wheelchairs are very effective means for achieving mobility, and many modular and customized designs are available. When cognitive abilities and upper-limb function permit, electric-powered wheelchairs with customized hand controls offer independent mobility.

54. **What is the natural history in spastic quadriplegia?**
The incidence of medical comorbidities is high, and there is excessive mortality from a variety of causes. Major surgical interventions must be approached cautiously, with rigorous efforts made to stabilize medical comorbidities and to care for these children in a supportive multidisciplinary team setting.

55. **Does correction of deformities in spastic quadriplegia improve function?**
Not usually. The majority of individuals with spastic quadriplegia have severely impaired gross motor function, with GMFCS IV or V. Progressive musculoskeletal deformities may further impair function, but correction of deformities rarely improves function as much as parents and caregivers would hope. Spastic hip dislocation may result in pain, loss of transfer ability, and impaired sitting. Reconstructive surgery to relocate the hip can, at best, return the individual to the predislocation functional level.

56. **What are the main orthopaedic issues in spastic quadriplegia?**
Given the severe impairment of gross motor function, comfortable sitting is of great importance to the quality of life. The prerequisites for comfortable sitting are a straight spine, a level pelvis, and flexible and enlocated hips. In spastic quadriplegia, spastic hip displacement and scoliosis are very common and progressive and may cause severe deformity and impair function and quality of life.

57. **What is the cause of hip displacement in CP?**
Gross motor function, according to the GMFCS, accurately predicts the risk of hip displacement (Table 79-2).

58. **What is meant by screening for spastic hip disease (SHD)?**
Hip development is normal in children with CP at birth. This is followed by silent hip displacement until severe subluxation or dislocation occurs. Screening refers to a program of

TABLE 79-2. RISK OF HIP DISPLACEMENT ACCORDING TO THE GROSS MOTOR FUNCTION CLASSIFICATION SYSTEM (GMFCS) LEVEL

GMFCS level	Description	Hip Displacement (MP >30%)
I	Near-normal gross motor function	0%
II	Walks without aids, limited running	15%
III	Walks with aids	41%
IV	Stands for transfers, walking is very limited	70%
V	Lacks head control and sitting balance	90%

MP = migration percentage.

regular clinical examinations and radiographs to detect hip displacement when it is early, asymptomatic, and easily corrected by preventative surgery. A radiograph of the hips should be obtained by age 24 months, or earlier if there are signs of restricted hip abduction. A further radiograph should be obtained every 6–24 months, according to the child's risk profile, especially considering the GMFCS level and the migration percentage (MP) on the most recent radiograph.

59. **Why is hip displacement treated?**
Hip displacement may progress from silent displacement to painful degenerative arthritis, especially in more severely affected children. The effects of untreated hip displacement or dislocation are pain, impaired function, and a diminished quality of life. Ambulatory children (GMFCS II and III) may suffer a loss of walking ability, fixed deformity, and pain from degenerative arthritis or gait asymmetry because of hip dislocation. Nonambulatory children (GMFCS IV and V) may develop a painful degenerative arthritis over time and lose the ability to stand for transfers and to sit comfortably. For these children, the role of hip reconstruction is controversial.

60. **What are the treatment options for hip displacement?**
It is better to prevent hip displacement by lengthening of the hip adductors and flexors than to try to treat established hip dislocation. Preventive surgery is more effective in younger children who are at least partially ambulatory and have mild-to-moderate degrees of displacement. It may promote more normal hip development when hip displacement is mild. More severe displacement or dislocation may require the use of femoral and/or pelvic osteotomies to correct both femoral antetorsion and coxa valga, angular or rotational abnormalities, and acetabular dysplasia. For the severely affected child (GMFCS V), dislocated hips with severe degenerative changes may present too late for reconstructive surgery, especially in centers where systematic screening is not available. Such a child may require some form of resection arthroplasty of the proximal femur. Complications are common and relief of pain is often incomplete. Arthrodesis or valgus osteotomy may be used in carefully selected cases.

61. **Is a cast necessary after hip surgery in children with CP?**
In the past, hip spica casts were widely used, but the current trend is to avoid casts or to use them for shorter periods. Casts can cause severe complications including pressure sores, increased respiratory complications, an increased burden of care, and psychosocial difficulties. They may contribute to an increased risk of avascular necrosis. No-cast surgery requires

complete correction of all deformities, good soft tissue balance, and precise osteotomies with stable internal fixation. Increased care from physical therapists is required after no-cast surgery to ensure optimal positioning, to avoid recurrent contractures, and to optimize rehabilitation.

62. **Which children develop scoliosis? What types of curves are seen?**

Scoliosis, like hip displacement, is frequent in nonambulant children and GMFCS IV and V but is rare in ambulant children. An idiopathic-type curve is occasionally seen in a child with hemiplegia, but severe neuromuscular curves are found only in severely involved children. Neuromuscular curves are long thoracolumbar curves with pelvic obliquity and a tendency to early onset and rapid progression. The curves are much more severe in the sitting position than in the recumbent position (i.e., there is collapse under the influence of gravity). Thoracic kyphosis is very common because of weakness and collapse into flexion during sitting in severely involved children (GMFCS V). Dorsal kyphosis can be controlled by appropriate seating in many children, but some will require surgical correction. Lumbar lordosis occurs in association with severe hip flexion contractures, mainly in marginally ambulant children (GMFCS IV).

63. **What is the relationship between hip displacement and scoliosis?**

Hip displacement and scoliosis are frequent in the same subset of nonambulant children with CP and GMFCS levels IV and V. There is sometimes a clear temporal relationship among unilateral hip dislocation, pelvic obliquity, and scoliosis. In other cases, the relationship is not so clear. When hip dislocation and scoliosis coexist, there should be a careful analysis of the interaction between suprapelvic (i.e., spinal) deformity and infrapelvic (i.e., hip) deformity. A comprehensive plan to deal with all deformities needs to be developed for each child.

64. **What are the effects of progressive scoliosis?**

The most important consequences of progressive scoliosis are loss of function and impaired quality of life. Given that severe curves occur in the most severely involved children, loss of function can be difficult to determine, and we lack good tools to measure quality of life, however these are currently being developed. The principal adverse effect of severe spinal deformity is loss of sitting ability, which can be devastating for the child and for the caregivers. Comfortable sitting improves communication, self-esteem, hand function, and ease of transportation; it also preserves respiratory function and shortens feeding time.

65. **What is the role of bracing?**

Severe neuromuscular curves are difficult to brace, and bracing is not effective. Seating modifications may be a better option than bracing prior to surgery.

66. **What are the indications for surgical correction of spinal deformity?**

Documented curve progression and loss of function are the important indications for surgery. Loss of sitting function may be documented by reports from parents and caregivers in relation to a decreased ability to sit, reduced time spent sitting at school, increased discomfort and need for repositioning in the chair, frequent chair modifications, and pressure areas over the sacrum, ischial tuberosities, or greater trochanters.

67. **What are the principles of scoliosis surgery in CP?**

The children with the largest curves have the poorest general health and require multidisciplinary assessment and intensive management to successfully negotiate spinal surgery. Preoperative respiratory assessment and care, nutritional supplementation, and seizure control may make the difference between a successful outcome and a protracted postoperative course or postoperative mortality. Long neuromuscular curves need long instrumented fusions, usually from T2 to the pelvis. Preoperative curve severity and stiffness assessments will determine the choice between single-stage posterior surgery and combined anterior and posterior surgery in one or two stages.

68. Why are insufficiency fractures common in spastic quadriplegia?

Osteopenia is very common because of diminished weight bearing, reduced physical activity, and reduced muscle mass. Nutritional deficiencies include poor intake of calcium, vitamin D, and protein. Some medications for epilepsy (e.g., Valproate) have an anti-vitamin D effect. The presence of severe spasticity and fixed deformities may result in high torsional forces on the skeleton during activities of daily living and transfers. Fractures range from metaphyseal buckle fractures to diaphyseal fractures, which are usually spiral, displaced, and unstable. Fractures in children with spasticity result in severe pain because of increased spasms, and they may impair function and independence.

69. How can fractures in children with CP be managed?

Long-bone fractures require prompt reduction and internal fixation, usually with flexible, intramedullary nails. Plates in osteopenic bone and spastic limbs are sure to fail. Buckle fractures can be managed by well-padded casts or splints. Good pain and spasticity management are part of optimal fracture care.

BIBLIOGRAPHY

1. Bax M, Goldstein M, Rosenbaum P, et al: Proposed definition and classification of cerebral palsy. Dev Med Child Neurol 47:571–576, 2005.

2. Gage JR: The treatment of gait problems in cerebral palsy. In Clinics in Developmental Medicine, 2nd ed. New York, MacKeith Press, 2004.

3. Graham HK: Classifying cerebral palsy (On the other hand). J Pediatr Orthop 25:127–128, 2005.

4. Miller F, Dabney KW, Rang M: Complications in cerebral palsy treatment. In Epps CH Jr (ed): Complications in Pediatric Orthopaedic Surgery. Philadelphia, JB Lippincott, 1996, pp 477–544.

5. Rodda J, Graham HK, Carson L, et al: Sagittal gait patterns in spastic diplegia. J Bone Joint Surg 86B:251–258, 2004.

6. Scrutton D, Damiano D, Mayston M: Management of the motor disorders of children with cerebral palsy. In Scrutton D, Damiano D, Mayston M (eds): Clinics in Developmental Medicine, 2nd ed. New York, Mac Keith Press, 2004, pp 105–129.

7. Soo B, Howard J, Boyd RN, et al: Hip displacement in cerebral palsy: A population based study of incidence in relation to motor type, topographical distribution and gross motor function. J Bone Joint Surg 64A:121–129, 2006.

8. Winters TF, Gage JR, Hicks R: Gait patterns in spastic hemiplegia in children and young adults. J Bone Joint Surg 69A:437–441, 1987.

CHAPTER 80

SPINA BIFIDA

Selim Yalçin, MD, and Nadire Berker, MD

1. **What is spina bifida (SB)?**

   Spina bifida means "cleft spine," which is an incomplete closure in the spinal column. It is an all-encompassing term describing a group of congenital defects characterized by incomplete development of the brain, spinal cord, or their protective coverings, caused by the failure of the fetal spine to close properly during the first month of pregnancy. The synonyms are *neural tube defects, myelodysplasia,* and *spinal dysraphism.*

2. **What are the types of SB?**

   SB is classified into aperta (i.e., visible or open) lesions and occulta (i.e., hidden or invisible) lesions. Infants born with **spina bifida aperta** have an open lesion on their spine, with significant damage to the nerves and spinal cord. In **spina bifida occulta,** there is a fusion defect in one or more of the laminae of the vertebrae without apparent damage to the spinal cord. It does not cause any symptoms in the vast majority of those affected. Often, people only become aware that they have SB occulta after a lumbar spine radiography is taken for an unrelated problem. There are few cases of SB occulta, such as diastematomyelia and lipomas, in which malformation of fat, bone, or membranes causes incomplete paralysis with urinary and bowel dysfunction.

3. **What are the types of SB aperta?**

   - **Meningocele:** The sac in the child's back contains the meninges and the cerebrospinal fluid; there are no neural elements inside. Meningocele causes mild disability, but it is the least common form of SB.
   - **Myelomeningocele:** The sac in the back contains the spinal cord and nerve roots. In some cases, sacs are covered with skin; in others, tissue and nerves are exposed. This is the most severe and the most common form of SB. Generally, the terms *spina bifida* and *myelomeningocele* are used interchangeably.

4. **Why does it occur?**

   The exact cause of SB is unknown. It is suspected that genetic, nutrition, and environment factors play a role. SB is often associated with maternal folic acid deficiency, other teratogens, and genetic abnormalities. Maternal valproic acid use also impairs folic acid metabolism, increasing the risk of SB. The risk of having a second child with SB is 2–3%.

5. **What is the incidence?**

   SB aperta occurs in approximately 1 per 1000 live births, but there is marked racial and geographic variation. The incidence is decreasing in countries where improved prenatal screening and early termination of pregnancy are available. Decreases in the prevalence of SB have been reported since folic acid fortification of grain products began in 1990s. In developing countries, the numbers are increasing due to a relative lack of prenatal diagnosis, together with improved neonatal care that enables babies born with SB to survive.

6. **How is it diagnosed?**
   Ultrasound screening will show SB aperta at as early as 12 weeks of gestation. Abnormally high levels of maternal serum α-fetoprotein (AFP), measured at 16–18 weeks of pregnancy, may indicate a neural tube defect. Elevated AFP and acetylcholinesterase levels in amniotic fluid are highly suggestive of an open neural tube defect.

7. **Can it be prevented?**
   The risk of SB may be minimized through preconception and periconception folic acid intake. Spinal cord defects occur in the first 28 days of pregnancy, before the mother is aware that she is pregnant. Therefore, all women of childbearing age should receive 0.4 mg folate before conception and during early pregnancy. Early detection of SB will enable the parents to choose to terminate the pregnancy.

8. **What are the clinical findings?**
   There are no clinical findings in most babies with SB occulta. In some babies, however, there is an abnormal tuft, a hairy patch, a small dimple, or a birthmark on the skin, indicating spinal malformation. Babies born with myelomeningocele have a visible sac protruding from the spinal cord at the back. There is muscle weakness or paralysis and loss of sensation below the lesion level and also loss of bowel and bladder control. A large percentage (70–90%) of babies with myelomeningocele have hydrocephalus and Chiari's malformation. In toddlers and preadolescents, tethering of the spinal cord may lead to progressive neurologic deficit. Urologic findings are incontinence, infections, and hydronephrosis, leading to chronic renal failure. Children have multiple deformities of the extremities and the spine; pathologic fractures and pressure sores are frequently encountered. Obesity, psychosocial problems, upper-extremity dysfunction, mental retardation, and spasticity may add to the clinical picture.

9. **What is the treatment of hydrocephalus?**
   Hydrocephalus is controlled by a ventriculoperitoneal shunt.

10. **What is Chiari's malformation?**
    Caudal displacement of the cerebellum, along with kinking and elongation of the fourth ventricle and medulla, is known as Chiari II malformation. Nearly all children with SB aperta have this problem.

11. **What is tethered cord? How is it treated?**
    Tethered cord syndrome is stretching of the spinal cord due to an inelastic structure anchoring the caudal end of the spinal cord to the spine. The symptoms are change in bowel and bladder function, deterioration of functional status, increased lumbar lordosis, back and buttock pain, spasticity, foot deformities, and scoliosis. Approximately 25% of children with SB will develop symptoms related to a tethered cord. Tethering of the spinal cord should be suspected if the child demonstrates progressive neurologic deficit. Surgical untethering is performed to reverse the neurologic deficits; retethering occurs in 11–20%.

12. **What is the early treatment?**
    Neonatal management focuses on closure of the defect as early as possible and stabilization of cerebrospinal fluid (CSF) flow. If the fetus is diagnosed to have an open neural tube defect by maternal ultrasound, the baby should be delivered by cesarean section to minimize injury to the sac in the medical center, where the surgical closure will occur. The sac must be closed as soon as possible, and hydrocephalus must be treated also. Any infections must be dealt with aggressively. All congenital orthopaedic deformities must be treated according to state-of-the-art principles.

KEY POINTS: PRINCIPLES OF MANAGEMENT IN SPINA BIFIDA

1. Prevention of a deformity is always easier and more efficient than surgical correction.

2. Do not attempt surgical correction if the parents are not compliant with treatment because recurrence is inevitable.

3. Do not correct deformities if surgery will not increase function or improve patient care.

4. Spina bifida causes flaccid paralysis; therefore, braces are necessary for ambulation. The role of the orthopaedic surgeon is to keep the extremity malleable for bracing. In case of a contracture, release everything and put it in a brace.

---

13. **What are the principles of urologic treatment?**
    Neurogenic bladder in the neonate is evaluated by physical examination and abdominal ultrasound. Voiding cystourethrogram should be performed after 6 months of age. Intermittent catheterization is necessary if postvoiding residual urine volume is more than 20 mL. The child should be evaluated at regular intervals for urinary infection and changes in bladder function.

14. **How is the level of paralysis defined?**
    The motor innervation level does not always correlate with the level of vertebral abnormality. Moreover, it is difficult to estimate the actual level of voluntary movement in the infant because of ongoing reflex activity. The physician can obtain clues to discover the level of paralysis by observing the baby, asking the family, and palpating the muscles. The level of neurologic involvement can be defined more clearly as the child grows.

15. **How is the neurologic level determined?**
    Neurologic deficit may be of three types: complete paraplegia, asymmetric paralysis, and skip lesions. Children with skip lesions have few functioning muscles in the distal parts of the paralytic extremities.
    Neurologic levels are defined according to the most distal functional muscle. Only the intercostal and proximal paravertebral muscles are functional in upper thoracal involvement. Abdominal muscles are spared in lower thoracal involvement. Iliopsoas and hip adductor muscles are active in the upper-lumbar level. Quadriceps muscle activity is present in mid-lumbar involvement. Tibialis anterior and medial hamstrings are functional in the lower-lumbar level. Ankle plantar flexors are active in the sacral level. Sensory levels do not often correlate with motor levels.

16. **What is the expected prognosis according to the level of the lesion?**
    Babies with thoracic and upper-lumbar-level paralysis become wheelchair-dependent adults. Mid-lumbar-level babies have the potential to be household ambulators with high braces and walkers. Lower-lumbar-level lesions are expected to become functional ambulators using ankle-foot orthoses (AFOs) and crutches. Lower-lumbar and sacral-level patients are generally able to live independently. Children will fulfill their expected potential with judicious treatment and follow-up.

17. **What is the significance of sensory loss?**
    The most important problem caused by loss of sensation is skin breakdown. Loss of deep sensation leads to problems with balance and movement. It is necessary to teach children to compensate for decreased sensation by substituting other sensory modalities such as vision.

18. **What are the principles of follow-up and treatment?**
Children with SB need treatment by a multidisciplinary team consisting of a neurosurgeon, a urologist, a pediatric orthopaedic surgeon, a physiatrist, a physiotherapist, an orthotist, and certain other allied health professionals, depending on the patient's specific problems. Evaluation and follow-up should be scheduled at 3- to 6-month intervals, according to the patient's needs. Patients without significant problems need yearly follow-up visits. Management includes monitoring of shunt function, neurologic status, urinary infection, and reflux control; prevention and correction of orthopaedic deformities; exercises to prevent deformity and to gain function; and bracing and providing efficient mobility.

19. **What are the aims of orthopaedic surgery?**
Orthopaedic surgeons try to prevent and correct deformities that lead to improper posture, that create problems with bracing, and that cause skin breakdown.

20. **Should all deformities be corrected?**
Correction of deformity is indicated if it will result in ease of patient care, prevent skin breakdown, facilitate sitting and standing balance, help brace fitting, and facilitate ambulation.

KEY POINTS: PREVENTABLE COMPLICATIONS OF SPINA BIFIDA

1. Hip external rotation deformity

2. Hip flexion deformity

3. Knee flexion deformity

4. Ankle plantar flexion deformity

5. Pressure sores

6. Obesity

21. **What are the principles of muscle-tendon surgery?**
Tenotomies are usually preferred over tendon lengthenings and transfers. Recurrence is common after Achilles tendon lengthening, whereas simple Achilles tenotomy provides more reliable results. Tendon transfers have not been successful in controlling deformity or in gaining function.

22. **What is the role of osteotomy?**
Corrective osteotomies are preferred in knee flexion contractures because recurrence is likely after soft tissue releases at the knee joint. Furthermore, skin complications are common during the postoperative casting period after soft tissue releases. Supramalleolar or calcaneal osteotomies correct varus-valgus deformities and help provide a plantigrade foot while keeping the foot flexible. Soft tissue releases are preferred over osteotomies for hip flexion contractures.

23. **Is arthrodesis indicated?**
There is a high rate of pseudoarthrosis after arthrodesis at the foot. Furthermore, a rigid foot is not desirable since it is prone to develop pressure sores; therefore, arthrodesis is usually not a treatment option in SB.

24. **What are the types of spinal deformity? When do they occur?**
Lumbar hyperkyphosis, congenital vertebral anomalies such as formation and segmentation defects, and neuromuscular scoliosis.

Lumbar hyperkyphosis is present at birth and is relentlessly progressive. Congenital kyphosis and scoliosis can be seen on radiographs at birth, but the clinical deformity becomes obvious after a few years. Neuromuscular scoliosis develops in adolescence.

25. **What are the treatment principles in spine deformity?**
Lumber hyperkyphosis decreases survival because it leads to major pressure sores over the hump. The respiratory and the gastrointestinal system functions are compromised because they are restricted by the deformity. Kyphosis must be corrected early. Treatment principles in congenital kyphosis and scoliosis are the same as in children without SB. Correction is attempted with anterior or posterior (or both) hemiepiphysiodesis, which should be performed at around 2–3 years of age in order to prevent the defective vertebrae from increasing the deformity. Pediatric spinal instrumentation may improve the results in congenital spinal deformity. Spinal instrumentation is the treatment of choice in neuromuscular scoliosis.

26. **Do spinal orthoses work?**
Orthoses are contraindicated in hyperkyphosis due to their potential for skin breakdown. They do not prevent progression of deformity in congenital kyphosis and scoliosis, where deformity increases as the child grows. The use of spinal orthoses in neuromuscular scoliosis is controversial as they lead to chest-wall restriction and discomfort for the child. Modifications of the wheelchair and seating systems may be better options.

27. **Is early spinal fusion indicated?**
Early fusion is usually the best treatment option since all spinal deformities are progressive. The most important disadvantage of early spinal fusion is inhibition of spinal growth; however, it is not important for the child's torso to remain short after surgery. On the contrary, this can be considered desirable since children with short stature can handle the crutches better and have better sitting balance in the wheelchair.

KEY POINTS: UNPREVENTABLE COMPLICATIONS OF SPINA BIFIDA

1. Spine deformity

2. Hip dislocation

3. Genu valgum

4. Pes calcaneus

5. Fractures

28. **What are the causes of deformity in the lower extremities?**
Postural deformity, muscle imbalance, instability, fractures, and congenital deformities (mainly at the feet) result in multiple deformities of the lower extremities.

29. **What is the importance of posture?**
A child with SB needs an extension posture in order to stand and walk with the least amount of energy expenditure. The pelvis must be level, the hip and knee in neutral, and the feet

in plantigrade position. Flexion posture increases the energy cost of walking, thus impairing walking ability. The child with flexion posture usually needs a wheelchair.

30. **What are the problems of the hip?**
Typical problems of the hip are postural external rotation deformity, flexion contracture, and dislocation. External rotation deformity is common in babies with high-level lesions, whereas hip flexion contracture occurs in older children. The prevalence of hip dislocation is 20% in the L5 level, 35% in L4, and up to 70% in higher levels of involvement.

31. **Should a hip dislocation be treated?**
Most bilateral hip dislocations do not interfere with walking ability and are painless. Unilateral dislocations causing limb-length discrepancy and pelvic obliquity need to be treated in ambulatory children.

32. **Is hip flexion contracture important?**
Hip flexion contracture interferes with extension posturing and makes ambulation difficult. Proper positioning and exercises are necessary to prevent the development of hip flexion contracture in young children. Soft tissue releases are performed in the ambulatory older child.

33. **What are the problems at the knee joint?**
Knee flexion contracture and valgus deformity are the main problems at the knee joint. Flexion deformities are usually treated with distal femoral extension osteotomies—mild deformities respond to soft tissue surgery. Postoperative casting must be closely monitored to avoid skin breakdown.

34. **What are the principles of treatment in foot deformity?**
The insensate foot with deformities is typical for children with SB. The aim of treatment is to achieve a flexible plantigrade foot that can tolerate long-term bracing and weight-bearing without developing pressure sores. Try to prevent deformities with early bracing, positioning, and exercise. Prefer tenotomies over tendon transfers or lengthenings.

35. **Can children with SB walk?**
Quadriceps is the key muscle for functional ambulation. Children with neurologic involvement at L4 and below are able to become independent functional ambulators. Children with upper-lumbar involvement become household or limited-community ambulators with knee-ankle-foot orthoses (KAFOs), hip-knee-ankle-foot orthoses (HKAFOs), or reciprocating gait orthoses (RGOs); most of these children prefer wheelchairs for means of primary mobility after adolescence. Children with thoracal involvement can use parapodiums and RGOs for therapeutic ambulation.

36. **What determines walking ability?**
The most important factor determining walking ability is the neurologic level of involvement. The motivation of the child and family, the correction of the deformity, and proper bracing are also crucial. All children, including those with high levels of involvement, can walk using extensive braces. The golden years of ambulation are between 6 and 10 years of age. Increase in body weight and size in adolescence results in greatly increased energy expenditure during walking in thoracal and upper-lumbar–level children. Therefore, most adolescents with lesions at L3 and above prefer the wheelchair.

37. **Are fractures common?**
Fractures are seen in 20% of children with SB aperta because of osteopenic bones. The femur is the most common site of fracture. In the ambulatory patient, the reason is generally a fall or similar trauma. There is generally no history of trauma in the nonambulatory patient: the

child is brought to the physician because of a painless swelling in the leg. The swelling, erythema, and heat over the fracture site are commonly mistaken for an infection or tumor.

38. Do fractures need surgery?
No. Fractures usually heal quickly with simple splints and do not need surgery; however, splints and casts need close monitoring for early signs of skin breakdown.

39. What are the rehabilitation methods?
Rehabilitation methods consist of exercises, bracing, assistive devices, and education of families and patients. Range-of-motion and stretching exercises are used to prevent deformity, strengthening exercises may improve muscle strength in partially involved muscles, and coordination exercises are given to improve balance. Bracing and assistive devices help increase walking ability. Education of the patient and the family about the nature of the problems enable better compliance with treatment.

40. Why do we prescribe braces?
Braces are used to prevent deformity, support normal joint alignment, control the range of motion during gait, and facilitate function. Children with high-level lesions need a device that provides body support while facilitating extremity movement. A parapodium, a swivel walker, or an RGO is used for this purpose. For children with mid- and lower-lumbar lesions, a KAFO is sufficient, and sacral level patients use various AFOs.

41. What should we teach the families?
Since SB is a chronic problem with many different complications, families need to learn how to cope with the various issues that arise during growth and development. Teach the families the signs and symptoms of shunt dysfunction and tethered cord. Show them how to perform clean intermittent catheterization and home exercises. Guide them to supervise the diet of their baby, to establish a bowel routine, to practice preventive measures for skin breakdown, and to handle the brace properly. Family cooperation is essential for the success of most treatments.

42. Why is skin breakdown common?
Pressure sores are very common: almost all children with SB aperta have one or more sores by age 20 years. Causes are pressure over anesthetic skin sites, burns, dermatitis, ill-fitting braces, and friction due to creeping on the ground. Patients with mental retardation, hydrocephalus, kyphosis, chronic incontinence, and orthopaedic deformities are at high risk for a pressure sore.

43. How can pressure sores be avoided?
Teach the child and the family to take care of the skin by inspecting it regularly, keeping it clean and dry, and avoiding injury. Keep braces and spinal orthoses clean, and be very careful when putting them on for the first time. Use total-contact lower-extremity bracing to distribute the load evenly over a wider body area to minimize pressure build-up. Always have the caregiver check water temperature before bathing the baby.

44. How common is latex allergy? Why does it occur?
Allergic reactions to latex are common in patients with SB. The incidence varies between 28% and 67%. Chronic and frequent exposure to latex products because of catheter use or multiple surgeries may be a cause of this problem. Patients with SB who require surgery should be protected by a latex-free environment.

45. Why are some of these children obese?
Paralysis of muscle results in a decrease in lean body mass and, therefore, reduced energy expenditure. The basal metabolic rate is low. Children with high-level lesions have markedly

decreased bodily activity and decreased body mass; therefore, they are more prone to obesity than children with low lumbar and sacral-level lesions. Weight reduction is extremely difficult; therefore, prevention by dietary intervention is absolutely necessary.

46. Is intelligence normal?
Children without hydrocephalus and infections have normal intelligence. Repeated central nervous system infections and shunt malfunction cause decreased mental function, particularly in children with high-level lesions. In general, the higher the level of lesion, the poorer the mental state.

47. Are the upper extremities normal?
Upper-extremity dysfunction may be present in children with SB because of several reasons. Children have to use their upper extremities for support and balance; therefore, they have difficulty manipulating and exploring with their hands. Chiari II malformation may result in cerebellar ataxia, and hydrocephalus causes pyramidal tract damage, both of which contribute to upper-extremity dysfunction.

BIBLIOGRAPHY

1. Broughton NS, Menelaus MB, Cole WG, Shurtleff DB: The natural history of hip deformity in myelomeningocele. J Bone Joint Surg 75B:760–763, 1993.

2. Carroll NC: Assessment and management of the lower extremity in myelodysplasia. Orthop Clin North Am 18:709–724, 1987.

3. Detrait R, George TM, Etchevers HC, et al: Human neural tube defects: Developmental biology, epidemiology, and genetics. Neurotoxicol Teratol 27:515–524, 2005.

4. Diaz-Llopis I, Bea Munoz M, Martinez Agullo E, et al: Ambulation in patients with myelomeningocele: A study of 1500 patients. Paraplegia 31:28–32, 1993.

5. Lintner SA, Lindseth RE: Kyphotic deformity in patients who have a myelomeningocele. Operative treatment and long-term follow-up. J Bone Joint Surg 76B:1301–1317, 1994.

6. Marshall PD, Broughton NS, Menelaus MB, Graham HK: Surgical release of knee flexion contractures in myelomeningocele. J Bone Joint Surg 78B:912–916, 1996.

7. Mazur JM, Shurtleff DB, Menelaus MB, Colliver J: Orthopaedic management of high level spina bifida: Early walking compared with early use of a wheelchair. J Bone Joint Surg 71A:56–61, 1989.

8. Molnar GE, Murphy KP: Spina bifida. In Molnar GE, Alexander MA (eds): Pediatric Rehabilitation, 3rd ed. Philadelphia, Hanley & Belfus, 1999, pp 219–244.

9. Noonan KJ: Myelomeningocele. In Morissy RT, Weinstein RT, Weinstein SL (eds): Lovell and Winter's Pediatric Orthopaedics, 6th ed. Philadelphia, Lippincott, Williams & Wilkins, 2006, pp 605–647.

10. Ozaras N, Yalcin S: Spina Bifida Tedavi ve Rehabilitasyon. Istanbul, Turkey, Avrupa Medical Publishing, 1999.

11. Schoenmakers MA, Gooskens RH, Gulmans VA, et al: Long-term outcome of neurosurgical untethering on neurosegmental motor and ambulation levels. Dev Med Child Neurol 45:551–555, 2003.

CHAPTER 81

MUSCULAR DYSTROPHY

Michael Sussman, MD

1. **What is Duchenne's muscular dystrophy (DMD)?**

   DMD is the most common heritable disease of muscle. Boys affected with this condition show progressive deterioration in motor function. They will cease walking in the preteen years and ultimately die of the disease by age 20. Characteristic histologic and immunohistochemical changes are seen in muscle tissue obtained from biopsy, and there is also a genetic marker for the disease. The basis for DMD is a complete absence of the protein dystrophin in muscle.

2. **What is Becker's muscular dystrophy (BMD)?**

   BMD is also a heritable muscular dystrophy and is allelic with DMD (i.e., the defect resides on the same gene). The muscle has similar histologic morphology to DMD on standard hematoxylin and eosin (H&E) and adenosine triphosphatase (ATPase) stains. Patients with BMD have a later onset of the disease process and a milder clinical course. In some cases, boys may retain the ability to walk throughout the second decade. There is much more heterogeneity in the age of onset and clinical course as compared with DMD. Although it is histologically indistinguishable from DMD using standard muscle stains, it can be distinguished by immunohistochemical staining for dystrophin and more precisely by a Western blot analysis of muscle tissue, which will show a complete absence of dystrophin in DMD and a reduced quantity of a smaller molecular weight dystrophin in BMD.

3. **What is the difference between Duchenne's and Becker's muscular dystrophy, limb-girdle muscular dystrophy, and other muscular dystrophies and myopathies?**

   The other muscular dystrophies have different clinical courses, sites of involvement, and prognosis, as well as different molecular and genetic basis. Dystrophin is normal in all other muscle diseases, although abnormalities in dystrophin associated proteins are responsible for other diseases, particularly limb girdle dystrophy. Myopathies are nonprogressive, whereas most dystrophies are progressive.

4. **What is the inheritance pattern in DMD?**

   It has been recognized since the 1950s that Duchenne's and Becker's muscular dystrophy affect only boys and are therefore both X-linked recessive conditions. There is a 15% spontaneous mutation rate. A female carrier will pass the disease to half of her male children and the carrier state to half of her female children. The incidence is 1:3500 male live births.

5. **What is the molecular basis of Duchenne's and Becker's muscular dystrophy?**

   Both Duchenne's and Becker's muscular dystrophy are due to abnormalities in or absence of the protein dystrophin. Dystrophin is one of a family of proteins that stabilize the muscle cell (i.e., myofiber) membrane. Dystrophin is a very large protein with a molecular weight of 427 kD (collagen is 300 kD), and its gene constitutes a full 1% of the X chromosome. Although the absolute quantity of dystrophin within the myofiber is relatively small compared to the actin and myosin muscle proteins, this small quantity of dystrophin provides a very important stabilizing function for the myofiber membrane. Several consequences result from the absence or abnormality of dystrophin, as follows:

- Dystrophin physically stabilizes the myofiber membrane. In its absence, muscle contraction, particularly eccentric contraction, causes the membrane to become disrupted, and cellular contents, including proteases, leak out into the extracellular space, inducing an inflammatory reaction and subsequent fibrosis. This process also leads to progressive necrosis of muscle fibers.
- In the absence of dystrophin, the metabolic activity of the cell is disrupted. Ultimately, myofibers work at decreased efficiency because of the inability to provide energy for the contractile mechanism.
- The regenerative capacity of muscle to replace necrotic muscle fibers is significantly diminished in the absence of dystrophin.
- A number of dystrophin-associated proteins (DAPs), including sarcoglycans, dystroglycans, and others, are critical for muscle cell function and the interaction of the myofiber with the structural connective tissue network. In the absence of dystrophin, these DAPs are not incorporated into the myofiber and extracellular matrix network, thereby further altering normal muscle function.

6. **What is the genetic basis for the abnormality of dystrophin in Duchenne's and Becker's muscular dystrophy?**
   Several types of gene mutations result in abnormalities in dystrophin, which in turn are responsible for DMD and BMD (which are called *dystrophinopathies*):
   The most common abnormality, which accounts for two thirds of the cases, is a large deletion from the genetic material of the dystrophin gene. In DMD, the deletions interrupt the normal triplet reading frame so that when the gene is respliced, all of the downstream sequence becomes nonsense and no dystrophin whatsoever is produced. In BMD, the deletions are usually in a noncoding region (i.e., an intron) and do not disrupt the reading frame. When the gene is respliced, the reading frame is maintained, but a reduced quantity of a smaller-than-normal dystrophin is produced. This truncated dystrophin protein has some function, but not normal function, accounting for the milder clinical course of patients with BMD.
   - In 15–20% of patients with DMD, a single point mutation within a coding sequence results in a premature stop codon, which causes cessation of dystrophin synthesis. This resultant incomplete protein is degraded, and no dystrophin whatsoever is produced.
   - Point mutations occur, which may alter splicing sequences within the gene, which in turn may result in either absence of dystrophin (thereby causing DMD) or synthesis of a shortened protein (thereby causing BMD). There may be also gene duplications in rare cases.

7. **How can the genetic abnormality be ascertained?**
   The specific genetic abnormality can be identified in 95% of cases by DNA analysis from a blood sample. Currently clinical laboratories at the University of Utah and Baylor University can provide deletion analysis as the first step, which will provide an absolute diagnosis for two thirds of patients. If nothing is found on this analysis, these laboratories then proceed to complete sequencing of the gene. Using this approach, 95% of patients with Duchenne's and Becker's dystrophy can be accurately diagnosed based on DNA analysis from a blood sample.

8. **What are the clinical signs of DMD?**
   Because of the relative rarity of this condition, the clinician must have a high index of suspicion in order to make the diagnosis. A positive family history should raise the index of suspicion, and the diagnosis will be made early in life. In patients without a family history, however, diagnosis may be significantly delayed. It has been shown by Read and Galasko that the mean delay between the time that patients present to the orthopaedic surgeon and the time of diagnosis averages 2 years. The disease should be suspected in the following circumstances:
   - A male child does not walk by the age of 18 months, with no other obvious reason, such as cerebral palsy, to explain delay in acquisition of this developmental milestone.
   - The patient shows not only delayed walking, but also delayed acquisition of other motor skills such as ascending and descending stairs.
   - The boy has enlargement of the calves, a condition known as *pseudohypertrophy*.

- The boy uses Gowers' maneuver in rising from the floor (see question 9).
- The boy is unable to do "wheelbarrow walking." This indicates significant weakness of the shoulder girdle and the proximal muscles of the upper extremities.
- Unlike neurologic diseases, in which deep tendon reflexes are lost relatively early in their course, in DMD, deep tendon reflexes continue to be present until the muscle becomes too weak to respond.

9. **What is Gowers' maneuver? What does it indicate?**
   Gowers' maneuver (Fig. 81-1) is the motor process used by a child with weak pelvic girdle musculature to arise from a sitting position on the floor. It involves several components, as follows:
   - The sitting child will assume the prone position, on hands and knees.
   - The child will then extend the knees and, with the hands still on the floor, will assume a quadruped or "bear" type of position.

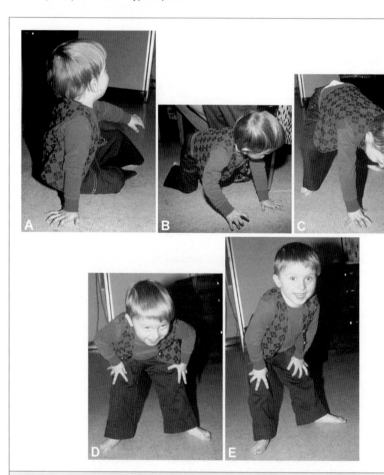

Figure 81-1. Gowers' maneuver. **A,** Patient is sitting on the floor. **B,** Patient rolls over into the prone position on the hands and knees. **C,** Patient rises in the "bear" position. **D,** Patient uses the upper extremities to keep the knees extended and to move the trunk upright on the lower body. **E,** Patient finally achieves the upright position.

- Following this, to bring the trunk into the upright position, as well as to help maintain knee extension, the child will use the hands to "walk up" the leg until the upright position is finally achieved.

It is difficult to do manual muscle testing in young children, and Gowers' maneuver is an excellent screening test for significant muscle weakness. It is found universally in boys with DMD; however, it is not specific for DMD and may be seen in other conditions causing weakness of the pelvic girdle muscles.

10. **If one suspects muscular dystrophy based on clinical findings, what laboratory studies can be used to confirm the diagnosis?**
    - **Creatine kinase (CK):** If muscular dystrophy is suspected, blood should be drawn and levels of CK should be measured. This is a universally available and inexpensive test. The normal range is 0–250 U/L, whereas in patients with DMD or BMD, levels will be 10,000 U/L or greater. Equivocal elevations of CK are not indicative of DMD or BMD but may indicate the presence of other dystrophies such as limb-girdle dystrophy. The CK test is not specific, and significant elevations may be found in some cases of limb-girdle dystrophy as well as in inflammatory myopathies such as dermatomyositis and polymyositis and in some forms of congenital muscular dystrophy.
    - **Other muscle enzymes:** Other muscle enzymes such as aspartate aminotransferase (AST) and lactate dehydrogenase (LDH) are also elevated in dystrophinopathies, and unnecessary liver studies should be avoided.
    - **DNA analysis:** If the CK is elevated to greater than 5000 and the clinical history is consistent with DMD or BMD, a blood sample should be drawn and sent for DNA analysis. If these studies are positive, no further diagnostic studies will be necessary.
    - **Electromyography (EMG) and nerve conduction studies (NCV):** These studies are no longer indicated in the diagnostic evaluation of children with suspected DMD or BMD. NCV may be indicated in patients with suspected peripheral neuropathy.
    - **Muscle biopsy:** This is no longer necessary for diagnosis in most patients but may be necessary in the 5% of cases that cannot be diagnosed by DNA testing. If a muscle biopsy is done, be certain that the specimen is flash frozen or sent immediately to a laboratory with experience in muscle disease. All specimens should have a Western blot done for dystrophin in addition to immunohistochemical stains (Figs. 81-2, 81-3).

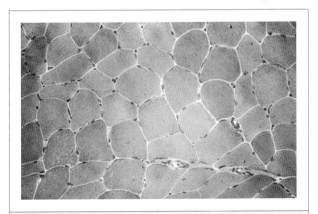

Figure 81-2. Section of normal muscle.

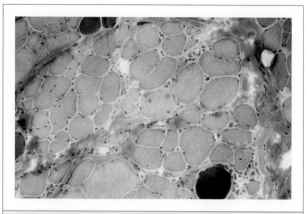

Figure 81-3. Section of muscle from a patient with relatively advanced Duchenne's muscular dystrophy (DMD) showing irregularity in the diameter of muscle fibers, central nuclei, evidence of necrosis, and intramuscular fibrosis.

11. **What is the differential diagnosis for a 3- to 5-year-old boy with significant muscle weakness?**
    - DMD
    - Childhood-onset type III spinal muscular atrophy (SMA)
    - Dermatomyositis
    - Emery-Dreifuss dystrophy
    - Limb-girdle muscular dystrophy
    - Other myopathies (various myopathies have characteristic changes on either standard histologic or ultrastructural studies, but they are generally nonprogressive)

12. **What is SMA?**
    SMA is an autosomal recessive condition due to an abnormality of the survival motor neuron genes, located on chromosome 5. In this condition, anterior horn cells are progressively lost, resulting in progressive flaccid muscle weakness. Patients with type III SMA walk until age 5–20 and have a variable life span thereafter, dependent on pulmonary function. Type III SMA is the second most prevalent disease causing progressive weakness in childhood and can usually be distinguished from DMD on clinical examination. SMA patients will show atrophy rather than pseudohypertrophy and will have loss of reflexes early in the course of the disease. In addition, because of muscle irritability, spontaneous contractions occur. These can be most readily seen in the tongue as constant fasciculations and in the fingers as a fine tremor at rest (they are seen on EMG as fibrillations).

13. **What is dermatomyositis?**
    Dermatomyositis is an inflammatory disease of the muscle of unknown cause. Unlike the insidious onset of DMD, dermatomyositis has a relatively acute onset of muscle weakness. It is associated with a malar rash, elevated serum CK, and an elevated erythrocyte sedimentation rate. Specific abnormalities will be seen on EMG. Absolute diagnosis may be made by skin and muscle biopsy, which will show the characteristic changes of perivascular inflammation and muscle necrosis. Many of these patients have spontaneous remission or respond to corticosteroid treatment, but some patients will continue to progress to severe and chronic involvement. This disease does not have any genetic association.

14. **What is Emery-Dreifuss dystrophy?**

    Patients with Emery-Dreifuss dystrophy may appear similar to those with DMD but will have normal dystrophin and will not show the characteristic changes on muscle biopsy of patients with DMD. They do not have calf enlargement (i.e., pseudohypertrophy) and present within the first decade of life with progressive weakness. The deterioration in function is slower than in patients with DMD. The hallmark of this condition is the early onset of flexion contractures at the ankles and elbows and extension contractures in the posterior cervical area, causing progressive neck extension with loss of neck flexion. This is also an X-linked condition, and it has been shown to result from abnormalities in the muscle-cell nuclear-membrane-associated protein emerin. A DNA test is available.

15. **What is limb-girdle muscular dystrophy?**

    Limb-girdle muscular dystrophy is actually a group of muscular dystrophies with different ages of onset and different rates of progression and outcome. Affected individuals will have a mildly to markedly elevated CK level, normal dystrophin, and dystrophic changes on muscle biopsy, but not those histologic changes characteristic of DMD. These patients may show abnormalities in other muscle-cell-membrane-associated proteins, such as adhalin and the sarcoglycans, which can be of diagnostic significance. These are usually autosomal recessive conditions, and about 50% can be more specifically diagnosed by detecting abnormalities of specific DAPs in the muscle.

16. **What is the natural history in the first decade of DMD?**

    Affected patients will walk late, usually after the age of 18 months, and will never walk completely normally. Patients will develop an abductor lurch and increasing lumbar lordosis as time progresses. Between age 7 and 9 years, increasing quadriceps weakness results in loss of the initial knee flexion wave, with weight acceptance best ascertained using computer-based gait analysis. This means that when the swing phase limb lands at the beginning of stance phase, there will be no flexion of the knee to absorb the shock and diminish the vertical motion of the pelvis. This adaptation accommodates for the weak quadriceps, which could not support body weight if knee flexion were allowed. The gait becomes slower, and ultimately the ability to walk is lost between the ages of 9 and 12 years.

17. **How can the end of walking ability be predicted?**

    Continued ability to walk can be determined by utilizing a 30-foot timed walk at the patient's maximum walking speed. McDonald and others have demonstrated that if this 30-foot walk requires more than 12 seconds, the patient will lose the ability to walk within 1 year. If the course takes between 6 and 12 seconds, the patient will lose walking ability within 2 years, and less than 6 seconds correlates with more than 2 years of walking ability left.

18. **How does joint contracture affect the ability to ambulate?**

    Most patients will develop Achilles tendon contracture by age 6 or 7 years, as indicated by limitation of passive dorsiflexion at the ankle only to neutral. Boys will walk in equinus, but this Achilles tightness provides a ground reaction force, which helps to maintain knee extension during stance phase. Mild to moderate degrees of equinus will help stance phase stability due to the knee extension moment created by the ground reaction force of the plantar-flexed foot. As patients reach the end of the ambulatory phase, they will develop minor degrees of knee flexion contracture, and the combination of weak quadriceps and knee flexion contracture may contribute to their loss of walking ability. All patients will also have significant degrees of hip flexion contracture and will accommodate to this by increasing their lumbar lordosis.

19. **Can functional walking be prolonged with bracing or surgery?**

In most cases, significant contractures do not develop until after the child no longer has the ability to ambulate. Therefore, contracture release is rarely beneficial in prolonging ambulation. Prophylactic surgery to lengthen hamstrings at age 6–7 years has been advocated, primarily in Europe, but the outcomes following this surgery do not appear to be significantly different than controls.

Knee-ankle-foot orthoses (KAFOs) have also been advocated and may be helpful for transfers in a few patients but are generally rejected as being too cumbersome and not providing a functional gait.

Rigid ankle-foot orthoses (AFOs) used at night will delay onset and progression of equinus deformity and are best instituted when passive dorsiflexion is limited to 10 degrees or less, which usually occurs between age 5 and 7 years. However, AFOs should not be recommended for daytime use in the ambulatory patient since, by constraining ankle motion, they will make walking much more difficult.

20. **What is the natural history of patients once they become full-time wheelchair users?**

At about age 9–12 years, most boys with DMD will lose the ability to walk and will become full-time wheelchair users. At this time, they should have a manual chair as well as a power chair for mobility. Because of upper-extremity weakness, a manual chair is not practical for independent use but is more easily transportable than a power chair for dependent mobility during trips in the community. A power chair provides independent mobility and should be obtained for all patients.

21. **When does scoliosis become a problem?**

At the time that patients become full-time sitters, they also begin to develop scoliosis. These curvatures progress despite any nonoperative intervention, including bracing and special seating, and will progress to severe degrees of deformity, resulting in loss of comfort and sitting balance, as well as compromise of pulmonary function.

22. **What is the best treatment for spinal deformity in patients with DMD?**

Since bracing and seating are not efficacious in preventing curve progression, and once curves appear they almost always continue to progress to a severe disabling degree, it is generally agreed that once patients begin to develop a curve and the curvatures reach the range of 20 degrees, spinal instrumentation and fusion should be undertaken to prevent further curve progression and to provide long-term sitting stability. Segmental fusion techniques should be used since the bone is osteoporotic, and attention should be paid to maintaining thoracic kyphosis, which will benefit head control. Although there is some controversy regarding the lowest level of fusion, several studies have demonstrated that fusion to L5 is sufficient in patients with mild curves <30 degrees associated with milder degrees of pelvic obliquity of <10 degrees.

23. **Do all boys with DMD develop scoliosis?**

No, 5–10% of boys with DMD will not develop scoliosis; in these patients, a total thoracolumbar lordosis pattern develops, which seems to stabilize the spine and protect it from the development of scoliosis.

24. **Once spinal fusions are done, what particular orthopaedic needs require attention?**

Following spinal fusion, patients may be taller and have difficulty getting in and out of the family van with a ramp because of the increased height. In addition, because the head is at a higher level and spinal mobility has been lost, some patients may have problems with self-feeding, and adaptations will need to be introduced to maintain the ability to self-feed.

25. **What is the usual cause of death?**
By age 17–18 years, the forced vital capacity (FVC) is usually in the range of 20–30%, and the expiratory pressure with cough is markedly diminished. Chronic pulmonary failure may occur due to hypoventilation. The usual situation is onset of a respiratory illness, which causes acute and rapid decompensation and death if the patient is not aggressively managed with intubation. Some patients and families, however, choose not to elect this treatment since, once intubated, most boys require continued positive pressure ventilation with a tracheostomy. Alternatively, ventilatory support may be provided by noninvasive techniques in boys experiencing chronic respiratory failure, as evidenced by hypoxemia and hypercarbia.

26. **What other organ systems are affected in DMD?**
In addition to skeletal muscle, dystrophin is found in cardiac muscle, smooth muscle, and brain tissue, which accounts for involvement in the following areas:
- Pulmonary function deteriorates due to weakness and contracture of the ventilatory muscles beginning in the early teen years.
- Cardiac function is affected, as documented by a decreasing ejection fraction beginning in the early teens.
- Gastric dilatation, as well as chronic constipation, may occur in teenagers, presumably due to smooth muscle dysfunction.
- Cognitive function overall is diminished, particularly in verbal expressive areas, although some patients may have normal or better cognition.

27. **Will any currently available medical intervention alter the natural history of DMD?**
Yes! Daily administration of corticosteroids will significantly and dramatically alter the natural history of DMD. This was initially demonstrated in the early 1990s by using prednisone at a dose of 0.75 mg/kg in a relatively short-term study that showed maintenance of muscle strength in the treated patients versus controls. A subsequent, much longer-term study showed that Deflazacort (which is similar to prednisone) at a dose of 0.9 mg/kg/day markedly alters the natural course of the disease. In this study, one third of treated patients continued to walk at age 18 years, whereas none of the untreated patients walked past age 12 years. The deterioration in pulmonary function was significantly reduced so that the FVC of treated patients was 73% at age 18 versus 33% in the controls. Alternate dosing patterns, such as reduced dosage and alternate-day doses, do not seem to be as effective as daily dosage in the prescribed amounts; however, there are ongoing studies using alternative dosing regimens in hopes of achieving a maximum benefit with reduced side effects. Administering higher-than-recommended dose does not have any greater beneficial effects. Deflazacort, although available in Europe, is not available in Canada or the United States.

28. **What are the side effects of corticosteroid administration?**
The major side effects of corticosteroid administration are weight gain, behavioral changes, and linear growth retardation resulting in reduction of adult height. Some patients gain significant amounts of weight, whereas others do not seem to show any influence on weight from the corticosteroids. As a group, however, the weight gain is much less for patients on Deflazacort than patients on prednisone, which seems to be the main advantage of Deflazacort. Patients started on Deflazacort beginning at age 7 years lose an average of 10 inches (23 cm) of height. Patients may also experience behavioral changes and exhibit aggressive behaviors. The behavioral effects may be minimized by giving the medication in the evening and tend to become less pronounced with time.

KEY POINTS: MUSCULAR DYSTROPHY

1. Duchenne's muscular dystrophy (DMD) is an X-linked, recessive disease resulting in progressive deterioration of muscle and replacement with fibrofatty tissue. The clinical course is very predictable, resulting in loss of ambulation between the ages of 10 and 12 years and death due to respiratory insufficiency, usually by age 20.

2. When the diagnosis of DMD is suspected by clinical examination, the creatinine kinase (CK) level in the blood should be checked. The diagnosis is likely if the level is >10,000 U/L and can be firmly established by DNA studies from a blood sample, which will provide an absolute answer in 95% of cases. Muscle biopsy and electromyography (EMG) are rarely, if ever, indicated for diagnosis.

3. The disease is due to an absence of the muscle-membrane-associated protein dystrophin, which in turn is due to an abnormality in the gene, located on the X chromosome. In two thirds of cases, this abnormality is inherited from an asymptomatic mother, and in one third it is a new mutation.

4. Scoliosis occurs in 90% or more of affected boys, with onset usually at the second decade. If untreated, curves will progress to life-altering degrees. The recommended treatment is early instrumentation and fusion before the curves become severe.

5. Corticosteroid treatment in pharmacologic doses can remarkably alter the natural history of DMD. Patients who receive regular doses of corticosteroid beginning in childhood may walk until the late teens and will have significant preservation of pulmonary and cardiac function. Side effects, however, are significant, the major ones being obesity, loss of height (up to 12 inches), behavioral changes, and, in some cases, asymptomatic cataracts.

---

29. **Does the use of corticosteroids reduce the risk of developing scoliosis?**
    Yes. In a study of 72 patients in Toronto, 91% of patients who were not treated developed significant scoliosis, whereas only 11% of Deflazacort-treated patients developed significant scoliosis. However, these patients need to continue to be followed to ensure that scoliosis does not develop in the later teenage years.

30. **Does the use of corticosteroids alter the accepted treatment paradigm for early surgical treatment of scoliosis in DMD patients?**
    Although it is not clear at this point, it would be the author's recommendation that patients with small curvatures continue to be followed through and past skeletal maturity without the early intervention strategy recommended for non-steroid-treated patients. Since pulmonary function seems to be well maintained in these patients, surgery, even at later stages of the disease, may be less risky.

31. **Does use of corticosteroids affect other organ systems?**
    Yes. Cardiac function and pulmonary function are significantly better in treated patients than in those not receiving corticosteroid treatment.

32. **Are other medications beneficial to DMD patients?**
    Lisinopril, which is an angiotensin-converting enzyme (ACE) inhibitor, also has been shown to significantly improve cardiac function in teenage patients with DMD.

33. **Are there other potential treatments that may become available in the foreseeable future?**

Yes. Two of these are in early clinical trials:

- **Myostatin inhibition:** Myostatin is a normally circulating cytokine that inhibits muscle cell proliferation. Currently under trial is an antibody to myostatin that blocks its activity, therefore allowing for enhanced muscle regeneration.
- **Stop code inhibition:** PTC-124, an analog of gentamycin, has been shown to inhibit certain premature stop codons in animal models and in some patients who have this genetic defect. Trials are currently under way to see if this approach may be effective in DMD patients.

  In addition, a variety of genetic approaches are under investigation:
- The use of antisense oligonucleotides to block the abnormal region of the gene, allowing resplicing and synthesis of a truncated, but partially functional, dystrophin
- Upregulation of utrophin, which is very similar to dystrophin and may substitute for it
- Introduction of a normal dystrophin gene: this is the ultimate goal and will provide a complete cure for DMD; however, given the large size of the gene, this presents great technical hurdles

34. **Are there other medical complications of which orthopaedic surgeons should be aware?**

Yes. A **malignant hyperthermia-like response to general anesthesia** may occur in DMD or BMD patients, so halogenated hydrocarbon anesthetics and succinylcholine should be avoided and intravenous sodium dantrolene should be available for treatment if a malignant hyperthermia event occurs.

35. **What is the Muscular Dystrophy Association (MDA)?**

The MDA is a charitable organization that has raised a tremendous amount of funds for both research and treatment of patients with DMD and BMD, as well as other neuromuscular diseases. One of their most important services to patients is a yearly week-long summer camp that is held at multiple sites throughout the United States for patients with these conditions. There are similar organizations in other countries.

BIBLIOGRAPHY

1. Alman BA, Raza SN, Biggar WD: Steroid treatment and the development of scoliosis in males with Duchenne muscular dystrophy. J Bone Joint Surg 86A:519–524, 2004.
2. Biggar WD, Harris VA, Eliasoph L, Alman B: Long term benefits of deflazacort treatment for boys with Duchenne muscular dystrophy in their second decade. Neuromuscular Disorders 16:249–255, 2006.
3. McDonald CM, Abresch RT, Carter GT, et al: Profiles of neuromuscular diseases: Duchenne muscular dystrophy. Am J Phys Med Rehabil 74(Suppl):S70–S92, 1995.
4. Moxley RT 3rd, Ashwal S, Pandya S, et al: Practice parameter: Corticosteroid treatment of Duchenne dystrophy: Report of the Quality Standards Subcommittee of the American Academy of Neurology and the Practice Committee of the Child Neurology Society. Neurology 64:13–20, 2005.
5. Read L, Galasko CS: Delay in diagnosing Duchenne muscular dystrophy in orthopaedic clinics. J Bone Joint Surg Br 68:481–482, 1986.
6. Sussman M: Duchenne muscular dystrophy. J Am Acad Orthop Surg 10:138–151, 2002.

CHAPTER 82

ARTHROGRYPOSIS MULTIPLEX CONGENITA

George H. Thompson, MD

1. **What is arthrogryposis multiplex congenita?**
   A congenital nonprogressive disorder in which there are multiple joint contractures. It is a diagnosis of exclusion as there are more than 150 different disorders or syndromes that have joint contractures as part of their manifestations. The term *amyoplasia*, or *amyoplasia congenita*, is frequently used to refer to those children with no abnormalities other than joint contractures.

2. **Describe the clinical criteria for diagnosis.**
   A characteristic limb appearance and position, a lack of visceral involvement, a lack of significant dysmorphic facial features, and a negative family history.

3. **Describe the typical features of the arthrogrypotic limb.**
   The extremities are featureless, with a tubular shape and absent skin creases. There can be either flexion or extension joint contractures.

4. **Describe the typical facial appearance in involved infants and children.**
   The head and face are usually not dysmorphic, but there may be micrognathia and microstomia due to lack of mandibular motion. The latter can result in difficulty in feeding, respiratory infections, and a failure to thrive. There is frequently a midline facial hemangioma, termed a *flame nevus* (Fig. 82-1).

5. **What viscera are involved?**
   There are no visceral abnormalities. There may be labial hypoplasia in females and an increased incidence of inguinal hernias in males.

6. **Describe the topographic classification of arthrogryposis multiplex congenita.**
   The topography of involvement is classified as quadrimelic (i.e., all four extremities), bimelic (i.e., the upper or lower extremities only), or monomelic (i.e., one extremity). Approximately two thirds of involved children have quadrimelic involvement (*see* Fig. 82-1). Bimelic lower-extremity involvement is the next most common topographic involvement. Bimelic upper-extremity and monomelic involvement are rare.

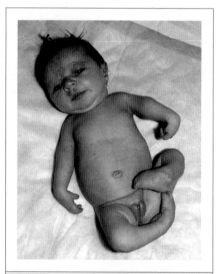

Figure 82-1. A 1-month-old girl with the quadrimelic form of arthrogryposis. Note the flame nevus of the forehead.

7. **What are the two neuromuscular forms of arthrogryposis multiplex congenita?**
This disorder can be divided into neuropathic and myopathic forms. The neuropathic form, which involves dysgenesis or dysfunction of the anterior horn cells, is the most common, accounting for 95% of cases. The myopathic form occurs in approximately 5% of cases.

8. **Describe the typical muscle histopathologic findings in the neuropathic form.**
The muscles are denervated and partially replaced by fat and fibrous tissue. The remaining muscle tissues will show fiber-type disproportion and an increase in the number of neuromuscular junctions. There will also be electron-microscopic abnormalities. There is periarticular fibrosis due to an increase in collagen formation. This leads to joint contractures.

9. **What form of arthrogryposis multiplex congenita has a genetic basis?**
Distal arthrogryposis, which includes involvement of the face, hands, and feet, is inherited as an autosomal dominant trait. All other forms of arthrogryposis are sporadic.

10. **What are the general concepts in the management of arthrogryposis multiplex congenita or amyoplasia?**
Physical and occupational therapy, orthotics, and surgery. The last includes both soft tissue releases and osteotomies. Usually, soft tissue releases are performed early, whereas osteotomies are performed in later childhood and adolescence.

11. **What is the characteristic posture of the shoulders?**
The shoulders are adducted and internally rotated. There is typically weakness of the deltoid muscles.

12. **Which is more common in the elbow: extension or flexion contracture?**
Extension contracture. This is due to weakness of the biceps and brachialis muscles and to a secondary posterior elbow and triceps contracture. Flexion contractures occur much less frequently.

13. **Describe the typical position of the wrist, fingers, and thumb.**
The wrist is typically flexed and in ulnar deviation due to contracture of the flexor carpi ulnaris. The thumb is adducted, assuming a thumb-in-palm position. There is a contracture of the adductor pollicis muscle and the first web space. The fingers are typically flexed at the metacarpophalangeal, proximal interphalangeal, and distal interphalangeal joints. Active and passive motion is limited.

14. **List the treatment goals for upper-extremity deformities.**
Self-care and mobility skills. Self-care typically involves feeding and toileting. It is usually best to have one extremity in flexion for feeding and the other in extension for toileting. The extremities should be able to meet in the midline for coordinated functions. Mobility skills include the use of crutches and wheelchairs and assistance in arising from a chair.

15. **What procedures are beneficial in the correction of shoulder adduction and internal rotation?**
Usually treatment of this deformity is not necessary since it produces minimal functional impairment. Occasionally, an internal derotation proximal humeral osteotomy can be performed to place the extremity in a more functional position.

16. **What procedures are beneficial in the correction of an elbow extension contracture?**
Posterior elbow capsulotomy and muscle and tendon transfer (of the triceps, pectoralis major, or latissimus dorsi) to the biceps tend to produce the best functional results. The muscle

selected depends on its strength. These transfers usually increase range of motion and elbow function. Occasionally, a distal humeral flexion and derotation osteotomy may be performed to salvage a very stiff extended elbow.

17. **What procedures are beneficial in the correction of wrist flexion and ulnar deviation deformities?**
Serial casting and splinting can be effective in infants. Flexor carpi ulnaris to extensor carpi radialis brevis transfer and a volar capsulotomy can be beneficial in improving the position of the wrist in young children. Occasionally, in very stiff deformity, a proximal row carpectomy can be performed. Wrist fusion can be considered in an adult.

18. **What procedures are beneficial in the correction of thumb-in-palm and finger flexion deformities?**
Adductor pollicis lengthening and deepening of the first web space can be useful for the thumb-in-palm deformity. A volar release and skin grafts are occasionally necessary for proximal interphalangeal joint contractures. This will not improve motion. Arthrodeses can also be considered.

19. **What is the incidence of teratologic hip dislocation in arthrogryposis multiplex congenita?**
Approximately two thirds of involved infants will have either hip dysplasia or dislocation. This is a teratologic disorder since the dislocation occurs prior to birth. The hip examination of an involved newborn will typically demonstrate flexion, abduction, and external rotation contractures.

20. **Which is the most common knee deformity: flexion or extension contracture?**
A flexion contracture is most common and occasionally is associated with a pterygium. This contracture is due to quadriceps weakness. Occasionally, the knees will be contracted in extension. This produces much less functional impairment, especially if the child is a walker. In nonwalkers, the extension contracture can be problematic and can interfere with sitting. This may require treatment.

21. **What is the most common foot deformity?**
Congenital talipes equinovarus (i.e., clubfoot) is the most common foot deformity. Other less common deformities include congenital vertical talus and calcaneovalgus foot.

22. **What are the treatment goals for lower-extremity deformities?**
Alignment and stability to achieve maximum ambulatory potential. Treatment is directed at joint stability and alignment in the upright or standing position.

23. **What treatment may be best for moderately flexible bilateral teratologic hip dislocations?**
This is controversial. Some authors prefer to leave the hips dislocated. Reduction may result in stiffness and subsequent difficulties in standing or sitting. Hip mobility is of major importance. Others, however, recommend extensive open reduction, possibly combined with a proximal femoral shortening and derotation osteotomy.

24. **Describe the management of unilateral teratologic hip dislocation.**
Closed reduction is usually unsatisfactory. Open reduction through a medial or an anterior approach is effective in young children. The anterior approach also allows an acetabuloplasty to be performed to correct coexistent acetabular dysplasia. In the older child, a pelvic osteotomy and a proximal femoral varus, shortening, and derotation osteotomy may be beneficial in achieving a stable hip.

25. **What procedures are beneficial in the treatment of knee flexion contractures?**
Initially, passive range-of-motion therapy and night-time splinting can be attempted. If this is unsatisfactory, hamstring release and posterior knee capsulotomy are commonly performed. An Ilizarov frame may be beneficial in severe cases. Extension supracondylar osteotomy of the distal femur can be considered. The deformity tends to recur with growth, however. In the older child or adolescent, anterior distal femoral hemiepiphysiodesis or stapling may be beneficial in achieving correction with growth.

26. **What procedures are considered in the correction of knee extension deformity?**
This deformity does not require treatment. Physical therapy will usually allow a satisfactory range of motion for comfortable sitting in nonwalkers. Occasionally, quadriceps lengthening in nonwalkers may be beneficial in achieving 90 degrees of knee flexion.

27. **At what age is talipes equinovarus best treated with a complete soft tissue release?**
Clubfeet are usually treated surgically at 12–18 months of age. It is important that the child be ready to assume an upright posture with or without orthoses shortly after the feet have been corrected. Early operative intervention predisposes to recurrent deformities.

28. **List three procedures for the treatment of recurrent clubfeet in young children.**
Repeat complete soft tissue release, talectomy, and Verbelyi-Ogston procedure (i.e., decancellation of the talus and cuboid). An Ilizarov frame may be a helpful adjunct in severe recurrences.

29. **What is the incidence of scoliosis in arthrogryposis multiplex congenita?**
Approximately two thirds of involved children will develop scoliosis. A single thoracolumbar curve is the most common pattern. Curves will be progressive in approximately one half of the patients with scoliosis.

30. **Describe the management of progressive arthrogryptotic scoliosis.**
Scoliosis in arthrogryposis multiplex congenita has the same general characteristics as other neuromuscular spinal deformities. The curves tend to progress steadily throughout growth and development. They respond poorly to orthotics. Early surgical intervention is the best method of management. This may consist of a posterior spinal fusion with segmental spinal instrumentation or, occasionally, a combined anterior and posterior spinal fusion with segmental spinal instrumentation.

KEY POINTS: ARTHROGRYPOSIS MULTIPLEX CONGENITA

1. Arthrogryposis multiplex congenita or amyoplasia is characterized by multiple contractures, usually involving all four extremities.

2. The most common deformity is rigid talipes equinovarus (i.e., clubfoot).

3. Hip dislocations are teratologic in origin and are best treated by open reduction.

4. Upper-extremity involvement in less common, but contractures can have a significant effect on activities of daily living.

5. Early management consists of physical therapy and splinting, and soft tissue surgery and osteotomies are commonly used in older children and adolescents.

BIBLIOGRAPHY

1. Akazawa H, Oda K, Mitani S, et al: Surgical management of hip dislocation in children with arthrogryposis multiplex congenita. J Bone Joint Surg Br 80:636–640, 1998.

2. Axt MW, Niethard FU, Doderlein L, Weber M: Principles of treatment of the upper extremity in arthrogryposis multiplex congenita type I. J Pediatr Orthop Part B 6:179–185, 1997.

3. Banker BQ: Neuropathologic aspects of arthrogryposis multiplex congenita. Clin Orthop 194:30–43, 1985.

4. Bernstein RM: Arthrogryposis and amyoplasia. J Am Acad Orthop Surg 10:417–424, 2002.

5. Brunner R, Hefti F, Tgetgel JD: Arthrogryotic joint contracture at the knee and the foot: Correction with a circular frame. J Pediatr Orthop Part B 6:192–197, 1997.

6. Cassis N, Capdevila R: Talectomy for clubfoot in arthrogryposis. J Pediatr Orthop 20:652–655, 2000.

7. Choi IH, Yang MS, Chung CY, et al: The treatment of recurrent arthrogrypotic club foot in children by the Ilizarov method: A preliminary report. J Bone Joint Surg Br 83B:731–737, 2001.

8. D'Souza H, Aroojis A, Chawara GS: Talectomy in arthrogryposis: Analysis of results. J Pediatr Orthop 18:760–764, 1998.

9. Ezaki M: Treatment of the upper limb in the child with arthrogryposis. Hand Clin 16:703–711, 2000.

10. Goldfarb CA, Burke MS, Strecker WB, Manske PR: The Steindler flexorplasty for the arthrogrypotic elbow. J Hand Surg 29A:462–469, 2004.

11. Gross RH: The role of Verebelyi-Ogston procedure in management of the arthrogrypotic foot. Clin Orthop 194:99–103, 1985.

12. Hall JG: Arthrogryposis multiplex congenita: Etiology, genetics, classification, diagnostic approach, and general aspects. J Pediatr Orthop Part B 6:159–166, 1997.

13. Legaspi J, Li YH, Chow W, Leong JC: Talectomy in patients with recurrent deformity in club foot. A long-term follow-up study. J Bone Joint Surg Br 83:384–387, 2001.

14. Murray C, Fixsen JA: Management of knee deformity in classical arthrogryposis multiplex congenita (amyoplasia congenita). J Pediatr Orthop Part B 6:186–191, 1997.

15. Niki H, Staheli LT, Mosca VS: Management of clubfoot deformity in amyoplasia. J Pediatr Orthop 17:803–807, 1997.

16. Smith DW, Drennan JC: Arthrogryposis wrist deformities: Results of infantile serial casting. J Pediatr Orthop 22:44–47, 2002.

17. Widmann RF, Do TT, Burke SW: Radical soft-tissue release of the arthrogrypotic clubfoot. J Pediar Orthop B 14:111–115, 2005.

18. Yau PW, Chow W, Li YH, Leong JC: Twenty-year follow-up of hip problems in arthrogryposis multiplex congenita. J Pediatr Orthop 22:359–363, 2002.

CHAPTER 83

POLIOMYELITIS

Hugh G. Watts, MD

1. **Since the vaccine was developed 40 years ago, poliomyelitis has disappeared Why do I need to read anything about it now?**

   Poliomyelitis has not disappeared by any means. The World Health Organization claims that in the Western hemisphere, there have been no new wild cases since the early 1990s, but in the rest of the world, particularly in Africa, poliomyelitis is widespread. An outbreak occurred in the Dominican Republic (thought to be a mutation of the attenuated Sabin virus). The most recent reports show about 100 new paralytic cases per day worldwide, and there is an estimate that only 1 in 10 cases is reported.

2. **I live in the United States and don't plan to practice outside, so why should I read this?**

   The world is a small place, made smaller by rapid airplane travel and immigration. This brings children who have had the disease to the United States. In November 2005, four nonimmunized children in Minnesota contracted the disease, probably from a traveler from southeast Asia. Furthermore, the use of the vaccine occasionally causes a clinical episode of poliomyelitis, either in the vaccinated child or in the vaccinated child's parents.

3. **What is poliomyelitis?**

   The poliomyelitis virus is an enterovirus (like the Coxsackie and echo viruses). When poliomyelitis is contracted, the anterior horn cells of the spinal cord may be destroyed, with permanent loss of muscle activity.

4. **What kinds of clinical poliomyelitis are there?**

   Clinical infections can be divided into the following:
   - **Abortive poliomyelitis:** This is a brief febrile illness with anorexia, nausea, vomiting, headache, and sore throat, as well as coryza, cough, pharyngeal exudate, and diarrhea.
   - **Nonparalytic poliomyelitis:** Children have the same symptoms as abortive poliomyelitis, but they also will have headache, nausea, and vomiting that are more intense and there will be soreness and stiffness of the muscles, particularly in the back of the neck and in the muscles of the trunk and limbs.
   - **Paralytic poliomyelitis:** Children will have all of the symptoms described above as well as weakness or paralysis of the trunk and extremities. The spinal form is the most common and involves the neck, trunk, and extremities. The bulbar form can involve one or more of the cranial nerves, or there may be a combination of the bulbar and spinal forms.

5. **Why don't we see more children with the bulbar form of the disease?**

   These patients frequently die from respiratory failure.

6. **How is the poliomyelitis virus spread?**

   Humans are the only natural host of the poliomyelitis virus, and it is spread from person to person by fecal and oral routes. Some epidemiologists have joked that "if saliva were red and feces were blue, the world would be purple." This is particularly so in the unhygienic world of the child.

7. **What is the pathophysiology of poliomyelitis?**

The poliomyelitis virus multiplies and kills off the anterior horn cells. Some of the injury to the nerve cells may be reversible. Adjacent nerves may sprout to reinnervate surrounding paralyzed muscles.

The neural lesions occur chiefly in the anterior horn cells of the spinal cord and, to a lesser extent, in the intermediate and dorsal horns and the dorsal root ganglia. The cerebral motor cortex (except the motor area) is spared, as is the cerebellum (except the vermis and the deep midline nuclei).

8. **When thinking about poliomyelitis, how would you divide the discussion of the disease?**

This is a really a "tell me what I am thinking" question. So I'll tell you what I'm thinking:

- We can look at the issues related to acute infection by the poliomyelitis virus. This is a topic more appropriate to a book on pediatrics or infectious diseases.
- We can look at the chronic problems that result from the paralysis due to poliomyelitis. This is really the purview of this chapter. But first, let us spend a little time on the features of acute infections and their prevention.

9. **What other diagnoses might be confused with an acute poliomyelitis infection?**

The most common by far is a postinfectious polyneuropathy better known as the Guillain-Barré syndrome. Generally, the headache and meningeal signs are less striking. The paralysis tends to be symmetrical, and sensory changes and pyramidal tract signs are common (but absent in poliomyelitis).

Guillain-Barré syndrome usually becomes apparent about 10 days following a nonspecific viral infection. Spontaneous recovery begins usually at 2–3 weeks and in most situations is complete. However, there is a chronic form or an intermittent recurrent form affecting about 7% of children. Children with this may be hard to distinguish from those with the chronic residua of poliomyelitis.

10. **What kind of vaccines are available to prevent poliomyelitis?**

There are two types: the oral, living, attenuated virus (i.e., Sabin) and the injectable, killed virus (i.e., Salk).

11. **Which poliomyelitis vaccine is best?**

Best for what? The living, attenuated vaccine is cheap and easy to administer and has the added advantage of secondarily spreading the vaccine through fecal contamination from actively vaccinated children. This makes it especially useful for gaining herd immunity in the event of an epidemic. But this vaccine is readily inactivated by heat, which makes the care and feeding of the vaccine more precarious. The oral vaccine, in addition, may cause a clinical case of paralytic poliomyelitis in about 1:5,000,000 children who are vaccinated (or in the children's parents: there is also the possibility of the parents contracting the disease from their child).

This is why the injectable vaccine is important. It is particularly indicated when inoculating pregnant women or for inoculating children who are compromised in their immune status due to some chronic illness. The current recommendation in the United States is to use the injectable killed virus.

12. **Let's turn to the issue of the chronic residua of poliomyelitis How would you divide the problems that a child with poliomyelitis would have?**

There are three problem issues: (1) muscle weakness, (2) growth, and (3) deformity.

13. **What sort of problems would you expect a child to have as a result of muscle weakness?**

Obviously, it is going to depend on how severe the muscle weakness is and which muscles are involved, as well as the balance between opposing muscles.

14. **How weak is "weak"? Just how do you test muscle strength?**
   Manual muscle testing was developed for the management of poliomyelitis. The possible strength of a muscle is divided into six grades, ranging from 0–5:
   - **Grade 0:** This is obvious, as there is no muscle twitch at all.
   - **Grade 1:** The muscle twitches and can be felt by your palpating hand, but no useful motion is generated.
   - **Grade 2:** The muscle is able to power the joint through a *full range of motion with gravity eliminated*. An example of this is if you hold your arm in front of you with your humerus parallel to the floor, your elbow bent at 90 degrees, and your forearm parallel with the floor. Your triceps can then straighten your elbow and, in doing so, carry your forearm through the range of extension, but with gravity eliminated.
   - **Grade 3:** The muscle is able to carry the joint through a *full range of motion against gravity*. Using the same example, you would hold your humerus out to the side, parallel with the floor, and your elbow bent at 90 degrees, but this time with your forearm dangling toward the floor. Your triceps would then be used to extend your elbow its full possible range of motion against gravity.
   - **Grade 4:** The muscle is able not only to go through a full range of motion against gravity, but also against added resistance.
   - **Grade 5:** The muscle functions normally.

15. **How reproducible is this grading system?**
   It really depends on the part of the scale that we are talking about. You can easily open the jar of pickles that your grandmother has difficulty opening or the jar of peanut butter that a 3-year-old cannot open. Yet, you are all probably "normal." There is clearly an age-related factor in determining what normal muscle strength is. The same goes for a grade of 4.
   However, below grade 4, the muscle testing is remarkably reproducible. One has to take care that, in assigning a grade of 2 or 3, the muscle is able to carry the limb through the *full* range of motion. If there are contractures that limit the range, then the strength is determined by the muscle's ability to carry the limb through the *possible* range.

16. **Does a grade of 3 (out of 5) mean the muscle is 50% of the strength of normal?**
   Definitely not! It depends, in part, on which muscle is in question. However, for the quadriceps, it takes about 10% of normal muscle strength to be able to extend the knee a full range of motion against gravity (i.e., grade 3). Again for the quadriceps, it takes about 5% of muscle strength to extend the knee its full range of motion with gravity eliminated (i.e., grade 2). This means that it only takes a small percentage loss of muscle strength to go from a situation where you can walk because your quadriceps can hold your knee straight to the point where you cannot walk without a brace.

17. **What does this tell you about the so-called "postpoliomyelitis syndrome," which can develop as you get older?**
   Do you think that you might lose a small percentage of strength in your quadriceps with age? Obviously, yes. You lose 1% of your muscle strength per year after the age of 30. This means that if you had poliomyelitis and grade 3 quadriceps as a teenager, you would be able to walk around without a brace, but as you got a bit older and lost an additional 5% of normal muscle strength, you would have to wear a brace in order to be able to walk. This has nothing to do with recrudescence of the virus; rather, it is an effect of getting older. (Maybe we should more usefully call this "postbirth syndrome.")

18. **What muscles do you need to keep your knee from giving way when you are walking?**
   Obviously, the quadriceps is the first muscle to come to mind, but if the quadriceps is absent, your gluteus maximus can take its place. The soleus muscle is the other muscle that can take its place.

19. **What do I mean by "Which muscles can take the place of the quadriceps?"**
To explain this, why don't you stand up. Now lean forward a bit at your waist and reach down and grasp your patella between your thumb and your index. As you lean forward, you can wobble your patella from side to side. What does this tell you? It means that your quadriceps is not doing any work. You are actually standing up without using your quadriceps.

20. **How does that work?**
Because your center of gravity falls in front of your knee joint, gravity is working to extend your knee. The ligaments at the back of the knee are preventing your knee from hyperextending, thereby supporting your weight. Now, with your thumb and index finger wobbling your patella, gradually bend your knees. You will see that you come to a point, when your knee is flexed at about 10–15 degrees, when you cannot move your patella. That is the point when the quadriceps start doing their work.

    You can see that anything that brings your center of gravity in front of your knees will allow you to stand on your leg without using your quadriceps. Now you can see that the gluteus maximus, by pulling the femur posteriorly, brings the knee behind your center of gravity. The same thing is true for the soleus.

    Conversely, a seemingly minor knee flexion contracture of, say, 20 degrees, in combination with a weak quadriceps, could make walking without a brace impossible.

21. **What happens if I have a weak gluteus maximus? How can I stand up?**
By leaning backward and getting your center of gravity behind the axis of the hip joint, the trunk wants to fall backward but cannot because of the tight ligaments in front of the hip joint. (You remember the Y-shaped ligament of Bigelow from first-year anatomy, of course.) These ligaments prevents your hip from hyperextending and allow you to stand up.

22. **What happens if both my gluteus maximus and my quadriceps are weak?**
Now you are in trouble. You need to lean forward to get your weight anterior to your knee, and you need to lean backward to get your weight posterior to your hip. With a little cleverness and a certain amount of breath-holding, you *can* precariously balance that way. But the smarter thing to do is to use a brace that prevents the knee from flexing and then stand by leaning backward at the hip. This kind of a brace we would call a knee-ankle-foot orthosis (KAFO). Please check out the chapter on braces for details.

23. **How does poliomyelitis affect the growth of a limb?**
When muscle activity across a joint is not normal, the cartilage cells of the physis are not stimulated to grow normally, and a short leg is a common result.

24. **What happens with a leg that is too short?**
For details on this matter, I direct you to the chapter on anisomelia (a fancy word for "one limb is shorter than the other"). Keep in mind that if the child has poliomyelitis, you do not necessarily want the legs to end up being equal in length. The weight of a brace, the thickness of the brace on the sole of the foot, and the muscle weakness may make it hard to swing the leg forward when walking if the legs are exactly equal. This is particularly true if the child is wearing a long leg brace (i.e., a KAFO) with the knee locked and fully extended.

25. **How does muscle weakness of poliomyelitis result in deformity?**
Deformities from muscle weakness can be a result of the imbalance of muscles or of fibrosis of the dead muscle. For an example of muscle imbalance, imagine a child in whom the posterior tibialis muscle of the leg is paralyzed and the peroneal muscles are normal. Soon the heel of the child's foot would be pulled into eversion, and if the foot is allowed to grow with this imbalance, the bones will gradually become misshapen. Lack of muscle pull can also alter the shape of a bone in other ways. For example, a weak gluteus medius will give less pull on the

apophysis of the greater trochanter, leading to a valgus shape of the upper end of the femur as growth progresses.

26. **How did the muscle become fibrotic?**
When the nerve to a muscle dies, the muscle gradually becomes atrophic and is replaced by fibrous tissue. This fibrous tissue can work as a very tough band, preventing a joint from going through its full range of motion. The most common example of this is the tensor fascia lata muscle and its extension down the leg (i.e., the fascia lata). The fibrosis of the tensor fascia lata muscle can cause an abduction contracture of the hip, and, since the muscle is anterior to the axis of the hip joint, it usually causes a hip flexion contracture as well. The continuation of the fascia lata to the tibia is posterior to the knee joint, and so fibrosis can lead to a flexion deformity in the knee. Furthermore, the fascia lata inserted laterally on the proximal tibia can lead to a rotational deformity as the tibia grows.

27. **Is there anything special about the physical examination of a child with poliomyelitis?**
The answer is obviously "yes," or I would not have asked the question. The mechanics of walking require a subtle alignment of the center of gravity in relation to the joints. What is happening at one part of the body, such as the ankle, can make a big difference in what happens in another part, such as the knee. A classic example is the effect of an equinus deformity (i.e., a plantiflexion contracture at the ankle) in helping to support the knee. Remember, we talked about keeping the axis of the knee joint posterior to the center of weight-bearing. The soleus muscle can do that, but so can an equinus contracture.

KEY POINTS: POLIOMYELITIS

1. Do not overlook this disease. Air travel makes everyone susceptible.
2. Because of the interdependence of the joints, you must evaluate the entire child. (Do not focus on an individual deformity.)
3. Set priorities.
4. Understand why the choice of vaccines is made.

28. **How does that happen?**
In a normal child, the ankle gradually plantarflexes as the heel strikes the floor. If the ankle is in equinus when the foot touches the ground, the weight of the body pushes the foot flat onto the ground. The tibia cannot move forward (because the ankle is fixed in equinus from the contracture) and is now angled posteriorly. As inertia carries the body forward, the knee remains posterior to the weight-bearing line. That may be obvious to you now, but its not always obvious to the surgeon who may decide to lengthen a tight heel cord and finds, to his or her dismay, that the child is now unable to stand and walk without using a long leg brace. This is what I mean about the importance of the inter-relationships of one part of the body to the rest. This means that a physical examination of *all* of the parts of the body, including a manual muscle test of the parts, is a necessary minimum for evaluating a child with poliomyelitis.

29. **Who should be treating a child with the residua of poliomyelitis?**
Most characteristically, the treatment falls to the orthopaedic surgeon. This is because the management often involves both bracing and surgery. The physical therapist is usually an

important member of the treating team. The orthotist (i.e., the brace maker) will usually be involved in the treatment.

30. **With so many different areas of weakness, I am overwhelmed. Where do I begin?**
The problem is best managed by setting priorities. Initially, the priority should be to get the child walking. This can be done with fairly simple bracing. Getting the child to fit into a brace may require some simple surgical releases at the hips, knees, or ankles.

The second priority is to correct the factors that are liable to create deformities with further growth. Later, one can focus on doing surgical treatments to reduce the extent of bracing or crutches that are needed. This is followed by attention to the loss of function in the upper extremities, and then finally to correcting problems in the spine (i.e., scoliosis).

31. **What can be done to correct contractures?**
If a child is very young—for example, under the age of about 3 years—exercises may be enough to stretch out contractures. As the child gets older and the joint contractures become stiffer, the contractures may be amenable to serial casting. *Serial casting* is where a cast is put on with the limb as straight as possible. Usually, over the next week or two, the contracture will relax a little bit while inside the cast, allowing a new cast to be applied with the joint about 10 degrees straighter than it was. Although this has the advantage of not requiring surgery, it can be a considerable hassle for the child and the child's family. It may be simpler to do soft tissue releases by surgery. In later years, during adolescence and young adulthood, it may be simpler just to correct the deformity by cutting the bone (i.e., an osteotomy) and straightening the limb.

32. **What can be done to correct an imbalance of muscle pulls across a joint?**
Sometimes this can be managed by providing a brace to replace the missing muscle strength. The simplest example of this would be in a child who has plantar flexors of the ankle but no dorsal flexors. This could be managed with a simple brace to hold the foot from going into equinus.

At other times, it may be possible to transfer a muscle so that its tendon insertion is put in a more advantageous location. For example, if a child has a weak gastrosoleus muscle but has intact peroneus muscles, it is possible to move the insertions of the peroneal tendons back to the os calcis to give sufficient strength. If this does not allow good push-off, at least it will prevent deformity in the growth of the shape of the os calcis.

33. **Is there any penalty to transferring a muscle?**
When a muscle is transferred, it characteristically loses one grade of strength. This means that when transferring a muscle that is grade 3, the muscle will probably end up with a strength of grade 2, meaning it will not do very much (except perhaps take away a deforming force).

In addition, moving a muscle may make the joint that it originally controls unstable. In the example above, in which the peronei are moved back to the os calcis, this movement may make the subtalar joint unstable. In that case, the problem might be managed by fusing that subtalar joint to take away the need for the peroneal muscles.

34. **Do you find that parental attitudes and social attitudes toward children with poliomyelitis are different from those toward some other chronic diseases of childhood?**
Yes. Because poliomyelitis does not affect mental status, nor does it affect the cerebellum, these children function remarkably well. Furthermore, because the disease is acquired, parents seem to feel that there is less reflection on the family genes than a situation in which the problems are a result of a congenital deformity. In addition, there have been prominent people who have had the disease. Probably the most well known in the United States is Franklin D. Roosevelt, the 32nd President (from 1933–1945).

BIBLIOGRAPHY

1. Cherry JD: Enteroviruses. In Behrman (ed): Nelson Textbook of Pediatrics, 14th ed. Philadelphia, W.B. Saunders, 1992, pp 823–831.
2. Herring JA (ed): Tachdjian's Pediatric Orthopedics, 3rd ed. Philadelphia, W.B. Saunders, 2002, pp 1321–1444.
3. Watts HG: Orthopedic techniques in the management of the residua of paralytic poliomyelitis. Techn Orthop 20:179–189, 2005.

CHAPTER 84

LIMB DEFICIENCY

John E. Herzenberg, MD, FRCSC, and Dror Paley, MD, FRCSC

1. **What is limb deficiency?**
   Part of a limb is missing. The missing part may be at the end of the limb (i.e., terminal deficiency; e.g., congenital amputation), leaving a simple stump. The proximal bones may be absent, with foreshortening of the limb, as in phocomelia (i.e., intercalary deficiency). Alternatively, there may be a deficiency along the length of the limb, as in the radius or fibula, with shortening and deformity of the hand, leg, or foot (also termed *paraxial deficiency,* which is subdivided into *preaxial* and *postaxial deficiencies*).

2. **What causes limb deficiencies?**
   The cause is usually unknown, especially in isolated single-limb anomalies in an otherwise normal child. The classic exception was multilimb deficiency caused by the drug thalidomide. There are other exceptions—particularly tibial defects, which are known to be heritable. Some rare syndromes involving limb deficiency and facial abnormality have been reported as being genetic, in some cases associated with maternal diabetes.

3. **How likely is it to happen again in the same family?**
   Very unlikely. An increasing number of reports of genetic transmission, however, make genetic counseling a reasonable recommendation. Children with radial clubhand, tibial hemimelia (TH), and multiple limb deficiencies should be referred to a geneticist. Most cases of congenital femoral deficiency (CFD) and fibular hemimelia (FH) do not require genetic evaluation.

4. **How is congenital limb deficiency classified?**
   Classification of congenital limb deficiency is confusing because of variable international nomenclature. Specific terms for the more common anomalies, such as CFD, TH, and FH, have been established in the literature.

5. **What is the most common type?**
   A left below-elbow transverse hemimelia (i.e., a congenital below-elbow amputation).

6. **Are limb deficiencies associated with other syndromes or congenital defects?**
   Radial deficiencies in particular are associated with a number of syndromes, including blood dyscrasia, Fanconi anemia, thrombocytopenic purpura (i.e., thrombocytopenia-absent radius [TAR] syndrome), congenital heart defect, Holt-Oram syndrome (i.e., anterior septal defect and radial clubhand, less commonly with tetralogy of Fallot), and vertebral and other defects, as in the VATER syndrome (vertebral defects, anal atresia, tracheoesophageal fistula with esophageal atresia, and radial and renal anomalies). These associations rarely occur in patients with other multilimb deficiencies.

7. **How early should these children be seen by a pediatric orthopaedist?**
   As soon after birth as possible, to allow the parents to have accurate information and reasonable expectations from the very beginning. In cases of congenital deficiencies, it is possible to predict both the ultimate limb-length discrepancy (LLD) and the height at skeletal

TABLE 84-1. MULTIPLIER METHOD FOR PREDICTING ULTIMATE LIMB-LENGTH DISCREPANCY (LLD) IN BOYS AND GIRLS

Lower Limb							
Multiplier for BOYS				Multiplier for GIRLS			
Age (yr + mo)	M	Age (yr + mo)	M	Age (yr + mo)	M	Age (yr + mo)	M
Birth	5.080	7 + 6	1.520	Birth	4.630	6 + 0	1.510
0 + 3	4.550	8 + 0	1.470	0 + 3	4.155	6 + 6	1.460
0 + 6	4.050	8 + 6	1.420	0 + 6	3.725	7 + 0	1.430
0 + 9	3.600	9 + 0	1.380	0 + 9	3.300	7 + 6	1.370
1 + 0	3.240	9 + 6	1.340	1 + 0	2.970	8 + 0	1.330
1 + 3	2.975	10 + 0	1.310	1 + 3	2.750	8 + 6	1.290
1 + 6	2.825	10 + 6	1.280	1 + 6	2.600	9 + 0	1.260
1 + 9	2.700	11 + 0	1.240	1 + 9	2.490	9 + 6	1.220
2 + 0	2.590	11 + 6	1.220	2 + 0	2.390	10 + 0	1.190
2 + 3	2.480	12 + 0	1.180	2 + 3	2.295	10 + 6	1.160
2 + 6	2.385	12 + 6	1.160	2 + 6	2.200	11 + 0	1.130
2 + 9	2.300	13 + 0	1.130	2 + 9	2.125	11 + 6	1.100
3 + 0	2.230	13 + 6	1.100	3 + 0	2.050	12 + 0	1.070
3 + 6	2.110	14 + 0	1.080	3 + 6	1.925	12 + 6	1.050
4 + 0	2.000	14 + 6	1.060	4 + 0	1.830	13 + 0	1.030
4 + 6	1.890	15 + 0	1.040	4 + 6	1.740	13 + 6	1.010
5 + 0	1.820	15 + 6	1.020	5 + 0	1.660	14 + 0	1.000
5 + 6	1.740	16 + 0	1.010	5 + 6	1.580		
6 + 0	1.670	16 + 6	1.010				
6 + 6	1.620	17 + 0	1.000				
7 + 0	1.570						

Mature Length = L × M.
Modified from Jonathan Paley, et al: J Pediatr Orthop 24:732–737, 2004.

maturity from a single visit by using the multiplier method (Tables 84-1, 84-2). Armed with this information, parents can better plan their long-term goals.

8. **Is there an indication for surgery for these cases?**
    With the exception of patients with simple transverse congenital amputations, who can be easily fitted with a prosthesis, most patients need some surgical modification to maximize function. Surgery falls into two broad categories:
    - Prosthetic reconstruction
    - Lengthening reconstruction

TABLE 84-2. MULTIPLIER METHOD FOR PREDICTING FINAL HEIGHT IN BOYS AND GIRLS

Height							
Multiplier for BOYS				Multiplier for GIRLS			
Age (yr + mo)	M	Age (yr + mo)	M	Age (yr + mo)	M	Age (yr + mo)	M
Birth	3.535	8 + 6	1.351	Birth	3.290	8 + 6	1.254
0 + 3	2.908	9 + 0	1.322	0 + 3	2.759	9 + 0	1.229
0 + 6	2.639	9 + 6	1.298	0 + 6	2.505	9 + 6	1.207
0 + 9	2.462	10 + 0	1.278	0 + 9	2.341	10 + 0	1.183
1 + 0	2.337	10 + 6	1.260	1 + 0	2.216	10 + 6	1.160
1 + 3	2.239	11 + 0	1.235	1 + 3	2.120	11 + 0	1.135
1 + 6	2.160	11 + 6	1.210	1 + 6	2.038	11 + 6	1.108
1 + 9	2.088	12 + 0	1.186	1 + 9	1.965	12 + 0	1.082
2 + 0	2.045	12 + 6	1.161	2 + 0	1.917	12 + 6	1.059
2 + 6	1.942	13 + 0	1.135	2 + 6	1.815	13 + 0	1.040
3 + 0	1.859	13 + 6	1.106	3 + 0	1.735	13 + 6	1.027
3 + 6	1.783	14 + 0	1.081	3 + 6	1.677	14 + 0	1.019
4 + 0	1.731	14 + 6	1.056	4 + 0	1.622	14 + 6	1.013
4 + 6	1.675	15 + 0	1.044	4 + 6	1.570	15 + 0	1.008
5 + 0	1.627	15 + 6	1.030	5 + 0	1.514	15 + 6	1.009
5 + 6	1.579	16 + 0	1.021	5 + 6	1.467	16 + 0	1.004
6 + 0	1.535	16 + 6	1.014	6 + 0	1.421	16 + 6	1.004
6 + 6	1.492	17 + 0	1.010	6 + 6	1.381	17 + 0	1.002
7 + 0	1.455	17 + 6	1.006	7 + 0	1.341	17 + 6	—
7 + 6	1.416	18 + 0	1.005	7 + 6	1.309	18 + 0	—
8 + 0	1.383			8 + 0	1.279		

Mature Height = Ht. × M.
Modified from Jonathan Paley, et al: J Pediatr Orthop 24:732–737, 2004.

9. **In general, what is the role of amputation and prosthetic fitting (i.e., prosthetic reconstruction surgery)?**

In the more severe lower-limb deficiencies, when reconstruction is not possible or when the necessary expertise or family or child cooperation is not available, the best functional result is obtained by amputation of the foot (which often is deformed) and prosthetic fitting. This is particularly true in cases of severe CFD, FH, and TH. An excellent functional and cosmetic result can be achieved by using this technique. Prosthetic reconstruction surgery usually is performed at age 9–12 months.

10. **What are the surgical principles of reconstructive amputation for limb deficiency?**
Reconstructive amputation should provide a good end-bearing stump to facilitate prosthetic replacement in an otherwise unreconstructable limb. This typically applies only to the lower limb, usually for FH, TH, and some cases of proximal focal femoral deficiency (PFFD). Amputation is almost never indicated for upper-extremity deficiencies. The overriding principle is never to amputate through the shaft (i.e., the diaphysis) of a bone but to disarticulate at the joint level (usually the ankle) to retain the distal epiphysis for growth and the ability to bear weight on the end of the stump, which greatly simplifies the prosthetic fitting. Another important advantage is the avoidance of terminal spiking. A specialized type of amputation called *rotationplasty* is used for severe CFD (see question 40).

11. **What are the principles of management of upper-limb versus lower-limb deficiencies?**
Prosthetic replacement of the upper limb is much less satisfactory than replacement of the lower limb. Almost any hand remaining is more functional than a prosthesis because a prosthesis is insensate. Despite improvements in myoelectric prostheses, upper-extremity amputees tend to reject prostheses unless they are bilateral. Amputation is never indicated for upper-limb deficiencies. However, surgery to improve function may be helpful. Occasionally, a short residual limb should be lengthened to improve prosthetic fitting.

12. **When can limbs be lengthened?**
In carefully selected cases by well-trained surgeons in specialized centers. Limb lengthening is challenging for both the patient and the surgeon and is very prone to complication. New methods to reconstruct the hip and knee for femoral deficiencies and the foot deformity for fibular deficiencies have made lengthening very feasible in these cases, and good final functional results can be achieved. High-grade tibial deficiency remains a formidable challenge to limb lengthening.

13. **When is amputation preferred to limb lengthening?**
See question 9. Limb lengthening requires a reconstructable deficiency, a surgeon with the required skills, and a motivated patient and family with the necessary financial and emotional resources to negotiate the prolonged treatment times associated with limb lengthening. If any of these factors is absent, amputation is preferred.

14. **What are the complications of amputation and prosthetic fitting?**
Very few. Other associated problems such as genu valgum, instability of the hip and knee, and acetabular insufficiency are not solved by amputation. These problems, when present, require separate consideration. The cost of the prosthesis and the need for regular replacement in the growing child can be a financial problem in some situations. Although the cost may be covered by certain childrens' hospital organizations, it can be problematic for adults. The long-term costs, amortized over a lifetime, may be higher for amputation than for lengthening.

15. **What functional result can be expected in a child with unilateral ankle disarticulation?**
Excellent. Walking is smoother than running, but these children have function close to normal and are capable of competing with their peers in most sports.

16. **What functional result can be expected in a child with a unilateral through-knee or above-knee amputation?**
Loss of the knee joint greatly diminishes function, but modern prosthetics allow a good walking gait with only a slight limp. Complete independence in school and work can be expected, but the higher energy costs of walking and running may limit sports participation, especially in

the absence of a functional knee joint. Appropriately timed epiphyseodesis can be considered to ensure that the end position of the prosthetic knee joint is symmetrical with the opposite normal side.

17. **What about functional expectations in a multilimb deficiency?**
Infinitely variable. A bilateral below-knee amputee can achieve independence. A bilateral through-knee amputee with normal upper limbs usually will have limited outside independence and will use a wheelchair for speed and distance. If all four limbs are seriously deficient, independence is lost and a great deal of help is needed. Toileting can be a special problem. Some children have no arms and are dependent on their legs and feet for feeding and grooming. In these cases, when the child has adapted well to the deficiency, great caution should be taken before embarking on a lower-extremity reconstruction plan. In such cases, children who were previously independent became dependent after well-meaning but misguided lower-extremity surgery.

18. **How good are prosthetic lower limbs?**
Generally excellent at below-knee levels and acceptable at through-knee levels. Better suspension, socket-lining technology, and prosthetic feet (e.g., Seattle and energy-storing) have improved function in recent years. Replacing the limb after a high-thigh or hip disarticulation remains less satisfactory. The congenital amputee may have ipsilateral hip and knee pathologic conditions that diminish their performance. These merit reconstruction when possible.

19. **How good are prosthetic upper limbs?**
Generally disappointing. The fine manipulative, proprioceptive, and sensory functions of the hand are irreplaceable. Children with a unilateral upper limb prosthesis often will reject it. Purely cosmetic hands may be accepted in later adolescence. Bilateral below-elbow amputees will often prefer a standard split-hook device for function and biofeedback.

20. **What are the advantages and disadvantages of myoelectric prostheses?**
The advantages are fairly good cosmesis and excellent grip strength. The disadvantages are weight, cost, breakdown, and the difficulty in cleaning and maintaining the glove. They are very useful to older unilateral below-elbow amputees in aiding bimanual work. For laborers, a standard split-hook device is more practical and durable.

21. **What are the psychologic effects of limb deficiency, amputation, and prosthetic reconstruction?**
The birth of a baby with a significant limb deficiency is devastating to the parents. Early consultation with an expert will help promote understanding and acceptance. In some cases, amputation as a therapeutic step will be rejected and well-chosen second opinions are necessary. Once surgery is over and function has been established, parents become very positive and proud of their child's achievements. For the most part, the children themselves are very accepting and untroubled by the limb defect, unlike children suffering amputation due to trauma or malignancy. Nonetheless, peers can be cruel, and child amputees may experience some degree of peer rejection and abuse.

22. **Is a child with a traumatic amputation different?**
Absolutely. The psychologic injury to both the child and the parents is severe and permanent. In North America, these injuries often are associated with a component of parental or guardian guilt, as in lawn mower, snowblower, and agricultural equipment accidents.

23. **What are the surgical issues associated with traumatic amputation in childhood?**

Preservation of length and growth. Children often heal so well that length can be maintained by patience, secondary wound closure, and skin grafting. Vacuum-assisted wound closure has been a significant advance in posttraumatic wound care. Great efforts to preserve distal epiphyses are worth it to provide growth and end bearing.

Terminal spiking is a process by which a transected bone end in young children elongates and becomes pointed, often protruding through the skin of the stump. Sometimes called *terminal overgrowth,* this unhappy state can lead to multiple stump revision procedures. The major reconstructive challenges after extremity-mutilating injuries usually are related to growth arrest, knee function, and angular deformities.

24. **Can anything be done to prevent terminal spiking?**

In some cases, yes. The most common incidence is in below-knee amputations because the fibula is particularly prone to overgrowing and protruding through the skin. Fusion of the end of the fibula to the tibia with free transfer of the proximal fibular epiphysis to the end of the tibia may prevent further spiking.

25. **What are the most common indications for lengthening reconstructive surgery in cases of limb deficiency?**

The indications for this type of surgery are CFD, FH, radial clubhand (i.e., radial hemimelia), and tibial deficiency (i.e., TH).

26. **What are the complications associated with limb lengthening?**

Unfortunately, there are many. Subluxation of joints, especially the knee and hip, and deformity and fracture of the lengthened bone are some of the more serious possible complications. Knee and ankle contracture, nerve palsy, and muscle weakness are also potential complications. However, most of the complications associated with limb lengthening are avoidable or treatable, provided the surgeon maintains careful awareness and control of the clinical situation. Successfully treated complications do not preclude a good end result. Often, 6–12 months of frequent follow-up visits are necessary, and the patient and family can face a great deal of stress.

27. **What can be done for radial clubhand?**

In ideal circumstances, the hand can be stabilized on the end of the ulna (i.e., ulnar centralization). Radialization moves the hand to the ulnar side of the ulna, and the ulna acts as a bony block to recurrence. Centralization, or radicalization, usually is done acutely, but it may also be done by gradual distraction with an external fixator. Tendon transfer helps to maintain the correction. Because these children always have a missing thumb, the index finger can be moved to function as a thumb by pollicization.

28. **What is the incidence of CFD?**

Approximately 1 in 50,000.

29. **What is the spectrum of CFD?**

There are confusing terminology and multiple classifications. Classically, the term *proximal femoral focal deficiency* has been loosely applied to all instances of short femur, ranging from mild shortening to total absence of the proximal two thirds of the femur. More recently, there has been a consensus to use the term *CFD* (congenital femoral deficiency) to refer to the entire spectrum.

30. **How do I classify CFD?**

Many classifications exist, including the Pappas, Aitken, Hamanishi, and, most recently, Paley classification (Fig. 84-1).

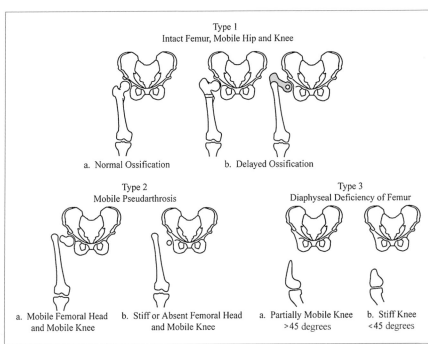

Figure 84-1. Paley's classification of congenial femoral deficiencies. (From Paley D: Lengthening reconstruction surgery for congenital femoral deficiency. In Herring JA, Birch JG [eds]: The Child with a Limb Deficiency. Rosemont, IL, American Academy of Orthopedic Surgeons, 1997, p 114.)

31. **What is the natural history of the unossified cartilage of the femoral neck in CFD?**
Most will ossify within a few years, although typically in a varus pattern. The soft cartilage anlage bends as the child bears weight. The shear forces cause further delay in ossification and make the varus worse.

32. **What hip deformities are associated with CFD?**
   - Coxa vara with abduction contracture of the hip (the gluteus medius and minimus)
   - Extension deformity of the femur with flexion contracture of the hip joint (the tensor fascia lata, rectus femoris, and psoas)
   - Retroversion of the hip (bony retroversion and contracture of the piriformis tendon)
   The proximal femur may have a region of delayed ossification in the subtrochanteric area or the femoral neck. This often may be misinterpreted as pseudoarthrosis.

33. **What knee deformities are associated with CFD?**
   - Absent anterior cruciate ligament (ACL) or posterior cruciate ligament (PCL) or both
   - Valgus due to hypoplastic lateral femoral condyle
   - A small patella
   - Patellar instability or dislocation (lateral)
   - Rotary subluxation (either posterolateral or anteromedial)
   - Flexion contracture (capsular plus biceps femoris and fascia lata)

34. **What other congenital anomalies are associated with CFD?**
FH, foot deficiency, and occasionally bilaterality.

35. **What is the differential diagnosis of bilateral PFFD together with FH?**
Camptomelic dysplasia, with its characteristic short angulated femur and tibia, may be confused with these two conditions when present together. It often is fatal because of pulmonary insufficiency.

36. **What are the treatment options for lengthening in cases of CFD?**
Limb lengthening is a viable treatment option for the Paley type 1a and 1b cases and some of the type 2 cases. Depending on the predicted LLD, two to four lengthenings are required, spread over the growing years from age 2–14 years. Epiphysiodesis can be combined with the lengthening for up to 5 cm of correction. Angular and rotational deformities can be simultaneously corrected.

37. **What are the indications for hip surgery for CFD?**
Before lengthening the femur, evaluate hip stability. If the center-edge (CE) angle is less than 20 degrees or the sourcil is not horizontal, consider Dega pelvic osteotomy. If there is excessive retroversion, consider proximal derotation osteotomy. If the neck shaft angle is less than 100 degrees, consider valgus osteotomy, usually in combination with extensive soft tissue realignment (i.e., a super-hip procedure). If the hip flexion contracture is greater than 15 degrees, a soft tissue release is indicated. We often perform these procedures in combination when the patient is age 18–36 months as a prelude to the first lengthening. During lengthening, it is sometimes necessary to release the proximal musculature (i.e., the tensor fascia latae [TFL] and rectus femoris) at the hip to allow continued lengthening and to facilitate knee motion. Milder degrees of hip varus and retroversion can be corrected during a second lengthening procedure.

38. **What is the best age to start lengthening for CFD?**
There are many psychologic and social considerations. Children between the ages of 2 and 4 years tolerate the lengthening very well. We prefer to begin at this age in cases of large LLD. If the child is older, we often wait until he or she is older than 6 years for psychologic reasons. One needs to consider whether multiple lengthenings will be needed.

39. **What age is best for amputation for CFD?**
Symes amputation may be done at age 1 year. For more complex Van Ness rotationplasty procedures, it is better to wait until the child is a little larger (i.e., age 2–3 years).

40. **What types of amputation can be done for CFD?**
Van Ness rotationplasty, if possible, because of the improved functionality of having a "knee" joint. Prerequisites include a mobile ankle. To improve the function of rotationplasty, the femoral remnant can be fused to the pelvis. Some families object to the appearance of the rotationplasty. Rotationplasty requires lower oxygen consumption than an above-knee amputation.

Traditionally, a Symes amputation is done. This works well for mild cases, in which there is little LLD and the patient's knee is at a functional level. The Symes amputation does not address the hip deformities. Hip reconstruction can be combined with a Symes procedure to improve function.

41. **What is the best level for lengthening the femur in CFD?**
Distal femoral metaphysis, where the bone is wide. There is typically a valgus deformity in the distal femur, so distal lengthening allows simultaneous correction of the valgus. Do not perform internal rotation correction distally! This would lead to lateral patellar subluxation. Although the proximal femur is a useful level for derotation, lengthening in this region leads to poor bone formation and a high risk of fracture.

42. **How do I prevent knee subluxation in CFD lengthening?**
    If there is any preoperative anteroposterior knee instability present, stabilize the knee by extending the femoral frame to the tibia, with hinges to constrain the motion to flexion-extension, disallowing subluxation. Adding a tibial frame with knee hinges also facilitates physiotherapy and night-time knee extension splinting. Intrinsic knee instability can be improved by reconstruction of the ACL and PCL, which can be accomplished with autogenous local tissue such as the fascia lata.

43. **What are the specific complications of femoral lengthening in cases of CFD?**
    Beyond the usual complications of lengthening (see Chapter 38 on anisomelia), special problems more commonly associated with CFD lengthening include knee and hip subluxation, knee contracture, malalignment of the limb, and refracture after frame removal.

44. **Who should perform limb lengthening for CFD?**
    Lengthening for CFD is fraught with serious complications. If performed incorrectly or if the surgeon does not know how to prevent or treat the complications associated with lengthening, the results of treatment can become worse than the natural history. For these reasons, this type of surgery should be performed only by pediatric orthopaedic surgeons who are very experienced in this type of treatment.

45. **What is the role of physical therapy in CFD lengthening?**
    Maintain full knee extension and at least 60 degrees of knee flexion. If knee flexion drops to 40 degrees, stop the lengthening! You can always lengthen again, but you cannot make a new knee joint.

46. **What is the safe range for lengthening?**
    For each lengthening, 5–7.5 cm seems to be reasonable. We do not think that the percent of lengthening is critical. We have not seen growth arrest or slowdown in isolated femoral lengthenings, even in toddlers. With multiple treatments of 5–7.5 cm each, spread over the entire childhood, it is possible to lengthen up to 25–30 cm.

47. **How do I predict limb-length deficiency in patients with congenital deficiencies such as CFD and FH?**
    Normal growth is predictable. Congenital deficiencies usually stay proportionate. For example, a 15% difference at birth will still be a 15% difference at maturity, although the absolute amount of LLD will increase. Using this concept and the Green-Anderson data, a Multiplier Table was developed by Paley et al to predict LLD in congenital deficiencies based on a single outpatient visit (*see* Table 84-1). An alternative method is the Moseley straight-line graph (*see* Chapter 38 on anisomelia).

48. **What is the incidence of FH?**
    Approximately 1 in 40,000.

49. **How do I classify FH?**
    The most commonly used classification is the Achterman-Kalamchi method, based on the appearance of the fibula (short, very short, absent), but an alternate method was recently proposed (i.e., Paley classification, Fig. 84-2) based on the status of the ankle joint. This method helps to guide surgical reconstruction.

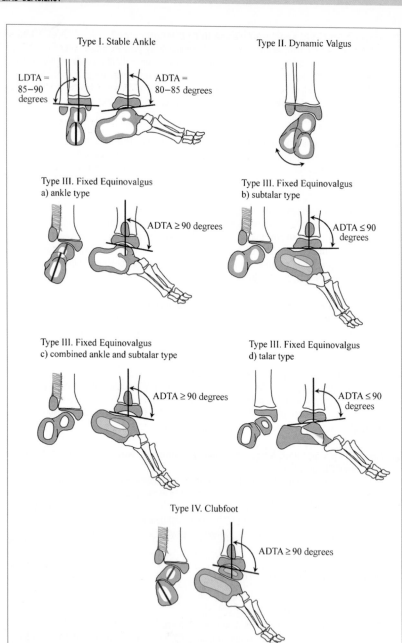

Figure 84-2. Paley's classification of fibular hemimelia, based on status of the ankle joint. LDTA = lateral distal tibial angle, ADTA = anterior distal tibial angle.

KEY POINTS: LIMB DEFICIENCY

1. Upper-extremity prosthetics are not as effective as lower-extremity prosthetics.

2. Limb lengthening is fraught with potential complications and should be performed only by experienced surgeons.

3. Common complications of limb lengthening include joint contracture, nerve damage, fracture after frame removal, pin infection, joint subluxation, and malalignment.

4. Predicting ultimate limb length and mature height can be done at the first patient visit with the multiplier method.

---

50. **What ankle and foot deformities are associated with FH?**
    - Equinus contracture
    - Valgus contracture
    - Ankle stiffness
    - Malorientation of the ankle joint into procurvatum and valgus
    - Talocalcaneal coalition
    - Absent lateral rays
    - Clubfoot (occasionally)

51. **What are the knee deformities associated with FH?**
    - Anterior cruciate ligament instability
    - Posterior cruciate ligament instability
    - Patellar instability
    - Occasionally knee flexion contracture
    - Rotary subluxation
    - Valgus

52. **What are the treatment options for FH?**
    Symes amputation versus lengthening and reconstruction.

53. **What are the indications for amputation in patients with FH?**
    This is controversial. Some sources recommend amputating all feet that have only three rays and feet in which the level is projected to be at the mid-calf region. A study from the Texas Scottish Rite Hospital found excellent long-term functional and psychologic outcomes for children with FH who underwent amputation. Other authors have achieved excellent results with lengthening reconstruction surgery (LRS) and find few indications for prosthetic reconstruction. Several studies that concluded that LRS is not as good as amputation based their conclusions on the high rate of recurrent equinovalgus foot deformity. The lengthening itself was not the problem. Most authors would not consider amputation for an equinovalgus foot deformity without an LLD or for an LLD without a foot deformity. We have mostly solved this problem with minimal recurrence by combining extra-articular soft tissue release with realignment osteotomy of the ankle or subtalar region. This is combined with lengthening at the same time as early as 18 months of age.

54. **What are the specific complications of tibial lengthening in FH?**
    Besides the usual litany of complications associated with general limb lengthening, patients with FH may experience recurrent ankle deformity and contracture, rebound tibial valgus (i.e., the

Cozen phenomenon), and fracture of the regenerate. Some claim that tibial growth arrest commonly occurs after tibial lengthening in cases of FH, but we have not observed this except in cases in which a second lengthening is done in the same bone within 2 years of the first lengthening procedure.

55. **What is the role of physical therapy in lengthening in cases of FH?**
The foot usually is included in the frame, so primary physical therapy efforts are directed at maintaining knee extension.

56. **What is the safe range for lengthening?**
In children under age 4 years up to 5 cm; in older children, 5–8 cm.

57. **What is the incidence of TH?**
One in 1,000,000. Considering that there are four types of TH, the incidence of each individual type is even less.

58. **How is TH classified?**
Four types exist based on the Lloyd-Roberts classification. Type 1 has no tibia, although some patients who appear to have no tibia develop an upper tibia during the first years of life (i.e., delayed ossification). Type 2 has an upper tibia, type 3 (which is very rare) has a lower tibia, and type 4 has congenital diastasis of the ankle. Recently, a new classification has been proposed, consisting of five types: absent tibia, absent distal tibia, distal joint and physis present, diastasis of the tibia and fibula, and overgrowth of the fibula (Fig. 84-3).

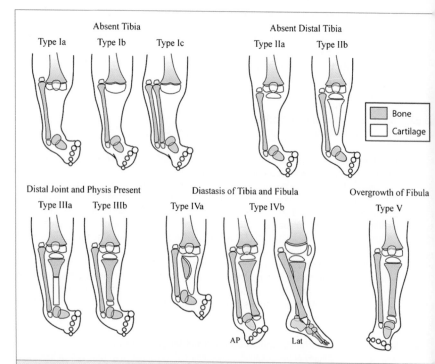

Figure 84-3. Classification of tibial hemimelia. AP = anteroposterior, Lat = lateral.

59. **What are the treatment options for type II TH?**
Amputation versus reconstruction and lengthening.

60. **For complete absence of the tibia, what is the best treatment?**
The Brown procedure to centralize the fibula has been largely abandoned. A new procedure described by Weber uses the patella to substitute for a proximal tibia and then puts the fibula under this modification.

61. **For congenital diastasis of the tibia, what is the best treatment?**
Maintain the ankle motion, but reorient the foot plantigrade and lengthen through a supramalleolar osteotomy during the first 3 years of life. Distal fibular epiphyseodesis may be required to prevent overgrowth of the fibula. Perform recurrent lengthening as needed and, when the patient is mature, shave the prominent bump of the medial malleolus. Another option is lengthening through the talus and calcaneus (i.e., Ilizarov U-osteotomy) to effectively raise the Spherion height (i.e., the distance from the medial malleolus to the floor).

BIBLIOGRAPHY

1. Achterman C, Kalamchi A: Congenital deficiency of the fibula. J Bone Joint Surg Br 61:133–137, 1979.

2. Bowen JR, Kumar SJ, Orellana CA, et al: Factors leading to hip subluxation and dislocation in femoral lengthening of unilateral congenital short femur. J Pediatr Orthop 21:354–359, 2001.

3. Brown KL: Resection, rotationplasty, and femoropelvic arthrodesis in severe congenital femoral deficiency. J Bone Joint Surg Br 83:78–85, 2001.

4. Buck-Gramcko D: Radialization as a new treatment for radial club hand. J Hand Surg 10A(6 Pt 2):964–968, 1985.

5. Catagni MA, Bolano L, Cattaneo R: Management of fibular hemimelia using the Ilizarov method. Orthop Clin North Am 22:715–722, 1991.

6. Choi IH, Kumar SJ, Bowen JR: Amputation or limb lengthening for partial or total absence of the fibula. J Bone Joint Surg Am 72:1391–1399, 1990.

7. Herring JA, Birch JG (eds): The Child with a Limb Deficiency. Rosemont, IL, American Academy of Orthopaedic Surgeons, 1997.

8. Herzenberg JE, Scheufele LL, Paley D, et al: Knee range of motion in isolated femoral lengthening. Clin Orthop Relat Res 301:49–54, 1994.

9. Jones E, Barnes J, Lloyd-Roberts GC: Congenital aplasia and dysplasia of the tibia with intact fibula: Classification and management. J Bone Joint Surg Br 60:31–39, 1978.

10. Manner HM, Radler C, Ganger R, Grill F: Dysplasia of the cruciate ligaments: Radiographic assessment and classification. J Bone Joint Surg Am 88:130–137, 2006.

11. McCarthy JJ, Glancy GL, Chang FM, Eilert RE: Fibular hemimelia: Comparison of outcome measurements after amputation and lengthening. J Bone Joint Surg Am 82:1732–1735, 2000.

12. Naudie D, Hamdy RC, Fassier F, et al: Management of fibular hemimelia: Amputation or limb lengthening. J Bone Joint Surg Br 79:58–65, 1997.

13. Nogueira MP, Paley D, Bhave A, et al: Nerve lesions associated with limb-lengthening. J Bone Joint Surg Am 85:1502–1510, 2003.

14. Paley D: Principles of Deformity Correction. Berlin, Springer-Verlag, 2002.

15. Paley D, Bhave A, Herzenberg JE, Bowen JR: Multiplier method for predicting limb-length discrepancy. J Bone Joint Surg Am 82:1432–1446, 2000.

16. Paley D, Herzenberg J: Distraction treatment of congenital and developmental deformities of the hand and foot. In Buck-Gramcko D (ed): Congenital Malformations of the Hand and Forearm. London, Churchill Livingstone, 1998, pp 73–117.

17. Paley J, Talor J, Levin A, et al: The multiplier method for prediction of adult height. J Pediatr Orthop 24:732–737, 2004.

18. Sabharwal S, Paley D, Bhave A, Herzenberg JE: Growth patterns after lengthening of congenitally short lower limbs in young children. J Pediatr Orthop 20:137–145, 2000.

19. Shapiro F: Ollier's disease: An assessment of angular deformity, shortening, and pathological fracture in twenty-one patients. J Bone Joint Surg Am 64:95, 1982.

20. Steel HH, Lin PS, Betz RR, et al: Iliofemoral fusion for proximal femoral focal deficiency. J Bone Joint Surg Br 69:837, 1987.

21. Weber M: A new knee arthroplasty versus Brown procedure in congenital total absence of the tibia: A preliminary report. J Pediatr Orthop 11B:53–59, 2002.

22. www.limblengthening.org: International Center for Limb Lengthening, Baltimore, MD.

SYNDROME EVALUATION

William G. Mackenzie, MD

CHAPTER 85

1. **What is a syndrome?**
   A syndrome is a group of birth defects that are considered together as a characteristic of a particular disease. Sometimes congenital anomalies occur together by chance alone, such as birthmarks and clinodactyly of the fifth finger, but these do not indicate an underlying syndrome. A syndrome is often present if all four extremities and the spine are involved, if limb deformities are symmetric, or if there is a typical dysmorphic face, associated nonorthopaedic anomalies, or a typical orthopaedic malformation such as a radial club hand (which is seen as a component of syndromes).

2. **What causes syndromes?**
   Dysregulation of important pathways in the development of a child may cause malformation of organs, resulting in uncommon abnormalities occurring together, producing a syndrome. These pathways can be dysregulated by genetic mutations of important parts of the pathway or by factors extrinsic to the fetus, such as toxins in the environment like alcohol, as in fetal alcohol syndrome. The clinical features in a syndrome may vary in their presence or severity in individuals with the same syndrome and even within a family that has a syndrome. This may be due to modifying genes or to fetal environmental factors.

3. **How do we classify syndromes?**
   A clinically useful way of classifying syndromes has been suggested by Alman and Goldberg, as follows:
   - **Mutation of genes encoding structural proteins:** Osteogenesis imperfecta, type II collagenopathy such as spondyloepiphyseal dysplasia and Kniest syndrome, Marfan's syndrome, Ehlers-Danlos syndrome, and homocystinuria
   - **Mutation resulting in dysregulation of cell proliferation and overgrowth:** Neurofibromatosis, Beckwith-Wiedemann syndrome, Russell-Silver syndrome, and Proteus syndrome
   - **Mutation of genes that encode proteins that are important in cell-signaling systems (i.e., coordinated cell proliferation, movement, and apoptosis):** Nail-patella syndrome, Goldenhar's syndrome, and Cornelia De Lange's syndrome
   - **Mutation in genes that encode for proteins that are important for nerve or muscle development and function:** Familial dysautonomia, Rett syndrome, muscular dystrophies, Charcot-Marie-Tooth disease, and others
   - **Mutation in genes that encode for enzymes:** Mucopolysaccharidoses
   - **Chromosomal abnormalities that involve large sections of DNA and multiple genes:** Down syndrome, Turner's syndrome, Noonan's syndrome, trichorhinophalangeal syndrome, Prader-Willi syndrome, and Rubinstein-Taybi syndrome
   - **Teratogenic agents:** Fetal alcohol syndrome and VACTERL association (vertebral abnormalities, anal atresia, cardiac abnormalities, tracheoesophageal fistula and/or esophageal atresia, renal agenesis and dysplasia, and limb defects)
   - **Contracture syndromes:** Arthrogryposis multiplex congenita, Larsen's syndrome, and popliteal pterygium syndrome

KEY POINTS: SYNDROME EVALUATION

1. Syndromes are characteristic groups of birth defects caused by dysregulation of pathways that lead to limb and organ development.

2. Syndromes may be due to genetic aberrations or due to fetal environmental factors.

3. A careful examination and history with an open mind by the observer can lead to an accurate diagnosis in many cases.

4. **Why is it important to make the diagnosis of a syndrome?**
There are many important reasons to make an accurate diagnosis. It makes it possible to have a discussion with the family about associated medical conditions and expected orthopaedic problems in the child's future. The associated medical abnormalities may be more important than the orthopaedic problems early in the child's life. An example of this is in Ellis-van Creveld syndrome, in which postaxial polydactyly is the most obvious problem, but these children should be checked closely for a structural cardiac defect and restrictive lung disease. Pulmonary, renal, or cardiac abnormalities may have a significant impact on anesthesia. An accurate diagnosis also allows the child to be included in research trials. In addition, early diagnosis allows the geneticist to have a discussion with the family about the risk of recurrence with subsequent pregnancies.

5. **How do you make the diagnosis of a syndrome?**
A thorough history and physical examination, as well as an open mind, will commonly result in an accurate diagnosis. Consultations by specialists in genetics and developmental medicine can be helpful to make the diagnosis and to provide counseling to the family.
   Radiographic evaluation can demonstrate characteristic features present in many dysplasias. A standard set of radiographs includes a flexion-extension lateral view of the cervical spine; standing anteroposterior (AP) and lateral views of the thoracolumbar spine; a standing AP view, hips to ankles, of both lower extremities; an AP view of one arm from the shoulder to the wrist; and a posteroanterior view of both hands and wrists.
   For most syndromes, the diagnosis can be made using clinical and radiographic findings. Standard laboratory testing may be helpful if one is trying to differentiate rickets from metaphyseal dysplasia or is making the diagnosis of hypophosphatasia or one of the mucopolysaccharidoses. Molecular genetic testing is not available for all syndromes, is extremely expensive, and is usually done to confirm a diagnosis rather than to make the diagnosis. Chromosome studies are appropriate when a child has multiple unrelated abnormalities together with a mental deficit or growth retardation.

6. **What skeletal abnormalities are present in orthopaedic syndromes?**
See Table 85-1.

TABLE 85-1. SKELETAL ABNORMALITIES IN ORTHOPAEDIC SYNDROMES

Abnormality	Syndrome
Short limb segments	
Short proximal segment (i.e., rhizomelia)	Achondroplasia, chondrodysplasia punctata, femoral hypoplasia, unusual facies syndrome
Short middle segment (i.e., mesomelia)	Leri-Weill syndrome, Robinow's syndrome
Short distal segment (i.e., acromelia)	Down syndrome, fetal warfarin syndrome
Disproportion between trunk and limb length	
Short trunk and short limbs	Kniest dysplasia, Morquio's syndrome, spondyloepiphyseal dysplasia
Short limbs and relatively normal trunk	Achondroplasia, spondyloepiphyseal dysplasia
Asymmetric limb size	Klippel-Trénaunay-Weber syndrome, Russell-Silver syndrome, hemihypertrophy
Absence of one or more skeletal elements	Tibial hemimelia, amniotic band sequence ectrodactyly, VACTERL association
Duplication of one or more skeletal elements	Trisomy 13, Ellis-van Creveld
Bone fragility, repeated fractures	Osteogenesis imperfecta (types I & II), hypophosphatasia, osteopetrosis
Multiple enlarged joints	Kniest syndrome, Stickler's syndrome
Joint contractures	Arthrogryposis (several types), Hurler's syndrome, oligohydramnios sequence, fetal alcohol syndrome, popliteal pterygium
Joint hypermobility and laxity	Down syndrome, Marfan's syndrome, Ehlers-Danlos syndrome

VACTERL = Vertebral abnormalities, anal atresia, cardiac abnormalities, tracheoesophageal fistula and/or esophageal atresia, renal agenesis and dysplasia, and limb defects.
Adapted from J. M. Aase, MD.

BIBLIOGRAPHY

1. Alman BA, Goldberg MJ: Syndromes of orthopedic importance. In Morrissy RT, Weinstein SL (eds): Lowell and Winters Pediatric Orthopedics. Philadelphia, Lippincott Williams & Wilkins, 2006, pp 205–250.

2. Canepa G, Maroteaux P, Pietrogrande V: Dysmorphic Syndromes and Constitutional Diseases of the Skeleton. Padua, Piccin Nuova Libraria, 2001.

3. Jones KL, Smith DW: Smith's Recognizable Patterns of Human Malformation, 5th ed. Philadelphia, W.B. Saunders, 1997.

CHAPTER 86

SHORT STATURE EVALUATION

Michael J. Goldberg, MD

1. **What is short stature?**

   Short stature is defined as a height below the third percentile line or greater than 2 standard deviations below the mean. Updated percentile charts for plotting height by chronologic age are available from the Centers for Disease Control and Prevention (CDC) and the National Center for Health Statistics and are reproduced in almost every pediatric text. Keep in mind that, by using this definition, 2.5% of normal children will be considered short. Furthermore, the standardized growth charts are based on the U.S. population and are less accurate for certain ethnic and racial groups.

2. **What are the causes of short stature?**

   Causes include endocrine disorders such as growth hormone deficiency or hypothyroidism; metabolic bone diseases such as rickets; and chronic diseases such as renal failure or congenital heart disease. Some children are small and fail to thrive because of nutritional, physical, or psychologic abuse. Short stature is also a feature of a number of well-recognized syndromes. These can be chromosome disorders (such as Turner's syndrome or Down syndrome), a single gene disorder (such as familial dysautonomia), or a dysmorphic syndrome in which the gene locus is suspected but the molecular pathology is not yet confirmed (such as de Lange's syndrome or Russell-Silver syndrome). Short stature may also be the result of a primary disorder of bone and cartilage growth. These are called *skeletal dysplasias*. Some children are short because they come from a short family. This is known as *constitutional* or *familial short stature*. Some 80% of so-called "short children" fall into this category, in which work-ups yield no specific cause of their short stature.

3. **How are children with short stature evaluated? (Fig. 86-1)**

   History is particularly critical and should include the height of the parents and family members; the age of the mother's menarche; the child's prenatal growth; whether the mother experienced infection, hypertension, or alcohol, tobacco, or drug exposure during pregnancy; the child's birthweight and length; the child's history of major illness, trauma, or surgery; and an estimate of the child's rate of growth. It is helpful to determine whether growth retardation began prior to birth (i.e., intrauterine growth retardation, a common occurrence in syndromes, and intrauterine infections), or whether the child was somewhat small at birth but then stayed very small, such as with skeletal dysplasias. Some children grow normally for a while and then fall below the growth curve, a phenomenon seen in some endocrine disorders. Although crossing a growth curve is normal prior to age 2 years, crossing such growth curves after that age can be the first sign of an underlying abnormality. The patient must have a careful and complete physical examination, noting not only an accurate height but also proportions and a search for dysmorphic features. Clinical examination includes assessing the signs and stages of puberty (i.e., the Tanner stages), which is somewhat easier to do in girls than in boys.

4. **How are children measured?**

   Height measurement by a flip-top bar mounted on a scale is too inaccurate to be of great value. An accurate measurement can be obtained by using a Harpenden stadiometer. In children

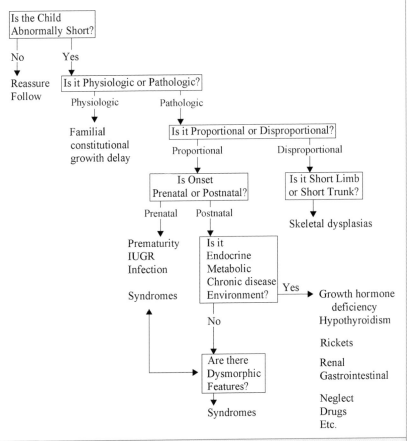

Figure 86-1. Series of clinical questions to attain a tentative diagnosis and to launch additional diagnostic steps as needed. IUGR = intrauterine growth retardation. (Adapted from Goldberg MJ, Yassir W, Sadeghi-Nejad A: Clinical analysis of short stature. J Pediatr Orthop 22:690–696, 2002, p 691.)

younger than 3 years, the child's length can be more easily measured supine. The normal rate of growth is dependent on the child's age, and even then it is not continuous, but rather is saltatory.

5. **What are proportional and disproportional short stature?**
   Children with normal stature exhibit some physiologic disproportion. Infants and young children have a long trunk and short limbs compared with adults. The ratio of trunk length to lower body segment length (i.e., the upper-to-lower [U:L] ratio) is 1.7 at birth and decreases to 1 in adults.

6. **Why is the ratio between trunk length and limb length important?**
   In general, children with short stature fall into two groups: proportionate and disproportionate. In children with proportionate short stature, the relationship between their trunk length and their limbs is identical to that of a child of normal stature except that these children are small. Proportionate short stature is typical of endocrine disorders such as absent growth hormone

and failure to thrive due to chronic disease. Disproportionate short stature is characteristic of skeletal dysplasias (i.e., dwarfism). Disproportionate short stature may be one of short limbs in relation to the trunk or a short trunk in relation to the limbs. Shortening of the extremities can be documented by measuring the U:L ratio and comparing it to age-appropriate standards. However, in the clinical setting, the determination of disproportionate short stature is often best done by simple inspection rather than by quantitative methods.

Clinical tip: Determining where the fingertips are with the arms held at the sides during upright standing assists in differentiating short-trunk from short-limb skeletal dysplasias. In short-limb dwarfism, such as achondroplasia, the fingertips come to just below the waist, whereas in short-trunk dwarfism, such as spondyloepiphyseal dysplasia, the fingers come almost to the knees.

7. **What laboratory and imaging studies help differentiate the various types of short stature?**

   Useful imaging and laboratory studies include hand and wrist radiographs for skeletal age; urinalysis; complete blood cell count; erythrocyte sedimentation rate; serum electrolytes; blood urea nitrogen and creatinine; calcium, phosphorous, and alkaline phosphatase; thyroid function studies; and a random growth hormone and insulin-like growth factor-I (IgF-I). If a **skeletal dysplasia** is suspected, a limited skeletal survey should include a lateral radiograph of the skull, a posteroanterior (PA) and lateral view of the thoracic and lumbar spine, an anteroposterior (AP) view of the pelvis, and an AP view of only one upper and one lower extremity.

8. **What is skeletal age?**

   The degree of bone maturation is due to factors other than just the age of the child. Hormones (thyroid, growth, and sex) have a significant effect on the maturation of bone. Thus, children with the same chronologic age may have different skeletal or bone ages. Greulich and Pyle obtained serial radiographs of the hands of children at various ages and established the most common radiographic appearance for each age. This is known as the *bone* or *skeletal age*. By comparing the patient's hand radiograph to the radiographs in the *Greulich and Pyle Atlas,* one can determine the patient's bone age. Thus, a child may have a chronologic age of 8 years but a skeletal age of only 5 years. Delayed bone age is typical of short stature secondary to endocrine disorders. Bone age corresponds well to the development of secondary sexual characteristics. There is considerable interobserver variability and, in addition, there is wide standard deviation (i.e., variation) among normal children, and different genetic populations have different rates of maturation.

   Clinical tip: An AP radiograph of the hand and wrist gives considerable information when evaluating a child for short stature. It not only gives the skeletal age, thus providing a clue to whether there is an endocrine basis for short stature, but also illustrates the morphology of the bone and any peculiarities of bone growth. The hand and wrist is a sensitive area for seeing the changes due to skeletal dysplasias and changes due to endocrinopathies.

9. **What is a skeletal dysplasia?**

   A skeletal dysplasia is a generalized developmental disorder that affects both bone and cartilage.

10. **What are the clinical findings in skeletal dysplasias?**

    The child is abnormally short, typically well below the third percentile. The child has disproportionate short stature and dysmorphic facial features. Since skeletal dysplasias affect both bone and cartilage, there are often abnormalities in the facial structures.

11. **How are children with short stature treated?**

    Treatment depends on the cause of short stature. For children with an endocrinopathy such as growth hormone deficiency, replacement therapy with genetically engineered recombinant human growth hormone is very effective. For children who are short due to a thyroid condition, treatment with thyroid replacement is helpful. Likewise, in children with metabolic bone disease (i.e., rickets), the management of the metabolic calcium, phosphorous, and vitamin D disorder often improves height. Management of height is less effective for children who have chronic diseases since the underlying disease often disrupts the growth hormone-somatomedin axis. Pharmacologic treatment of children with skeletal dysplasias and with most syndromes is usually ineffective.

12. **In what conditions is growth hormone treatment effective?**
    In addition to use in treating children with growth hormone deficiency, growth hormone has a positive effect on both the rate of growth and the eventual height of children with intrauterine growth retardation, chronic renal failure, and Turner's syndrome. There is some evidence that growth hormone may be effective in familial hypophosphatemic rickets, prematurity, and certain syndromes such as Prader-Willi, Noonan's, and Russell-Silver. Growth hormone has been tried and was not proven to be effective in a number of conditions such as skeletal dysplasias, physiologic short stature, and chronic diseases other than renal.

13. **How is growth hormone administered? What are its adverse side effects?**
    Growth hormone is administered subcutaneously daily. A slow-release preparation administered once every 2–3 weeks is approved by the Food and Drug Administration (FDA), but the daily subcutaneous administration is believed by many clinicians to be more effective. Orthopaedic adverse side effects include slipped femoral capital epiphysis, avascular necrosis, and progression of scoliosis.

KEY POINTS: SHORT STATURE EVALUATION

1. By answering a series of questions, the clinician can arrive at a tentative diagnosis and can launch additional studies as needed:
   - Is the child abnormally short?
   - Is it physiologic or pathologic?
   - Is it proportional or disproportional?
   - Is onset prenatal or postnatal?
   - Is it endocrine, metabolic, or chronic disease?
   - Are there dysmorphic features?

2. Establishing the etiology of the short stature is critical to understanding what interventions may or may not be effective in trying to gain more height.

14. **How can the stature of children with skeletal dysplasias be increased?**
    There is no evidence that children with skeletal dysplasias are deficient in growth hormone or have other endocrine or metabolic abnormalities. Children with skeletal dysplasias can be made taller by elongation of the long bones (i.e., the femur and tibia) followed by the elongation of the humerus so that the child looks in proportion. Gradual distraction of the femur and tibia using special fixators can result in substantial elongation of up to 30 cm. The technique involves performing an osteotomy through the long bone and then distracting the bone slowly as new bone callus is formed in the gap. Distraction is at the rate of 1 mm a day, so the procedure takes considerable time.

15. **Why is skeletal elongation controversial?**
    The proponents of skeletal elongation argue that disproportionate short stature poses both physical and emotional handicaps for the child; the person is stigmatized and impaired in

activities of daily living because of the standard height of countertops and workbenches. Elongation offers psychologic benefits and a more normal appearance. In addition, angular malalignment of the legs, present in many skeletal dysplasias, can be straightened. This realignment of the joints may prevent precocious arthritis. In certain dysplasias such as achondroplasia, skeletal elongation of the femur appears to improve the swayback (i.e., lumbar lordosis) characteristic of this disorder. Those opposed to skeletal elongation argue that average adult height is rarely achieved and that a normal proportional ratio of limbs to trunk is very difficult to accomplish. In addition, they argue that, from the child's perspective, undergoing a prolonged surgical procedure results in the child feeling psychologically rejected by the parents. The procedure takes substantial time and is carried out in a child who usually has no symptoms. Often, there is significant loss of school time and socialization. In addition, experimental lengthening in immature dogs has demonstrated damage to the growth plate from compressive forces as well as compression across the articular cartilage, predisposing to arthritis. The procedure is expensive and fraught with complications. There are no long-term outcome studies that establish the benefits of lengthening procedures in children with dwarfism.

BIBLIOGRAPHY

1. Dimeglio A: Growth in pediatric orthopaedics. J Pediatr Orthop 21:549–555, 2001.
2. Goldberg MJ, Yassir W, Sadeghi-Nejad A: Clinical analysis of short stature. J Pediatr Orthop 22:690–696, 2002.

CHAPTER 87

OSTEOCHONDRODYSPLASIA

Mohammad Diab, MD

1. **Distinguish *dwarf* from *midget, dysplasia* from *dysostosis, deformity* from *malformation,* and *syndrome* from *disease.***
   - A midget demonstrates proportionate short stature, whereas in dwarfism there is disproportionate affection of parts of the body.
   - Dysplasia represents systemic disease of bones, whereas dysostosis indicates involvement of a single bone or a group of physically or functionally related bones.
   - Malformation describes primary disease, whereas deformity occurs as a secondary phenomenon.
   - Syndrome, used by Galen as a compound of Greek *sun* (meaning *with* or *together*) and *dromos* (meaning *a course, race,* or *running*) signifies a concurrence of signs in or the clinical presentation of a disease.

2. **How are the osteochondrodysplasias classified anthropometrically? How are they classified radiographically?**
   Disproportionate involvement of the trunk is known as *microcormia,* from the Greek *mikros* (meaning *small*) and *kormos* (meaning *trunk*). Disproportionate involvement of the limbs is known as *micromelia,* from the Greek *melos* (meaning *limb*). Micromelia may be subdivided into the following categories:
   - **Rhizomicromelia:** From the Greek *riza* (meaning *root*), indicating that the humerus or os femoris is affected
   - **Mesomicromelia:** From the Greek *mesos* (meaning *mid*), indicating that the radius and ulna or the tibia and fibula are affected
   - **Acromicromelia:** From the Greek *akros* (meaning *end*), indicating that the hands or feet are affected

   The **radiographic classification** is based on the region of bone principally affected, such as epiphysis versus metaphysis versus diaphysis. The convenience of this system has led to its wide adoption by clinicians. However, it is simplistic, bears no relationship to morbidity, and frequently suggests a connection between entities where there is none.

3. **Define *collagen*.**
   Collagen, derived from the Greek *kola* (meaning *glue*) and the suffix *-gen* (meaning *giving rise to*), is the name given to a family of proteins that compose the principal constituents of the extracellular matrix of the tissues of the musculoskeletal system.

   The collagen molecule is composed of three polypeptide chains, each assigned the Greek letter α, and is therefore a trimer. Although the primary structure of each polypeptide chain differs among collagen types, a repeating three-amino-acid sequence is strictly preserved, represented by the formula $(Gly-X-Y)_n$. Every third residue is a glycine (Gly). X and Y can vary; however, a high proportion of amino acids at the X position tend to be proline (Pro), and a high proportion at the Y position tends to be hydroxyproline (Hyp).

   Portions of a collagen chain that follow this typical sequence are helical and are known as collagenous domains (COL); those that do not are termed *noncollagenous domains* (NC). The individual chains may be identical, encoded by the same gene, in which case they form a **homotrimer,** or they may be different gene products, forming a **heterotrimer.**

Cleavage of amino-terminal and carboxyl-terminal propeptides during or after secretion converts procollagen to collagen. The tertiary structure of each collagen chain is a left-handed helix, and the three chains wrap around one another to form a right-handed superhelical molecule.

At least 20 genetically distinct types of collagens have been identified. Each is given a Roman numeral indicative of the order of discovery. Bone contains types I and V. The hyaline cartilage of diarthrodial articulations contains types II, IX, and XI. The hypertrophic zone of epiphyseal cartilage contains type X. In the anulus fibrosus of the intervertebral disk, type I predominates, whereas in the nucleus pulposus, type II predominates. Skin contains types I and III. Blood vessels contain types I, III, and V. Type III also occurs at tendon insertion into bone.

4. **Define *proteoglycan*.**
Proteoglycans (PGs), formerly known as *protein polysaccharides* or *mucoproteins,* refer to a molecule of "protein and sugar." PGs have three components:
- **Glycosaminoglycan (GAG):** Formerly known as *mucopolysaccharide,* this represents an unbranched chain of repeating disaccharide units, of which one is an amino sugar. With the exception of hyaluronic acid, the GAGs carry a high negative charge on account of the sulfate and carboxyl groups added to their sugar residues.
- **Link protein:** This interacts noncovalently to stabilize the bond formed between each GAG and
- **Protein core**

PG monomers interact specifically, although noncovalently, with hyaluronate to form very high molecular weight aggregates. The major proteoglycan of cartilage is aggrecan, of which the protein core may have covalently attached as many as 100 chondroitin sulfate and 50 keratan sulfate GAGs. Cartilage also contains small nonaggregating proteoglycans including **decorin**, which decorates the surface of type II collagen fibrils, and **biglycan**, of which the core protein bears two chondroitin sulfate GAGs.

The molecular structure and negative charge of PGs enables them to occupy a large volume for mass and to attract water according to the Gibbs-Donnan equilibrium. They form a porous hydrated gel that resists compression and regulates the passage of molecules and cells through the extracellular matrix. By contrast, collagen fibrils form a scaffold that maintains the structural integrity of the extracellular matrix and primarily resists tensile forces.

5. **What is the clinical ramification of epiphyseal diseases compared with those that affect the metaphyses and diaphyses of long bones?**
Epiphyseal diseases result in osteoarthritis.

6. **Describe the four principal type II collagenopathies. Give the characteristic features of this group of disorders.**
Type II collagen is a homotrimer of polypeptides encoded by the COL2A1 gene of chromosome 12. The principal tissues of distribution are hyaline cartilage and vitreous humor; therefore, the phenotypic expression of mutations in COL2A1 are primarily osseous and ocular. The four type II collagenopathies of most clinical relevance are as follows:
- Premature osteoarthritis with mild short stature
- Stickler's syndrome
- Spondyloepiphyseal dysplasia
- Kniest dysplasia

They can be considered to distribute on a spectrum of increasing severity. **Osseous abnormalities** include:
- Spinal deformity, including kyphoscoliosis, hyperlordosis, and hypoplasia or aplasia of the dens axis with atlantoaxial instability
- Epiphyseal degeneration, leading to premature osteoarthritis of the proximal os femoris to coxa vara

- Clubfoot
- Varying degrees of short stature
  Ocular abnormalities include the following:
- Vitreous degeneration
- Myopia
- Retinal detachment
- Cataract
  Other anomalies also may be present, including:
- Sensorineural and conductive hearing loss
- Cleft palate
- Inguinal and umbilical hernias

7. **Give three characteristic features of diastrophic dysplasia. What mutation has been identified in diastrophic dysplasia? For what other osteochondrodysplasias is this mutation responsible?**

   The term *diastrophic*, from the Greek *dia* (meaning *throughout, in different directions, thoroughly,* or *completely*) and *strophe* (meaning *a turning, twisting,* or *crookedness*) was suggested to describe the severe twisting of the spine and feet. Characteristic features include:

   - Spinal deformity, including kyphoscoliosis, hypoplasia or aplasia of the dens axis with atlantoaxial instability, and cervical kyphosis
   - Clubfoot
   - Calcification of the auricular cartilage, producing cauliflower ears, and of costal cartilage
   - Shortening and abduction of the first metacarpal, producing hitchhiker thumb
   - Periarthric contractures associated with osteoarthritis
   - Cleft palate
   - Hearing loss

   Diastrophic dysplasia is caused by a mutation in the solute carrier family 26 member 2 (SLC26A2) gene on human chromosome 5q32–33.1. The gene encodes a novel sulfate transporter (ST), and fibroblasts from diastrophic individuals demonstrate significantly diminished sulfate uptake.

   Although the disease affects principally cartilage and bone, the sulfate transporter is ubiquitously expressed. This may reflect the high sulfate requirement of chondrocytes, compared with other cell types, for the synthesis of proteoglycans, of which the sulfate groups confer a negative charge essential to their function in the extracellular matrix. Abnormality of type IX collagen has been observed in hyaline cartilage from a diastrophic individual. Several forms of type IX collagen have been identified. One bears a chondroitin sulfate glycosaminoglycan on the $\alpha 2$ chain and is therefore a proteoglycan.

   Mutations in the SLC26A2 gene have been identified in atelosteogenesis type II (AO II) and achondrogenesis type IB (ACG-IB). In both, abnormal sulfation of proteoglycans has been demonstrated.

   The following theory has been advanced to explain the above findings. Diastrophic dysplasia, AO II, and ACG-IB represent different phenotypic expressions of mutation in the same gene, ACG-IB being the null allele. This resembles the type II collagenopathies (see above).

   Disease severity is inversely related to diastrophic dysplasia ST activity and the degree of proteoglycan sulfation. This is supported by the fact that in ACG-IB, mutations occur in both alleles and tend to be premature stop codons; in AO II, both alleles are affected but by less-damaging mutations, and in diastrophic dysplasia, one allele is spared.

8. **Define *fibroblast growth factor receptor* (FGFR). Name three osteochondrodysplasias caused by FGFR mutations.**

   Nine genetically distinct fibroblast growth factors (FGFs) have been identified in mammals. Their pleiotropic effects, which include mitogenesis, differentiation, and chemotaxis, are mediated by

FGFRs. Four FGFRs have been identified in mammals. They belong to the tyrosine kinase family of receptors. Their common structural features include a split intracellular tyrosine kinase domain, a transmembrane domain, and two or three extracellular immunoglobulin-like domains. FGFRs are expressed at different stages of development and are located on the surface of several cell types including chondrocytes during endochondral ossification and cells of the embryonic central nervous system.

Four types of FGFRs have been identified, designated 1 through 4. In general, mutations in the FGFR3 gene affect predominantly bones that develop by endochondral ossification, whereas dominant mutations involving FGFR1 and FGFR2 principally cause syndromes that involve bones arising by membranous ossification. As a result, mutations in FGFR1 and FGFR2 cause syndromes involving craniosynostosis, and the dwarfing syndromes are associated with FGFR3 mutations. Examples of the former are Pfeiffer syndrome (caused by FGFR1 mutation), Apert's syndrome, and Crouzon disease (caused by FGFR2 mutations). Examples of the latter dwarfing syndromes include achondroplasia, thanatophoric dysplasia, and hypochondroplasia.

9. **What is achondroplasia?**
Achondroplasia is the most common osteochondrodysplasia, occurring once in every 15,000 live births. It is an autosomal-dominant disorder with complete penetrance. Eighty percent of cases are new mutations, and $\geq$99% of the mutations are in the G380R region of FGFR3. Features include:
- **Facies:** Frontal bossing, midface hypoplasia, and a low nasal bridge
- **Limbs:** Rhizomelic shortening; relative overgrowth of the clavicle, producing broad shoulders; relative overgrowth of the fibula, producing ankle varus; genu varum; brachydactyly; a deep cleft between the longest and ring fingers; equalization of the length of the fingers, producing a trident hand; and limited elbow and hip extension
- **Joints:** Ligamentous laxity
- **Spine:** Thoracolumbar kyphosis in infancy, lumbar hyperlordosis, and lumbar spinal stenosis due to short pedicles and progressive interpedicular narrowing in the lumbar spine
- **Pelvis:** Constriction at triradiate cartilage with a flat acetabular roof and relative flaring of the ilia, producing champagne pelvis; and coxa vara
- **Neural:** Hydrocephalus; occasional foramen magnum stenosis, producing brainstem compression

10. **What is thanatophoric dysplasia?**
Thanatophoric dysplasia is so named because it is death-bearing in the perinatal period. Features include:
- Kleeblattschädel (meaning *clover-leaf skull*) as a result of hydrocephalus and sutural synostosis
- A narrow thorax with short horizontal ribs and hypoplastic scapulas
- Telephone-receiver ossa femorum
- Platyspondyly

11. **What is hypochondroplasia?**
This presents a spectrum ranging from severe, which is indistinguishable from achondroplasia, to mild, which approaches the normal. FGFR3 additionally, and FGFR4 solely, have been implicated in oncogenesis.

12. **By what sclerosing bone dysplasia is the French impressionist painter H. M. R. de Toulouse-Lautrec Monfa said to have been affected? Describe the clinical and radiographic features of this disorder. What is the underlying mutation?**
Pyknodysostosis, or "the condition of bad bones that are thick and dense," from the Greek *puknos* (meaning *close-packed, dense,* or *thick*). This is characterized by the following features:
- **Skull:** Delayed suture closure, frontal bossing, micrognathia, narrow palate, hypodontia, and caries

- **Chest:** Aplasia or hypoplasia of the clavicle
- **Spine:** Scoliosis, spondylolysis, and spondylolisthesis
- **Hands:** Brachydactyly, acro-osteolysis of the distal phalanges, and onychodysplasia

Pyknodysostosis shares several features with osteopetrosis including generalized sclerosis, which leads to cortical thickening and increased osseous density on röntgenogram, as well as a propensity to fracture.

In pyknodysostosis, there is normal demineralization but abnormal degradation of the organic component of bone by osteoclasts. The disease maps to chromosome 1q21, to which cathepsin K localizes. Cathepsin K belongs to the papain cysteine protease superfamily, among which it is unique in having an expression restricted to a specific cell type—namely, the osteoclast. Actions include collagenolysis, elastinolysis, and gelatinolysis during skeletal remodeling. Finding the mutation in the gene that encodes cathepsin K and deficiency of the enzyme leading to pyknodysostosis has implications for the treatment of diseases characterized by excessive bone loss, such as osteoporosis. Downregulation of the gene or inhibition of the enzyme may retard morbid osseous resorption.

KEY POINTS: OSTEOCHONDRODYSPLASIAS

1. The osteochondrodysplasias are classified variably, based upon clinical and radiographic characteristics.

2. Basic scientific investigations are unveiling mutations in extracellular matrix proteins and regulatory pathways that eventually will reorganize and clarify our approach to these disorders.

3. Spinal deformities pose the greatest surgical challenge in the osteochondrodysplasias.

4. The management of other deformities in these disorders must be influenced by patient demands, which may support a less aggressive approach.

13. **Define type IX collagen Give three characteristic features of the osteochondrodysplasia for which a mutation in its gene is responsible.**

Type IX collagen is a heterotrimer of genetically distinct $\alpha 1$, $\alpha 2$, and $\alpha 3$ chains. Each chain consists of four NC and three COL domains, designated NC1, NC2, NC3, NC4, COL1, COL2, and COL3, respectively. The chains are linked together by intrachain (in NC4) and interchain (in NC1, NC2, and NC3) disulfide bonds between cysteinyl residues located in the noncollagenous domains. The trimeric type IX collagen molecule is kinked at the NC3 domain, which is five amino acids longer in the $\alpha 2$ chain than in the other two chains. In some forms, the $\alpha 2$(IX) NC3 domain gives rise to a chondroitin sulfate side chain, making the type IX collagen molecule a proteoglycan. Type IX collagen molecules are covalently linked to type II collagen molecules in hyaline cartilage, where the former may serve as a regulator of the fibrillar organization of the latter.

COL9A1 maps to 6q12-q13, COL9A2 to 1p33-p32.2, COL9A3 to. Mutations in all three genes have been identified in one form of multiple epiphyseal dysplasia (MED). MED is characterized by the following features:

- **Stature:** Mild shortening
- **Spine:** Irregularity of vertebral endplates
- **Long bones:** Delayed ossification of small and irregular epiphyses, premature osteoarthritis, coxa vara (producing Trendelenburg gait), osteonecrosis of femoral head, and osteochondritis dissecans

Symmetric involvement of femoral capital epiphyses and a stable clinical presentation in the setting of other epiphyseal irregularities distinguishes MED from Legg-Calvé-Perthes disease. Relative sparing of the spine contrasts with spondyloepiphyseal dysplasia, whereas relative sparing of the pelvis contrasts with pseudoachondroplasia.

MED also is caused by mutation in cartilage oligomeric matrix protein (see below), which in turn also produces pseudoachondroplasia (see above).

Mutation in COL9A2 has been identified in a Finnish subpopulation with intervertebral disk disease associated with sciatica.

14. **Define type X collagen Give three characteristic features of the osteochondrodysplasia for which a mutation in its gene is responsible.**

Type X collagen is a disulfide-linked homotrimer, $\alpha1(X)_3$, encoded by the gene COL10A1 on 6q21-q22.3. It is produced by hypertrophic chondrocytes found in zones of cartilage destined for matrix mineralization, such as the growth plate and the cartilage bridge formed in delayed fracture healing or pseudarthrosis. These chondrocytes also synthesize type II collagen. By contrast, chondrocytes in the proliferative zone synthesize type IX collagen as well as types II and X. Collagen-type-X gene expression is modulated in response to body calcium levels and by pro- as well as antimineralization agents such as calcium β-glycerophosphate and levamisole. These findings suggest a role for type X collagen in endochondral ossification.

Mutation within the gene encoding type X collagen, COL10A1, causes metaphyseal chondrodysplasia, type Schmid (MCDS). Features of this disorder include the following:

- **Stature:** Mild to moderate shortening
- **Long bones:** Metaphyseal cupping and flaring, coxa vara (producing Trendelenburg gait), and femoral and tibial bowing, producing genu varum and ankle varus

Unlike epiphyseal dysplasia, osteoarthritis is not a prominent feature. The hands and spine are relatively spared. Several mutations in COL10A1 that result in a reduction of type X collagen synthesis do not cause MCDS, which argues against haploinsufficiency as the underlying mechanism. Based upon *in vitro* experiments and studies of type X null and transgenic mice, a dominant gain of function effect has been proposed: abnormal type X collagen chains are incorporated into trimers, which are thereby damaged, or they are unable to assemble into larger aggregates but are directly injurious to chondrocytes.

15. **Define *cartilage oligomeric matrix protein* (COMP). Give three characteristic features of the osteochondrodysplasia for which a mutation in its gene is responsible.**

COMP belongs to the thrombospondin family of extracellular calcium binding proteins, which interact with structural components of the extracellular matrix and are involved in the regulation of cellular migration, adhesion, and proliferation. It is a pentameric glycoprotein of identical subunits that are made up of four epidermal growth factor (EGF)-like and seven calmodulin-like tandem repeats and are linked centrally by disulfide bonds between amino termini. COMP is expressed in the territorial matrix surrounding chondrocytes in articular, tracheal, and nasal cartilage, and in tendon surrounding type I collagen fibrils.

Mutations in the COMP gene, located on 19p13.1, cause pseudoachondroplasia (PSACH) and MED. COMP-null mice do not develop PSACH or MED, suggesting that the phenotypes are produced by synthesis of abnormal COMP (i.e., dominant negative) rather than a reduction of the amount synthesized (i.e., haploinsufficiency). PSACH resembles achondroplasia (see above) except for the following features:

- **Skull:** Relative sparing
- **Spine:** Odontoid hypoplasia, producing atlantoaxial instability

That the phenotype MED is produced by mutations in COMP and type IX collagen, together with identification of a MED family unlinked to either locus, demonstrates the genetic heterogeneity of MED. That PSACH and MED are linked to mutations within the COMP gene suggests an allelic relationship between these phenotypes, the latter being a milder clinical expression of the former.

16. **Define *parathyroid hormone-related protein (PTHrP), parathyroid hormone/ parathyroid hormone-related protein (PTH-PTHrP) receptor, and Indian hedgehog (Ihh).* Give three characteristic features of the osteochondrodysplasia for which a mutation in its gene is responsible.**

On account of a homology between amino-terminal domains, parathyroid hormone (PTH) and parathyroid hormone-related protein bind the same receptor (the PTH-PTHrP receptor), through which they exert similar effects on calcium and phosphate homeostasis and skeletal development and turnover. The PTH-PTHrP receptor is a heterotrimeric guanosine triphosphate-binding protein (i.e., G-protein)-coupled transmembrane receptor located on 3p22-p21.1. It is expressed by cells within the proliferative zone of the growth plate that are destined for hypertrophy.

Ihh belongs to a family of conserved molecules that serve as signals during organogenesis in the embryo. Ihh is expressed in committed prehypertrophic chondrocytes. It is targeted at perichondrium, where it induces expression of a second signal, PTHrP. Ihh and PTHrP participate in a negative feedback loop that controls the temporal and spatial sequence of differentiation of chondrocytes from the proliferative to hypertrophic state during endochondral ossification.

Mutation in the gene encoding the PTH-PTHrP receptor has been identified in metaphyseal chondrodysplasia, type Jansen (MCDJ) and multiple enchondromatosis of Ollier. MCDJ is characterized by the following features:

- **Skeleton:** Osteopenia and morbid fracture
- **Joints:** Contracture, especially flexion of the hips and knees
- **Kidneys:** Stones
- **Head and neck:** Deafness and nasal dysplasia
- **Laboratory abnormalities:** Hypercalcemia, hypophosphatemia, hypercalciuria, hyperphosphaturia, increased urinary excretion of cyclic adenosine monophosphate (cAMP), elevated 1,25(OH)2 vitamin D3, elevated alkaline phosphatase, reduced PTH, and reduced PTHrP

The skeletal manifestations resemble those of hyperparathyroidism. The underlying mechanism in MCDJ involves ligand-independent activation of PTH-PTHrP receptor, leading to abnormal endochondral ossification. Several other such constitutively activating receptor mutations have been identified, including rhodopsin in retinitis pigmentosa, thyrotropin receptor in hyperfunctioning thyroid adenomata, and luteinizing hormone receptor familial male precocious puberty.

17. **Give three characteristic spinal deformities in achondroplasia.**

- **Reduction in interpedicular distance in the lumbar spine:** This may lead to clinically significant spinal stenosis. Affected children assume positions in which the lumbar spine is flexed to obliterate lordosis and to expand the capacity of the spinal canal. Low back pain with radiculopathy or other neural compromise necessitates operative intervention. This consists of wide decompression, including facet joints and pedicles, with long arthrodesis to avoid postdecompression instability, especially kyphosis.
- **Thoracolumbar kyphosis:** This is evident in the sitting child and, in the majority of cases, is a manifestation of ligamentous laxity. With walking, the majority of such deformities resolve spontaneously. Those that persist (beyond age 5 years) and are significant (i.e., > 40 degrees) require arthrodesis with instrumentation. Because of a high rate of spinal stenosis, consideration must be given to decompression in conjunction with arthrodesis. This in turn may necessitate a circumferential approach to achieve fusion.

- **Narrowing of the foramen magnum occipitale:** This produces compression of the upper part of the cervical division of the spinal cord. Symptoms and signs include respiratory compromise, motor retardation, and sleep apnea. Work-up includes sleep apnea study and consultation of published standards for the size of foramen magnum occipitale in achondroplasia. Decompression is the standard operative treatment.

18. **What spinal anomaly has the greatest potential for morbidity in spondyloepiphyseal dysplasia?**

In spondyloepiphyseal dysplasia, hypoplasia of the dens axis leads to atlantoaxial instability. This necessitates posterior arthrodesis: atlantoaxial or, in the event that the posterior arch of the atlas has not ossified, occipitoaxial.

BIBLIOGRAPHY

1. Beighton P: McKusick's Heritable Disorders of Connective Tissue. St. Louis, Mosby-Year Book, 1992.
2. Bellus GA, McIntosh I, Smith EA, et al: A recurrent mutation in the tyrosine kinase domain of fibroblast growth factor receptor 3 causes hypochondroplasia. Nat Genet 10:357–359, 1995.
3. Briggs MD, Hoffman SMG, King LM, et al: Pseudoachondroplasia and multiple epiphyseal dysplasia due to mutations in the cartilage oligomeric matrix protein gene. Nat Genet 10:330–336, 1995.
4. Diab M, Wu J-J, Eyre DR: Collagen type IX from human articular cartilage: A structural profile of intermolecular cross-linking sites. Biochem J 314:327–332, 1996.
5. Gelb BD, Shi G-P, Chapman HA, et al: Pycnodysostosis, a lysosomal disease caused by cathepsin K deficiency. Science 273:1236–1238, 1996.
6. Hästbacka J, de la Chapelle A, Mahtani MM, et al: The diastrophic gene encodes a novel sulfate transporter: Positional cloning by fine-structure linkage disequilibrium mapping. Cell 78:1073–1087, 1994.
7. Hästbacka J, Superti-Furga A, Wilcox WR, et al: Atelosteogenesis type II is caused by mutations in the diastrophic dysplasia sulfate transporter gene (DTDST): Evidence for a phenotypic series involving three chondrodysplasias. Am J Hum Genet 58:255–262, 1996.
8. Muragaki Y, Mariman ECM, van Beersum SEC, et al: A mutation in the gene encoding the $\alpha2$ chain of the fibril-associated collagen IX, COL9A2, causes multiple epiphyseal dysplasia. Nat Genet 12:103–105, 1996.
9. Rousseau F, Saugier P, Le Merrer M, et al: Stop codon FGFR3 mutations in thanatophoric dwarfism type 1. Nat Genet 10:11–12, 1995.
10. Schipani E, Kruse K, Jüppner H: A constitutively active mutant PTH-PTHrP receptor in Jansen-type metaphyseal chondrodysplasia. Science 268:98–100, 1995.
11. Shiang R, Thompson LM, Zhu Y-Z, et al: Mutations in the transmembrane domain of FGFR3 cause the most common genetic form of dwarfism, achondroplasia. Cell 78:335–342, 1994.
12. Spranger J, Winterpacht A, Zabel B: The type II collagenopathies: A spectrum of chondrodysplasias. Eur J Pediatr 153:56–65, 1994.
13. Supert-Furga A, Hästbacka J, Wilcox WR, et al: Achondrogenesis type IB is caused by mutations in the diastrophic dysplasia sulphate transporter gene. Nat Genet 12:100–102, 1996.
14. Thomas JT, Lin K, Nandedkar M, et al: A human chondrodysplasia due to a mutation in a TGF-β superfamily member. Nat Genet 12:315–317, 1996.
15. Vortkamp A, Lee K, Lanske B, et al: Regulation of rate of cartilage differentiation by Indian hedgehog and PTH-related protein. Science 273:613–622, 1996.
16. Wallis GA, Rash B, Sykes B, et al: Mutations within the gene encoding the $\alpha1(X)$ chain of type X collagen (COL10A1) cause metaphyseal chondrodysplasia type Schmid but not several other forms of metaphyseal chondrodysplasia. J Med Genet 33:450–457, 1996.

CHAPTER 88

NEUROFIBROMATOSIS

Alvin H. Crawford, MD, FACS, and Elizabeth K. Schorry, MD

1. **What is neurofibromatosis (NF)?**
   Neurofibromatosis type 1 (NF1), also called *von Recklinghausen's disease* and *peripheral neurofibromatosis,* is a multisystemic disease that primarily affects cellular growth of neural tissue. It is an autosomal dominant disorder.

2. **How common is NF?**
   NF1 has been found to affect 1 in 4000 people. It is one of the most common dominantly inherited gene disorders in humans. The NF1 gene in humans is located on chromosome 17 and codes for a protein called *neurofibromin*.

3. **What are the causes?**
   Approximately 50% of all cases are new mutations, which is one hundredfold higher than the usual mutation rate for a single locus and may reflect the huge size of the NF1 locus (estimated at 350,000 base pairs). The other 50% of cases are familial, with an affected parent.
   The manifestations of NF1 vary from one person to another, but each individual who carries the gene will eventually show some clinical features of the disease, the penetrance of NF1 being close to 100%.

4. **What is the pathophysiology?**
   The majority of features of NF1 are related to changes in activation of Ras, a protein involved in cell cycle regulation. Mutations in neurofibromin cause Ras to change to an activated state, resulting in cell proliferation and tumor growth. In this respect, NF1 acts as a typical tumor-suppressor gene. It is not yet well understood how Ras affects the orthopaedic manifestations of NF1.

5. **What are the criteria for diagnosis?**
   The consensus development conference on NF1 held at the National Institutes of Health in 1987 concluded that the diagnosis of NF1 could be assigned to a person with two or more of the following criteria:
   1. More than 6 café-au-lait spots, at least 15 mm in their greatest diameter in adults and 5 mm in children
   2. Two or more neurofibromas of any type or one plexiform neurofibroma
   3. Freckling in the axillary or inguinal regions
   4. Optic glioma
   5. Two or more Lisch nodules (i.e., iris hamartomas)
   6. A distinctive bony lesion, such as sphenoid wing dysplasia or thinning of the cortex of a long bone, with or without pseudarthrosis
   7. A first-degree relative with NF1
   These criteria have been shown to be very useful, even in young children. Since the consensus panel meeting, specific kinds of learning disabilities and magnetic resonance imaging (MRI) abnormalities (especially in children) have also been specifically associated with NF1. The pediatric orthopaedist encounters other conditions associated with café-au-lait spots, namely, Watson syndrome, fibrous dysplasia (i.e., McCune-Albright syndrome), LEOPARD

(lentigines, electrocardiogram [EKG] abnormalities, ocular hypertelorism, pulmonary stenosis, abnormalities of genitalia, retardation of growth, and deafness) syndrome, and Noonan syndrome. Only the gene for Watson syndrome has been linked to the NF1 locus.

6. **What are the different types of NF?**
   There are two distinct genetic types of NF. The most common is NF1, which can be clearly distinguished from central NF (NF2). NF2 is also an autosomal dominant disorder but occurs less frequently (it is estimated to affect 1 in 40,000 people). Characteristically, in NF2, there are bilateral schwannomas of the vestibular portion of the eighth cranial nerve, resulting in hearing loss; schwannomas of other peripheral nerves, meningiomas, and ependymomas are also common. Eighth cranial nerve tumors are not found in NF1. The gene for NF2 is located on chromosome 22 and encodes a protein named *merlin*. Segmental NF is another form of NF in which features of NF1 (i.e., café-au-lait spots, freckling, and neurofibromas) are seen in only one segment of the body. This is thought to be due to somatic mosaicism for the NF1 gene mutation. A final form, schwannomatosis, has recently been described and involves multiple deep and painful schwannomas. It may be genetically distinct from NF1 and NF2. NF2 will not be discussed further in this chapter.

7. **What happens if the condition is not treated?**
   NF1 is a progressive disorder. Additional features and complications often develop with increasing age. Orthopaedic manifestations of NF1 often show progressive deterioration over time. If treatment is not effective, significant disability occurs.

8. **What are the clinical features?**
   - **Café-au-lait spots:** The dermatologic features include café-au-lait spots, which are present in more than 90% of patients with NF1. The pigmentation is melanotic in origin and is located both in the basal layers of the epidermis and in melanocytes of upper layers. Axillary and inguinal freckles are diffuse small hyperpigmented spots of 2–3 mm in diameter. They are uniquely found in the axillary and inguinal regions, areas not exposed to sunlight, and, if present, are helpful diagnostic criteria. About 40% of children with NF1 have axillary freckling.
   - **Cutaneous neurofibromas:** Formerly called *fibroma molluscum,* these are small neurofibromas in the subcutis. Neurofibromas are mixed-cell tumors rich in Schwann cells but also include fibroblasts, endothethial cells, and glandular elements. The primary cell responsible for tumor formation is unknown. Cutaneous neurofibromas often begin to appear around the time of puberty and increase in numbers with age. Some adults may have hundreds or even thousands of them.
   - **Plexiform neurofibroma:** This is a type of neurofibroma that has a "bag of worms" feeling and is very sensitive. It is often found underlying an area of cutaneous hyperpigmentation. When the pigmentation approaches or crosses the posterior midline of the body, it appears that the tumor may be aggressive and may originate from the spinal canal. In contrast to cutaneous neurofibromas, plexiform neurofibromas are thought to be congenital lesions and usually become first evident in early childhood. Plexiform neurofibromas have the potential to become malignant, developing a malignant peripheral nerve sheath tumor (MPNST) within the plexiform tumor.
   - **Elephantiasis:** Another rare dermatologic manifestation of the disease, this is characterized by large soft tissue masses with a rough, raised, villous type of skin. Attempts to resect sizable portions of the soft tissue have met with limited success. There is dysplasia of the underlying bone when the lesions occur in an extremity.
   - **Verrucous hyperplasia:** This is an infrequent and unsightly cutaneous lesion of NF1. There is tremendous overgrowth of the skin with thickening, but also with a velvety, soft, papillary quality. The lesion is geographic, develops most often in a unilateral fashion, and is considered to be one of the most grotesque cutaneous lesions found in humans.

- **Ophthalmologic Lisch nodules:** These are slightly raised, well-circumscribed hamartomas in the iris and are present in more than 50% of patients with NF1 who are 6 years of age or older; the incidence increases to 90% by adulthood. The lesions are thought to be specific for NF1.
- **Optic gliomas:** Although optic gliomas account for only 2–5% of all brain tumors in childhood, as many as 70% of these are found in persons with NF1. About 15% of NF1 patients will have an optic nerve glioma. In many patients, these tumors change little in size over many years and do not affect vision; a small percentage will eventually result in visual impairment.
- **Additional features of NF1:** These include a high incidence of learning disabilities and attention deficit hyperactivity disorder (ADHD), which may significantly impact a child's performance in school.

9. **What should be asked in the history?**
The primary questions are whether there is a family history of the clinical manifestations of NF1 and whether there are relatives with significant birthmarks similar to the dermatologic examples just listed. The parent may only have dermatologic lesions without orthopaedic or neurologic manifestations, whereas the child and siblings may show all the manifestations of NF1.

10. **What spinal deformities are associated with neurofibromatosis?**
The primary spinal deformity is scoliosis (Fig. 88-1), which appears to be the most common osseous defect associated with NF1. It may vary in severity from mild, nonprogressive forms to

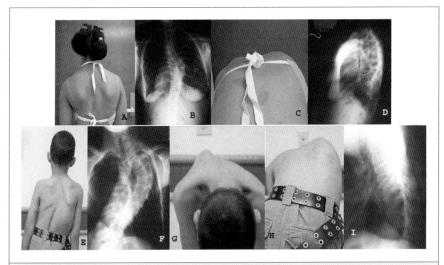

Figure 88-1. Two children with neurofibromatosis type I and scoliosis. One has the nondystrophic type of scoliosis, and the second has the characteristic dystrophic scoliosis felt to be associated with neurofibromatosis type I. *A,* Clinical photograph of a child who presented with multiple café-au-lait spots, referred from her pediatrician because of a positive Adam's bend scoliosis test. This is a nondystrophic, idiopathic-appearing curvature. She had a 45-degree curvature and was recommended for corrective surgery. *B,* Standing posteroanterior (PA) thoracolumbar x-ray. The curvature cannot be distinguished from idiopathic scoliosis. *C,* Clinical photograph of Adam's bend test from behind shows a minor rib hump, but note multiple café-au-lait spots. *D,* The lateral thoracolumbar x-ray is indistinguishable from idiopathic scoliosis. *E,* Clinical photograph of a 13-year-old boy with dystrophic scoliosis. There is truncal imbalance to the right. *F,* PA x-ray showing short, segmented, sharply angulated curvature of the cervicothoracic region with significant rotation. *G,* Clinical photograph of Adam's bend test seen from head down. Note the sharp angulation of the right rib cage. *H,* Clinical photograph of Adam's bend test seen from behind, illustrating the sharp rotation of the rib cage as well multiple café-au-lait spots. *I,* Lateral thoracolumbar sacral spine x-ray showing thoracic lordosis.

severe curvatures. The cause of dystrophic NF1 spinal deformity is unknown, but it has been suggested to be secondary to osteomalacia, a localized neurofibromatous tumor eroding and infiltrating bone, endocrine disturbances, or mesodermal dysplasia.

In a general orthopaedic clinic, 2% of the population with scoliosis will have NF1, whereas in a population with NF1, perhaps 10–20% of patients will have some disorder of the spine. The majority of patients will have nondystrophic spinal deformities. The dystrophic or classic spinal deformities of NF1 include short, segmented, sharply angulated curvatures. Dystrophic radiographic findings include scalloping of the vertebral margins, severe rotation of the apical vertebrae, widening of the spinal canal, enlargement of the neural foramina, an occasional widening of the interpediculate distance, defective pedicles, the presence of a paraspinal mass, spindling of the transverse process, and rotation of the ribs, resembling a twisted ribbon. *There is no site, side, or gender predilection for the curvature.* There is invariably thoracic lordosis associated with this deformity.

There may also be nondystrophic spinal deformities, not unlike idiopathic scoliosis. These nondystrophic idiopathic-appearing deformities have the tendency to become dystrophic (i.e., modulation) with time or following spinal fusion. Pseudarthrosis is not uncommon following spinal surgery in NF1, and, as a result, there is a growing trend toward performing anterior and posterior fusion in these patients to prevent pseudarthrosis.

Cervical spine deformities as well as kyphotic deformities and spondylolisthesis secondary to pathologic involvement of the pedicles and pars interarticularis are seen somewhat uncommonly in NF1. Most often, the deformity or appearance of dysplasia has to do with bone erosion from adjacent neurofibromas or **dural ectasia.**

All patients with NF1 who undergo surgery *requiring* endotracheal anesthesia and halo traction or who present with neck tumors should undergo a cervical spine x-ray series. Widening of the neural foramina on oblique views may represent "dumbbell lesions" characteristic of neurofibromas as they extrude from the spinal canal. If there is any suspicion of subluxation, computed tomography (CT) scans and MRI are appropriate studies. Other reasons for obtaining cervical spine x-rays include torticollis and dysphagia.

Dural ectasia, meningocele, pseudomeningoceles, and dumbbell lesions are all related to the presence of neurofibromas or abnormal pressure phenomena in and about the spinal canal neuraxis. High-volume myelography or MRI should be used in the investigation of all dystrophic curves prior to initiating treatment.

11. **What tibial disorders are seen?**
    Tibial dysplasia is a rare problem that occurs in 1:140,000 liveborn children but in 2–5% of children with NF1. The bowing associated with NF1 is always anterolateral. *Because not all patients present initially with pseudarthrosis, we prefer the term* congenital tibial dysplasia *(CTD).* The deformity may present before other manifestations such as café-au-lait spots. It is usually evident within the first year of life, with a fracture not uncommonly occurring before 1–3 years of age. The management is frustrating, fracture and refracture are common, and limb-length inequality is frequent.

    There are two types of bowing: nondysplastic and dysplastic. In nondysplastic (type I) bowing, there is anterolateral bowing with increased bony density and sclerosis of the medullary canal. This type may convert to dysplastic bowing following osteotomy to correct the angulation. In dysplastic (type II) anterolateral bowing, there is a failure of medullary canal tubulation, anterolateral bowing with cystic prefracture or canal enlargement due to previous fracture, and frank pseudarthrosis and atrophy with "sucked candy" narrowing of the ends of the two fragments.

    The most effective treatment to date has been chronic bracing initiated at the time of diagnosis. Other forms of treatment include pulsating electromagnetic fields, surgical bone grafting, vascularized autogenous graft, Ilizarov callotasis (i.e., compression, transplantation, and distraction histogenesis), and amputation.

The quality of life associated with numerous unsuccessful operative procedures makes chronic bracing the reasonable alternative. The previously reported high incidence of central nervous system (CNS) neoplasms associated with CTD has not been substantiated in multidisciplinary NF clinics. The National Neurofibromatosis Foundation International Database (NNFFID, including 25 clinics) reported 5% of NF1 patients to have CTD, whereas 50–80% of patients with CTD have NF1; 43% had fibular dysplasia without tibial involvement. The average number of surgeries was 2.9 (0–13), and 16% underwent amputation.

The European Pediatric Orthopaedic Society study resulted in six papers published in the *Journal of Ped Orthop B* in 2000. Of the 340 cases, there was detailed follow-up on 172. NF1 was seen in 54.7% of the patients. They recommend two main treatments: the Ilizarov procedure and vascularized fibular grafting. Efforts were made to avoid surgery before age 3 years.

The current author recommends early continuous bracing. Regardless of the operative procedure performed, some form of internal (i.e., medullary canal) and external bracing is recommended to prevent refracture. Amputation remains a successful method of treatment for those patients who have undergone multiple failed attempts at synostosis. Corrective osteotomy for cosmesis has been associated with failure to unite, even in type I lesions.

Posterior medial congenital bowing (i.e., kyphoscoliosis tibia) is a benign condition associated only with occasional limb-length inequality. Tibial bowing associated with skin dimples, bilateral presentation, ring constrictions, and foot deformities is rarely associated with NF1.

12. What are the disorders of bone growth?

- Segmental hypertrophy
- Subperiosteal bone growth and proliferation

Overgrowth of an extremity is a well-known complication of NF1 and may be related to changes in the soft tissues (i.e., hemangiomatosis, lymphangiomatosis, elephantiasis, or beaded plexiform neuromas). The overgrowth in bone and soft tissue is usually unilateral, involving the upper or lower extremities or the head and neck. These osseous changes characteristically cause the bone to elongate with a wavy irregularity or a thickening of the cortex. There is a higher incidence of neoplasia associated with this segmental hypertrophy than with other lesions.

Subperiosteal bone proliferation is another of the protean manifestations of NF1. Most cases are initiated by minor fractures with subperiosteal bleeding followed by osseous dysplasia of the subperiosteal hematoma. The early onset of subperiosteal hematoma may be identified on technetium bone scanning by the presence of a "doughnut sign," a peripheral rim of increased activity surrounding a relatively photopenic center appearing in the blood pool and in delayed imaging. Aggressive aspiration of the lesion may prevent the development of the dysplasia.

13. What type of imaging is useful?

For scoliotic lesions, the primary imaging modality is posteroanterior and lateral thoracolumbar spine films. If there is evidence of significant dysplasia or neurologic clinical involvement, then MRI is recommended. As previously stated, soft tissue neurofibromas and spinal cord dural ectasia or hydrostatic expansion of the dural sac may be responsible for some of the bony deformities. These could be identified more readily with a contrast MRI. If there is significant deformity, the MRI may not be successful and high-volume CT myelography may be more informative. A three-dimensional (3-D) reconstructed CT is extremely helpful for surgical planning of the severely deformed dysplastic curves. It is not uncommon to have subluxation of the costotransverse articulation with penetration of the rib head into the spinal canal in some of the more severely deformed dysplastic curves. Please look for them.

Plain x-rays are usually utilized to determine the characteristics of the anterolateral tibial bowing associated with CTD. MRI has recently been used to determine whether healing is occurring in the area of pseudarthrosis.

For disorders of bone growth, plain x-rays and radioisotope scintigraphy (i.e., bone scan) are usually adequate to identify the lesions and their level of activity.

KEY POINTS: NEUROFIBROMATOSIS

1. Neurofibromatosis type I (NF1) is a progressive, multisystem disease that will lead to significant disability if not treated. A team approach is most effective in managing the multidimensional problems of this condition.

2. Almost 50% of all cases of neurofibromatosis are new mutations.

3. Patients with NF1 have an increased risk of malignant nerve sheath tumors and other malignancies.

4. Patients with NF1 who are scheduled for surgery requiring endotracheal intubation or who present with neck tumors should have cervical spine x-rays before surgery to rule out cervical spine involvement.

---

14. **Are laboratory studies useful?**
    Mutation analysis using DNA sequencing is available for the NF1 gene and is a highly reliable test with 95% sensitivity. Testing is usually not needed to confirm the diagnosis in a patient who meets the National Institutes of Health (NIH) diagnostic criteria; however, it can be quite helpful in cases in which the diagnosis is in question. Prenatal diagnosis for NF1 is also available by amniocentesis and chorionic villous sampling, but it is infrequently requested.

15. **With what other conditions may NF be confused?**
    McCune-Albright syndrome, Watson syndrome, and Proteus syndrome. The contour of café-au-lait spots associated with Albright's fibrous dysplasia has historically been identified as irregular as opposed to the smooth edges in NF1. This finding does not always bear out clinically. The Elephant Man, who was initially speculated to have NF, has been determined to instead be affected with Proteus syndrome, another overgrowth disorder. Watson syndrome, an association of café-au-lait spots and pulmonic stenosis, has been found to be due to mutations in the NF1 gene and is not a separate disorder.

16. **Does the condition require treatment?**
    All of the conditions associated with NF1 require monitoring for evidence of progression. If there is progression, active treatment is recommended.

17. **Who should manage the problem?**
    Since NF1 is a multisystemic, multidimensional problem, it is most important that the patient be managed by a team. We propose that the team consist of a developmental pediatrician, a geneticist, an orthopaedist, a neurologist, and a social worker. Consultation should be readily available with ophthalmology, general surgery, oncology, and neurosurgery. The condition can best be managed by recognition of the manifestations of the disease and a complete evaluation of the patient and family, with involvement of a multidisciplinary team according to the nature of lesions present. Most important is specific treatment of individual lesions based on careful judgment, especially concerning radical operative procedures. Thereafter, continuing observation of the patient for the remainder of life is required.

18. **What is the prognosis?**

Long-term studies have shown that about two thirds of individuals with NF1 have mild-to-moderate involvement throughout their lifetime; one third will have severe complications related to NF1. There is little doubt that NF1 predisposes one to an increased risk of certain malignancies. Under-recognition of this relationship may occur when the cutaneous signs of NF1 are overlooked or are not yet apparent in young children. Lifetime risk for MPNST, formerly called *neurofibrosarcoma,* is reported between 5–8%. Other malignancies including childhood leukemia (i.e., juvenile chronic myelogenous leukemia [CML]), rhabdomyosarcoma of the urogenital tract, pheochromocytoma, and Wilms' tumor have been reported.

19. **What should I tell the family?**

The family should be informed of the multifaceted nature of NF1 when the child is first diagnosed. A good basic physical examination is essential. There is controversy in the field regarding the value of routine screening studies. Our center routinely performs an MRI of the brain at initial diagnosis to evaluate for optic nerve glioma and screening chest x-rays every 3 years. The family should be informed of the possibility of progression of the features of NF1 and emphatically encouraged to maintain continuous follow-up. They should be counseled about the genetic etiology of the disorder and its recurrence risk.

20. **What are the complications?**

Although there are significant osseous as well as neurologic complications associated with NF1, the majority of patients do not have severe complications. Our NF1 multidisciplinary center likely has attracted more severe involvement of musculoskeletal problems because of our interest in complex cases.

It is important to be aware that 25% of all affected patients with NF1 have café-au-lait spots as the only manifestation of the disease and less than 10% of NF1 patients will ever require orthopaedic treatment.

BIBLIOGRAPHY

1. Cohen MM Jr: Further diagnostic thoughts about the elephant man. Am J Med Genet 29:777–782, 1988.
2. Crawford AH: Neurofibromatosis. In Weinstein SL (ed): Pediatric Spine: Principles and Practice. New York, Raven Press, 1994, pp 619–649.
3. Crawford AH: Neurofibromatosis in children. Acta Orthop Scand 218:1–60, 1986.
4. Crawford AH: Orthopaedic complications of von Recklinghausen's disease in children. Curr Orthop 10:49–55, 1996.
5. Crawford AH, Schorry EK: Neurofibromatosis in children: The role of the orthopaedist. J Am Acad Orthop Surg 7(4):217–230, 1999.
6. Goldberg NS, Collins FS: The hunt for the neurofibromatosis gene. Arch Dermatol 127:1705–1707, 1991.
7. Grill F, Vollini G, Dungle, et al: Treatment approaches for congenital pseudarthrosis tibia: Results of the EPOS multicenter study. European Paediatric Orthopaedic Society (EPOS). J Pediatr Orthop 9(2):75–89, 2000.
8. Mandell GA, Harcke HT: Subperiosteal hematoma another scintigraphic "doughnut." Clin Nucl Med 11:35–37, 1986.
9. National Institute of Health Consensus Development Conference Statement: Neurofibromatosis. Neurofibromatosis 1:172, 1988.
10. Riccardi VM: Type I neurofibromatosis and the pediatric patient. Curr Probl Pediatr 22:66–106, 1992.
11. Sirois JL, Drennan JC: Dystrophic spinal deformity in neurofibromatosis. J Pediatr 10:522–526, 1990.
12. Stevenson DA, Birch PH, Friedman JM, et al: Descriptive analysis of tibial pseudarthrosis in patients with neurofibromatosis one. Am J Med Genet 84:413–419, 1999.

CHAPTER 89

OSTEOGENESIS IMPERFECTA

Paul D. Sponseller, MD

1. **What is osteogenesis imperfecta (OI)?**

   OI is a genetically transmitted disease resulting in fragility of the entire skeleton. Ligamentous laxity is another theme. It is seen with varying degrees of severity, from an infant with multiple fractures to a child who has only a few fractures before maturity. The clinical variation is due to differences in the mutation. The incidence of OI is about 1 in 20,000 in the population. Intelligence is not affected.

2. **How is the diagnosis made?**

   It is usually a clinical diagnosis, made by a combination of physical and radiographic findings. In most cases, OI is not readily confused with other entities. The patients usually have short stature. The sclerae are blue in many (but not all) cases. The dentin of the teeth may be abnormally thin in some cases. Deformities of the long bones on both sides of the body usually develop. The ligaments are usually slightly lax. Hearing may be impaired owing to defects in the bones of the middle ear. There may be a positive family history.

   Radiographically, the bones usually demonstrate osteopenia. In most patients, this is evident from inspection of the films, but in even the mildest cases of OI, densitometry studies show a decrease in mineralization. The bone cortices are usually thin, and trabecular patterns are not well developed. The long bones may be thin and bowed. The pelvis may show acetabular protrusion. The vertebrae may be biconcave.

   In questionable cases, diagnosis may be confirmed by DNA testing.

3. **What is the cause of OI?**

   OI has been identified as a defect in type I collagen in 90% of cases. Type I is the collagen that makes up most of the organic scaffolding for bone. It is a triple helix, composed of two α-I chains and one α-II chain. Glycine, the smallest amino acid, constitutes every third amino acid, and its small size is critical to the coiling of the collagen chains. Mutations of various amino acids result in OI of varying degrees of severity, depending on how much collagen exists and how functional it is. Since glycine is so crucial to the structure of collagen, mutations involving substitution of cystine for glycine often produce severe forms of OI. Other mutations have been found, however. Since type I collagen also plays a role in other components of connective tissue such as ligaments and tendons, it is not surprising that patients with OI have ligamentous laxity as well. Type I collagen is also a constituent of dentin and sclerae, thus explaining involvement of these tissues in some patients with OI.

4. **Is there a test for OI?**

   Genetic analysis of collagen from dermal fibroblasts will many times identify an abnormality in type I collagen. There are many false-negative findings with this test, however. It is not routinely recommended, especially since clinical examination is diagnostic in many cases. DNA-based testing is available both *in utero* and later in life but is not routinely clinically useful in so-called "classic" cases.

5. **How are the various forms classified?**

   There are many different classification systems. The most commonly used is that of Sillence, which included four types. It has been expanded with the finding of three new types.

- **Type I:** Mild OI; blue sclerae and normal teeth; autosomal dominant; the most common type
- **Type II:** Perinatally lethal OI; patients rarely survive infancy
- **Type III:** Severe, progressively deforming OI; dentinogenesis imperfecta; neonatal fractures
- **Type IV:** Moderately severe OI; sclerae fade from blue to white
- **Type V:** Radial head dislocation, hyperplastic callus, and white sclerae; normal type I collagen
- **Type VI:** White sclerae; excessive osteoid on biopsy
- **Type VII:** Abnormality on the short arm of chromosome 3; described in the Native Canadian population

Most mutations causing Sillence type I OI are those causing a null allele effect, in which the mutated RNA is degraded intracellularly, which results in production of half of the normal amount of collagen type I. Mutations causing types II, III, and IV are those in which there is synthesis of abnormal α-chains, which are incorporated into bone and function abnormally. Since there are more than 300 known mutations in type I collagen that cause OI, it is natural that this classification does not fully capture the true variability in OI.

6. **What is the differential diagnosis?**
On *in utero* ultrasonography, the reduced size and limb flexion of camptomelic dysplasia or diastrophic dysplasia may resemble OI. At birth, hypophosphatasia and chondroectodermal dysplasia may have some similarities to OI. Congenital syphilis may present with bowing of the long bones. In infancy, nonaccidental injury, or child abuse, is the most important thing to rule out. Malabsorption syndromes such as celiac disease may produce osseous fragility, as may scurvy or endocrinopathies such as hyperthyroidism and hyperparathyroidism. Also note that juvenile osteoporosis may present with spontaneous or pathologic fractures but is usually a transient, self-limited disorder. Fibrous dysplasia may exhibit bone deformities and fractures, but the bones are not as tapered and thin as in OI, and many of the bones in an affected patient are totally free of the disease. A patient with leukemia or lymphoma may occasionally present with pathologic fractures.

7. **How is child abuse distinguished from OI?**
Usually on clinical grounds; rarely by diagnostic tests. Clinically, a witnessed injury caused by low force and the presence of abnormalities of the teeth, sclera, or hearing may suggest OI. A skeletal survey should be done, looking for thin, gracile diaphyses of long bones, wormian (i.e., inclusion) bones in the cranial sutures, acetabular protrusion, or multiple vertebral compressions (i.e., codfish vertebrae). The pattern of fracture is not diagnostic, unfortunately. In some cases, a fibroblast biopsy may be helpful if positive. A negative test, however, does not rule out OI. A specialist with expertise in OI, such as a geneticist or an endocrinologist, can be invaluable in ruling in or ruling out the diagnosis.

8. **What are the gross and histologic characteristics of bone in OI?**
In general, the bone in OI is coarse in external texture. It is not cylindrical in shape like normal bone, but rather is flattened or irregular in cross section. It often has a crumbling, pumice-like texture. The cortices are thin. The medullary cavity may be flattened or obliterated, which explains the difficulty sometimes encountered with rod stabilization. Histologically, the trabecular network is often random and poorly developed. The bone is highly cellular. The trabeculae have been compared to Chinese letters. The bone is mostly woven in nature, with little lamellar bone, especially in the more severe varieties of OI.

9. **What is the natural history?**
Most babies with type II of Sillence die in early infancy. Most patients with other types live indefinitely. Intelligence is not affected, and most patients are quite resourceful. The use of powered personal transportation has greatly increased mobility. Most patients are employed and independent. Medical problems that may cut short the life span of a person with OI include restrictive lung disease as well as brain stem compression or basilar invagination.

10. **Is there a medical treatment for OI?**

    Many different agents have been attempted, but none is widely accepted. Excess calcium and phosphorus intake has no beneficial effect. Growth hormone and calcitonin have been shown to increase bone mineral density. Growth hormone may increase the height of persons with OI by a minimal amount.

    Bisphosphonates act by decreasing osteoclastic resorption of bone, therefore halting the excessive turnover seen in OI. The net effect is to increase bone mass. Bisphosphonates have been clinically demonstrated to increase bone density and to decrease fracture rates in children. The agents most commonly used are pamidronate and alendronate. Patients using pamidronate will usually manifest lines of increased bone density for each administration (Fig. 89-1). Bone marrow transplant is being investigated for the most severe cases in young infants. In the long run, an effective medical treatment seems likely. In the short term, the best advice is to consider bisphosphonates, to think preventively, and to eat a regular diet.

11. **What are the main orthopaedic sequelae?**

    Bowing of the long bones due to fractures and microfractures, scoliosis, basilar invagination, spondylolisthesis, protrusion acetabulae (Fig. 89-2), and degenerative joint disease. Ligamentous laxity exists and may cause pes planus and laxity of the knee joints. Limb-length inequality may develop owing to asymmetric fractures.

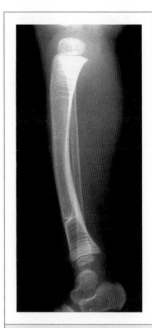

Figure 89-1. Tibia of a 2-year-old patient with type I osteogenesis imperfecta (OI). Note stress fracture on the tension cortex of distal tibia. Also note evenly spaced bands in the upper and lower metaphysis from pamidronate infusion every 3 months.

12. **Does orthotic treatment play a role in the management of OI?**

    Braces for the lower extremities may help young patients to stand before they are able to do so on their own. Lightweight hip-knee-ankle-foot braces or pneumatic trousers may prevent fractures in patients who are at risk but who have not had rod stabilization. Ankle-foot orthoses may help those with unstable or valgus ankles. Bracing for scoliosis or basilar invagination has a small but definite role.

KEY POINTS: OSTEOGENESIS IMPERFECTA

1. Bisphosphonates improve (but do not normalize) bone density and improve function in children.

2. Bone density improves spontaneously at puberty, and the fracture rate declines.

3. When internal fixation is needed, rods are superior to plates because they are load-sharing and do not produce stress risers.

4. Basilar invagination occurs as the skull settles around the upper cervical spine and may produce spasticity, respiratory depression, and cranial nerve dysfunction.

13. **Is bone healing in OI delayed or normal?**

Bone healing is usually biologically normal. It may be disturbed by mechanical factors, however, such as severe bowing at the site of fracture, which leads to tension in the callus. In one survey, more than 20% of OI patients had at least one nonunion. Therefore, the fractures in these patients should be treated by effective immobilization or internal fixation, as clinically appropriate. The surgeon should be especially aware of the need to internally fix avulsion fractures of the olecranon.

14. **What are the indications for straightening and rodding the long bones?**

Straightening the bowed long bones may be indicated in patients with severe diaphyseal bowing that prevents standing. Usually, this involves anterolateral bowing of the femur and anterior bowing of the tibia. Another indication is the occurrence of multiple fractures in a given region, which the rods can help markedly reduce. The technique may also be used effectively in the upper extremities, with rods inserted in the humerus or the ulna.

Rods are superior to plates because they are load-sharing and can internally bridge nearly the entire bone. Bailey and Dubow developed a telescoping pair of rods that could be anchored in each epiphysis of a long bone and would then expand with growth. A newer modification, the Fassier-Duval rod, has been developed for the femur, which has better anchorage in the epiphysis and does not usually require arthrotomy of the knee (Fig. 89-3).

A prerequisite for this procedure is a reasonable size of the bones and the presence of at least a visible cortex, which some patients do not have.

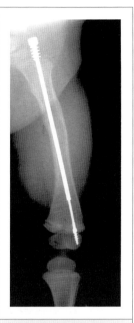

Figure 89-2. Expandable rods in the femur of a patient with osteogenesis imperfecta (OI).

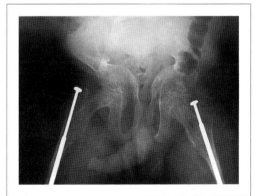

Figure 89-3. Severe protrusion acetabula in a 10-year-old child with type III osteogenesis imperfecta (OI). Limitation of motion and constipation were the results.

15. **What adjuncts are available for patients with very thin diaphyses or comminution?**
    Allograft bone applied circumferentially around the native bone may help to control rotation
    and length. It incorporates well in OI.

16. **When and how is scoliosis treated in OI?**
    Scoliosis curves exceeding about 50 degrees in patients with reasonable bone cortices
    may benefit from surgical stabilization (Fig. 89-4). Segmental fixation with rods
    that are not excessively rigid is recommended. The curve should not be corrected
    aggressively or else hooks will cut through bone and all will be lost. Special care should be
    taken not to correct much kyphosis. Some authors have recommended the use of methyl
    methacrylate to reinforce the vertebrae or the hook purchase sites. The rods should be
    slightly flexible to allow assembly without undue stress on the hooks. The surgeon
    should prepare for more bleeding than is seen in idiopathic scoliosis. Mean long-term
    correction is less than in idiopathic scoliosis, but the important goal is to prevent or minimize
    progression.

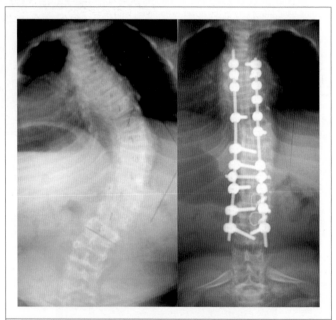

Figure 89-4. *Left*, A 9-year-old girl with type III osteogenesis imperfecta (OI) and a
severe progressive 66 degree curve. *Right*, 1 year after posterior fusion and
instrumentation.

17. **What is basilar invagination?**
    Basilar invagination or impression is the settling of the cranium upon the cervical spine,
    producing an infolding of the base of the skull with pressure on the neurologic structures in this
    region. It occurs owing to mechanical forces, with the deformable bone of OI unable to
    withstand the increasing weight of the head. Compressive structures include the ring of the
    atlas, the clivus, and the odontoid process (Fig. 89-5). Basilar invagination is present if the tip of
    the odontoid extends more than 7 mm above McGregor's line (drawn from the hard palate

posteriorly to the lowest point on the occiput). It is present radiographically in up to one quarter of patients with OI. Surprisingly, it is most common in the mild type IV B. Symptoms may include cranial nerve palsies, headaches, respiratory depression, spasticity, nystagmus, and weakness. It may be responsible for some of the early mortality seen in young adults with OI.

18. **How is basilar invagination treated?**
    There is no completely satisfactory treatment for this condition. Conservative treatment has been reported, with full-time use of a brace (the sternomandibular-occipital variety) followed by partial relief of symptoms. Surgical therapy is also an option. For very mild, early cases of symptomatic basilar invagination, if the compression is not significant anteriorly, posterior decompression and fusion *in situ* with posterior instrumentation may possibly be effective in preventing future subsidence if an abundant base of support is constructed posteriorly.

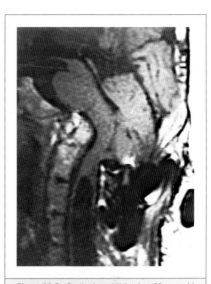

Figure 89-5. Basilar invagination in a 25-year-old man with type osteogenesis imperfecta (OI). Note compression from both anterior and posterior edges of the foramen magnum. Anteriorly, the compression is due to the clivus, atlas, and dens. Note also the hydrosyringomyelia of the cervical spinal cord. The patient had spasticity, weakness, and apneic spells.

If significant bony compression anteriorly is seen, anterior transoral decompression must be considered. This is done as a combined effort by a neurosurgeon, an otolaryngologist, and an orthopaedic surgeon. The tongue, mandible, and maxilla may be divided for exposure, and resections may be performed on the clivus, anterior atlas, and odontoid. Then, posterior fusion with plate fixation is performed from the occiput to the upper or middle cervical spine. Posterior decompression may be needed as well.

19. **Are other neurologic problems common in OI?**
    Hydrosyringomyelia and communicating hydrocephalus are seen in a significant minority of patients. Macrocephaly is common. Seizures are more common than in the general population.

20. **Are patients with OI prone to chronic pain?**
    Chronic pain is seen with increasing frequency as age increases. The cause may be multifactorial. There may be a biochemical reason for the pain. Treatable orthopaedic causes should be ruled out (Fig. 89-6), such as stress fractures and degenerative joint disease. If none can be found, bisphosphonates or physical modalities may be helpful. Antidepressants may be needed. Referral to a multidisciplinary pain clinic is justified, wherein a combination of behavioral therapy, counseling, and long-acting analgesics can be worked out.

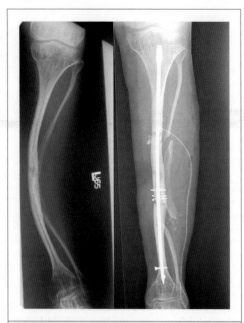

Figure 89-6. Osteotomies and intramedullary fixation to improve pain with standing in osteogenesis imperfecta (OI).

BIBLIOGRAPHY

1. Cole WG: Advances in osteogenesis imperfecta. Clin Orthop 401:6–16, 2002.

2. Glorieux FH, Bishop NJ, Plotkin H, et al: Cyclic administration of pamidronate in children with severe osteogenesis imperfecta. N Engl J Med 339:947–952, 1998.

3. Luhmann SJ, Sheridan JJ, Capelli M, Schoenecker PL: Management of lower-extremity deformities in osteogenesis imperfecta with extensible intramedullary rod technique: A 20-year experience. J Pediatr Orthop 18:88–94, 1998.

4. Marini JC, Gerber NL: Osteogenesis imperfecta: Rehabilitation and prospects for gene therapy. JAMA 277:746–750, 1997.

5. Ring D, Jupiter JB, Labropoulos PK, et al: The treatment of deformity of the lower limb in adults who have osteogenesis imperfecta. J Bone Joint Surg 78A:220–225, 1996.

6. Sawin PD, Menezes AH: Basilar invagination in osteogenesis imperfecta and related osteochondrodysplasias: Medical and surgical management. J Neurosurg 86:950–960, 1997.

7. Seikaly MG, Kopanati S, Salhapb N, Herring JA: Impact of alendronate on quality of life in children with osteogenesis imperfecta. J Pediatr Orthop 15:786–793, 2005.

8. Stott NS, Zionts LE: Displaced fractures of the apophysis of the olecranon in children who have osteogenesis imperfecta. J Bone Joint Surg 75A:1026–1103, 1993.

9. Zionts LE, Ebramzadeh E, Stott NS: Complications in the use of the Bailey-Dubow extensible nail. Clin Orthop 348:186–195, 1998.

CHAPTER 90

RICKETS AND METABOLIC DISORDERS

James Aronson, MD, and Elizabeth A. Aronson, APN, MNSc

1. **What is metabolic bone disease?**

   Impairment in the shape, strength, and composition of bone due to altered bone mineral homeostasis. The major factors affecting this homeostasis can be thought of as the "three 3s": the intra- and extracellular levels of three ions (calcium, phosphorus, and magnesium), which are regulated by three hormones (parathyroid hormone [PTH], calcitonin, and 1,25-dihydroxyvitamin D) and act upon three tissues (bone, intestine, and kidney). Of course, other minerals, hormones, and target tissues are involved as well, making this disease category a complex interaction of many exogenous and endogenous factors, calling for a team approach in coordinating care. Frequent clinical features include electrolyte disturbances, fractures, bone deformity, abnormal gait, and short stature.

2. **What are common forms of metabolic bone disease in children?**

   The most commonly encountered forms of metabolic bone disease in children are the various types of rickets and renal osteodystrophy. Nutritional rickets, the historical counterpart, is much less commonly seen today due to improved diets and supplementation of foods with calcium and vitamin D; however, it can occur in socially depressed areas such as inner cities and in children of parents of certain religious affiliations with strict dietary practices. Other less common but important pediatric metabolic conditions include osteoporosis, immobilization, anticonvulsant therapy, celiac disease and other malabsorption syndromes, and other inherited diseases including hypophosphatasia, X-linked hypophosphatemia, and various forms of vitamin D–dependent rickets.

3. **What is the pathophysiology of the bone disease in these metabolic disorders?**

   Although there are multiple types of rickets, the basic pathogenesis is a relative decrease in calcium or phosphorus (or both) of large enough magnitude that it interferes with physeal growth and normal mineralization of the skeleton of the growing child. This decrease in calcium or phosphorus may be due to inadequate intake or impaired absorption of phosphorus or vitamin D, decreased conversion of vitamin D to its active form, end-organ insensitivity, impaired release of calcium from bone, or phosphate wasting. In addition, there is evidence that insufficient vitamin D may interfere with mineralization independent of calcium and phosphate levels.

   In **renal osteodystrophy,** glomerular damage leads to phosphate retention, and tubular injury causes decreased production of the active form of vitamin D (i.e., 1,25-dihydroxyvitamin D) due to lack of 1-hydroxylase activity. These two factors severely inhibit intestinal calcium absorption and reduce plasma ionized calcium. The resultant hypocalcemia triggers secondary hyperparathyroidism, which remains ineffective in increasing intestinal absorption of calcium. Therefore, the body's only means of increasing serum calcium levels is by bone resorption. Untreated or undertreated metabolic acidemia may worsen bone resorption.

   In patients with **osteoporosis,** the bone is made normally but is reduced in overall amount. In children, osteoporosis may be idiopathic, as in juvenile osteoporosis, or may be due to disuse or chronic corticosteroid administration. The pathophysiology of idiopathic juvenile osteoporosis is unclear, but various theories include increased bone resorption versus decreased bone formation (possibly due to deficient 1,25-dihydroxyvitamin D or calcitonin or due to a fundamental disturbance in the transduction of mechanical forces that stimulate new bone formation). In disuse osteoporosis, the lack of stress across bone results in a net decrease in bone mass. The precise link between mechanical force and cell physiology is not clear, however. Glucocorticoids decrease bone mass through suppression of osteoblast function (secondary to decreased cell numbers) and by promoting apoptosis of osteoblasts, as well as through decreased intestinal absorption of calcium, resulting in increased PTH secretion and enhanced osteoclast activity.

Hypophosphatasia results from a genetic error in the synthesis of alkaline phosphatase, an enzyme necessary for the maturation of the primary spongiosa in the physes. This results in normal production of bone (osteoid) but inadequate mineralization, with resultant skeletal deformities that mimic rickets.

4. **How much do I have to know about calcium, vitamin D, and phosphorus metabolism to be able to effectively manage the orthopaedic needs of these patients?**
    Just the basics. Healthy bone requires constant calcium and phosphorus concentrations within the serum. These concentrations are normally maintained in a steady state through an elaborate system involving the kidney, gut, and skeleton. Low levels of calcium stimulate the release of PTH, which stimulates the synthesis of the active form of vitamin D (i.e., 1,25-dihydroxyvitamin D). Together, these two hormones act to increase intestinal absorption, renal tubule reabsorption, and bone resorption of calcium, with a resultant increase in serum levels. Activated vitamin D is a necessity in facilitating calcium transportation across the gut. Chronic stimulation by PTH can also work independently to stimulate osteoclasts to resorb bone. The net effects on the skeleton are decreased mineralization, a decreased amount of bone, and altered structure and integrity of bone. Calcitonin works in the opposite way to decrease serum calcium concentrations.

    Normal serum calcium and phosphorus levels are required to maintain bone homeostasis. Hypocalcemia will result in (and potentially cause) metabolic bone disease if there are abnormalities in any of the following:

    ■ **Calcium:** Inadequate dietary intake, insufficient intestinal absorption (due to either deficient activated vitamin D or PTH or, in cases of steatorrhea, calcium binding with free fatty acids and forming an insoluble compound that cannot be absorbed), or reduced renal reabsorption

    ■ **Vitamin D:** Lack of sufficient amounts of the activated form. This deficiency can occur secondary to insufficient dietary intake (i.e., nutritional rickets), decreased intestinal absorption (as with steatorrhea, since vitamin D is fat soluble), or in certain genetic forms of rickets in which the end-organ gut cell is insensitive to vitamin D. It can also occur due to insufficient conversion of vitamin D to its active form owing to lack of ultraviolet light exposure, hepatic disease, or, especially, renal tubule dysfunction, since the sequential and essential sites of conversion are the skin, the liver, and the kidney. The ingested provitamin ergosterols are stored in the skin and, in the presence of ultraviolet light, are converted to ergocalciferol (i.e., vitamin D2) and cholecalciferol (i.e., vitamin D3). After transportation to the liver, they are converted to 25-hydroxyvitamin D. The final and most critical conversion occurs in the kidney, where 25-hydroxyvitamin D is converted to either the less-active 24,25-hydroxyvitamin D or the highly active 1,25 hydroxy form.

    ■ **Phosphorus:** Hyperphosphatemia, which occurs in renal osteodystrophy due to glomerular damage, "turns off" the system that actively transports calcium out of the gut into the extracellular space, resulting in inability to absorb calcium from the intestinal tract. It also shunts renal conversion of 25-hydroxyvitamin D into the less active 24,25-hydroxy form. Conversely, hypophosphatemia, which occurs in several forms of rickets, also causes skeletal abnormalities since adequate phosphorus is absolutely required for normal mineralization.

5. **What are the differences among rickets, osteomalacia, and renal osteodystrophy?**
    Anatomically, rickets and osteomalacia are both characterized by the presence of excessive amounts of unmineralized osteoid, resulting in skeletal deformity. **Rickets** occurs only in the growing skeleton, however, and is further characterized by deficient mineralization and excess cartilage accumulation in the growth plates at the site of enchondral bone formation. **Osteomalacia** is the adult counterpart of rickets, occurring only after the physes have closed. It lacks the growth abnormalities observed in childhood rickets.
    Osteodystrophy is a syndrome of four pathologic entities, as follows, that occur in response to the profound hypocalcemia of renal disease:
    - **Rickets or osteomalacia:** With deficient mineralization of osteoid
    - **Osteitis fibrosa cystica:** A condition associated with severe lytic changes in the skeleton due to overproduction of PTH
    - **Osteosclerosis:** Occurs in about 20% of patients with osteodystrophy (especially in the spine and occasionally in the long bones), due to increased numbers of bony trabeculae rather than increased mineralization
    - **Ectopic calcification or mineralization:** Occurs secondary to precipitation of calcium salts (in the corneas, conjunctivae, skin, arteriolar walls, and periarticular soft tissues) if calcium levels increase to normal with dietary indiscretion, spontaneous improvement, or dialysis

6. **Are X-linked (i.e., hypophosphatemic) and vitamin D–resistant rickets the same thing?**
    This is a trick question. First, hypophosphatemia is a common denominator in many forms of rickets. Second, although *X-linked* and *vitamin D–resistant* are terms often used interchangeably to describe a relatively common inherited form of rickets, there are many other types of vitamin D–resistant rickets. This common form of vitamin D–resistant rickets has also been called *refractory rickets, familial hypophosphatemia, familial vitamin D–resistant rickets,* and *phosphate diabetes.* It is caused by a genetic (X-linked–dominant) error in phosphate transport, probably located in the proximal nephron, although there is increasingly strong evidence that the defective tubular reabsorption of phosphate in this disease is not intrinsic to the kidney but is instead due to an unidentified circulating humoral agent. Several studies suggest that the PHEX gene is affected in many families expressing this disorder. It is fully expressed in hemizygous male patients. Isolated hypophosphatemia may signify the presence of the trait in heterozygous females. With full expression, the condition consists of hypophosphatemia, lower-limb deformities, and stunted growth. Although the hypophosphatemia is present shortly after birth, the skeletal deformities and short stature really do not become evident until the child begins walking and the deformities progress beyond the physiologic range.

7. **How does the nonorthopaedic management vary among the different types of rickets?**
    For children with renal phosphate wasting, the mainstay of medical management is replacement of phosphate and, often, administration of vitamin D, most commonly in the form of calcitriol (i.e., 1,25-dihydroxyvitamin D3). For children with renal osteodystrophy, administration of calcium, either as a dietary supplement or as a phosphate binder, along with calcitriol or other vitamin D analogues, is common. The role of bisphosphonates in treating steroid-induced osteoporosis in children is currently under investigation. Bisphosphonates appear to be useful treatment for other types of pediatric bone disease such as osteogenesis imperfecta.

8. **What are the clinical features of rickets?**
    - **General:** Irritability or apathy, short stature (often under the third percentile), muscle weakness, and signs and symptoms of hypocalcemia in severe cases
    - **Skull:** Frontal bossing and enlargement of the suture lines
    - **Dental anomalies:** Delayed dentition, enamel defects, and extensive caries

- **Trunk:** Enlargement of the costal cartilages (i.e., rachitic rosary), long thoracic kyphosis (i.e., rachitic catback deformity), and protuberant abdomen
- **Extremities:** Ligamentous laxity; long-bone deformities including bowing and shortening; and apparent enlargement of the elbows, wrists, knees, and ankles. General guideline: if the disease manifests during the stage of physiologic bowing (from age 1–2 years), the result will be varus, whereas active disease during the stage of physiologic genu valgus (from age 2–4) produces valgus (Fig. 90-1)

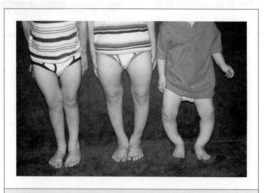

Figure 90-1. Three brothers with vitamin D–resistant hypophosphatemic rickets, demonstrating typical skeletal deformities. Note the valgus deformity in the oldest child and varus in the youngest boy. The two older children have previously undergone ostotomy for severe deformity.

9. **What other conditions should be considered in the differential diagnosis of rickets?**

   Physiologic genu varus or valgus; Blount disease; metaphyseal, epiphyseal, or other skeletal dysplasias; achondroplasia or hypochondroplasia; fibrous dysplasia; and enchondromatosis.

10. **What should be asked in the history?**
    - **Past medical:** Renal or hepatic abnormalities, use of anticonvulsants, growth and development, previous fractures, and reduced sunlight exposure
    - **Dietary:** Malabsorption syndromes, milk allergy, or other reasons for reduced dietary intake of calcium
    - **Family:** Short stature, lower-limb deformities, frequent fractures, or bone dysplasias
    - **Dental:** Delayed eruption or excessive caries

11. **What imaging studies are useful?**

    Plain radiographs are the most useful, with classic findings seen in florid rickets. In milder forms of rickets, radiographic findings may be subtle. A bone scan may be useful in these cases to delineate increased activity over the shafts of long bones, ribs, and the skull, and especially at the sites of fracture.

12. **What findings can be seen on the plain radiographs?**

    General findings include osteopenia, thin cortices, and small trabeculae with overall decreased bone mass. The osteopenia is more marked in the metaphyses, contributing to a "washed-out" appearance. The cortices, vertebral end plates, and trabeculae often appear fuzzy and indistinct. Classic findings, most often seen with florid rickets, include irregular widening or cupping of the physes (Fig. 90-2). Looser's lines (also known as Milkman's pseudofractures) are ribbon-like radiolucencies extending transversely from one cortex across the medullary canal. They represent areas of weakening or incomplete fracture and are pathognomonic for rickets and osteomalacia. The most common sites include the concave side of long bones, especially the femoral neck, ischial and pubic rami, ribs, clavicles, and axillary borders of the scapulae.

13. **What laboratory tests can be useful to screen for rickets?**
The main tests are serum calcium, phosphate, alkaline phosphatase, serum 25-hydroxyvitamin D (which is low in vitamin D–deficient rickets), 1,25-dihydroxyvitamin D3, and PTH levels. In infancy, abnormal laboratory values may be the only findings in a child with rickets. In vitamin D–resistant (i.e., hypophosphatemic) rickets, abnormal laboratory findings include normal or slightly low serum calcium, low serum phosphate, low serum alkaline phosphatase, and elevated urine phosphate levels. Administration of vitamin D does not produce a response in these individuals. PTH levels are high in vitamin D deficiency and normal or only slightly increased in other forms of rickets. Alkaline phosphatase levels are almost always elevated in active rickets.

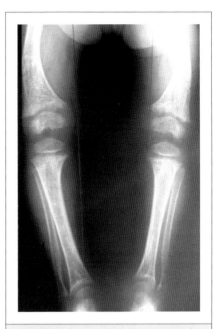

Figure 90-2. Classic radiographic appearance of the lower extremities in rickets. Note the widened physes, cupped metaphyses, and diaphyseal bowing.

14. **When is orthopaedic treatment (i.e., bracing or surgery) indicated?**
In the presence of fracture or when deformity exceeds the physiologic range and predisposes the individual to progressive deformity, altered mechanical alignment, or degenerative joint disease. With advances in medical management of this condition, orthopaedic intervention in the form of bracing or surgery is much less commonly needed.

15. **If surgery is needed, what can I expect regarding bony healing in patients with rickets?**
With adequate medical management, bony healing occurs, although some studies have found it to be delayed. After surgery, these patients should be watched carefully since the prolonged immobilization due to hospitalization or casting may lead to hypercalcemia.

16. **After orthopaedic treatment of rachitic deformities, what can I tell the parents about the prognosis and the risk of recurrence?**
With all forms of rickets, the likelihood of recurrence is increased in cases of inadequate medical control. Compliance must be stressed since lapses in the medication regimen will result in recurrent rickets and skeletal deformities. With X-linked hypophosphatemic rickets, recurrent deformity and short stature are more common despite adequate medical management and may necessitate reosteotomy or growth hormone therapy. Continued medical management

(i.e., phosphate and vitamin D replacement) after physeal closure is controversial since rachitic deformities of the skeleton do not tend to occur in adulthood and continued treatment carries a risk of nephrocalcinosis. Proponents of phosphate and vitamin D replacement in adult patients with rickets believe that it may reduce the risk of bone pain, stress fractures, osteoarthritis, and dental abscesses.

KEY POINTS: RICKETS AND METABOLIC DISORDERS

1. The major factors affecting bone mineral homeostasis can be thought of as the "three 3s": intra- and extracellular levels of three ions (calcium, phosphorus, and magnesium), which are regulated by three hormones (parathyroid hormone, calcitonin, and 1,25-dihydroxyvitamin D) and act upon three tissues (bone, intestine, and kidney).

2. Although there are multiple types of rickets, the basic pathogenesis is a relative decrease in calcium, phosphorus, or both, of large enough magnitude that it interferes with physeal growth and normal mineralization of the skeleton of the growing child.

3. This decrease in calcium or phosphorus may be due to inadequate intake or impaired absorption of phosphorus or vitamin D, decreased conversion of vitamin D to its active form, end-organ insensitivity, impaired release of calcium from bone, or phosphate wasting.

4. Plain radiographs are the most useful diagnostic tool, with classic findings seen in florid rickets. In milder forms of rickets, radiographic findings may be subtle. A bone scan may be useful in these cases.

17. **What are some radiographic findings in renal osteodystrophy that differentiate it from rickets and osteomalacia?**
    - Changes due to osteitis fibrosa cystica are unique to renal osteodystrophy and include "salt-and-pepper" skull, absence of the cortical outline of the outer centimeter of the clavicles, and subperiosteal resorption of the ulnas, terminal tufts of the distal phalanges, and medial proximal tibias.
    - Brown tumors appear as expanded destructive lesions and are usually round or ovoid, with indistinct margins. They are due to secondary hyperparathyroidism and are most common in cases of severe and long-standing renal osteodystrophy. Brown tumors may be present in the long bones or pelvis and, when associated with thinning or expansion of the cortex, may be the site of pathologic fractures. These lesions sometimes resemble primary or metastatic bone tumors.
    - Slipped epiphyses are noted.

18. **What are the most common sites of epiphyseal slipping in renal osteodystrophy?**
    The proximal femur is by far the most common site. Other reported sites include the proximal humerus, the distal femur, and the distal tibia. Slippage of the distal radial and ulnar epiphyses occurs almost exclusively in older (i.e., prepubertal and adolescent) children and may lead to ulnar deviation of the wrists.

19. **What is the cause of the epiphyseal slipping in this disease?**
    It is due to profound hyperparathyroidism, which results in resorption of metaphyseal bone. This weakening of the metaphyseal area, in combination with the chronic nature of the disease, results in epiphysiolysis. Studies have shown that the risk of slippage is increased during

periods of rapid growth or in cases of untreated renal disease and severe hyperparathyroidism. Treated renal disease with more-normal PTH levels does not cause epiphyseal slippage.

20. **What are the clinical features of idiopathic juvenile osteoporosis?**
Bone and joint pain in previously healthy children, with onset usually between the ages of 8 and 14 years. Later symptoms include growth arrest, osteopenia of varying severity, collapse of the vertebral bodies, metaphyseal fractures, and metatarsal stress fractures. The condition may be limited to the spine or may also involve the long bones, with bone loss more marked in the metaphyses than the diaphyses.

21. **What differential diagnoses should be considered before making the diagnosis of idiopathic juvenile osteoporosis?**
Because this is a rare disorder and a diagnosis of exclusion, other conditions resulting in osteopenia and bone fragility must be ruled out. These include malnutrition, type I osteogenesis imperfecta, hematologic malignancies, hyperthyroid disorders, Cushing's disease, steroid-induced osteopenia, and disuse osteopenia. Rapid progression after many years of normality differentiates idiopathic osteoporosis from osteogenesis imperfecta.

22. **What studies are useful in evaluating idiopathic juvenile osteoporosis?**
Laboratory and histomorphometric studies are difficult to interpret and are not very helpful in evaluating this condition. Radiographs demonstrate decreased bone mass (i.e., osteopenia), especially in the metaphyseal regions; quantitative computed tomography and dual-photon densitometry can help measure decreases in bone density, but age-appropriate controls are limited. For children, a z score, not a T-score, should be used to interpret information generated by dual-energy x-ray absorptiometry (DEXA) scanning.

23. **What is the natural history of idiopathic juvenile osteoporosis?**
This is a self-limited disorder that tends to resolve spontaneously within 2–4 years or after puberty. The completeness of the resolution depends on the age of onset and is related to the amount of growth potential remaining after the process stops. It has been difficult to demonstrate the efficacy of any treatment regimen in altering the natural history of this disease. Prolonged disuse or immobilization can worsen the osteoporosis and clinical symptoms, however. Adequate nutritional intake of vitamin D and calcium should be strongly encouraged.

24. **Which anticonvulsants cause osteomalacia, rickets, and calcium metabolism disturbances?**
Primarily phenytoin. Carbamazepine alone does not seem to cause significant osteomalacia or calcium metabolism disturbances, but when used in conjunction with valproate or phenytoin, it may enhance their adverse effects. Data are conflicting regarding valproate, with some studies showing no effect on the skeleton and others demonstrating clear decreases in bone density with valproate therapy. Phenobarbital does not affect hepatic metabolism of vitamin D but has been shown in some studies to reduce bone density; other studies have shown that overall plasma levels are not reduced and the skeleton is not affected. Clinically significant effects on bone due to anticonvulsants are very rare in noninstitutionalized, normally active patients. Rarely, Fanconi syndrome with renal phosphate wasting has been ascribed to anticonvulsant use.

25. **How are the orthopaedic problems associated with anticonvulsants managed?**
Although the exact pathogenesis of the osteomalacia or rickets varies with different drugs, most anticonvulsants appear to increase the daily vitamin D requirement. The orthopaedic manifestations of this increased requirement are more severe in patients with already-reduced vitamin D levels (such as in institutionalized patients with reduced sunlight exposure or dietary supply) or in those with concomitant disuse osteopenia. Treatment is aimed at prevention of

orthopaedic problems and includes ensuring adequate sunlight exposure and normal dietary intake of vitamin D, avoidance of disuse osteopenia through weight-bearing activites, and, when possible, switching to an anticonvulsant with fewer skeletal manifestations. Administration of additional vitamin D may improve biochemical abnormalities in calcium metabolism but has not been shown to reverse cortical bone loss. The use of prophylactic vitamin D in patients receiving anticonvulsants remains controversial.

26. **Which endocrine problems commonly cause orthopaedic manifestations in the pediatric population?**
See Table 90-1.

TABLE 90-1. ENDOCRINE PROBLEMS THAT COMMONLY CAUSE ORTHOPAEDIC MANIFESTATIONS IN CHILDREN		
Hormone	**Excess or Deficiency**	**Orthopaedic Manifestations in Childhood**
Parathyroid	Excess	Increased osteoclast activity with bone resorption and skeletal pain
	Deficiency	Increased bone density and soft tissue calcification; main clinical symptoms are systemic due to hypocalcemia (i.e., seizures)
Thyroid	Excess	Osteopenia
	Deficiency	Delayed bone age and growth retardation, late appearance of the secondary ossification centers with occasional stippling, slipped capital femoral epiphyses, and a large posterior fontanel in newborns
Androgens	Excess	Precocious puberty, with initial accelerated growth but early growth plate closure and, ultimate, short stature
	Deficiency	Initial delayed bone age but late physeal closure and a final height above average
Estrogen	Excess	Enhanced epiphyseal maturation with reduced cell proliferation, resulting in short stature
	Deficiency	Increased bone resorption and osteoporosis; in rare cases of complete loss of estrogen action, tall stature is observed due to extreme delays in growth plate closure
Glucocorticoids	Excess	Suppression of growth hormone synthesis with short stature, profound and irreversible osteopenia with possible vertebral and other compression fractures, and osteonecrosis of the secondary ossification centers

Acknowledgments

The authors wish to thank A. Michael Parfitt, MD, Thomas Wells, MD, and John Fowlkes, MD, for their expert advice in the preparation of this chapter.

BIBLIOGRAPHY

1. Apel DM, Millar EA, Moel DI: Skeletal disorders in pediatric renal transplant population. J Pediatr Orthop 9:505–511, 1989.

2. Chung S, Ahn C: Effects of anti-epileptic drug therapy on bone mineral density in ambulatory epileptic children. Brain Dev 16:382–385, 1994.

3. Favus MJ (ed): Primer on the Metabolic Bone Diseases and Disorders of Mineral Metabolism, 4th ed. Philadelphia, Lippincott, Williams & Wilkins, 1999.

4. Gough H, Goggin T, Bissessar M, et al: A comparative study of the relative influence of different anticonvulsant drugs, UV exposure and diet on vitamin D and calcium metabolism in out-patients with epilepsy. Q J Med 59:569–577, 1986.

5. Latta K, Hisano S, Chan JCM: Therapeutics of X-linked hypophosphatemic rickets. Pediatr Nephrol 7:744–748, 1993.

6. Mankin HJ: Rickets, osteomalacia and renal osteodystrophy: An update. Orthop Clin North Am 21:81–96, 1990.

7. Sheth RD, Wesolowski CA, Jacob JC, et al: Effect of carbamazepine and valproate on bone mineral density. Pediatrics 127:256–262, 1995.

8. Stanitski DF: Treatment of deformity secondary to metabolic bone disease with the Ilizarov technique. Clin Orthop 301:38–41, 1994.

9. Zaleske DJ, Doppelt SH, Mankin HJ: Metabolic and endocrine abnormalities of the immature skeleton. In Morrissey RT (ed): Lovell and Winter's Pediatric Orthopaedics, 3rd ed. Philadelphia, J.B. Lippincott, 1990, pp 203–261.

CHAPTER 91

HEMATOLOGIC DISORDERS

Ryan C. Goodwin, MD

HEMOPHILIA

1. **What is the genetic picture of hemophilia and von Willebrand's disease?**
   A sex-linked (expressed mainly in males) recessive gene located on the X chromosome causes this disease. The incidence of hemophilia is 1 in 10,000. von Willebrand's disease is a genetic deficiency of factor VII with associated platelet dysfunction. It carries an autosomal dominant inheritance pattern and should be considered in the differential diagnosis of female children with bleeding disorders.

2. **How is hemophilia diagnosed?**
   Partial thromboplastin time (PTT) and specific factor assays are the definitive diagnostic laboratory studies. The blood level of the factors VIII and IX (or their percent activity of the normal) is divided according to the severity of the clinical manifestations, as follows:
   - **50–200% activity:** Within the normal limits
   - **25–50% activity:** Essentially normal
   - **5–25% activity:** Mild form
   - **1–5% activity:** Moderate form
   - **1% of normal factor level:** Severe hemophilia

3. **What are the common musculoskeletal manifestations in hemophilia?**
   The characteristic musculoskeletal manifestations in hemophilia are most common in patients with deficits of either factor VIII (i.e., classic hemophilia, or hemophilia A) or factor IX (i.e., Christmas disease, or hemophilia B). Musculoskeletal complaints typically relate to bleeding. Recurrent hemarthroses produce joint pain, stiffness, and arthropathy. Patients with moderate hemophilia experience only mild arthropathy. With severe factor deficiency, spontaneous bleeding into joints or tissues may occur. With the moderate form, bleeding usually follows minor trauma, and patients with mild factor deficiency will rarely develop hemarthrosis after major trauma or surgical interventions.

4. **What is the advantage of magnetic resonance imaging (MRI) in the work-up and treatment of hemophilic arthropathy?**
   MRI presents details of soft tissue and articular cartilage better than plain radiographs. It is also helpful in decision making regarding surgical synovectomy. Its ability to demonstrate early stages of cartilage or synovial alternations can assist in therapy planning.

5. **Which are the commonly affected skeletal sites in hemophiliacs? How is this related to the patient's age?**
   The knee, ankle, and elbow are most commonly affected. In small children, the ankle is the most commonly affected due to frequent jumping. The knee is most commonly affected in children over the age of 5 years. Of great concern are the deep soft tissue hemorrhages, occurring particularly in the calf, thigh, iliopsoas muscle, and upper extremities.

6. **What are the physical findings of minor hemarthrosis?**
   Swollen and warm joints. In the older child, pain or discomfort can precede the swelling.

7. **What are the modes of treatment in major hemarthrosis?**
    Major hemarthrosis is the result of major trauma or recurrent bleeding into a joint already affected with synovitis. The treatment of painful minor intra-articular hemorrhage begins with early aspiration at the same time as or shortly after factor transfusion. This is followed by short-term compression dressing and splinting in the most comfortable position, rehabilitation exercises (with splints in between), and continuous concentrate transfusions to reduce the risk of synovitis. The most crucial therapeutic measure is the evacuation of the intra-articular massive bleeding by aspiration. It can prevent potential synovitis and recurrent hemarthrosis. Joint decompression leads to dramatic relief of pain. It also reduces the likelihood of infection by removing the clot or blood that may serve as a medium for bacterial growth. Transfusion of factor is critical for successful treatment, along with analgesic medications.

8. **What is "treatment on demand" for hemophilia?**
    "Treatment on demand" is just that; transfusion of factor at the time of hemarthrosis and for an additional 2–3 days, with avoidance of aspirin and nonsteroidal anti-inflammatants. The therapeutic goal is factor levels of 30–50 international units (IU) per dL. Treatment given on demand or as secondary prophylaxis appears to be inefficient in ultimately preventing hemophilic arthropathy.

9. **What are the indications for prophylactic transfusions for hemophiliacs?**
    Ongoing prophylaxis with continuous administration of factors VIII and IX from the first years of life as a primary prophylaxis regimen has been shown to decrease the incidence of hemarthrosis when compared to treatment on demand. An inherent significant increase in cost for the factor administration with this technique is a disadvantage. Prophylactic administration of factor is individualized and should be directed by a hematologist as the dosing varies by patient age, weight, and factor levels. Increasing plasma levels of factor to 30–40% of normal is therapeutic.

10. **What is the role of synovectomy in hemophiliacs?**
    Synovectomy reduces the incidence of chronic or recurrent hemarthrosis. Its use is controversial in hemophiliacs because of an uncertain influence on the progression of the arthropathy, and it is undecided whether to use arthroscopic synovectomy, an open synovectomy, or medical synovectomy. The use of continuous passive motion (CPM) after arthroscopic synovectomy has improved the results, but arthroscopy is demanding and lacks hemostasis, and it is usually not possible to perform a total synovectomy. The open technique is more comprehensive. Medical (chemical or radioactive) synovectomy has historically been less effective than surgical synovectomy, but it is simple and safe. More recent studies suggest that radionuclide synovectomy may be as effective as surgical synovectomy, without the morbidity.

11. **What are the advantages and disadvantages of radioactive synovectomy?**
    Radioactive synovectomy is the only option for patients with factor VIII inhibitors. Its advantages include low cost, the use of outpatient facilities, and only short-term transfusion of the expensive concentrates. The disadvantages include possible chromosomal changes, the toxic effect on the articular surface, and a higher rate of recurrent hemarthrosis than that following surgical synovectomy.

12. **What are the indications for synovectomy?**
    Patients with severe recurrent hemarthrosis (i.e., 2–3 episodes per month) are candidates for synovectomy. Advantages of open synovectomy include more experience with the technique and the ability to perform a more thorough synovectomy. Disadvantages include the morbidity of an open approach and a greater risk for postoperative stiffness. Arthroscopic synovectomy is

probably best reserved for patients with minimal degenerative changes. It is extremely difficult to perform a complete synovectomy through the arthroscope.

13. **How is elbow synovectomy performed in children and adolescents?**
Whereas elbow synovectomy usually includes radial head excision in older adolescents and adults, this is contraindicated in children for whom arthroscopic synovectomy is the treatment of choice. Open synovectomy without radial head excision can be considered in children in whom arthroscopic synovectomy becomes too technically challenging.

14. **What are the clinical features and sites of muscle hemorrhages in hemophiliacs?**
Muscle hemorrhages are common in severely affected hemophiliacs and are usually the result of minor trauma or occur spontaneously. They occur mainly in the calf, forearm, iliopsoas, and quadriceps. Bleeding is characteristically deep and within the body of the muscle. Presenting symptoms can range from vague pain on motion to pain at rest. The significant hemorrhages into the compartments may result in fibrosis, contractures of muscles, bony bridge, and stiffness of the joints across which the muscles act. To prevent compartment syndrome and contractures, treatment is primarily nonsurgical and includes physiotherapy, ice packs, elevation, compression, dressings, and splints.

15. **What is a hemophilic pseudotumor?**
A hemophilic pseudotumor occurs only in a severe hemophiliac. It is a result of uncontrolled hemorrhage into a confined space. As the cavity expands, pressure necrosis occurs with erosion of the surrounding tissues. An expanding pseudotumor with periosteal attachment may cause erosion and cortical thinning of bone. The result may be a fracture of the involved bone or impingement on vital structures. Findings of pseudotumor include a soft tissue mass, calcifications, cortical thinning, bone destruction, and new bone formation. The differential diagnosis includes osteomyelitis, aneurysmal bone cyst, and bone sarcomas. The femur and pelvis are affected with the highest incidence in adults. Bones of the hand, forearm, calcaneus and foot, leg, cranial vault, and mandible were also reported to be affected. Computed tomography (CT) and MRI are helpful in confirming the diagnosis. It is essentially an expanding hematoma and should not be aspirated or drained, especially in the absence of factor transfusion.

16. **What are the treatment modalities for compartment syndrome after muscle bleedings in hemophiliacs with or without inhibitors?**
General treatment includes appropriate replacement treatment and physical therapy to restore the normal range of motion and to avoid fibrosis of the muscles. In patients with compartment syndrome and no inhibitors, the factor must first be raised to 100%, and then an appropriate surgical procedure such as fasciotomy is carried out. (It is highly recommended that this be done within 24 hours.) In patients with high titer inhibitors, treatment, consisting of alternative transfusions, must be initiated as early as possible.

17. **What is the treatment for equinus contracture following hemorrhage into the gastrocnemius soleus muscle?**
Hemorrhage into the calf muscles can result in an equinus deformity. Aggressive treatment with serial casting and splinting is recommended as soon as possible after a single factor replacement transfusion. The ankle joint is held in a cast in a maximum dorsiflexion position. Surgery may be indicated in resistant deformity.

18. **How are iliopsoas hemorrhage and hemarthrosis of the hip joint differentiated?**
A patient with an iliopsoas hemorrhage presents with vague symptoms of lower abdominal pains or upper thigh discomfort. The hip is flexed and externally rotated. The hip cannot be

extended on examination because of pain, but internal and external rotation of the hip joint are normal. In hemarthrosis of the hip joint, the rotational movements are painful and limited.

19. **What is a common complication of iliacus hemorrhage? How it is treated?**
Extension of hemorrhage of the iliacus muscle distally underneath the inguinal ligament may compress the femoral nerve. This can progress to complete femoral neuropathy in 60% of iliacus bleeding. The treatment of choice is bed rest and analgesics, physical therapy to avoid hip flexion contracture, and continuous factor replacement to the level of at least 50% for 7–14 days.

20. **What is a significant complication of knee flexion contracture, and what is the best way to treat it?**
Severe and long-lasting knee contracture can result in posterior subluxation of the tibia. In such patients (mainly in those with inhibitors), traction and serial casting and wedging are aimed at reducing the knee flexion contracture. The correction is maintained with long-term bracing and physiotherapy. Another effective optional treatment of knee flexion contracture is hamstring release and posterior capsulotomy. Bony procedures such as extension supracondylar osteotomy are also used.

21. **What and where are typical fractures in hemophiliacs? How are they treated?**
Fractures occur most frequently in the lower extremities, with femoral supracondylar and femoral neck fractures being the most common. Immediate adequate factor replacement, open reduction, and internal fixation may be used when indicated as for nonhemophilic patients. When a fracture can be treated noninvasively, transfusion protocol is individualized, depending on the fracture location and the estimated amount of bleeding.

SICKLE CELL ANEMIA

22. **What is sickle cell (SC) disease?**
SC disease is a genetic blood disorder that causes a malformation of the normal adult erythrocyte to assume a sickle shape under decreased oxygen tension. These cells are dysfunctional and do not transport oxygen effectively and efficiently, resulting in a variety of clinical symptoms. Blacks are predominantly affected, although the condition has been seen in Caucasians, Indians, and people of Mediterranean descent.

23. **What is the genetic transmission of sickle cell disease?**
An autosomal dominant gene results in the formation of hemoglobin S (HgS), which differs from the normal adult hemoglobin (HgA) by the substitution of valine for glutamic acid in the sixth amino acid position in each of the two β-polypeptide chains. HgS results from an abnormal b-globulin gene on chromosome 11. A homozygous state for the abnormal HgS (HgS-S) produces the classic SC anemia. It is a chronic hemolytic anemia. The heterozygous genotype produces a sickle trait (HgS-A). These patients have no clinical manifestations under physiologic conditions but can transmit the disease (in a homozygous state) to their offspring.

24. **What is the ethnic distribution of the gene for HgS? What is the resultant incidence of SC anemia?**
The gene for HgS occurs in 8–10% of blacks in the United States, in up to 40% in some ethnic groups in Central Africa, and in 0.8% in non-black persons. An SC trait appears in about 20% of the populations of Central Africa, and SC anemia appears in approximately 1–2%. In the black population in the United States, SC anemia is less frequent and occurs in

14 per thousand of the population. The incidence of SC disease and its variants is 7.7% in the African-American community.

25. **What is sickling of the erythrocytes, and what initiates the process?**
Sickling is a result of HgS polymerization, which changes the soluble HgS into a gel. This results in distorted and fragile erythrocytes that are more rigid and viscous and are rapidly destroyed. Low oxygen tension or reduced blood flow are the most common conditions initiating these pathologic changes.

26. **What are the clinical results of the hemolytic changes?**
These changes will result in increased hemolysis and in small vessel occlusion and infarcts. Two separate pathologic abnormalities cause the clinical manifestations in SC disorders:
- Sickling of the red cell, producing vaso-occlusion and thromboembolic bone infarcts
- Increased destruction of SC red cells, producing hemolysis, an increased erythroblastic activity, and expansion of the bone marrow activity.

27. **What musculoskeletal problems result from (1) vaso-occlusion in SC disorders and (2) hemolytic anemia?**
1. Dactylitis, avascular necrosis (AVN) (particularly in the femoral head), osteomyelitis, retardation of height and growth, septic arthritis, reactive arthritis, and leg ulcers
2. Hyperplasia of the bone marrow will result in increased size of the medullary cavity, osteoporosis, thinning of the bone cortices, and biconcavity of the vertebrae. It accounts for the tendency to spontaneous fracture.

28. **What are the causes and incidence of dactylitis (i.e., hand-foot syndrome) in SC disorders? What is a characteristic expression?**
Dactylitis is usually manifested between 6 and 12 months of age, when hemoglobin F (fetal) is replaced by HgS. The syndrome affects the short tubular bones of the hands and feet. A typical case is a child below the age of 2 years with a swollen, tender, and painful hand or foot. The symptoms are usually triggered by cold weather and last for 1–2 weeks. The incidence of dactylitis was reported to be 45% in patients with SC disorders, and 41% of the affected patients suffer from recurrent episodes. The hands and feet are spared after the age of 6 years due to the disappearance of the hematopoietic marrow activity in them.

29. **What other conditions may be confused with dactylitis? How are they best recognized?**
Osteomyelitis resembles dactylitis since both present clinically as localized soft tissue swelling and tenderness, with systemic fever and leukocytosis. Radiographs yield similar findings in the two conditions, such as patchy areas of bone destruction, subperiosteal bone reaction, and, finally, bone reformation. Aspiration of the affected bone is the best way to differentiate between the two; bone scan is not adequately informative. MRI can also be used to identify and an abscess, if present. The bony resolution after 4–8 weeks differs in the self-limiting nature of dactylitis from osteomyelitis.

30. **Describe the most common cause and site of extremity pain in SC anemia.**
SC crises, usually occurring between 3 and 4 years of age and lasting from 3–5 days, cause the accumulation of sequestrated SCs in the vascular canals leading to a localized area of bone marrow infarction or soft tissue crisis. The secondary inflammatory response will contribute to the process by causing a rise in the intramedullary pressure and its resulting severe pain. The most common sites are the long bones, such as the humerus, tibia, and femur, whose growing ends are particularly involved. The physical findings are mild swelling, limitation of the range of motion, and low elevation of temperature.

31. **How often do SC crises that require intravenous (IV) steroid therapy occur?**
The rates are 0.8 per year in SC anemia (SS), 1.0 per year in the Sb8, and 0.4 per year in SC and Sb1. When HgF is elevated, the rate of crisis is low. High doses of intravenous corticoids significantly reduce the severity of the pain and its duration.

32. **Are growth disturbances common in SS children?**
Yes. Retardation of growth is common. In children with SS, weight and height are significantly low before 2 years of age. Skeletal maturity is also significantly retarded in children with SS, and pubertal development is delayed. Chronic anemia, infections of the epiphysis, and osteomyelitis can be the possible etiologic factors.

33. **What are the common radiographic features in SC disease?**
In the skull, the calvarium is thickened, the diploic space is widened or ballooned, and the bony texture has an agranular appearance. These changes occur in one third to one half of the patients with SC disease. Granular osteoporosis, pelvic demineralization, and rib broadening are nonspecific. Foci and microfoci of avascular necrosis can be identified by MRI and CT scan.
  In the long bones, there is patchy osteosclerosis with focal radiolucency, cortical thinning, widening of the medullary canal, and mild periosteal elevation. Cortical bone infarction with dense, amorphous, chalky zones and sclerosis are among the most common and typical radiologic feature of SC disorders. The combination of new layers of repair bone with an infarcted cortex occasionally creates a "bone within a bone" pattern. Vertebral deformity occurs in as many as 70% of the patients. Typically, the center of the subchondral bone plate is compressed and forms a sharp dip (i.e., a step deformity), whereas the periphery retains its normal contour. These changes usually occur in children older that 10 years of age, and they differ from osseous disk herniation, osteoporotic fractures, or changes in multiple myeloma.

34. **What is the etiology of the increased infection rate seen in SC disorders?**
Patients with SC disorders are more susceptible to infection because of hyposplenism, reduced liver functions, interference with the reticuloendothelial system functions, suppressed clearing of the organisms from the blood, and abnormal opsonizing and complement functions. The infarcted bone marrow will add to the risk by serving as a preferred site for colonization. The ongoing inflammatory state between painful crises involving neutrophil activation, as well as an abnormality of cytokine-regulated neutrophil function, may compromise host defenses against certain microorganisms.

35. **What are the most common bacterial organisms that cause osteomyelitis in patients with SC anemia?**
Although *Salmonella* and its related species are commonly implicated in musculoskeletal infections in SC patients, *Staphylococcus aureus* is the most commonly isolated organism. Younger patients are more likely to acquire *Salmonella* organisms than older children. Capillary occlusion secondary to intravascular sickling may infarct the bowel and permit the spread of the gram-negative bacterial agents. When empirical antibiotic therapy is initiated, coverage for both *Staphylococcus* and *Salmonella* species should be included. Of course, organism-directed therapy is ideal when an organism is ultimately identified.

36. **What is the rate of polyostotic involvement? Why is this significant?**
The rate of multifocal osteomyelitis, often symmetric, can range from 12–47%. It can be associated with some life-threatening disorders.

37. **Why is it difficult to differentiate bone infarction from osteomyelitis?**
■ The clinical manifestations of fever, pain, and swelling can overlap.

- The initial radiographs do not show abnormalities in either disorder.
- The erythrocyte sedimentation rate (ESR) is unreliable in SC disorders because of the change in the shape of the erythrocytes.
- Bone scan with technetium-99m or gallium-47 does not distinguish between them.
- Both may involve multiple long bones.
- Boys are more susceptible in both.
- SC crisis is 50 times more common than bacterial osteomyelitis.

38. **What clinical tools are helpful in differentiating between these two pathologies, and what are their limitations?**

   Combined technetium and gallium scintigraphy and technetium sulfur colloid bone marrow scan and gadolinium-data-enhanced MRI may help distinguish osteomyelitis from infarction in patients with SC.

   Unfortunately, patterns of infarction may not differ from osteomyelitis after 7 days from the onset of symptoms. The scintigraphic studies are useful in locating all areas of suspected osteomyelitis. The role of ultrasound (US) is to confirm the presence of a subperiosteal fluid collection, to guide aspiration (which may differentiate between a hematoma and an abscess), and to allow percutaneous drainage. A finding of 4-mm depth or more of subperiosteal fluid requires further imaging or aspiration to establish the diagnosis of osteomyelitis. An ill-appearing patient with fever, pain, and swelling should lead to aspiration or biopsy of the area, bypassing diagnostic studies (mainly radiographs and bone scan) that may be unreliable. MRI has been used increasingly in confirming the presence of osteomyelitis or abscess and is replacing the use ultrasound in many institutions.

39. **When and why is surgery indicated?**

   As in the treatment of any musculoskeletal infection, surgery is indicated to either obtain an organism for diagnosis or to drain an abscess and debride devitalized tissue. The procedure is coupled with long-term parenteral antibiotic therapy. Some recommend that the wound be left open when there is an extensive abscess, whereas others advise an immediate wound closure with closed suction perfusion irrigation or vacuum dressing. Aggressive treatment with incision, drilling of bone, drainage, and organism-specific antibiotics for at least 6 weeks is required to keep the incidence of chronic osteomyelitis low in these compromised patients.

40. **What is the most common complication of long-bone osteomyelitis in SC patients?**

   Pathologic fractures are the most common complication of osteomyelitis in long bones. In patients with SC disorders (in about 10% of the patients with osteomyelitis), these fractures are usually complicated by nonunion, delayed union, and malunion and joint stiffness.

41. **Can septic arthritis be expected in SC disorders?**

   Septic arthritis is uncommon in SC, but the knee joint is most often involved when it is present. The causative organism is usually not *Salmonella*. Septic arthritis carries a poor prognosis and typically requires aggressive surgical intervention. It can be complicated by AVN or dislocation in the hip joint.

42. **How can the spine be involved in sickle patients?**

   Bone marrow hyperplasia can result in radiographic changes. Collapse of vertebrae can occur as intervertebral disks can bulge into the endplates. Compression fractures may occur and can lead to kyphosis or trunk shortening. This may also occur if AVN of the vertebral body occurs. Vertebral osteomyelitis should always be considered in the differential diagnosis when spine-related symptoms occur, as happened in up to 24% of cases in one center.

43. **What are the typical features of reactive arthritis in children with SC anemia? What is the treatment?**

Reactive arthritis usually presents as an acute joint pain and moderate effusion in one or more joints (i.e., polyarthritis), and severe muscular spasm and tenderness may also accompany it. Analysis of the joint fluid reveals a low-grade inflammation (i.e., less than 20,000 leukocytes per mm^3). The arthritis can last from a few days to 2 months. During the phase of acute arthralgia, the treatment is nonoperative, consisting of molded splints and analgesics.

44. **What is the incidence and the prognosis of femoral head osteonecrosis in SC anemia, and on what factors does it depend?**

The prevalence and incidence of osteonecrosis in patients with SC disorders older than 5 years of age was found to be 9.8%. (In another, smaller study, the prevalence was significantly greater, at 41%.) Prevalence depends upon the age of onset and the different variants of the SC disorders. Bilaterality occurred in 54% of the patients with osteonecrosis, without relation to the type of SC disorder. Patients with frequent painful crises are at highest risk for femoral head osteonecrosis. The prognosis is better in young children because of their superior potential for healing, but it is guarded in older children.

45. **How useful is MRI in demonstrating AVN in SC?**

MRI can be useful in identifying changes in the femoral head prior to sclerosis and collapse on plain films. It is also helpful in identifying the extent of the osteonecrosis and the developmental sequence of the different femoral head segmental infarctions. Contrast enhancement may allow distinction between acute infarct and osteomyelitis and also recognition of osteomyelitis superimposed on bone infarction.

46. **What primary finding determines the management of AVN? What are the treatment options?**

The identification of the lateral pillar is crucial for selecting treatment of femoral head osteonecrosis. If the lateral pillar is intact, conservative treatment is effective. In total head involvement and deficiency of the lateral pillar, surgical management is indicated, such as Petrie casting, proximal femoral osteotomy, pelvic osteotomy, or core decompression. Attempts at femoral head containment are similar to those employed in the treatment of Perthes' disease (i.e., idiopathic osteonecrosis).

Total hip replacement yields poor results and prognosis because of the risks of infection, high blood loss, early aseptic loosening, and intraoperative femoral fracture and perforation. Intraoperative consideration includes the use of tourniquets, oxygenation, maintenance of blood volume, and avoidance of hypothermia. Postoperative considerations are the maintenance of intravascular volume and appropriate oxygenation.

47. **Which is the second most common location of osteonecrosis in patients with SC?**

Osteonecrosis of the humeral head. The incidence rate of radiographic evidence for the osteonecrosis is 5–6%. As for the femoral head, the prevalence rates are related to the child's age and the type of SS. Bilateral involvement was recorded in 67% of the patients with humeral osteonecrosis. Involvement of the non–weight-bearing shoulder leads to less disability and pain, and 79% of the patients are asymptomatic at diagnosis. The typical radiographic appearance includes the crescent sign and collapse of the humeral head, which usually begins in the superior medial quadrant. Further fragmentation will lead to pain and stiffness. Good function can be often sustained in 12–24 months, and there is no need for joint replacement.

48. **How common is cerebral infarction in SC anemia?**

The incidence of cerebral infarction is about 8% of the patients with SC disorders. It may result in spastic hemiplegia in children.

49. **What are the differences between Perthes' disease and AVN in SC disorders?**
Perthes' disease occurs in young children between 3 and 10 years old, whereas AVN in SC disorders usually occurs in the second decade of life or later. Perthes' disease is 10 times more common in white children and 5 times more common in boys. Hemoglobinopathic AVN has equal distribution between the sexes and is common among the black race. In Perthes' disease, the metaphysis is involved, whereas in SC disorders the metaphysis is almost never involved.

THALASSEMIA

50. **What are the pathology and the clinical features in thalassemia major (also known as Cooley's anemia, -thalassemia, and Mediterranean anemia)?**
The severe form of this disease is secondary to homozygous mutation of the β-globulin gene. The result is absent or severe deficiency of the β-polypeptide chain. The hemoglobin molecule is mainly composed of unpaired α-chains. This molecule is insoluble and causes intracellular precipitates. The hematologic findings include severe hypochromia, distorted erythrocytes, target cells, microcytosis, and very low hemoglobin levels. There are large HgF molecules in the red cells. The clinical manifestations are severe anemia (i.e., less than 5 gm/dL), growth and development retardation, hepatosplenomegaly, and bone marrow expansion with related skeletal changes secondary to the intense hematopoietic activity. Bone marrow transplantation in thalassemia represents the only form of radical cure of this disease.

Infants with severe anemia who are not treated during their first months of life will die before 5 years of age from infections and cardiac failure.

Advances in antenatal diagnosis, intrauterine intervention, and postnatal treatment have resulted in extended survival of children whose disease, until recently, was considered invariably fatal. Transfusion and chelation therapy and bone marrow transplantation provide long-term treatment and potential curative options.

51. **What are the characteristic skeletal involvements and most common complications in thalassemia?**
The main skeletal abnormalities are secondary to the hyperplasia and intramedullary excessive hematopoietic activity that cause expansion and widening of the marrow space, rarefaction of the bone trabeculae, resorption of the central bone, thinning of cortical bone, perpendicular periosteal spicules, and severe osteoporosis. The earliest changes are in the hands and feet: the marrow cavities are widened in the metacarpals, metatarsals, and phalanges. There are several abnormalities in the skull, such as osteopenia overgrowth of facial bones, widening of the diploic space, and radial striations, which give a "hair standing on end" appearance. The long bones demonstrate cortical thinning with multiple circumscribed osteolytic areas, which have a punched-out appearance.

Aseptic necrosis of the femoral head can complicate thalassemia. Fractures are a frequent complications and usually occur after minor trauma at an average age of 10–16 years. High prevalence of scoliosis (up to 40%) is another skeletal feature. The most frequent complaints are arthralgia and low back pain (30% and 25% of patients, respectively). A hypertransfusion regimen with chelation therapy reduces osteoporosis, decreases the incidence of this complication, and strengthens the bone. The treatment is also helpful in reducing the time needed for healing the fracture, a process that is improved with the supplement of vitamin C. Chelation therapy may induce bone dysplasia associated with height reduction. Reduction of the doses may improve bone growth.

52. **What is the rate of premature physeal closure in thalassemia?**
Premature closure of the physis is seen in 15–20% of the patients and is responsible for the high incidence of deformities. It is very common in the proximal humeral physis. Its pathogenesis

is obscure. It is more severe and frequent in patients older than 12 years in whom there has been a delay in initiating treatment with transfusions.

GAUCHER'S DISEASE

53. **What is Gaucher's disease? How common is it?**
    Gaucher's disease is a lysosomal storage disorder, with an incidence of 1:40,000. It is caused by a deficiency of the enzyme glucocerebroside β-glucosidase. The deficient enzyme results in reduced degradation and hydrolization of the glucocerebroside (an essential component of the cell wall), thus leading to its gradual accumulation in the macrophages of the reticuloendothelial system. These abnormal accumulations of Gaucher cells result in organ dysfunction. The major elements of bone pathology in Gaucher's disease are failures of osteoclast and osteoblast function, resulting in osteopenia and osteonecrosis.

54. **What are the different types of Gaucher's diseases?**
    There are three distinct clinical forms, as follows:
    - **Type I:** The chronic non-neuronopathic and most common type, the hematologic findings are mostly confined to viscera (the spleen and liver), and bone involvement dominates the clinical picture. Growth retardation in childhood and delay of puberty are characteristic of Gaucher's type I and are more frequent in those with severe disease. There is a spontaneous catch-up later. Enzyme replacement therapy apparently normalizes growth and possibly also the onset of puberty. Most (60%) of the patients are Ashkenazi Jews.
    - **Type II:** An acute neuropathic disease or infantile type; rare. The severe involvement of the central nervous system leads to an early death (before 2 years of age). In Gaucher's type II, there is a significant phenotypic and genotypic heterogeneity.
    - **Type III:** A subacute neuronopathic (juvenile) type, it is a mixture of types I and II.

55. **How is the genetic pathology correlated with the clinical presentation?**
    The genotype causes a variable deficiency of the enzyme, and it is best correlated with clinical severity and age at presentation. The most common symptom at presentation is a bleeding tendency (i.e., epistaxis and ease of bruising) from thrombocytopenia, which is the result of hypersplenism. The clinical signs include skin pigmentations, deposits in the sclera, hepatosplenomegaly, anemia, and bleeding disorders. Growth retardation is a prominent feature. Bone pain caused by small bone infarcts is usually reported in the femur or proximal tibia.

56. **How common is skeletal involvement?**
    Bone involvement is common; 75–90% of the patients have skeletal changes.

57. **What are the typical skeletal changes seen in Gaucher's disease?**
    The most frequent and characteristic one is the Erlenmeyer flask deformity of the distal femur. Its characteristic radiographic appearance is an abnormal expansion of the distal femoral metaphysis. The pathology is a result of fusiform widening of the relatively thin metaphyseal cortices by the Gaucher cell infiltrate and failure of trabeculation and remodeling. The typical metaphyseal flaring can also occur in the proximal tibia and proximal humerus. In addition, there may be loss of bone density (i.e., osteopenia), thinning of the cortex, medullary expansion, loss of the normal trabeculations, patchy myelosclerosis, bone crisis (infarct), osteonecrosis, bone marrow hemorrhagic cysts mixed with sclerotic areas, and pathologic fractures. These skeletal involvements are secondary to Gaucher cell infiltration of the bone marrow in the medullary cavity. The frequent occurrence of bone pain is due to vaso-occlusive crisis. The osteopenia is mainly located in the vertebrae and the long bones of the proximal limbs (i.e., the femora and humeri), where there is major hematopoietic activity. The infiltration of the marrow by Gaucher

cells produces osteopenia, cortical thinning, and weakening of the bone, which can lead to the complication of pathologic features.

58. **What is the pathophysiology of Gaucher's crisis? What are the presenting signs and symptoms?**

Gaucher's crisis, or pseudomyelitis, is the product of an intramedullary hemorrhage of a large bone segment that can also affect the subperiosteal space. Accumulation of blood under the confinements of the bony, nonexpanding walls creates excessive pressure, which can explain the intense pain of the crisis. The skeletal complaint of Gaucher's crisis is usually acute onset of severe pain localized to the distal femur, proximal tibia, and proximal femur. Other localized signs are heat, redness, swelling, tenderness, and limited function and motion of the affected limb. The leukocyte count and the ESR are elevated. These signs and symptoms are very similar to those of osteomyelitis.

59. **What are the typical radiographic and bone scan findings during the different stages of Gaucher's crisis?**

In the initial stage, the elevated intramedullary pressure creates ischemia of the bone. Radiographs are therefore normal, whereas the bone scan demonstrates reduced uptake. A few weeks following the crisis, the remodeling and reconstitution of bone will be presented radiographically as periosteal elevation and lytic changes in the medullary canal. The radioisotope uptake of the lesion in the bone scan at this stage is increased and surrounds the photopenic sites. When the bone recovers several months later, the bone scan is normal again, and radiographs show patchy myelosclerosis or osteonecrosis in the femoral head, tibial plateau, femoral condyles, or humeral head. Cold vertebral body on bone scan was reported in patients with Gaucher's disease and bone crisis.

60. **What characterizes osteomyelitis in Gaucher's disease?**

Secondary infection of the bony infarct can lead to the rare complication of osteomyelitis in Gaucher's disease. The diagnosis is usually delayed, and the causative bacteria is aerobic. Neither laboratory nor radiographic investigations can distinguish between the bone crisis and osteomyelitis. A biopsy or aspiration by strict aseptic technique can be helpful. Administration of antibiotics must be delayed until the bacteriologic diagnosis is made. A prolonged period of systemic antibiotics is required in Gaucher's infections because the infection is usually located in avascular bone.

61. **Where do pathologic fractures usually occur in children with Gaucher's disease?**

In the sites where bone crisis has altered the bony texture: the distal femur, proximal tibia, and femoral neck. Delayed union and nonunion are frequent complications because of the change in the normal quality of bony repair. Treatment is usually conservative.

62. **What are the causes for back pain in Gaucher's disease?**

Severe back pain can result from bone crisis or pathologic fracture of the spinal vertebrae. Mild back pain can be secondary to osteopenia. Kyphotic deformity, with or without neurologic compromise, may require anterior spinal release with fusion and posterior spinal fusion with segmental instrumentation. In cases of cord compromise, decompression may also be performed. Routine surveillance for spinal deformity is necessary.

63. **Where does osteonecrosis usually occur in Gaucher's disease? How is it treated?**

The femoral head. Other sites are the femoral condyles, tibial plateau, and humeral head. In young patients, conservative treatment with bed rest and no weight-bearing is recommended. Containment abduction bracing can be indicated when there is no collapse of the femoral head.

In older adolescents or adults, if collapse has occurred, partial or total hip replacement can be considered. Treatment of AVN in the shoulder is conservative unless the humeral head is destroyed.

64. **What are the considerations before surgical intervention in Gaucher's disease?**
Significant perioperative bleeding has to be considered. The thrombocytopenia secondary to hypersplenism and the clotting defects secondary to the liver involvement can be responsible for the bleeding.

65. **What is the role of enzyme replacement therapy (ERT)? What technique is most appropriate to assess ERT response?**
At high doses and long administration, ERT reverses almost all the systemic manifestations in patients with type III Gaucher's disease. Low-dose high-frequency ERT prevents fractures without complete suppression of painful bone crisis in patients with severe juvenile-onset type I Gaucher's disease. The use of ERT may lead to resolution of skeletal findings in type I and the changes in the bone marrow.

LANGERHANS CELL HISTIOCYTOSIS (I.E., HISTIOCYTOSIS X AND EOSINOPHILIC GRANULOMA)

66. **What are the three clinical entities of Langerhans cell histiocytosis? Which are most common?**
   - Eosinophilic granuloma (EG) of bone
   - Hand-Schuüller-Christian (HSC) disease
   - Letterer-Siwe (LS) disease

   Isolated EG of bone accounts for around 80% of cases, and multiple EGs of bone compose another 10% of cases. HSC-disseminated disease is present in around 9%, and LS in around 1% of cases. The incidence in children has been estimated at 3–4 per million.

67. **What are the clinical findings in HSC disease and LS disease?**
The clinical findings of polyuria, exophthalmos, and bone lesions in membranous bones are present in HSC disease. This constitutes one of the disseminated forms of the disease. LS is a similar, more-severe disorder with multisystem involvement, including bone, that occurs in younger children and has a poor prognosis.

68. **How is Langerhans cell histiocytosis classified?**
The classification is based on the presence of solitary or multiple bone involvement without soft tissue involvement, bone and soft tissue involvement, or soft tissue involvement alone. Organ dysfunctions (based on individual criteria) are determined and added to the classification.

69. **What is the proposed etiology and pathology in these conditions?**
Although the exact etiology is poorly understood, suspected theories include immunologic stimulation of Langerhans cells, resulting in uncontrolled proliferation and accumulation of the cells. Thoughts are that this does not represent a true malignancy but rather a defect in immune regulation. No hereditary pattern has yet been described.

70. **What are the common sites of soft tissue involvement, and what is the prognostic significance?**
The skin, lungs, liver, spleen, pituitary gland, and bone marrow. Systemic skin involvement is a poor prognostic sign. The involvement of lungs, liver, spleen, and bone marrow can be lethal.

Death can occur when the disease begins before 2 years of age but also may occur in late childhood or even in adulthood.

71. **How common are skeletal lesions, and what are the common sites in Langerhans cell histiocytosis?**
From 80–97% of the patients have bony involvement, and 50–77% are free of visceral involvement. The typical skeletal sites are the skull, pelvis, spine, ribs, and femur. The incidence of vertebral involvement varies between 7.8% and 25%.

72. **What are the presenting symptoms in patients with solitary bony lesions? What are the measures needed to rule out expanding involvement?**
In solitary bone lesions, the presenting complaints are swelling, pain, or limping. The possible expanding involvement can be detected by monitoring for the typical symptoms of the various organ dysfunctions and physical examination with special assessment of the liver, spleen, spine, skull, and extremities. Lateral skull radiographs are a good screening test, and there should be an additional survey of the chest skeleton. Laboratory tests are also useful for early detection of organ dysfunction.

73. **What are the typical radiographic appearances of the different bony lesions?**
In the skull, the typical appearance is punched-out lesions. In the spine, the vertebrae are collapsed (i.e., vertebra plana) with normal adjacent disk spaces. There is also metaphyseal or diaphyseal lytic with cortical thinning, widening of the medullary canal, endosteal scalloping, and occasional periosteal elevation.

74. **How specific are bone scanning, MRI, and CT in diagnosing bony lesion in Langerhans cell histiocytosis?**
Bone scan may detect early bony involvement not seen radiographically, but it bears a high false-negative rate. MRI bears the difficulties of differentiating EG from osteomyelitis and Ewing's sarcoma. MRI, CT, and bone scan can help in detecting the site of a lesion that may cause unexplained pain or spinal cord involvement.

75. **What is the unique structural aspect of Langerhans cells?**
The tubular or racket-shaped granules seen under electron microscopy.

76. **What is the histopathology of the classic bone lesion?**
The classic bone lesion contains histocytes with acute and chronic inflammatory cells. The typical granules of Langerhans cells are found in 2–79% of the histocytes.

77. **What is the necessary measure to confirm the suspected diagnosis of Langerhans cell histiocytosis?**
Tissue biopsy is necessary to confirm the diagnosis. The skin lesions are the best sites for the biopsy. In bony lesions, Craig needle transcutaneous aspiration is optimal. Open biopsy is used when curettage of the lesion is indicated. Biopsy is not indicated in patients with well-defined multifocal radiographic involvement. The radiographic and scintigraphic findings in subacute hematogenous osteomyelitis may be similar to those in EG.

78. **What are the ways to differentiate between the mature lesions of Langerhans cell histiocytosis and subacute or chronic osteomyelitis?**
The mature lesions of Langerhans cells histiocytosis include foci of necrosis, granulomatous changes with fibrosis, and Langerhans histiocytes. Differentiation is based on the use of electron microscopy, which may demonstrate the typical granules.

79. **What is the prognosis in the different types of patients with Langerhans cell histiocytosis?**
Patients with solitary bony lesions at presentation have the best prognosis, with no fatal dissemination. Patients with organ dysfunction at disease onset have a 30–70% mortality rate. Twenty percent of patients with multisystem involvement have a progressive disease course despite treatment. Multiple bone involvement without soft tissue involvement has a good prognosis. Evolution of soft tissue involvement, usually as diabetes insipidus, can occur in this group of patients. The mortality rate is low.

80. **What is the treatment of bone lesions? What is its influence upon healing?**
Methods of treatment for bony lesions without visceral involvement include observation, curettage, or steroid injection. The mode of treatment has no influence on the healing rate. In patients with painful lesions or with the imminent risk of fractures, bone graft can be added to the protocol of curettage and open biopsy.

81. **What are the clinical and radiographic features of spinal lesions? What is the treatment? What is the treatment of EG of the spine with neurologic deficit?**
Spinal lesion is usually accompanied by pain and postural changes such as torticollis, kyphosis, or scoliosis. The typical radiographic changes are vertebra plana with intact posterior elements. In spinal involvement without neurologic deficit, conservative treatment with immobilization by plaster casts or braces is sufficient.

In the rare event of neurologic involvement, MRI and clinical examinations are needed for evaluation of nerve root or spinal cord compression. In nerve root involvement, the treatment is usually rest, immobilization, and occasional steroid block. Surgical decompression is indicated in spinal cord compression. Radiotherapy may be the treatment of choice in disseminated spinal involvement.

For treatment of single or dual spinal lesions, observation with or without bracing seems to be sufficient. In patients with multifocal lesions, chemotherapy produces good results. For treatment of neurologic deficit, low-dose radiotherapy is favored.

Patients who underwent surgery, especially curettage and anterior fusion, had the worst outcome.

82. **What is the earliest radiographic finding seen in the healing of skeletal lesions?**
The earliest sign is the return of the trabecular structure of the affected bone. This change can be detected 6–10 weeks after diagnosis, and complete healing is obvious after 36–40 weeks. Radiography is recommended after 2 and 6 months from diagnosis. If no healing is evident after 4 months, additional therapy is indicated. Additional radiologic surveys and physical examination are recommended every 6 months for 2 years or more.

LEUKEMIA

83. **How common is leukemia among children?**
Leukemia is the most common form of childhood cancer, accounting for 34% of the malignancies in white children and 24% in black children in the United States. The most common type is acute lymphoblastic leukemia (ALL), which accounts for 70–80% of the leukemias in children.

84. **What are the musculoskeletal features of leukemia?**
Bone and joint pain is the most common presenting complaint and is the presenting complaint in 18% of ALL patients. Bone pain is diffuse, nonspecific, and asymmetric; it most frequently appears in the metaphyseal region and may extend to the adjacent joints, hips, knees, ankles,

and wrists. The incidence of these skeletal symptoms ranges from 10–32%. Back pain secondary to osteopenia, bone marrow infiltration, or fracture of the vertebral body can be the initial complaint. Necrotizing fasciitis is another rare feature. Children presenting with bone and joint complaints can be misdiagnosed as having rheumatic fever, septic arthritis, osteomyelitis, juvenile rheumatoid arthritis, or polymyositis.

85. **How common are radiographic changes, and what are their characteristic findings? Which radiographic sign is most significant for the correct diagnosis of leukemia?**

Children with leukemia may have significant symptoms and radiographic signs with a normal peripheral smear at the time of their presentation (10%). The radiographic changes of all patients with ALL at the initial stage of the disease, with an incidence from 44–57%, are about twice as frequent as are the presenting musculoskeletal complaints. The percentage is higher in children below 1 year of age and is significantly lower after 10 years of age. The skeletal changes are most common in the long bones and skull. The characteristic findings are focal ("moth-eaten") or diffuse osteolytic lesions, mainly in the form of bone resorption in the metaphysiodiaphyseal region, destruction and elevation of the periosteum with new bone formation, localized and generalized osteoporosis, radiolucent metaphyseal leukemic lines (bands), cortical defects, osteosclerosis, mixed osteolysis and sclerosis, a permeated pattern of destruction, widening of the cranial sutures of the skull, and subcortical radiolucent zones in the vertebral body. Osteopenia is the most common radiographic finding in the spine and is the most significant sign for making the correct diagnosis. None of the radiographic findings is pathognomonic or typical to leukemia. Bone scan was not found to correlate with the clinical presentation and is unreliable in leukemia.

Osteoporosis can be the first presenting sign of leukemic relapse in the adolescent.

KEY POINTS: HEMATOLOGIC DISORDERS

1. Hemophilia A, due to factor VIII deficiency, accounts for 80% of cases of hemophilia and affects males only (i.e., it is X-linked recessive).

2. Hemophilia B (i.e., Christmas disease), due to factor IX deficiency, accounts for 15% of cases of hemophilia and also affects males only (i.e., it is X-linked recessive).

3. von Willebrand's disease, due to factor VIII deficiency and platelet dysfunction, affects both males and females (i.e., it is autosomal dominant).

4. Sickle cell disease, due to abnormal formation of red cells, mainly affects African Americans (i.e., it is autosomal recessive).

5. Leukemia should be considered in the differential diagnosis of any ill child with bone pain or musculoskeletal complaints.

6. Langerhans cell histiocytosis is characterized by tubular or racket-shaped granules seen under electron microscopy in histiocytes.

7. Children are living longer with human immunodeficiency virus (HIV) and acquired immunodeficiency syndrome (AIDS). Long-term treatment strategies should be employed.

86. **What is the debate about bone involvement at the onset of diagnosis being a prognostic factor?**
Most authors report no prognostic significance for the presence of pathologic vertebral fracture or skeletal involvement at the onset of the disease. Other studies claim that children without radiographic skeletal involvement and those with five or more skeletal lesions will have the same poor outcome as with an aggressive form of leukemia, whereas those with one to four lesions were considered to have an indolent form of short-duration leukemia. Another study found no significant correction between the survival time and the extent of skeletal involvement.

87. **What are the possible musculoskeletal complications of chemotherapy?**
   - Steroid-induced osteopenia
   - Steroid-induced osteonecrosis
   - Pathologic fractures
   - Bone and soft tissue infections
   - Peripheral neuropathies
   - Toxic epidermal necrolysis
   - Paraparesis after lumber puncture

ACQUIRED IMMUNODEFICIENCY SYNDROME (AIDS)

88. **What causes AIDS? What is the major source of AIDS in children today?**
The condition is caused by a retroviral infection with the human immunodeficiency virus (HIV). Currently, most of the affected children are those born to HIV-infected mothers (i.e., vertical transmission). Children delivered by cesarean section carry one half the risk of those delivered vaginally to HIV-infected mothers. Perinatal antiretroviral therapy has dramatically reduced rates of vertical transmission. The majority of children infected with HIV are in sub-Saharan Africa. The rate of transmission of HIV in North America by blood product transfusion has been drastically reduced due to improved screening efforts.

89. **What is the most common musculoskeletal manifestation in HIV-infected children?**
Progressive or static encephalopathy can occur following glial cell HIV infection. The condition occurs more rapidly in children than in adults. Treatments are similar to those employed in children with cerebral palsy and other conditions producing extremity spasticity. Surgery is not contraindicated but should be planned carefully, with optimization of antiretroviral agents and precautions for potential nosocomial infections postoperatively. Musculoskeletal opportunistic infections are surprisingly uncommon in children with HIV. Any unusual infection might be a clue to making the diagnosis of HIV. With the advance of antiretroviral agents, children are living longer with HIV infection, and long-term musculoskeletal treatment strategies should be utilized and not avoided in these children.

BIBLIOGRAPHY

1. Adekile AD, Gupta R, Yacoub F, et al: Avascular necrosis of the hip in children with sickle cell disease and high Hb F: Magnetic resonance imaging findings and influence of alpha-thalassemia trait. Acta Haematol 105(1):27–31, 2001.

2. Aguilar C, Vichinsky E, Neumayr L: Bone and joint disease in sickle cell disease. Hematol Oncol Clin North Am 19:929–941, 2005.

3. Altarescu G, Hill S, Wiggs E, et al: The efficacy of enzyme replacement therapy inpatients with chronic neuronopathic Gaucher's disease. J Pediatr 138:539–547, 2001.

4. Altarescu G, Schiffmann R, Parker CC, et al: Comparative efficacy of dose regimens in enzyme replacement therapy of type I Gaucher disease. Blood Cells Mol Dis 26(4):285–290, 2000.

5. Anand AJ, Glatt AE: Salmonella osteomyelitis and arthritis in sickle cell disease. Semin Arthritis Rheum 24(3):211–221, 1994.

6. Azouz EM, Oudjhane K: Disorders of the upper extremity in children. Magn Reson Imaging Clin North Am 6:677–695, 1998.

7. Benetrt OM, Namnyak SS: Bone and joint manifestations of sickle cell anemia. J Bone Joint Surg Br 72:494–499, 1990.

8. Chambers JB, Forsythe DA, Bertrand SL, et al: Retrospective review of osteoarticular infections in a pediatric sickle cell age group. J Pediatr Orthop 20:682–685, 2000.

9. Crowley JJ, Sarnaik S: Imaging of sickle cell disease. Pediatr Radiol 29:646–661, 1999.

10. De Sanctis V, Pinamonti A, Di Palma A, et al: Growth and development in thalassemia major patients with severe bone lesions due to desferrioxamine. Eur J Pediatr 155:368–372, 1990.

11. Gallagher DJ, Phillips DJ, Heinrich SD: Orthopaedic manifestations of acute pediatric leukemia. Orthop Clin North Am 27:635–644, 1996.

12. Giardini C, Lucarelli G: Bone marrow transplantation for beta-thalassemia. Hematol Oncol Clin North Am 13:1059–1064, 1999.

13. Greene WB: Diseases related to the hematopoietic system. In Morissy RT, Weinstein SL (eds): Lovell and Winter's Pediatric Orthopaedics, 5th ed, vol 1. Philadelphia, Lippincott-Raven, 2000, pp 379–426.

14. Hamouda O: HIV/AIDS surveillance in Germany. J Acq Immun Def Syndr 32(suppl 1):S49–S54, 2003.

15. Hermann G, Pastores GM, Abdelwahab IF, et al: Gaucher disease: Assessment of skeletal involvement and therapeutic responses to enzyme replacement. Skel Radiol 26:687–696, 1997.

16. Hernigou P, Bachir D, Galacteros F: Avascular necrosis of the femoral head in sickle-cell disease. J Bone Joint Surg Br 75:875–880, 1993.

17. Howarth DM, Gilchrist GS, Mullan BP, et al: Langerhans cell histiocytosis: Diagnosis, natural history, management, and outcome. Cancer 85:2278–2290, 1999.

18. Ida H, Rennert OM, Kato S, et al: Severe skeletal complications in Japanese patients with type 1 Gaucher disease. J Inherit Metab Dis 22(1):63–73, 1999.

19. Kocher MS, Hall JE: Surgical management of spinal involvement in children and adolescents with Gaucher's disease. J Pediatr Orthop 20:383–388, 2000.

20. Koseoglu V, Kutluk MT, Cila A: Severe bone involvement with Langerhans cell histiocytosis. J Pediatr 133:711, 1998.

21. Levin C, Zalman L, Shalev S, et al: Legg-Calve-Perthes disease, protein C deficiency, and beta-thalassemia major: Report of two cases. J Pediatr Orthop 20:129–131, 2000.

22. McLaurin TM, Bukrey CD, Lovett RJ, et al: Management of thrombocytopenia-absent radius (TAR) syndrome. J Pediatr Orthop 19:289–296, 1999.

23. Meehan PL, Viroslav S, Schmitt EW Jr: Vertebral collapse in childhood leukemia. J Pediatr Orthop 15:592–595, 1995.

24. Moran MC: Osteonecrosis of the hip in sickle cell hemoglobinopathy. Am J Orthop 24(1):18–24, 1995.

25. Nathan DG, Orkin SH (eds): Nathan and Oski's Hematology of Infancy and Childhood, 5th ed. Philadelphia, W.B. Saunders, 1998.

26. Onur O, Sivri A, Gumruk F, et al: Beta thalassemia: A report of 20 children. Clin Rheumatol 18(1):42–44, 1999.

27. Overturf GD: Infections and immunizations of children with sickle cell disease. Adv Pediatr Infect Dis 14:191–218, 1999.

28. Rivard GE, Girard M, Belanger R, et al: Synoviorthesis with colloidal 32P chromic phosphate for the treatment of hemophilic arthropathy. J Bone Joint Surg Am 76:482–488, 1994. (Comment in J Bone Joint Surg Am 77:807–808, 1995.)

29. Schneider P, Farahati J, Reiners C: Radiosynovectomy in rheumatology, orthopaedics, and hemophilia. J Nucl Med 46 (Suppl 1):48S–54S, 2005.

30. Schreuder HW, Pruszczynski M, Lemmens JA, et al: Eosinophilic granuloma of bone: Results of treatment with curettage, cryosurgery, and bone grafting. J Pediatr Orthop B 7(4):253–256, 1998.

31. Sidhu PS, Rich PM: Sonographic detection and characterization of musculoskeletal and subcutaneous tissue abnormalities in sickle cell disease. Br J Radiol 72(853):9–17, 1999.

32. Siegel HJ, Luck JV Jr, Siegel ME: Advances in radionuclide therapeutics in orthopaedics. J Am Acad Orthop Surg 12(1):55–64, 2004.

33. States LJ: Imaging of metabolic bone disease and marrow disorders in children. Radiol Clin North Am 39:749–772, 2001.

34. Timsit MA, Bardin T: Metabolic arthropathies. Curr Opin Rheumatol 6:448–453, 1994.

35. Titgemeyer C, Grois N, Minkov M, et al: Pattern and course of single-system disease in Langerhans cell histiocytosis data from the DAL-HX 83- and 90-study. Med Pediatr Oncol 37(2):108–114, 2001.

36. Umans H, Haramati N, Flusser G: The diagnostic role of gadolinium enhanced MRI in distinguishing between acute medullary bone infarct and osteomyelitis. Magn Reson Imaging 18(3):255–262, 2000.

37. Vichinsky EP: The morbidity of bone disease in thalassemia. Ann N Y Acad Sci 850:344–348, 1998.

38. Vichinsky EP, Neumayr LD, Haberkern C, et al: The perioperative complication rate of orthopedic surgery in sickle cell disease: Report of the National Sickle Cell Surgery Study Group. Am J Hematol 62(3):129–138, 1999.

39. William RR, Hussein SS, Jeans WD, et al: A prospective study of soft-tissue ultrasonography in sickle cell disease patients with suspected osteomyelitis. Clin Radiol 55:307–310, 2000.

40. Wong AL, Sakamoto KM, Johnson EE: Differentiating osteomyelitis from bone infarction in sickle cell disease. Pediatr Emerg Care 17(1):60–64, 2001.

41. Yeom JS, Lee CK, Shin HY, et al: Langerhans' cell histiocytosis of the spine. Analysis of twenty-three cases. Spine 24:1740–1749, 1999.

INDEX

Page numbers in **boldface type** indicate complete chapters.